fourth edition

Introduction to
Human Disease

Thomas H. Kent, MD
Emeritus Professor of Pathology
University of Iowa
Iowa City, Iowa

Michael Noel Hart, MD
Professor and Chair of Pathology
University of Wisconsin
Madison, Wisconsin

Appleton & Lange
Stamford, Connecticut

Notice: The authors and the publisher of this volume have taken care to make certain that the doses of drugs and schedules of treatment are correct and compatible with the standards generally accepted at the time of publication. Nevertheless, as new information becomes available, changes in treatment and in the use of drugs become necessary. The reader is advised to carefully consult the instruction and information material included in the package insert of each drug or therapeutic agent before administration. This advice is especially important when using, administering, or recommending new or infrequently used drugs. The authors and publisher disclaim all responsibility for any liability, loss, injury, or damage incurred as a consequence, directly or indirectly, of the use and application of any of the contents of this volume.

Copyright © 1998 by Appleton & Lange
A Simon & Schuster Company
Copyright © 1993 by Appleton & Lange
Copyright © 1979 by Appleton-Century-Crofts

98 99 00 01 02 / 10 9 8 7 6 5 4 3 2 1

www.appletonlange.com

Prentice Hall International (UK) Limited, *London*
Prentice Hall of Australia Pty. Limited, *Sydney*
Prentice Hall Canada, Inc., *Toronto*
Prentice Hall Hispanoamericana, S.A., *Mexico*
Prentice Hall of India Private Limited, *New Delhi*
Prentice Hall of Japan, Inc., *Tokyo*
Simon & Schuster Asia Pte. Ltd., *Singapore*
Editora Prentice Hall do Brasil Ltda., *Rio de Janeiro*
Prentice Hall, *Upper Saddle River, New Jersey*

Library of Congress Cataloging-in-Publication Data

Kent, Thomas H. (Thomas Hugh), 1934–
    Introduction to human disease / Thomas H. Kent, Michael Noel Hart. — 4th ed.
      p.   cm.
    Includes index.
    ISBN 0-8385-4070-8 (case : alk. paper)
    1. Pathology.   2. Allied health personnel.   I. Hart, Michael Noel, 1938– . II. Title.
    [DNLM: 1. Pathology QZ 4 K37i 1998]
    RB111.K45   1998
    616.07—dc21
    DNLM/DLC
    for Library of Congress   97-48337
                                           CIP

Acquisitions Editor: Lin Marshall
Production Service: Jennsin Services
Art Coordinator: Eve Siegel
Art Work: ElectraGraphics
Designer: Libby Schmitz

ISBN 0-8385-4070-8

90000

9 780838 540701

PRINTED IN THE UNITED STATES OF AMERICA

CONTENTS

Preface ....*v*

Acknowledgments ....*vii*

Section I. An Overview
1. Introduction to Pathology 1
2. Most Frequent and Significant Diseases 11
3. Diagnostic Resources 21

Section II. Basic Disease Processes
4. Injury, Inflammation, and Repair...33
5. Hyperplasias and Neoplasms 69
6. Cancer 85
7. Genetic and Developmental Diseases......................................97

Section III. Major Organ-Related Diseases
8. Heart 117
9. Vascular System 141
10. Hematopoietic System 169
11. Bleeding and Clotting Disorders 195
12. Lung 209
13. Oral Region, Upper Respiratory Tract, and Ear.........................237
14. Alimentary Tract 253
15. Liver, Gallbladder, and Pancreas......................................285
16. Kidney, Lower Urinary Tract, and Male Genital Organs..................305
17. Female Genital Organs 331
18. Breast 347
19. Skin 359
20. Eye 391
21. Bones and Joints 409

22. Skeletal Muscle and Peripheral Nerve.......................441
23. Central Nervous System 457
24. Mental Illness...489
25. Endocrine System...505

Section IV. Multiple Organ System Diseases

26. Infectious Diseases..531
27. Immunologic Diseases 577
28. Physical Injury...605
29. Chemical Injury..617
30. Nutritional Disorders and Alcoholism 629

Index 639

PREFACE

Introduction to Human Disease is a textbook of pathology for health science students other than medical students. We have noticed, however, that medical students use it to obtain basic concepts before reading the more detailed and encyclopedic text designed for them. We have also noted that our family members use it to get types of information desired by lay people. This broad usage pleases us because it was our intent to provide a text that covers all aspects of human disease with minimal requirements for prerequisite knowledge.

We are gratified by the continued use of the first, second, and third editions by instructors who teach pathology courses to a wide variety of health science students including dental, pharmacy, physician assistant, pathology assistant, dental assistant, medical technology, nursing, physical therapy, occupational therapy, nutrition, and graduate students. We feel that all health science workers have a need for a common vocabulary and a broad understanding of human disease. For this reason, we define terms as clearly and specifically as possible and describe all of the common and important diseases of humans, including mental illnesses.

The fourth edition contains considerable new material. Overall 32 new terms have been introduced, 18 of these representing diseases that have not been discussed in the first three editions. Twenty-five of the 30 chapters have undergone more than minimal revision with ten undergoing extensive rewriting. Each chapter was reviewed by at least one outside reviewer for content and the entire text was critiqued by four reviewers. The numerous changes made in the fourth edition reflect the suggestions of the reviewers plus any omissions from the third edition as compiled by the authors.

The text is divided into four sections. Section I provides the most fundamental vocabulary and concepts, a broad analysis of the most common and significant diseases, and a discussion of the tools and process of diagnosis.

Section II provides a framework for the basic types of human disease: reactions to injury, neoplasia, genetically determined disease, and intrauterine injury.

Section III approaches disease from the most common viewpoint, by organ system. Within each chapter we view the most important anatomy and physiology, provide an overview of the most frequent and important diseases encountered, discuss diagnostic techniques (symptoms, signs, laboratory tests, and radiological and clinical procedures), profile the diseases, and discuss the consequences of failure of the organ to function.

Section IV presents diseases that tend to affect multiple organs and that share causative mechanisms within each group. Topics included are infections, immune reactions, external injury by physical and chemical agents encompassing environmental diseases, and disorders caused by nutritional deprivations and excesses. We have found that these chapters are easier to learn after the diseases of the organs have been studied. They can, however, be inserted earlier in a course without any prerequisites other than Sections I and II.

Each chapter contains review questions that address the most important aspects of the chapter. They can be considered the learning objectives. We have not included any references. We recommend any of the standard textbooks of pathology or internal medicine for additional reading. These texts contain an abundance of citations for the student who wishes to pursue any topic in greater depth.

ACKNOWLEDGMENTS

We would like to thank the following individuals who reviewed chapters for the fourth edition:

Edward Adickes, Sylvia Asa, James Brennan, Nancy Chiarantona, Teresa Darcy, Zsuzsanna Fabry, Dan Farrell, Thomas Farrell, Christina Iyama-Kurtycz, Ned Kalin, Dennis Maki, Terry Oberley, Jan Pollock, Catherine Reznikoff, Daniel Vandersteen, Annette Schlueter, Marta Voytovich, Donald Wiebe, Eliot Williams, Andrew Woodard, and especially Karen Fitzsimmons who reviewed a number of chapters and was particularly helpful with her suggestions.

Most of the line drawings were made by Jo Ann Reynolds for the first edition.

AN
OVERVIEW

The purpose of this section is to give you (1) the general vocabulary used to discuss and classify disease, (2) a feeling for the general frequency and significance of disease so that you can separate the forest from the trees, and (3) a perspective of the resources commonly used in diagnosis so that you can bridge the gap between their scientific basis as learned in the basic sciences and their pratical application in the care of patients.

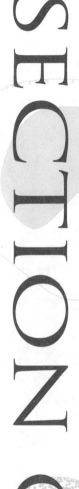

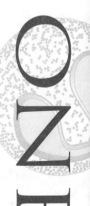

SECTION ONE

1.

Introduction to Pathology

PATHOLOGY

DISEASE

MANIFESTATIONS OF DISEASE

STRUCTURAL DISEASES

FUNCTIONAL DISEASES

CAUSES OF DISEASE

THE CARE OF PATIENTS

REVIEW QUESTIONS

PATHOLOGY

The term *pathology* has several meanings. In the broadest sense, pathology is the study of disease. All health scientists are lifelong students of pathology because, in one way or another, all are interested in altering the course of disease through better understanding of its nature.

A course in pathology, such as the one you are undertaking, provides a concentrated study of the nature of disease and lays the foundation for further study of disease within specific disciplines.

Pathology is also a name applied to one of the disciplines of medicine, one that deals with analysis of body fluids and tissues for diagnostic purposes and with teaching and research relating to fundamental aspects of disease. The roles of pathologists are outlined in Table 1–1.

TABLE 1–1. ROLES OF A PATHOLOGIST

Role	Subject
Experimental pathology	Research
Academic pathology	Teaching, research, anatomic and/or clinical pathology
Anatomic pathology	Morphologic examinations
Autopsy pathology	Postmortem study of the body
Surgical pathology	Biopsies and resected tissues
Cytopathology	Individual cells removed by scraping or washing
Molecular diagnosis	Nucleic acid (DNA and RNA) analysis
Clinical pathology	Laboratory tests
Chemistry	Chemical analysis
Microbiology	Microorganisms
Hematology	Blood and bone marrow, blood clotting
Blood banking	Blood transfusion services
Immunopathology	Antigen and antibody detection
Molecular diagnosis	Nucleic acid (DNA and RNA) analysis

Pathologists usually practice laboratory medicine or study basic aspects of disease within a department of pathology associated with a hospital and/or medical school. Sometimes pathologists subdivide themselves on the basis of special interests into experimental pathologists, anatomic pathologists, or clinical pathologists. Experimental pathologists are basic scientists who spend the majority of their time investigating the causes and mechanisms of disease. Anatomic pathologists perform autopsies, examine all tissues removed from live patients (surgical pathology), and examine cell preparations used to screen for cancer cells (cytology or cytopathology). Clinical pathologists analyze various specimens removed from patients, such as blood, urine, feces, spinal fluid, or sputum, for chemical substances, microorganisms, antigens and antibodies, nucleic acids, blood cells, and coagulation factors. Most pathologists in community medical centers practice both anatomic and clinical pathology. In health science teaching centers, pathologists are likely to combine teaching and experimental pathology with an interest in one or more of the special areas of anatomic or clinical pathology and are often referred to as *academic pathologists.*

DISEASE

Disease is a structural or functional change within the body judged to be abnormal. Minor changes that are of no importance may be judged to be variations of the normal state rather than disease. Pathology not only includes the study of basic structural and functional changes associated with a disease, but also includes the study of causes that lead to the structural and functional changes and the manifestations that result from them. Furthermore, pathology is concerned with the sequence of events that leads from cause to structural and functional abnormalities and finally to manifestations. This sequence is referred to as the *pathogenesis* of disease. The term *etiology* means the study of causes. It is commonly misused as a synonym for cause.

Diagnosis is the process of assigning a name to a patient's condition. The name applied (the noun) is also called the *diagnosis*. If possible, a diagnosis should be the name of the disease that the patient has, e.g., multiple sclerosis. Assigning this name implies that the illness will follow a course similar to that of other patients with the same disease. A diagnosis is a generalization (oversimplification) used for convenience of communication and thinking. Sometimes the findings cannot be expressed in terms of a disease, e.g., paralysis of unknown cause. In such cases, the clinical problem is used as the diagnosis until the patient's disease becomes evident. Clusters of findings commonly encountered with more than one disease are called *syndromes*. For example, leakage of protein into the urine, low serum protein, and edema are a common set of findings in long-standing diseases of the renal glomerulus. This constellation is called the nephrotic syndrome because it is not one disease, but a set of findings common to several diseases. Therefore, the patient may be diagnosed as having the nephrotic syndrome until the specific disease is known.

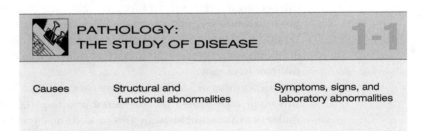

PATHOLOGY:
THE STUDY OF DISEASE

1-1

| Causes | Structural and functional abnormalities | Symptoms, signs, and laboratory abnormalities |

MANIFESTATIONS OF DISEASE

We will use the term *manifestations* to refer to the data that can be gathered about an individual patient, namely, symptoms, signs, and laboratory abnormalities (Table 1–2). *Symptoms* are evidence of disease

TABLE 1–2. MANIFESTATIONS OF DISEASE

Type of Manifestation	Nature of Data	Name for Collection of Results
Symptoms	Patient's perceptions	History
Signs	Examiner's observations	Physical examination
Laboratory abnormalities	Results of tests and special procedures	Laboratory findings

perceived by the patient, such as pain, a lump, or diarrhea. The written description of symptoms in the patient's record is referred to as the *history*. *Signs* are physical observations made by the person who examines the patient, such as tenderness, a mass, or abnormal heart sounds. Signs are recorded under *physical examination*. *Laboratory abnormalities* in the broad sense refers to the observations made by tests or special procedures, such as x-rays, blood counts, or biopsies.

STRUCTURAL DISEASES

Structural diseases are those diseases characterized by structural changes within the body as the most basic abnormality. They are also referred to as *organic diseases*. Structural changes are called *lesions* and may be biochemical or morphologic (visible). The term *lesion* is most often used in reference to morphologic change whether it be at the gross (naked eye), microscopic, or electron microscopic level. Three broad categories suffice to classify most structural diseases (Table 1–3), although some diseases fall into more than one category and some are difficult to classify.

Genetic and developmental diseases are defined for the purposes of this book as diseases that are caused by abnormalities in the genetic makeup of the individual (genes or chromosomes) or abnormalities due to changes in utero (during embryonic and fetal development).

TABLE 1–3. MAJOR DISEASE CATEGORIES

Genetic and developmental diseases
Acquired injuries and inflammatory diseases
Hyperplasias and neoplasms

The range of abnormalities in this category is very broad, extending from deformities present at birth (congenital anomalies) to biochemical changes caused by genes but influenced by environment so they appear later in life, e.g., diabetes mellitus. Due to overlap in classification schemes, many genetic and developmental diseases can also be classified as injuries, inflammations, proliferations, or even neoplasms.

Acquired injuries and inflammatory diseases are diseases due to internal or external forces or agents that destroy cells or intercellular substances, deposit abnormal substances (foreign bodies or materials produced by the body), or cause the body to injure itself by means of the inflammatory process. External agents of injury include physical and chemical substances and microbes. The major internal mechanisms of injury are vascular insufficiency, immunologic reactions, and metabolic disturbances. The direct effects of injury are referred to as *necrosis* if cells are killed in the injured area and *sublethal cell injury* if the injured cells are capable of recovery. Sublethal cell injury may also be called *degeneration,* but this term has many other vague connotations. The few types of necrosis have myriads of causes. Acute sublethal cell injury tends to appear similar regardless of cause or cells involved, but chronic sublethal cell injury has many variations. There are two general reactions to injury: inflammation and repair. *Inflammation* is a vascular and cellular reaction that attempts to localize the injury, destroy the offending agent, and remove damaged cells and other materials. *Repair* is the replacement of damaged tissue by new tissue of the same type and/or by fibrous connective tissue. Inflammation is a stereotyped response with several important variations. Unlike necrosis and inflammation, repair is greatly influenced by the type of tissue or organ that has been injured.

Hyperplasias and neoplasms is a category used to describe diseases characterized by increases in cell populations. Repair also may involve increases in cell populations, but the purpose is obviously to replace that which has been lost. In hyperplasia and neoplasia, the cell increase is beyond normal. *Hyperplasia* is a proliferative reaction to a prolonged external stimulus and will usually regress when the stimulus is removed. *Neoplasia* is presumed to result from a genetic change producing a single population of new (neoplastic) cells, which can proliferate beyond the degree allowed by the mechanisms that normally govern cell proliferation. Neoplasms are divided into two groups, benign and malignant, based on whether they will remain localized (benign) or will continue to grow and spread (malignant). *Cancer* is synonymous with malignant neoplasm. The situation is made more complicated by certain types of hyperplasias that slowly evolve, presumably through a series of genetic changes induced by external agents, into malignant neoplasms.

FUNCTIONAL DISEASES

Functional diseases are those diseases in which the onset begins without the presence of any lesions (biochemical or morphologic). The basic change is a physiologic or functional change and is referred to as a *pathophysiologic change*. Some long-standing functional diseases may, however, lead to secondary structural changes. The examples in Table 1–4 illustrate how either organic or functional diseases can have manifestations that are either structural or functional in nature.

Many mental illnesses are considered functional disorders, although some may have a genetic or other organic basis. The more mental illnesses are investigated, the more it is appreciated that there is likely to be an organic basis (on a biochemical level) to many of them. The most common functional disorders are tension headache and functional bowel syndrome, disorders that may be due to unconscious stimulation of the autonomic nervous system.

CAUSES OF DISEASE

Diseases are initiated by injury, which may be either external or internal in origin. Agents acting from without are termed *exogenous*, those acting from within are referred to as *endogenous*.

External causes of disease are divided into physical, chemical, and microbiologic (Table 1–5). Direct physical injury by an object is called *trauma*. Other physical agents causing disease include heat and cold, electricity, atmospheric pressure changes, and radiation (electromagnetic and particulate). Chemical injuries are generally subdivided by

TABLE 1–4. EXAMPLES OF VARYING EFFECTS OF STRUCTURAL AND FUNCTIONAL DISEASES

Disease	Type of Disease	Nature of Manifestations
Tension headaches	Functional (muscle spasm)	Functional (pain)
Benign tumor of the breast that produces a mass	Structural (tumor)	Structural (mass)
Exogenous obesity caused by craving for food	Functional (hunger)	Structural (obesity)
Cancer of the esophagus that prevents eating	Structural (cancer)	Functional (inability to eat)

TABLE 1–5. EXTERNAL CAUSES OF DISEASE

Physical injury
  Trauma
  Heat-cold
  Electricity
  Pressure
  Ionizing radiations
Chemical injury
  Poisoning
  Drug reactions

Microbiologic injury
  Bacteria
  Fungi
  Rickettsia
  Viruses
  Protozoa
  Helminths

the manner of injury into poisoning (accidental, homicidal, or suicidal) and drug reactions (toxic effects of prescription or proprietary drugs taken to treat disease). Microbiologic injuries are usually classified by the type of offending organism (bacteria, fungi, rickettsia, viruses, protozoa, and helminths) and are called *infections.*

Internal causes of disease fall into three large categories (Table 1–6). Vascular diseases may involve obstruction of blood supply to an organ or tissue, bleeding (hemorrhage), or altered blood flow such as occurs with heart failure. Immunologic diseases are those caused by aberrations of the immune system. Failure of the immune system to work when it is needed results in immunodeficiency disease. Overreaction or unwanted reactions of the immune system cause allergic (hypersensitivity) diseases. Metabolic diseases encompass a wide variety of biochemical disorders that may be primarily genetically determined or secondary effects of acquired disease. Metabolic diseases are most commonly categorized as abnormalities primarily involving lipids, carbohydrates, proteins, minerals, vitamins, and fluid. Some large categories of disease cannot be classified according to internal or external causes because the

TABLE 1–6. INTERNAL CAUSES OF DISEASE

Vascular
  Obstruction
  Bleeding
  Deranged flow
Immunologic
  Immune deficiency
  Allergy

Metabolic
  Abnormal metabolism or deficiency of:
    Lipid
    Carbohydrate
    Protein
    Mineral
    Vitamins
    Fluids

cause is not known, e.g., most neoplasms. Diseases of unknown cause are termed *idiopathic.* Adverse reactions resulting from treatment by a health specialist produce *iatrogenic* disease. *Nosocomial* diseases are those acquired from a hospital environment.

THE CARE OF PATIENTS

The "workup" of a patient encompasses three major steps: (1) History taking involves talking to the patient (or relatives) to ascertain the patient's symptoms and reviewing any other past or present medical problems that might relate to them; (2) physical examination involves systematic looking, feeling, listening, and sometimes even smelling the accessible parts of the body for signs of illness; and (3) when needed, laboratory tests and radiologic and clinical procedures are ordered to detect chemical and physiologic abnormalities which aid in establishing a diagnosis.

When the workup is completed, a diagnosis is made. As we have seen, this may be a disease, a prominent manifestation, or a syndrome. The diagnosis applied to a patient's illness plays the major role in selection of treatment. It also serves to indicate the likelihood of a favorable or unfavorable outcome. The expected outcome of a disease is called its *prognosis.*

The application of treatment to a patient is an attempt to alter the natural course of the patient's disease whether it be prevention of death, lessening the destructive effects, shortening the illness, or reducing symptoms. Follow-up of patients is important to determine whether the desired outcome has occurred or whether treatment has failed to control the disease or whether complications have developed. *Complications* are secondary problems known to occur with a disease in some but not all instances.

Diagnosis of specific diseases is not only useful to the patient for determining treatment and prognosis, but is also useful to future patients. It is through collection of data by disease category that our knowledge of prognosis, effectiveness of treatment, and frequency of complications is derived. Sometimes these data also further our understanding of the cause of a disease. This is particularly true when the distribution of the disease gives clues to possible causative factors. Major breakthroughs in our understanding of the causes of disease, however, tend to come from experimentation and/or technical advances that allowed finer definition of the body's structure and function.

The application of the process of patient care described above is limited by the availability of resources, by the nature of disease, and our ability to understand disease. The greatest effects on health care have come from knowledge of cause leading to preventative measures, particularly through improved nutrition, control of infectious diseases, and avoidance of toxic substances. New knowledge of this type is difficult and expensive to obtain with only occasional major breakthroughs. Application lags behind current knowledge and ability; for example, underdeveloped countries have, for educational and economic reasons, poor prevention of infectious disease. On the other hand, developed countries fail, for social reasons, to prevent the effects of tobacco and alcohol. In the United States, a great deal of effort is being directed toward the effects and complications of disease. For example, cancer is attacked with complex surgical, radiologic, and chemical techniques; surgical techniques are used to circumvent arteries obstructed by atherosclerosis; and organs that have failed are replaced by transplants from other individuals.

Economic considerations play an important role in the care of patients. The cost of diagnosis and treatment must be weighed against possible benefits. The concentration of serious disease in the elderly complicates cost/benefit decisions because of their already limited life expectancy. The cost of diagnosis may be small or large. If the cost is large, the benefits of each of the possible diagnoses must be weighed against the cost. Only through knowledge of disease can cost/benefit decisions be made about individual patients. In many cases the knowledge needed is highly technical and specific to the diseases under consideration. However, it is important to have a broad foundation of knowledge about the more common diseases, such as is presented in this book, before becoming enmeshed in the details of one's own area of specialization.

Review Questions

1. What is pathology?
2. What do pathologists do?
3. What categories of information are useful to describe a disease?
4. What is the major difference between a functional and an organic (structural) disease?
5. What are the fundamental characteristics of the three major forms of organic disease?
6. What are the six major types of causes of disease? Which causes are external and which are internal in origin?
7. What do the following terms mean?

    Benign
    Cancer
    Complications
    Congenital anomaly
    Diagnosis
    Etiology
    History
    Hyperplasia
    Iatrogenic
    Idiopathic
    Infection
    Inflammation
    Lesion
    Malignant
    Necrosis
    Neoplasia
    Nosocomial
    Pathogenesis
    Pathophysiology
    Prognosis
    Repair
    Sign
    Symptom
    Syndrome
    Trauma

2.
Most Frequent and Significant Diseases

CAUSES OF DEATH (MORTALITY)

CAUSES OF DISABILITY (MORBIDITY)

MEASURES OF MORTALITY AND MORBIDITY

FREQUENCY OF ACUTE DISEASES

FREQUENCY OF CHRONIC DISEASES

DISEASE FREQUENCY RELATED TO VISITS TO
FAMILY PHYSICIANS

AGING

REVIEW QUESTIONS

CAUSES OF DEATH (MORTALITY)

Diseases causing death are described in terms of mortality rate (number per 100,000 population dying per year). These statistics are compiled by government agencies from death certificates, which must be filled out by a physician at the time of death. More than 70 percent of all deaths in the United States are accounted for by the five most frequent causes (Table 2–1).

Heart disease accounts for nearly four out of every ten deaths in the United States. The vast majority of these deaths are caused by atherosclerosis—a degenerative disease of arteries that over a course

TABLE 2–1. LEADING OVERALL CAUSES OF DEATH, 1990

Heart Disease	720,000
Malignant Neoplasms	505,000
Cerebrovascular Disease (Stroke)	144,000
Accidents	92,000
Chronic Obstructive Pulmonary Disease	87,000
Pneumonia and Influenza	80,000
Diabetes	48,000
Suicide	31,000
Chronic Liver Disease	26,000
AIDS	25,000

From Health United States DHHS Pub. No. (PHS) 95-1232, 1994.

of many years obstructs the coronary arteries by the development of lipid-rich thickenings in the arterial lining. These areas of thickening are called *atherosclerotic plaques.* At some point, the blood supply suddenly becomes inadequate, and as a result a portion of the heart muscle is killed. The area of dead muscle is called a *myocardial infarct.* Myocardial infarcts are more frequent and occur at an earlier age in men than in women.

Cancers (malignant neoplasms) are the second leading cause of death in the United States accounting for one out of every five deaths. Cancer of the sex organs (breast, uterus, ovary, prostate), gastrointestinal tract, and lung account for 60 percent of all cancer deaths. The frequency of cancer increases dramatically between ages 50 and 80.

Stroke (cerebrovascular disease) is the third leading cause of death in the United States, accounting for 1 out of every 11 deaths. *Stroke* is the common name for cerebral vascular accident, which is caused by injury to an area of the brain, usually resulting from vascular obstruction or bleeding into the brain. Strokes, like heart disease, are most often due to obstruction of arteries resulting from atherosclerosis. Atherosclerosis of the arteries leading to the brain leads to death of a portion of the brain called a *cerebral infarct.* Strokes caused by bleeding usually result from high blood pressure (hypertension) or rupture of an aneurysm (a dilated outpouching of an artery). Strokes are most common in the elderly and commonly present with weakness of one side of the body or difficulty with speech.

Trauma caused by accidents is the fourth leading cause of death in the United States, accounting for 1 out of every 18 deaths. Automobile accidents are the most common cause of traumatic death. It is estimated that 50 percent of drivers responsible for automobile accidents are under the influence of alcohol. The young and elderly are most commonly affected by accidents.

Chronic obstructive pulmonary disease is the fifth leading cause of death, with most of these deaths due to emphysema caused by cigarette smoking.

CAUSES OF DISABILITY (MORBIDITY)

Another way diseases may be significant is in terms of disability. Disabilities are health problems that interfere with a person's normal physical, mental, or emotional functions. Health problems are what motivate the patient to seek health care. The frequency of disability within a population is called *morbidity*. The term *prognosis* refers to the outcome of a disease. Prognosis includes both morbidity and mortality estimates.

MEASURES OF MORTALITY AND MORBIDITY

The frequency of disease can be measured at a given point in time or over a period of time. Whichever method is used, the observations should be made on a predetermined population so that the results will not be biased. Examples of predetermined populations are all of the people living in one state, or all of the men in one state, or all of the women in the state aged 50 to 59.

Mortality rate is a measure of the number of people dying in a given time period. It is usually expressed as the number dying per 100,000 population per year. *Incidence* is a measure of the number of newly diagnosed patients in a given time period, usually a year. Persons who had the disease diagnosed before the year began are not counted. Incidence is a useful measure for those diseases of short duration where the persons with the disease either get well soon or die. Such diseases are easy to count over a year's time.

Prevalence refers to the number of persons with a disease at any one point in time. It is more difficult to measure because the population must be surveyed at one time, and it may be difficult to decide whether a person has the disease or not. For example, does a person who recently had a cancer removed still have cancer? One cannot always tell. Prevalence is best used as a measure of long-standing diseases that are neither cured nor lead to death within a few years.

Other measures derived from mortality rate, incidence, and prevalence data are often useful for comparative purposes. The relative incidence of a group of conditions, e.g., various cancers of a particular organ, can be expressed as a percentage of the total. Survival rate is the percentage of people with a particular condition that live for a given period of time after diagnosis; e.g., the 5-year survival rate of breast cancer is the percentage of all women with breast cancer who were alive 5 years after diagnosis, regardless of whether they still have cancer or not. The age adjusted or relative survival rate adjusts the rate for those who might have died from other causes based on their age.

FREQUENCY OF ACUTE DISEASES

Acute diseases are those that last a short period of time, usually a few days to a few weeks. Any health condition that causes the patient to seek medical consultation or to miss work or school or prevents normal daily activities is classified as a disease (illness). Almost half of acute diseases are respiratory illnesses, mostly acute viral diseases (Figure 2–1). Approximately one-sixth of acute diseases result from injuries of various types. The other one-third of acute diseases are about equally divided among nonrespiratory infections and a variety of noninfectious, noninjury type diseases. Acute conditions are best measured in terms of the number of diagnosed cases per population per year (incidence).

The frequency of acute illnesses decreases with age. For example, in one survey, children under 6 years of age had three acute illnesses per year compared to one per year for persons over age 44.

FREQUENCY OF CHRONIC DISEASES

Chronic diseases are those that last for a long time, often for the patient's lifetime. Unlike acute disease, the frequency of chronic disease dramatically increases with age. Prevalence is a good measure of chronic disease, because it indicates the proportion of the population that has the condition at any one time. The most prevalent chronic disease is periodontal disease (inflammation of the gums), which

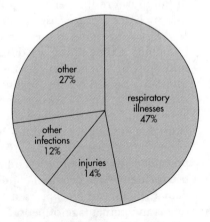

Figure 2–1. Frequency of acute diseases.

TABLE 2–2. PREVALENCE OF CHRONIC DISEASES (NUMBER OF CASES PER 1000 PERSONS)

Condition	All Ages
Chronic sinusitis	134
Arthritis	129
Deformities	129
Hypertension	108
Hay fever	101
Heart disease	86
Hearing impairment	86
Visual impairment	58
Asthma	56
Chronic bronchitis	54
Hemorrhoids	36
Dermatitis	35
Diabetes	30
Indigestion	27
Back ailments	23

Data from Vital and Health Statistics, U.S. Department of Health and Human Services; DHHS Publication No. (PHS) 96-1521, 1995.

affects about one-third of persons between 45 and 65 and about one-half of persons over 65. Patients often do not report periodontal disease as a disabling condition, so it is not listed in the comparative data given below. Mental diseases are also quite prevalent but are not accurately reported, because criteria for diagnosis vary and social stigma inhibit reporting.

Most of the leading causes of chronic disease reported in a national survey are associated with aging (Table 2–2). Arthritis occurs predominantly in the elderly. Diabetes mellitus, back ailments, hearing impairments, and visual impairments are other common chronic diseases that increase in frequency with age. Two chronic conditions that are about equally frequent in the young and old are chronic bronchitis and asthma.

DISEASE FREQUENCY RELATED TO VISITS TO FAMILY PHYSICIANS

Common conditions encountered in a family practice office are listed in Table 2–3 in approximate order of frequency. Upper respiratory

TABLE 2–3. TOP 20 REASONS FOR VISITS TO A FAMILY PHYSICIAN

1. Unspecified
2. Supervision of normal pregnancy
3. Routine infant or child health check
4. Routine general medical examination
5. Gynecologic examination
6. Vaccination
7. Acute upper respiratory infection
8. Essential hypertension
9. Depressive disorder
10. Acute sinusitis
11. Acute otitis media
12. Cystitis
13. Acute bronchitis
14. Initiation of contraceptive measures
15. Backache
16. Acute pharyngitis
17. Abdominal pain
18. Pain in joint (arthralgia)
19. Unspecified disorder of skin
20. Asthma

infections, sinusitis, otitis media, asthma, pharyngitis, bronchitis, cystitis, and abdominal pain comprise the acute conditions.

AGING

Humans, like other species, have a finite lifespan. This lifespan is determined by the process of aging, a normal process affecting all individuals that is progressive and irreversible. The human lifespan is about 85 years for females and a few years less for males. The lifespan is that age at which 50 percent of the population will die from the effects of aging.

The aging process begins at physical maturity (age 17) but does not have a marked influence on death rate until much later in life. The mechanism of death from aging is increased susceptibility to disease. For example, aged individuals will die from respiratory infections, accidents, or exposure to cold that would not have killed them at a younger age. Although medical care can protect an elderly person against a potentially fatal disease such as influenza, increased susceptibility to disease may soon be expressed by death from another cause.

There is no simple explanation of aging. Both genetic and acquired factors are involved. From a genetic standpoint, each species has a maximum lifespan that is attained by a few individuals. The maximum lifespan of about 110 years for humans has not changed during the time that the average life expectancy has risen from the 20 to 85 years of age. Some families or inbred groups of people tend to live longer than others, perhaps due to a lesser tendency to develop certain diseases. On the other hand, individuals with the rare genetic disease called *progeria* show the changes of aging at a very young age. From an experimental standpoint, cells in culture will undergo a limited number of cell divisions before dying out. The exact significance of this observation is unknown, although cell metabolism and cell turnover rates do decrease somewhat with age.

Evidence for the accumulation of acquired injuries as the cause of aging relate to alterations in cells and intercellular substances. Mutations, damage to DNA, and cell death due to radiation or the formation of free radicals may account for decreased cell turnover and decreased cell function that is observed with aging. Cross-linking of collagen and other long-lived connective tissue substances makes them more rigid and less functional leading to changes such as degenerative arthritis, wrinkling of the skin, and cataracts.

Diseases that increase in frequency with age can be roughly divided into those that are age dependent and those that are age related. Age-dependent diseases occur to some extent in all individuals with time. Examples include senile degeneration of the skin, degenerative arthritis, osteoporosis, presbyopia, endocrine changes associated with atrophy of ovaries and testes, and hyperplasia of the prostate. Age-related diseases are not part of the aging process itself, since all individuals are not affected. Examples include many types of cancer, actinic and seborrheic keratoses, atherosclerosis, hypertension, Alzheimer's disease, diverticulosis of the colon, and cataracts. Still another group of diseases accumulate in frequency with age, although their onset is not age related. Examples include chronic lung disease from smoking and gallstones.

There is considerable variation in the degree to which various body systems are affected by aging. Decrease in immunity is not overtly obvious, but is expressed by an increased susceptibility to and severity of infections in the elderly and by an increased rate of development of cancer, due to a failure to reject cancer cells as foreign. Manifestations of aging in the endocrine system include impaired glucose tolerance that predisposes to diabetes mellitus, decreased thyroid function, and decreased gonadal function leading to osteoporosis and other changes. Neuronal loss is part of the aging process, but its most severe form (Alzheimer's disease) may have a specific cause. The musculoskeletal system and skin are particularly affected by aging as can be readily seen in aged individuals. Decrease in function of the heart, lungs, liver, and kidneys can be demonstrated, but the direct changes of aging have relatively little effect compared to the major diseases of these organs, some of which are age related. The intestines show little morphologic evidence of aging, but decreased motility is frequently manifested by constipation and diverticulosis in the elderly.

The aims of a good health care system are to alleviate disability and prolong life. The evidence is clear that lifespan is finite and determined by the aging process. Some individuals reach the species limit; others die earlier due to acute or chronic disease. In the society with primitive-health care, there is high infant mortality, uncontrolled serious infections, and high death rate from accidents. The improvement in survival in a society with modern medical care is due to good maternal-infant health care, vaccination against serious infections, and high recovery rate from infections and accidents. Further gains could be made toward an ideal health care system where all deaths would be due to the consequences of aging.

In the United States, the diseases that are responsible for most of these "early" deaths are heart disease, stroke, and cancer. There is also a distinct potential for preventing the early mortality by eliminating poor maternal-infant care, which occurs in selected portions of our society.

Heart disease and stroke deaths are in part due to aging itself, but there is also an environmental factor (presumably diet) that causes accelerated atherosclerosis in the United States as compared to societies with a low-cholesterol diet such as in Japan. Japanese, like Americans, die from the effects of aging on the vascular system, but they rarely die at an early age from myocardial infarcts. This evidence suggests that some gain toward the ideal health curve could be made by a change in diet. The gain that might be expected from preventing cancer is less than the gain that might be expected from retarding the progress of atherosclerosis. This is so because cancer causes fewer deaths than atherosclerosis, and most cancer deaths occur near the time that death would occur from aging itself, regardless of the nature of the final insult.

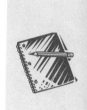

Review Questions

1. What are the leading causes of death? What percentage of people die from each?

2. How are incidence, prevalence, and mortality rates defined? Can you calculate them if given appropriate data?

3. What is the relative frequency of the leading causes of acute disease and how does this relate to age?

4. What are the most common chronic diseases? Which ones are age related?

5. Which acute and chronic diseases most frequently bring patients to their family physician?

6. How does aging relate to the causes of death?

7. What factors determine the limits of life expectancy?

8. What is the meaning of the following terms?
    Acute
    Age-dependent disease
    Age-related disease
    Aging
    Chronic
    Morbidity
    Prognosis

Diagnostic Resources 3.

APPROACH TO PATIENT CARE
  Symptomatic Disease
  Asymptomatic Disease
  Potential Disease

SCREENING

DIAGNOSTIC TESTS AND PROCEDURES
  Clinical Procedures
  Radiologic Procedures
    Diagnostic Radiology • Radiation Therapy • Nuclear Medicine
  Anatomic Pathology Tests and Procedures
    Surgical Pathology • Cytology • Autopsy
  Clinical Pathology Tests and Procedures
    Chemistry • Hematology • Microbiology • Immunopathology
    • Blood Bank
  Forensic Pathology
  Public Health Laboratories

REVIEW QUESTIONS

APPROACH TO PATIENT CARE

Symptomatic Disease

The most common approach to disease is to wait for the patient to seek help because of symptoms of disease. The health practitioner, presented with a sick patient, proceeds in a systematic fashion to help the patient by the steps outlined in Table 3–1. This process may take

TABLE 3–1. STEPS IN CARE OF SYMPTOMATIC DISEASE

1. Gather facts
   History
   Physical examination
   Laboratory tests
2. Interpret the facts and attach a summarizing label (diagnosis)
3. Treat the patient, if feasible
4. Follow up on results of treatment

minutes or weeks, depending on the complexity of the disease. Most diagnoses can be made from the history with physical examination and laboratory tests providing confirmatory evidence.

Asymptomatic Disease

Another approach to disease is to try to discover the disease in its asymptomatic stage, that is, before the patient notices it. Early diagnosis allows treatment to be started at an early stage of the disease. This approach can be applied to the individual through regular checkups such as regular dental appointments, well-baby examinations, and periodic physical examinations. This approach is also applied to defined populations through procedures such as tuberculosis testing of school children, school physicals, and army physicals. The attempt to discover disease in its early stage is called *screening*. The goal of screening is to either cure a disease by catching it early (e.g., cancer) or to begin treatment early to delay the progression of the disease (e.g., hypertension). It is of limited value to screen for diseases that cannot be treated or to spend large sums of money to find rare diseases.

Potential Disease

A third and obviously most desirable approach to disease is the prevention of its occurrence. The discipline that deals with prevention of disease is called *preventive medicine*. Most of the classic infectious diseases that formerly killed a significant proportion of the population (smallpox, plague, typhoid fever, typhus, measles, diphtheria, whooping cough) now fall into the category of potential diseases that are preventable by immunization and good sanitation. Other outstanding examples of preventable diseases are dental caries and periodontal disease, which have been greatly reduced by use of fluorides and preventive dentistry. We also know that reduction in alcoholism would prevent deaths from liver disease and accidents. Reduction in smoking would prevent many cancers (particularly lung cancer) and chronic obstructive pulmonary disease from developing. It is also likely that alteration of the types of lipids in the diet would lead to reduced atherosclerosis.

SCREENING

The techniques of screening for asymptomatic disease include history, physical examination, and laboratory tests. Screening by history involves a checklist of symptoms that may suggest further investigation. Examples of screening by physical examination include dental examination for caries, palpation of breasts for lumps, and listening to a baby's heart to detect murmurs. Some of the more important and widely used screening tests and procedures are listed in Table 3–2 along with their purpose.

DIAGNOSTIC TESTS AND PROCEDURES

Test is used here to refer to an analysis performed on a specimen removed from a patient. A *procedure* involves doing some manipulation of the patient beyond that usually done during physical examination.

TABLE 3–2. SCREENING TESTS AND PROCEDURES

Test or Procedure	Purpose
Cervical (Pap) smear	Early detection of uterine cancer
Blood count	Detection of anemia
Urinalysis	Detection of urinary infection or kidney disease
Fecal occult blood test	Detection of hidden bleeding from colon cancer
Serum lipids (especially cholesterol)	Detection of tendency to have atherosclerosis
Serology	Detection of syphilis prior to pregnancy
Dental x-rays	Finding caries (cavities)
Chest x-ray	Detection of tuberculosis or lung cancer
Mammography	Detection of breast cancer
Visual acuity tests	Detection of visual problems in preschool children and automobile license applicants
Audiograms	Detection of hearing problems in school children
Tuberculin skin test	Detection of children who might have tuberculosis
Electrocardiogram	Detection of asymptomatic myocardial infarcts
Sigmoidoscopy	Detection of colon cancer

Some procedures are done to obtain specimens for a test. Most tests are performed by or supervised by a pathologist. Procedures are performed by various types of physicians, including radiologists and pathologists.

Clinical Procedures

Primary health care practitioners may perform some common or simple tests and procedures themselves. For example, laboratory tests such as urinalysis, blood counts, and throat cultures may be done in a physician's office. Manipulative procedures such as sigmoidoscopy may be done by the primary care physician, or the patient may be referred to a specialist for more complex procedures. One function of the various medical specialists is the performance of specific manipulative procedures to detect disease in hidden areas of the body. For example, the urologist looks in the bladder with a cystoscope and the gastroenterologist looks into the stomach with an endoscope. Other procedures will be mentioned in the chapters that deal with diseases of the various organs.

Radiologic Procedures

Radiology is the discipline of medicine performed by radiologists and includes diagnostic radiology, nuclear medicine, and radiation ther-

TABLE 3–3. RADIOLOGIC PROCEDURES

Test or Procedure	Lesions Commonly Detected
Dental x-rays	Caries
Sinus films	Sinusitis
Chest x-ray	Any lesion that replaces normally air-filled lungs
Upper gastrointestinal series	Defects or tumors of the esophagus, stomach, and upper small intestine
Barium enema	Tumors, ulcers, and diverticula of the colon
Gallbladder series	Gallstones
Intravenous urogram	Decrease in kidney function, obstruction of the urinary tract
Bone films	Any lesion that destroys bone; fractures
Myelogram	Obstruction of the space surrounding the spinal cord
Arteriogram	Obstruction or displacement of arteries
Computerized tomography	Tumors and other lesions
Ultrasound	Gallstones, cysts, twin pregnancy
Magnetic resonance	Tumors and other lesions
Nuclear isotope scans	Tumors, altered tissue uptake of specific substances

apy. Some of the more common radiologic procedures used for diagnosis are listed in Table 3–3.

Diagnostic radiology involves x-ray and other imaging procedures such as ultrasound and magnetic resonance imaging that are used to locate and describe morphologic lesions in a living patient.

X-ray procedures are dependent upon differing absorption properties encountered in the x-ray path to produce images of the tissue. In conventional x-ray techniques, the net amount of x-radiation that passes through the body exposes film to produce a *roentgenogram* (colloquially called an x-ray). Radiodense material, such as barium, or radiolucent material, such as air, can be introduced into body passageways to provide contrast with tissue. Alternatively, the x-rays that pass through the body may be viewed with a fluoroscope, an instrument that uses a fluorescent plate to detect x-rays. A roentgenogram is a static image; a fluoroscopic image is dynamic and allows the radiologist to watch movements such as the passage of barium down the esophagus. A chest roentgenogram of a patient with advanced tuberculosis (Figure 3–1) shows radiodensity in the diseased left lung and radiopacity of the air-filled right lung.

Computerized tomography (CT) is a sophisticated x-ray technique in which the x-ray absorption patterns through planes of tissue are analyzed and recorded by computer for each point in the plane. The computerized images can be translated into printed images or viewed on a screen. Because computerized tomography looks at a

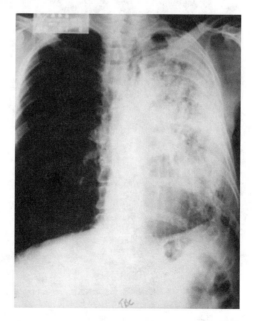

Figure 3–1. Chest roentgenogram, tuberculosis of left lung (right side of picture).

single plane at a time, lesions can be more sharply defined and precisely localized. As with conventional x-ray techniques, contrast materials can be used to outline hollow organs. Lesions that are hidden deep in the body such as the kidney cancer with spread to the liver (Figure 3–2) are well delineated by computerized tomography.

Magnetic resonance imaging (MRI) is similar to computerized tomography in its use of a computer to record tissue characteristics in tissue planes, but differs in that it does not use x-rays. The image is produced by displacing protons in atomic nuclei with radiofrequency signals while the body is surrounded by a strong magnet. The affected protons release a similar radiofrequency signal that can be evaluated by computer to produce images of a section through the body. Different physical characteristics of protons among the elements allow production of two types of images. T1 images give a strong signal for lipid and T2 images give a strong signal for water. Because of cost, the use of magnetic resonance is limited to major medical centers. It is very useful for locating lesions, especially neoplasms. The anatomic detail provided is illustrated in Figure 3–3.

Ultrasound examination measures the reflection of high frequency sound waves as they pass through body tissues. The greatest contrast is provided by interfaces of soft tissues and liquids; therefore, this technique has its greatest usefulness in studying cystic structures

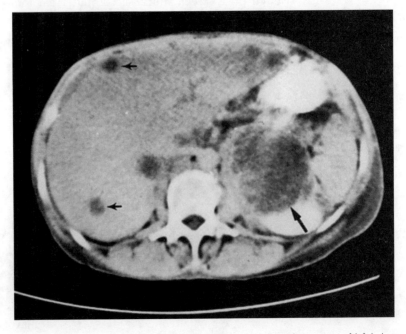

Figure 3–2. Abdominal cross-section by computerized tomography, cancer of left kidney (*large arrows*) with metastases to liver (*small arrows*).

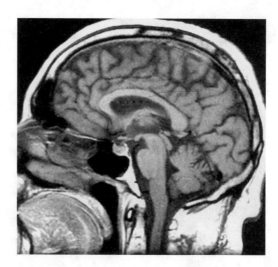

Figure 3–3. Normal head, including brain, by magnetic resonance imaging.

such as gallbladder, kidney, and gravid uterus. It is the procedure of choice for detecting gallstones. In pregnancy, it can be used without risk of radiation to the fetus. Twins and ectopic pregnancies are easily detected (Figure 3–4).

The subspecialty of nuclear medicine involves the injection of various radioactive materials into the bloodstream and subsequently determining their degree of localization within tissue. The body is scanned externally for radioactivity and the results recorded as a *nuclear isotope scan.* Areas of decreased concentration within an organ suggest a space-occupying lesion such as a neoplasm (negative image); some neoplasms exhibit an increased uptake of isotope (positive image) (Figure 3–5). The functional activity of an organ can also be evaluated; for example, the amount of radioactive iodine taken up by the thyroid gland reflects thyroid function.

Radiation therapy is the branch of radiology involved in treatment of cancer and other conditions with x-rays and gamma rays. Some cancers may be cured by radiation; others are treated to slow the progress of the disease and delay complications. When cure is not expected, the therapy is referred to as *palliative.*

Anatomic Pathology Tests and Procedures

Surgical pathology involves the diagnosis of lesions in pieces of tissue removed from a patient. Diagnosis is based on gross (naked-eye) and microscopic examination and interpretation by a pathologist. *Biopsy* is the procedure for obtaining small specimens. Partial (incisional)

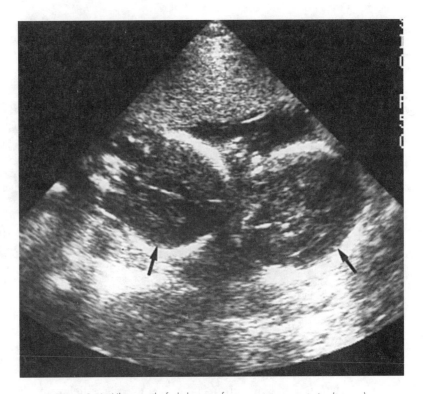

Figure 3–4. Ultrasound of abdomen of pregnant woman, twins (*arrows*).

biopsy specimens include only part of the lesion and are done primarily for diagnosis. Needle biopsy, which involves the insertion of a needle into a solid organ and aspiration of a core of tissue, is widely used for the diagnosis of liver, kidney, and prostate disease. Fine-needle aspiration (FNA) is a technique that uses a small caliber needle to obtain aspirated tissue for cytologic examination. Fine-needle aspiration is faster and less expensive than open biopsy for the diagnosis of certain cancers, but may not always provide a specimen that is adequate for diagnosis. Excisional biopsy specimens include the entirety of a small lesion and are done for both diagnosis and treatment. The removal of large specimens in the operating room is called *resection.* Resected specimens are usually removed primarily for treatment purposes. Biopsy specimens ordinarily require 1 to 2 days for preparation of microscopic slides by histotechnicians and then microscopic examination and diagnosis by a pathologist. When more rapid diagnosis is needed (as a basis for immediate therapeutic decision), a frozen section can be prepared in a few minutes for interpretation by the pathologist.

All tissues removed from a patient are examined by a pathologist to insure accuracy of diagnosis. Gross examination is sufficient for

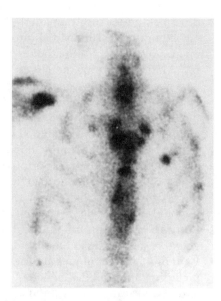

Figure 3–5. Nuclear isotope bone scan demonstrating spread of a breast cancer to bone (*dark areas*).

some specimens such as teeth, placentas, varicose veins, and tonsils from children. All other specimens are examined microscopically.

Cytology specimens contain cells sloughed or scraped from body surfaces. These are used primarily to detect cancer cells, and the majority of cytology specimens are from the uterine cervix (Pap smears). Ordinarily the stained smears are examined by a cytotechnologist, and any abnormalities are interpreted by a pathologist. Any body fluid, such as urine, sputum, cerebrospinal fluid, and pleural fluid, can be used for cytologic study. The vast majority of cytologic examinations are done to detect cancer.

An autopsy is the postmortem examination of a body. Organs of the neck, chest, abdomen, and cranium are ordinarily examined to make a final evaluation of the nature and extent of disease and to determine the probable cause of death. Biochemical, microbiologic, and immunologic tests can be performed if needed. The autopsy is performed by a pathologist with the help of a trained technician or a mortician. An autopsy requires advance permission of the next of kin. In the case of unexpected death or suspicion of homicide, the medical examiner or coroner may authorize an autopsy.

Clinical Pathology Tests and Procedures

Clinical pathology or *laboratory medicine* is the branch of pathology that performs laboratory tests on tissues and fluids other than those already described under surgical pathology and cytology. The clinical pathology laboratory is subdivided into sections of chemistry, hematology, microbiology, immunopathology, and blood bank. Biochemical tests on blood account for the largest number of tests done. Biochemical tests may be used to evaluate organ function or to detect relatively specific abnormalities. A complete blood count (CBC) is the most common hematologic test and consists of measurement of hemoglobin, counting of white and red blood cells, and microscopic evaluation for morphologic changes in the blood cells. Special hematologic tests are available for evaluation of various types of anemia and evaluation of blood coagulation. Blood banking or transfusion medicine involves the procurement, typing, testing, processing, storage, and administering of blood components as well as evaluation of adverse reactions to transfusion therapy. Immunopathology involves the detection of antigens and antibodies in blood and tissue and the study of lymphocytes. Immunologic techniques are used to detect a wide variety of diseases including immunodeficiencies, allergic (hypersensitivity) diseases, and certain cancers. Bacterial culture is the most common test performed in the microbiology laboratory because bacteria are easily grown and can be tested for their sensitivity to antibiotics. The ease and means of detection of other types of microbes such as parasites and viruses is variable.

Forensic Pathology

Forensic pathologists are pathologists specially trained to investigate accidental and criminal deaths. There are relatively few forensic pathologists in the United States, and most work in large metropolitan areas. In most communities, the investigation of accidental, sudden, or suspected criminal deaths is carried out by the county medical examiner or coroner, who may be any physician appointed to the office. When an autopsy is needed, the county medical examiner calls upon a general pathologist to perform the autopsy. In unusual cases, a forensic pathologist may be brought in to help.

Public Health Laboratories

Public health laboratories are established by governments to help in the control of communicable diseases. For this reason, they perform many microbiologic tests, such as blood tests for syphilis, rabies tests, and viral cultures to identify epidemics of virus infection. Water testing is another important aspect of community health. State health laboratories may serve as a reference laboratory and provide a link with the National Communicable Disease Laboratory in Atlanta, Georgia. Certain highly contagious diseases require reporting to state authorities.

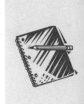

Review Questions

1. What strategies do health care practitioners use to deal with symptomatic disease, asymptomatic disease, and potential disease?

2. Which diseases are commonly detected by screening? What screening test or procedure is used for each?

3. What types of diagnostic tests and procedures are performed or directed by each of the following?
   - Forensic pathologist
   - Medical specialist
   - Pathologist
   - Primary care physician
   - Public health laboratory
   - Radiologist

4. What is the meaning of the following terms?
   - Biopsy specimen
   - Excisional biopsy
   - Fine-needle aspiration
   - Incisional biopsy
   - Needle biopsy
   - Procedure
   - Resected specimen
   - Test

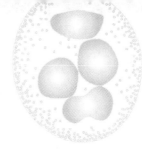

BASIC DISEASE PROCESS

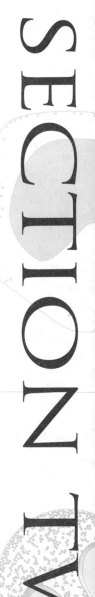

The purpose of this section is to give you a clear picture of the fundamental mechanisms of disease. The knowledge learned here will apply to almost every disease presented throughout the rest of the book. We have chosen to present this material rather concisely so that we can spend more time on individual diseases. We recommend that you study these chapters very thoroughly, review them as you progress through the book, and consult other texts to broaden your understanding of these topics.

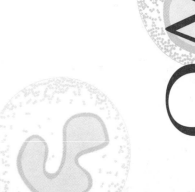

Injury, Inflammation, and Repair

REVIEW OF STRUCTURE AND FUNCTION
Cell Structure and Function • Classification of Cells and Intercellular Substances • White Blood Cells • Connective Tissue Structure • Regulation of Tissue Fluids • Physiologic Replacement of Cells

EVENTS FOLLOWING INJURY

INJURY
  Acute Injury and Necrosis
  Chronic Injury: Atrophy and Accumulations

INFLAMMATION
  Acute Inflammation
  Chronic Inflammation
  Granulomatous Inflammation
  Exudates and Transudates
  Gross Inflammatory Lesions
    Abscess • Cellulitis • Ulcer

REPAIR
  Regeneration
  Fibrous Connective Tissue Repair (Scarring or Fibrosis)
  Wound Repair

REVIEW QUESTIONS

REVIEW OF STRUCTURE AND FUNCTION

The body is made up of cells and intercellular substances that are capable of undergoing dynamic change to carry out body functions, including self-renewal. One or several of the more than 100 cell types, along with appropriate intercellular substances, comprise a tissue. The term *tissue* is usually used to refer to a functional grouping of cells and intercellular substances at the microscopic level. An *organ* is one or more tissues arranged into a tissue mass that carries out a major body function. For example, liver tissue forms one massive organ called the liver, whereas, loose connective tissue is a general type of tissue that may be a part of many organs. The cells that carry out the main function of an organ, and are usually most abundant and often unique to the organ, are called parenchymal cells. For example, hepatocytes, renal tubular epithelial cells, cardiac muscle cells, and osteocytes are the parenchymal cells of their respective organs (liver, kidney, heart, and bone).

Typical components of a cell are illustrated in Figure 4–1. The nucleus is surrounded by a nuclear membrane and contains loosely arranged chromatin, which stains with basic dyes such as hematoxylin because of its high content of deoxyribonucleic acid (DNA). During cell division, the chromatin aggregates into discrete strands, or chromosomes, which replicate and separate to form two daughter cells. The nucleus is vital to the cell because the genetic code in its DNA is

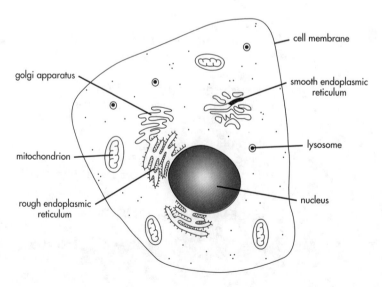

Figure 4–1. Components of a cell.

the ultimate regulator of cell function. Histologically, changes in the nucleus are used as indicators of cell death.

The cytoplasm of a cell consists of the cell membrane, cytoplasmic organelles, and a soluble phase called the cytosol. The cell membrane protects the cell from physical injury and selectively regulates the entrance and exit of various ions and nutrients, such as amino acids and sugars. Movement of water to and from the cell is dependent upon movement of ions and nutrients. When the regulation of water movement fails, the cell may swell or shrink. Cytoplasmic organelles include structures such as mitochondria, rough and smooth endoplasmic reticulum, Golgi apparatus, and lysosomes. Mitochondria are complex, membranous structures that generate energy for use by the cell. Injuries that interfere with energy production often cause the mitochondria to swell and later condense. The endoplasmic reticulum is a tortuous set of membranes. Rough endoplasmic reticulum is lined by small basophilic granules called *ribosomes* because of their high content of ribonucleic acid. Proteins produced under the enzymatic control of ribosomes are carried along the rough endoplasmic reticulum to the Golgi apparatus, where they are stored for secretion. The smooth endoplasmic reticulum also serves to transport materials through the cell and is the site of production of many biochemical substances other than proteins. Lysosomes are membrane-bound packets of digestive enzymes. Lysosomes may coalesce to surround and digest foreign substances that have been engulfed (phagocytosed) by the cell. Worn out or injured parts of the cytoplasm may also be digested by lysosomes, a process known as autophagocytosis.

A simple classification of tissue components is shown in Table 4–1. The two most varied classes of cells are epithelial cells and connective tissue cells. The distinction between these two classes of cells is very important in pathology because they react quite differently in disease situations. Epithelial cells work with each other in tight clusters to carry out specialized functions, such as protection of body surfaces, secretion of specific products, and special metabolic functions. Injury interferes with their specialized function and causes them to revert to a more primitive stage for purposes of reproduction to replace cells that have been killed. Connective tissue cells are more loosely arranged and are involved in general support functions, such as providing physical support and promoting the appropriate movement of fluids and nutrients. An example of the arrangement of the various cell types into a tissue is shown in Figure 4–2.

White blood cells (leukocytes) are very mobile nonepithelial cells that are specialized to aid in attacking foreign substances. Each type has a characteristic morphologic appearance (Figure 4–3). *Neutrophils*, also called *polymorphonuclear leukocytes* or *polys*, and *monocytes* can engulf (phagocytose) and digest foreign materials such as bacteria. When

TABLE 4–1. STRUCTURAL ELEMENTS OF TISSUES

Cells
  Epithelium
  Connective tissue cells
    Fixed: Fibrocytes, chondrocytes, osteocytes, endothelial cells
    Motile: Blood cells
  Muscle cells
  Nervous tissue cells
Intercellular substances
  Basement membranes
  Ground substance
  Collagen
  Elastin
  Cartilage
  Bone

monocytes leave the bloodstream and enter tissue they are called *macrophages* or *histiocytes*. Lymphocytes direct the attack against persistent foreign materials by remembering the chemical structure of the foreign materials. Lymphocytes release substances (lymphotoxins) that kill cells in the area of the foreign material and other substances that attract macrophages to the area. The macrophages, in turn, can phagocytose both the foreign material and dead cells to prevent further spread of the foreign substance. Some lymphocytes (B-cells) also transform into plasma cells to produce antibodies. Antibodies attach to the unique chemical structure of the foreign substance (antigen) to

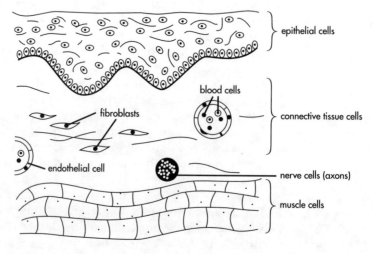

Figure 4–2. Comparative features of major cell types in the wall of the oral cavity.

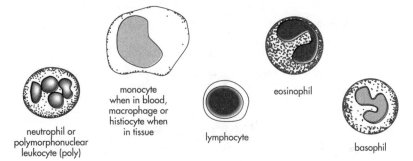

neutrophil or
polymorphonuclear
leukocyte (poly)

monocyte
when in blood,
macrophage or
histiocyte when
in tissue

lymphocyte

eosinophil

basophil

Figure 4-3. Types of white blood cells.

aid in neutralizing or destroying the foreign substance. The other two types of white blood cells, basophils and eosinophils, are much less abundant. Both are involved in allergic reactions and are discussed in Chapter 27.

The connective tissue structure of the body involves physical support and transportation. Gross tissues for physical support include bone, cartilage, tendons, fascia, and other fibrous tissues. At the microscopic level, connective tissues contain ground substance, which allows passage of fluid and nutrients. Basement membranes surround epithelial clumps and allow passage of fluid and nutrients to and from the epithelial cells. Collagen is the most abundant component of connective tissues. The amount of collagen relates to the strength and fibrous nature of the connective tissue. Thus, loose connective tissue contains little collagen and dense connective tissue contains much collagen. Vessels course through the supporting connective tissue to allow fluids to be carried close to epithelial cells and other active tissues such as muscle.

Regulation of tissue fluids is a function of movement of water in and out of small blood vessels (capillaries and venules) and uptake of fluid by lymphatics. Fluid and nutrients pass out of the small blood vessels and diffuse through the ground substance and basement membranes so that exchange with cells can occur. Reverse movement can occur back into blood vessels or into lymphatic vessels. The most important factors in this regulatory process are the pressure in the vessels, the osmotic pressure difference between tissue and blood due to the relative amount of large protein molecules present, and the size of the pores between endothelial cells in the lining of small vessels. This regulatory process is important in situations of injury, because larger amounts of fluid and nutrients are needed to react to the injury.

Physiologic replacement of cells is a normal process that closely relates to the repair of injuries to be discussed later in this chapter. Certain body cells wear out rapidly and are continually being replaced.

These include blood cells and cells lining body surfaces such as skin and intestinal mucosa. Most glandular epithelial cells and cells that form the supportive connective tissue undergo very slow replacement but are capable of more rapid replacement if necessary. Other types of cells, such as cardiac muscle cells and neurons, cannot be replaced.

EVENTS FOLLOWING INJURY

The events following injury are a continuum of necrosis, inflammation, and repair. Necrosis is the death of cells or tissue in a localized area of the body due to injury, either exogenous or endogenous. *Necrosis* consists of the direct effects of the injury plus the changes that occur in cells after they die. Mild forms of injury may produce sublethal cell injury without necrosis, changes that may be referred to as *degeneration.* We will avoid use of the word degeneration and use the term necrosis with the realization that lethal and sublethal cellular changes occur together in varying proportions. *Inflammation* is the vascular and cellular response to necrosis or sublethal cell injury and is the body's mechanism of limiting the spread of injury and removing necrotic debris. *Repair* refers to the body's attempt to replace dead cells, whether by regeneration of the original tissue or replacement by connective tissue.

Another type of cell death is *apoptosis,* often referred to as "programmed cell death." Apoptotic cell death ocurrs during embryogenesis when not all cells generated are needed. It is also the mechanism of ridding the body of excess lymphocytes following resolution of an inflammatory or immune event, of hormone-dependent cell death after the hormonal stimulus has been removed, of tumor cell death, and of cell death following injury from a variety of agents that might cause necrosis under other conditions. Apoptosis is referred to as programmed because it results from the activation of specific genes following appropriate stimuli. In tissue sections, it differs in appearance from necrosis in that the cell shrinks, the nuclear chromatin condenses into dense masses, blebs form in the cytoplasm, and the apoptotic cells are phagocytized by macrophages or adjacent parenchymal cells. Importantly, apoptosis does not elicit inflammation. Mainly for the latter reason, further discussion of cell death in this chapter will concern necrosis.

The relative intensity of necrosis, inflammation, and repair depends on the magnitude of the injury, the duration of injury, and, to some extent, on the location within the body and the nature of the injury. Some examples of how necrosis, inflammation, and repair vary with intensity and duration of injury are shown in Figure 4–4. In general, inflammation begins shortly after the effects of cell injury are

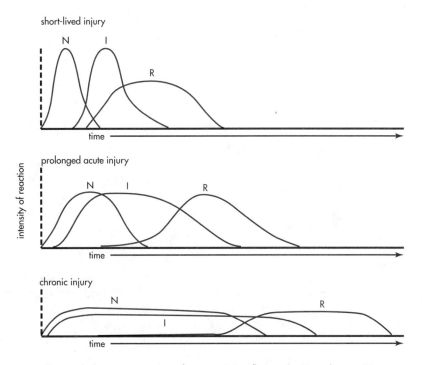

short-lived injury

prolonged acute injury

chronic injury

Figure 4–4. Time sequences of necrosis (N), inflammation (I), and repair (R).

evident. Repair is usually not well established until necrosis ceases, although in very chronic injuries, all three processes are likely to occur together. Inflammation itself, when intense, is a cause of necrosis. The body, in a sense, sacrifices some of its own tissue to isolate an injurious agent.

INJURY

The critical difference between sublethal (reversible) cell injury and necrosis is whether the cell can recover or is already dead. Certain changes in the nucleus, as seen in microscopic sections, indicate cell death. Nuclear changes may include condensation of the nucleus (*pyknosis*), fragmentation of the nucleus (*karyorrhexis*), and lysis or fading of the nucleus (*karyolysis*). These nuclear changes take a number of hours to develop, so cells that have died and are fixed in formaldehyde may not show these changes. For example, a person who has a myocardial infarct (heart attack) may die within 12 hours and not show these histologic changes of necrosis. If the patient had lived, some of the myocardial cells would have developed the histologic changes of necrosis whereas others may have developed reversible changes and then recovered. Reversible cell injury is characterized by preservation of the nucleus and variable changes in the cytoplasm such as swelling or condensation. These histologic changes reflect biochemical changes in the cell. There is no exact biochemical end point that determines cell death, but depletion in the cell's energy system and alteration of cell membrane permeability are important events in cell death. Once the nucleus is destroyed or the cell membrane disrupted, the cell cannot recover. After cell death, enzymes released from the cell's own lysosomes begin to digest the remains of the cell. Other events associated with necrosis include influx of calcium, dissolution of ribosomes, clumping of DNA followed by its enzymatic digestion, and finally rupture of the cell membrane.

Acute changes resulting from sudden injury to a cell or tissue lead to cell death or recovery within a short time. Necrosis is often associated with acute injury. Chronic injury (mild continuous injury) leads to cumulative effects on the cells and the tissues. Necrosis is not usually prominent and may be of such a low degree as to be imperceptible in histologic sections.

Acute Injury and Necrosis

The effects of acute injury have their most prominent effect on cells, because cells are more susceptible to injury than are the noncellular connective tissue elements. Cells may be injured by any of the exogenous and endogenous causes discussed in Chapter 1.

Lack of oxygen (anoxia) or reduced oxygen (hypoxia) is one of the most common causes of acute injury and necrosis. Cells are vulnerable to hypoxia in proportion to their oxygen requirements; thus metabolically active cells are selectively vulnerable. Selective vulnerability is well illustrated by cases of systemic anoxia from such causes as carbon monoxide poisoning, blood loss, or suffocation. In these situations, neurons in the brain and the kidneys' tubular epithelial cells are more vulnerable to necrosis than other types of cells. Localized hypoxia due to poor blood flow is called *ischemia*. When severe, ischemia leads to necrosis of the cells in the area of the deranged blood supply. An area of ischemic necrosis is called an *infarct*. Infarcts are most commonly due to obstruction of arteries, especially arteries that supply a defined segment of tissue. As noted in Chapter 2, atherosclerotic plaques that obstruct coronary arteries and lead to myocardial infarcts are responsible for a high percentage of all deaths. Atherosclerotic obstruction is also important in producing infarcts of the brain, legs, kidneys, and other sites.

Thrombi and emboli are also important causes of ischemic necrosis (infarcts). A *thrombus* is a blood clot that forms during life in a blood vessel due to activation of the coagulation mechanism. It is composed of layers of fibrin and entrapped blood cells. An *embolus* is any particulate object that travels in the bloodstream from one site to another and is most commonly a thrombus, but may be composed of other substances such as bone marrow, fat, air, or cancer tissue. Thrombotic emboli most commonly originate in the leg veins with spread through the vena cava and right heart to the pulmonary arteries or from the left side of the heart with spread through the aorta to various organs such as brain, legs, kidneys, spleen, and intestines. Bone marrow and fat emboli occur from trauma to bones; when severe, the fat globules pass through the pulmonary vessels and gain access to the systemic circulation where they may cause obstruction of the small vessels of the brain.

Trauma, infection, and hypersensitivity are other common causes of acute injury and necrosis. Trauma disrupts cells by direct physical force; the effects are dependent on the site injured and nature of the force applied. Although there are many types of infections and the degree of injury varies widely, most of the damage is produced by the body's own inflammatory reaction to the invading microorganism. The basic mechanisms of this process will be discussed; a much more detailed account of the reactions to the major groups of offending organisms and specific pathogens can be found in Chapter 26. Immunologic mechanisms are an important part of the inflammatory reaction and also contribute to the damage produced by inflammation, but the immune damage is usually less than the potential damage that could be inflicted by the offending agent. When an immunologic or presumed immunologic reaction occurs only in certain individuals (those that are sensitive), the reaction is called a hypersensitivity reaction or *allergy*. Poison ivy, hay fever, hives, and contact dermatitis are common examples. Sometimes the body's immune system reacts to its own tissues (*autoimmune reaction*) producing destructive diseases such as rheumatoid arthritis, lupus erythematosus, and thyroiditis. Chapter 25 details the mechanisms and classification of immunologic disease. It would be helpful at this time to examine the first portions of Chapters 26 and 27, which describe the common types of physical and chemical injuries.

The morphology of reversible cell injury and necrosis is a continuum (Figure 4–5). If the injury is mild and functional changes following the injury go away in a few hours, we can anticipate that the cells involved underwent sublethal changes with return to normal. If functional changes persist, it is likely that at least some cells underwent necrosis; recovery will then depend upon regeneration, a process discussed later in the chapter. Study of biopsy specimens or tissues

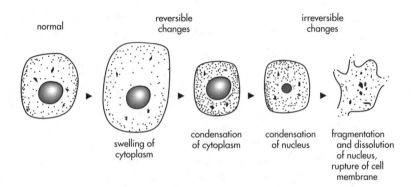

Figure 4–5. Cellular changes leading to cell death.

removed at autopsy allows the pathologist the opportunity to evaluate the extent of injury. Changes in reversibly damaged cells will be limited to the cytoplasm; necrotic cells will have both cytoplasmic and nuclear changes. Typically, the early change is cytoplasmic swelling producing enlarged cells with pale cytoplasm. Later the cytoplasm may be shrunken and more densely eosinophilic than normal. The development of nuclear changes—pyknosis, karyorrhexis, or karyolysis—indicates progression to necrosis. Thus, when reversible changes predominate, a tissue will be enlarged; when necrosis predominates, a tissue will be of normal size or shrunken.

Necrotic tissue takes on different gross and microscopic appearances depending on circumstances; recognition of these differences allows prediction of the cause of the necrosis. *Coagulation necrosis* is most commonly caused by anoxia, whether it be generalized or ischemic. The involved tissue undergoes slow disintegration with denaturation of cellular protein by the dead cells' own lysosomal enzymes. In many tissues, the coagulation process evolves slowly over a number of days producing the characteristic preservation of cell and tissue outlines until the later stages of the process. The pathologist can recognize the coagulation necrosis of an infarct by its pale yellow color and solid but soft texture. The location, size, and shape of the infarct will be dependent on the area supplied by the blocked artery.

Liquefaction necrosis is most commonly caused by certain types of bacteria, known as pyogenic bacteria. Pyogenic bacteria attract neutrophils into the area and the enzymes released by the neutrophils liquefy the dead tissue producing a thick, creamy mixture of dead tissue and neutrophils called *pus* or *purulent exudate*. When cut into, an area of liquefaction necrosis will exude pus and leave a hole in the tissue.

Caseous necrosis is most commonly caused by *Mycobacterium tuberculosis* (the bacteria that causes tuberculosis) or by certain types of fungi. Caseous necrosis looks different because it is necrosis of diseased tissue. The causative organisms are attacked by large numbers of lipid-containing macrophages. Necrosis of these macrophages produces a solid, amorphous, cheesy mass. Microscopically, a confluent mass of red cytoplasm with scattered nuclear dust remains. The alert pathologist, however, will use special staining techniques to demonstrate the causative organisms in the caseous material and sometimes the organisms can be cultured.

Enzymatic fat necrosis, which occurs in the pancreas and surrounding adipose tissue due to leakage of that organ's digestive enzymes, produces chalky, yellow-white nodules somewhat resembling caseous necrosis. The location, however, is limited to the pancreas and surroundings.

Gangrenous necrosis (gangrene) is coagulation necrosis with superimposed decomposition by saprophytic bacteria. It is similar to postmortem decomposition except that only a portion of the body is dead. In *gas gangrene,* however, the organisms causing the gangrene include a strain of bacteria of the genus *Clostridium* that produces gas and a necrotizing toxin. The toxin of gas gangrene can spread to normal tissue and produce lethal effects.

Chronic Injury: Atrophy and Accumulations

Chronic injury may produce a decrease in tissue size (atrophy) or accumulation of material within cells or between cells. Atrophy may be due to a decrease in the size of cells or a decrease in the number of cells or both. A gradual loss of cells is the most common mechanism. Some of the types of atrophy will be briefly discussed.

Senile atrophy is caused by aging. As persons age, their tissues often become smaller and decrease in functional capacity, presumably as a natural part of the aging process. For example, the brains of elderly people become smaller, while decreased memory and slowed thought processes provide some evidence of decreased cellular function.

Disuse atrophy occurs when the cells unable to carry on their normal function undergo atrophy. For example, when an arm or leg is placed in a cast, the muscle cells become smaller and show a decreased ability to contract.

Pressure atrophy results from steady pressure on tissue, such as might be produced by the mass of an expanding tumor. Bedsores are another common example. They occur in chronically bedridden patients due to continued external pressure on the skin.

Endocrine atrophy is due to decreased hormonal stimulation. Certain organs are maintained in a functional state by the action of hormones upon them. Insufficient hormone results in atrophy in the respective organ. For example, the decrease in estrogen and progesterone at the time of menopause results in atrophy of the breasts and the uterus.

Chronic injuries associated with accumulation of substances are quite different from atrophy. Many times, cells will slowly accumulate their own metabolic products or exogenous materials, with resultant decrease in cell function over a period of time. The storage of these materials may even result in an enlarged cell, albeit with decreased function. These types of chronic cell or tissue degeneration are classified according to the type of material accumulated.

Accumulation of lipid within cells is called *fatty change* or *fatty metamorphosis*. Fatty change should be distinguished from adiposity. In adiposity, there is an increased storage of fat in fat cells; in fatty change, fat droplets appear as an abnormality in parenchymal cells. Fatty change may be either acute or chronic, and characteristically occurs in cells involved in fat metabolism, especially the liver. The liver takes in lipid in the form of triglycerides (from dietary absorption) and free fatty acids (from adipose tissue stores or absorption). Triglycerides and free fatty acids are metabolized in the liver to lipoprotein, a much more soluble form of lipid that can be exported for use by other tissues. Droplets of triglyceride may form in hepatocytes due to decreased production of lipoprotein or increased uptake of lipid from the blood. Causes of fatty liver include mobilization of more fat than the liver can handle such as occurs in diabetes mellitus, excess dietary intake as in obesity, chemical injury as in alcoholism and carbon tetrachloride poisoning, and acute starvation where there is depletion of the proteins needed to form lipoproteins. In chronic alcoholism, the liver may become more than twice normal size due to the accumulation of fat in hepatocytes. In diabetes mellitus, there is decreased uptake of fat in adipose tissue and increased accumulation in the liver. Alcoholism is the most common cause of clinically significant fatty liver in affluent societies.

Glycogen storage is an example of accumulation of carbohydrate. It occurs in rare genetic conditions where specific enzymes for glycogen breakdown are missing. The glycogen accumulates in various organs and eventually causes malfunction.

Accumulations of excess protein become compacted, producing a dense, homogeneous, eosinophilic deposit called *hyalin*. Excess collagen and compacted fibrin clots are the most common causes of hyalinization. Amyloid is a hyalin deposit of protein that has a crystalline chemical structure, which polarizes light and stains with the dye Congo red. Certain small proteins leak from the blood and crystallize to form extracellular deposits of amyloid. Examples of proteins that can form amyloid include immunoglobulin light chains derived from abnormal proliferations of plasma cells, serum amyloid-associated protein produced by the liver in prolonged chronic inflammations, and beta protein deposited in the brain in Alzheimer's disease. Amyloid deposits develop very slowly, affect organ function late in the course of disease, and are not reversible.

Accumulations of minerals and pigments include calcification, hemosiderosis, and brown atrophy. In some situations, the deposition of minerals or pigments is associated with obvious tissue injury, but in others it is difficult to prove that excessive accumulation of a given pigment or mineral is deleterious to that tissue. Calcification is of two types. Excessive blood calcium, which may result from certain metabolic disorders, leads to calcium accumulation in tissues, especially those that excrete acid from the body such as renal tubules, lung, and gastric mucosa. This is termed *metastatic calcification.* As noted above, dying cells take on calcium. When this calcium remains as a deposit in the area of necrosis, it is known as *dystrophic calcification.* Most dystrophic calcification causes no problem in itself, but since calcium is radiopaque, it allows the radiologist to spot areas of disease. For example, foci of caseous necrosis in the lung caused by tuberculosis will remain evident to the radiologist for years or a breast cancer with focal calcification due to areas of necrosis may be discovered by mammography.

Hemosiderosis and *hemochromatosis* are terms applied to excessive iron accumulation in tissues; the former term implies iron accumulation in tissues; the latter term implies a more serious condition associated with tissue damage. Normally, the absorption of iron from the intestines is carefully regulated so that the body has enough for production of red blood cells and other needs, but not too much. Excessive iron may be introduced into the body by blood transfusion or excessive absorption may occur due to genetic causes, dietary overload, or increased need produced by hemolytic anemias (anemias caused by excessive destruction of red blood cells). The excess iron in the form of ferritin combines with protein to form hemosiderin, a brown pigment that accumulates in cells, especially macrophages and hepatocytes. Hemochromatosis is usually due to a genetic defect in regulation of iron uptake and its damaging effects are most felt in the liver and pancreatic islets with resultant cirrhosis of the liver and

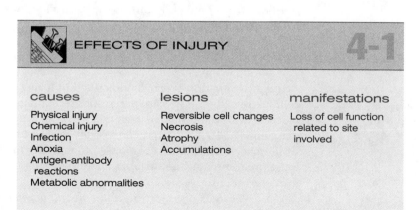

EFFECTS OF INJURY   4-1

causes	lesions	manifestations
Physical injury	Reversible cell changes	Loss of cell function
Chemical injury	Necrosis	related to site
Infection	Atrophy	involved
Anoxia	Accumulations	
Antigen-antibody reactions		
Metabolic abnormalities		

diabetes mellitus. Periodic withdrawal of blood lowers body iron stores and reduces the progress of this disease.

Brown atrophy is an old term applied to the brown color of the heart and the liver that develops with aging from the accumulation of *lipofuscin* pigment in myocardial fibers and hepatocytes. This poorly defined pigment, composed of lipid, carbohydrate, and protein, is the residue of lysosomal digestion of cellular debris and has no clinical significance other than being a marker for aging or increased cellular damage.

INFLAMMATION

Inflammation is the protective response that the body mounts in response to injury. The term is appropriate in that an inflamed lesion, such as a burn, is red, hot, and painful like fire. As we have seen, necrosis reflects the destructive effects of injury to cells. Inflammation focuses on materials—fluid, chemicals, and cells—brought to the injured area and how these materials limit the injury and remove necrotic debris. The process of inflammation involves very complex chemical and, to a lesser extent, neural mechanisms that serve to turn the "fire fighters" on quickly and mobilize more reserves, but also to turn the process off so that the cellular and chemical fire fighters do not destroy any more normal tissue than is necessary to control the spread of injury.

The nature of the inflammatory response is stereotyped; the degree and duration vary depending on the cause and time course of the injury. The stereotyped response is described under acute inflammation and the variations produced by prolonged injury and certain agents are described under chronic inflammation. Although inflammation is described as a protective response, it also has its damaging effects. The potential for drugs to modify the inflammatory response has stimulated continued research to unravel its complex biochemical control mechanisms.

Acute Inflammation

Acute inflammation is usually described in terms of the vascular and cellular response. The vascular response consists of an increase in blood flow to the inflamed area and increased vascular permeability that allows leakage of water, electrolytes, and serum proteins into the tissue spaces. The cellular response refers to the movement of leukocytes, predominantly neutrophils and monocytes, from the blood into the tissue (Figure 4–6).

These events produce the *cardinal signs of inflammation*: redness, swelling, heat, pain, and loss of function. The increased blood flow in dilated vessels is called *hyperemia* and causes *redness*. The leakage of

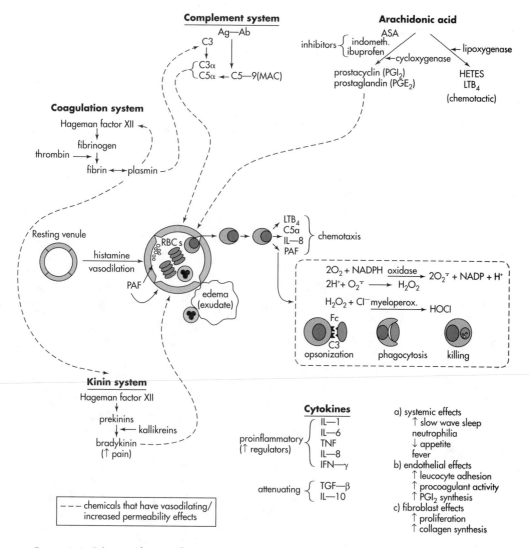

Figure 4–6. Schemae of acute inflammation indicating the roles played by the major chemical mediators.

fluid into the tissue is called *edema* and causes *swelling*. If the lesion is on the body surface, the increased blood in the area causes *heat* because the temperature of the skin is normally less than that of the blood. *Pain* results from the pressure of the swelling and the action of kinins on nerve endings. *Loss of function* results from the attempt to protect the painful, swollen lesion.

The effects of inflammation will be to destroy or limit the spread of the causative agent and to clean up the debris in preparation for repair. In simple injuries, such as a burn, a cut, or a chemical injury where the chemical has been diluted away, the causative agent is no longer a threat and the inflammatory reaction will be proportional to the amount of tissue damage. Tissue damage itself will incite a mild inflammatory reaction, enough to bring leukocytes to digest and remove the debris from the dead cells and increase lymph flow to carry away fluid from the lesion. Both neutrophils and macrophages engulf particulate matter, a process called *phagocytosis.*

Phagocytes (neutrophils and macrophages) play a key role in the inflammatory process. They move from their normal central location in the bloodstream to the periphery as the vessel dilates and the bloodstream slows—a process called *margination.* The leukocytes then stick to the endothelial cells (*adhesion*) due to complementary molecules on the leukocytes and endothelial cells that are activated by various chemical mediators of the inflammatory process. Once chemically stuck to the endothelial cell, leukocytes crawl between endothelial cells into the tissue (*emigration*). Neutrophils *migrate* faster from the vessel to the injured site, arriving within minutes and accumulating over hours. Macrophages are slower moving and peak later than neutrophils. Neutrophils may die soon after arrival at the injured site to liberate their powerful digestive enzymes or they may phagocytose and digest cellular debris and foreign material before dying.

Neutrophils are particularly important in certain types of bacterial infections such as those caused by *Staphylococcus aureus,* various streptococci (including pneumococcus), gonococcus, meningococcus, coliform bacteria, anaerobic bacteria from the intestines, and other organisms. These organisms are responsible for a large number of infections because many are part of the normal flora of the skin, mouth, respiratory tract, and intestines, and they are ever ready to cause infection whenever host defense mechanisms break down at these sites. Neutrophils engulf bacteria like they do with other particulate matter, but they also can recognize and move toward certain unknown chemicals contained in bacteria by the process of chemotaxis. *Chemotaxis* is the movement of white blood cells in response to a chemical gradient; it may be positive or negative. Bacteria have evolved mechanisms of resisting phagocytosis such as the thick polysaccharide capsule of some strains of pneumococcus (*Streptococcus pneumoniae*); the host can counter by producing antibodies that attach to the capsule of the pneumococcus and are easily recognized by phagocytes. Such phagocytosis-promoting antibodies are called *opsonins.* Opsonins come into play with organisms that have been previously encountered or when antibodies have been artificially induced by immunization such as is sometimes done in patients who are particularly susceptible to pneumococcal pneumonia. The brisk neutrophil reaction to these bacteria often results in the death of many neutrophils and much tissue breakdown to produce pus; for this reason the organisms are referred to as pyogenic (pus forming).

Macrophages arrive later and are hardier than neutrophils; they carry the major load in cleaning up the inflammatory debris including the dead neutrophils. The relative numbers of neutrophils and macrophages will depend on the amount and nature of the dead tissue and whether highly chemotactic foreign substances, such as pyogenic bacteria, are present. A staphylococcal infection will have lots of neutrophils; injured adipose tissue from trauma will have mostly macrophages gobbling up the spilled lipid. Macrophages also predominate in reactions to large inert foreign particles such as talc or suture material. They surround the foreign material and often form multinucleated giant cells and remain for a long time.

Phagocytosis by neutrophils and macrophages entails sequestration of a bacterium or other foreign particle into a cytoplasmic compartment where killing occurs mainly by the conversion of hydrogen peroxide (H_2O_2) to a lethal hydroxyl halide ($HOCl^-$) and also by the production of other free radicals that are also efficient at killing. Digestion of the particles follows release of hydrolases and other enzymes.

The role of noncellular elements in the inflammatory focus is more difficult to visualize. The increased fluidity of the lesion facilitates movement of cells and chemicals and also promotes increased lymph flow to carry fluid debris away from the area. It may also serve to dilute offending agents such as toxins and antigens. Fibrinogen is a soluble blood protein that may leak into the inflamed site and be converted to a stringy polymer, fibrin. This process involves several enzymes and is activated by exposure to tissue. The formation of fibrin serves as a barrier to the spread of injury; for example, the scab formed over a scrape of the skin is composed largely of fibrin and serves to keep bacteria out and fluid in. Because fibrinogen is a very large protein, it leaks into tissue only when the increase in vascular permeability is severe; even then some of the fibrin that is formed is lysed by the enzyme fibrinolysin. These control mechanisms prevent the formation of fibrin in mild injuries when it is not needed.

Patients who lack the ability to mount the acute inflammatory reaction succumb to infections that are easily warded off by a normal person, so the reaction is obviously very important. The acute inflammatory reaction can also be very damaging, so its control is important. It must be activated quickly and turned off when no longer needed. The control mechanisms are complex. We will outline them here mentioning the major elements involved. Much more detail is given in standard pathology textbooks. Refer to Figure 4–6 for an overview of acute inflammation, including the vascular and cellular responses, chemotaxis, opsonization, phagocytosis, and the chemical mediators of inflammation, all describe below.

The inflammatory reaction is initiated by local factors in the injured tissue. Stimulation of small nerve endings causes arteriolar dilatation, but this reaction is not an essential or prominent event. The release of histamine from mast cells is the most important initial event. Mast cells are scattered throughout the connective tissue of the body and release histamine when injured. Histamine diffuses from the injured site to cause vasodilatation and increased permeability of small venules. The venules leak plasma proteins, particularly albumen, drawing water into the tissue by osmotic pressure. Mast cells become depleted and the released histamine is diluted and inactivated, so the inflammatory reaction cannot be sustained by histamine. Parenthetically, it should be noted that histamine can be released from mast cells by two types of immunologic reactions: atopic allergy and immune complex reactions (see Chapter 27 for details). If the injury involves pyogenic bacteria, another important initiating factor is the chemotactic factor released from these organisms.

Once initiated, the inflammatory reaction can be quick and greatly amplified by chemicals circulating in the blood. Three chemical systems are involved: the kinin system, the complement system, and the coagulation system. In each case, an inactive protein precursor is activated by a series of enzymatic steps, with products of the reaction itself acting as catalysts to further speed the reaction. To counter the dangers of accidental triggering of these reactions, there are inhibitors, enzymes that destroy products of the reactions, and the dilutional effect of the bloodstream.

When kinins leak through the venule made permeable by histamine, they are activated to become bradykinin. Bradykinin itself causes increased vascular permeability and is thought to be the major factor in sustaining the flow of fluid and chemicals to the inflammatory site by a self-perpetuating reaction. Bradykinin also acts on nerve endings to cause pain. At some point, bradykinin will be deactivated faster than it forms and the vascular response will gradually subside.

When fibrinogen leaks through the permeable vessels along with other blood coagulation factors, the coagulation (clotting) system is activated to polymerize fibrinogen to fibrin. The role of fibrin has already been mentioned. Both the kinin and coagulation systems are initiated by a tissue factor known as the Hageman factor or Factor XII.

The splitting of complement into several active factors is initiated by complexes of antigen and antibody (see Chapter 27 for details) and by an alternate pathway by bacterial endotoxins and some normal tissue proteins. Complement fragment C5a is an important mediator of chemotaxis and fragments C3a and C5a have components known as *anaphylatoxins* that cause increased vascular permeability by stimulating release of histamine from mast cells and blood platelets.

The exact role of each of these reactions in a particular inflammatory lesion is difficult to evaluate and we have not discussed many of the chemical intermediates that have varying degrees of inflammatory and catalytic activity. It is more important to appreciate that the blood plays a sophisticated role in the regulation of the inflammatory reaction.

In addition to the chemicals from the plasma, neutrophils bring products that help amplify and sustain the reaction. Neutrophil enzymes can activate the complement and kinin systems, but perhaps more importantly they provide essential products for synthesis of prostaglandins.

Prostaglandins and leukotrienes are metabolites of arachidonic acid that are produced locally by cells and act as short-range hormones. The chemistry of these compounds is complex and the number of compounds produced and their effects are confusing. Suffice it to say that prostaglandins and leukotrienes are produced in response to inflammation and act locally to sustain the reaction. They are involved in producing vasoconstriction, vasodilatation, increased vascular permeability, chemotaxis, and fever. The anti-inflammatory action of aspirin and indomethacin, at least in part, appears to be due to inhibition of prostaglandin synthesis.

In addition to the three chemical systems just discussed, a variety of polypeptide *cytokines* serve to up- and down-regulate inflammation. Tumor necrosis factor (TNF), interleukin-1 (IL-1), IL-8, and IL-6 are produced by leukocytes and endothelial cells; they enhance the acute inflammatory process locally by increasing leucocyte adhesion to endothelium, increasing blood coagulation properties, and stimulating the further production of prostaglandins. Systemically, these cytokines elicit fever and neutrophilia, increase sleep, and decrease appetite—all recognizable signs of an acute infection. Other cytokines, such as IL-10 and TGF have a down-regulating effect and consequently aid in the resolution of acute inflammation.

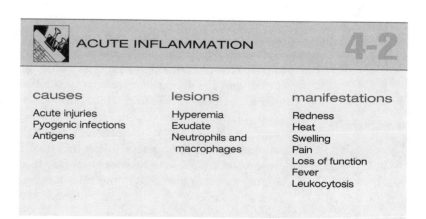

ACUTE INFLAMMATION   4-2

causes	lesions	manifestations
Acute injuries	Hyperemia	Redness
Pyogenic infections	Exudate	Heat
Antigens	Neutrophils and	Swelling
	macrophages	Pain
		Loss of function
		Fever
		Leukocytosis

We have already noted some important variations in the inflammatory process. Reactions with lots of neutrophils cause tissue destruction but are important in containing pyogenic bacteria and antigen–antibody complexes. Macrophages will be prominent when there is dead tissue to remove or foreign substances to surround or engulf. Edema will predominate when lots of histamine is released as in atopic allergy and immune complex reactions. Fibrin will form a protective barrier on injured surfaces. More variations will be described under chronic inflammation.

Chronic Inflammation

Chronic means persistent for a long time. In that sense, chronic inflammation may result from acute inflammation that persists because the cause is not completely eliminated or it may be associated with a cause that never was acute but is continuing at a low level for a long time.

The term *chronic inflammation* is also used as a label for the histologic picture typically associated with prolonged inflammation. As will be noted later, some chronic inflammations have a more specific appearance (e.g., granulomatous inflammation) and some clinically acute inflammations mimic chronic inflammation histologically. Let us first describe the typical appearance of chronic inflammation and then deal with the variations and their pathogenesis.

Since the injury in chronic inflammation is usually low grade, edema and hyperemia are less pronounced than in acute inflammation and few or no neutrophils are present. The area is infiltrated predominantly with lymphocytes, plasma cells, and less conspicuously with macrophages (Figure 4–7). Plasma cells are often prominent and easily recognized. They are derived from B lymphocytes in the tissue and their primary function is to produce antibodies. Presumably the antibodies produced by the plasma cells attach to foreign material in the area and allow the neutrophils and macrophages to phagocytose this material. The lymphocytes, which are mostly nucleus with a small rim of cytoplasm, play a much larger role than their innocuous appearance suggests. We know that different types of lymphocytes can perform various functions. They can recognize foreign materials, kill host cells in the area of foreign antigens to isolate the foreign substance, transform into plasma cells to produce antibody, and direct the traffic of other inflammatory cells, especially macrophages. However, histologically, we cannot tell which lymphocytes are doing what and why. Macrophages may play the same role as they do in acute inflammation (phagocytosis and digestion of debris), but they may also become directly cytotoxic to host cells under certain conditions.

Another hallmark of chronic inflammation, regardless of type, is the laying down of new fibrous tissue in the area. Whenever there

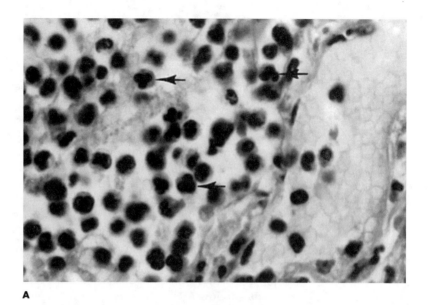

A

Figure 4–7 A. Microscopic appearance of acute inflammation characterized by presence of neutrophils (*arrows*).

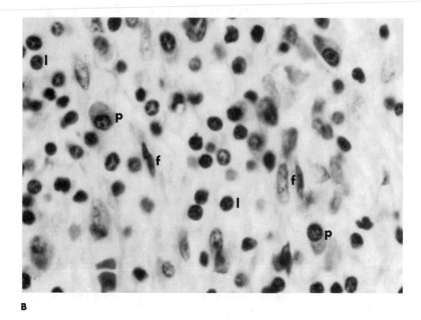

B

Figure 4–7 B. Microscopic appearance of chronic inflammation characterized by the presence of lymphocytes (l), plasma cells (p), and fibroblasts (f).

is tissue injury in the presence of chronic inflammation, there is a fibrous tissue proliferation that tends to wall-off the injured area and provide strength to the defective area. By judging the extent and the age of the new fibrous tissue, one can estimate the chronicity of the inflammation. The process of fibrous repair is discussed in the section on Repair.

Grossly, chronic inflammation has the same features as acute inflammation—edema, redness, heat, pain, and loss of function—but these features are much less pronounced and more variable in their intensity. Contraction of the developing fibrous tissue may distort the lesion and surrounding tissue and give the lesion a variegated, firm, glistening, gray appearance.

The pathogenesis of chronic inflammation involves persistence of the causative agent and a host reaction that is predominantly immunologic in nature. The immune response, which may be of one or several types, produces a more varied picture than the acute inflammatory response. A discussion of several patterns of chronic inflammatory responses follows.

Chronic inflammation due to persistent acute inflammation is usually caused by pyogenic bacteria. Foreign bodies and necrotic tissue provide a haven for these organisms to proliferate and cause continuing foci of acute reaction. The superimposed chronic inflammation is characterized by many plasma cells, which are producing antibodies to help fight the festering bacterial infection, and by fibrous tissue, which is attempting to wall-off the area. The reaction to a splinter is typical of this situation.

If the splinter (foreign body) is removed, the acute inflammatory reaction will eliminate the bacteria and digest the small amount of necrotic tissue. But, if the splinter is not removed, bacteria will often lurk in the foreign body and continue the inflammatory process into a chronic stage. Large amounts of necrotic tissue produce an even greater effect. Necrotic tissue is an ideal culture media for bacteria and is not accessible to the body's vascular transport system that delivers inflammatory cells and antibiotics. Consequently, the offending bacteria will gain the upper hand until the necrotic tissue is removed, either surgically or more gradually by the inflammatory reaction. In these types of chronic inflammation, there will usually be a focus of acute inflammation near the source of infection surrounded by a zone of chronic inflammation. Such lesions are sometimes called subacute inflammation or combined acute and chronic inflammation. Therapy should be directed at the removal of the cause; antibiotics are often of limited help because they cannot reach the offending organisms.

Another pattern of chronic inflammation is the persistence of low-grade injury without an initial acute phase. Agents include microorganisms, antigens, and, less frequently, chemicals. The variable patterns produced by these diverse agents and the several immunologic mechanisms involved tend to produce specific diseases rather than the stereotyped, nonspecific reaction of acute and persistent acute inflammation. Syphilis, hay fever, contact dermatitis, and viral infections will serve as examples to illustrate the diversity of chronic inflammation. Many others can be found in Chapters 26 to 29. The common denominator of these chronic inflammatory reactions is that they employ T lymphocytes to attack the offending agent (cellular immunity) and/ or B lymphocytes to produce antibody to it (humoral immunity). Consequently, lymphocytes and plasma cells predominate in the lesions.

The spirochete of syphilis (a bacterium) enters the skin and proliferates with little or no acute inflammation. Ten to 90 days later, the initial lesion at the site of entry develops as a chronic inflammatory lesion. It is slightly red, swollen, and firm with little or no pain and soon ulcerates. Histologically, there are many plasma cells, macrophages, fibroblasts, and new capillaries—hallmarks of chronic inflammation. Soon after the lesion develops, the body is loaded with antibody to the organism and the lesion gradually resolves, presumably because the antibodies allow the macrophages to remove the organisms. This is an example of an organism that produces little tissue damage itself and is not chemotactic to neutrophils. Damage to tissue is associated with development of the immune response, but the mechanism of injury is poorly understood. Killing the organisms with penicillin stops the process; failure to do so may be followed much later by serious chronic inflammatory lesions of the aorta or central nervous system.

In hay fever, the patient has a predisposed sensitivity to airborne allergens such as ragweed pollen, molds, or house dust. Immunoglobulin E (IgE) antibodies to the offending agent attach themselves to mast cells, and, when they encounter the antigen, cause the mast cells to release the contents of their cytoplasmic granules, including histamine and other substances, which in turn increase vascular permeability and secretion of mucus. Although the mechanism of this reaction is similar to the one occurring in acute inflammation, the prolonged exposure to the allergen causes it to be chronic. Antibody production is associated with an increase in plasma cells in the nasal mucosa and an infiltrate of eosinophils is also typical of inflammations involving IgE antibodies. Eosinophils are thought to degrade substances produced by certain types of allergic reactions. Therapy can be directed toward avoidance of exposure to the antigen, toward desensitizing the immune response, or toward suppressing the inflammatory reaction with antihistamines and vasoconstrictor drugs.

Contact dermatitis, another type of allergy in which the individual's hypersensitivity to an environmental antigen is involved, may be acute or chronic, depending on the dose of antigen and duration of exposure. Prolonged, low-grade exposure might occur with sensitivity to a cosmetic or metal in a watch band, thus producing a chronic, slightly edematous, mildly red lesion that may itch. It is characterized histologically by a lymphocytic infiltrate, spotty necrosis of epidermal cells, and a mild, prolonged chronic inflammatory reaction to the necrotic cells. In this situation, the antigen entering the epidermis is recognized by a small population of T lymphocytes. Upon encountering the antigen, these sensitized T lymphocytes recruit cytotoxic lymphocytes or macrophages that kill the host cells containing the antigen, either directly or by elaboration of toxic proteins called lymphotoxins. By sacrificing the host cells, the spread of antigen is limited. In contact dermatitis, the immune system of the susceptible person is fooled into recognizing an antigen that is harmless to nonallergic individuals.

The delayed hypersensitivity reaction is an important mechanism involved in the production of many chronic diseases. It is associated with a variety of allergies as illustrated by contact dermatitis, in protection against many microorganisms, in several types of autoimmune diseases, and in rejection of tissues transplanted from one individual to another. All of these situations are associated with lymphocytic infiltration and killing of host cells, producing the histologic picture of chronic inflammation. Lymphocytes usually predominate over plasma cells.

Viral infections often elicit cellular immune reactions of the delayed hypersensitivity type. These can develop abruptly, producing a clinically acute illness with a chronic inflammatory reaction histologically. For example, in many viral infections the organisms grow intracellularly in selected cells in the body. During the incubation period (10 to 14 days), some of the antigen from the virus is complexed with the surface of the infected cell. T lymphocytes recognize this antigen complex, become sensitized to it, and then recruit cytotoxic lymphocytes and macrophages to destroy the infected cells, thus eliminating the necessary environment for the virus. The cost of this protective reaction is the necrosis of host cells with release of cytokines that produce fever and other systemic manifestations. The onset of illness occurs suddenly as sensitized T lymphocytes reach the infected cells; recovery is gradual as injured host cells recover or are replaced. It should be noted that delayed hypersensitivity is not the only mechanism in viral-induced injury, and delayed hypersensitivity is involved in a variety of other types of infections.

The above examples make it clear that many, if not most, of what are considered chronic inflammatory reactions are really immune reactions. Both humoral and cellular immune reactions can be accelerated by previous immunization. Antibodies are important in preventing antigens from entering the body and in helping neutrophils

CHRONIC INFLAMMATION		4-3
causes	**lesions**	**manifestations**

Prolonged injury
Prolonged infection
Certain types of
  infection
Antigens
	Less exudate than
	  acute
	Lymphocytes and
	  plasma cells
	Occurs with fibrous
	  repair
		Same as acute, but
		  less severe and
		  more variable

and macrophages destroy them immediately after entry. When sensitized lymphocytes are already present, they can destroy an infected site in a day or two; the organisms do not have time to proliferate and spread. Smallpox has been eradicated from the world by making sure that all exposed persons were immunized. At the opposite extreme, suppression of the immune response is desirable in autoimmune diseases such as rheumatoid arthritis and with organ transplants where the effects are undesirable.

The above examples are only a sample of the diversity of chronic inflammatory diseases that will be expanded upon throughout the book. A knowledge of the agent and its distribution and dose, along with the type of immunologic reaction induced by the agent, serve to more easily understand the disease produced by the agent and to direct therapy and future research. The pathogenesis of many chronic inflammatory diseases is still incompletely understood. As you progress through the book, refer to Chapter 25 for more information on immunologic mechanisms.

Granulomatous Inflammation

Granulomatous inflammation is a specific type of chronic inflammation characterized by focal collections of closely packed, plump macrophages (Figure 4–8). Granulomatous inflammation occurs in response to certain indigestible organisms and other foreign materials and involves an element of cell-mediated immunity to the foreign material. In granulomatous inflammation, T lymphocytes become sensitized to the offending agent and recruit large numbers of macrophages that engulf the antigenic agent. These macrophages are called *epithelioid cells* because their abundant cytoplasm and close approximation to each other in aggregates make them resemble epithelial cells.

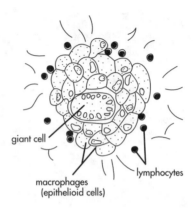

giant cell

lymphocytes

macrophages
(epithelioid cells)

Figure 4–8. A granuloma.

The macrophages in a granuloma often form a few giant cells, which makes them easily recognizable. Granulomas often become large enough to produce grossly visible pale, yellow nodules and in tuberculosis and fungal infections may become quite large and undergo caseous necrosis. Small granulomas heal by fibrosis. Large caseous granulomas are walled off by a fibrous rim and calcify.

The classic cause of granulomatous inflammation is tuberculosis. See Chapter 12 for more details on tuberculosis. Other microorganisms, particularly the fungi causing histoplasmosis, coccidioidomycosis, blastomycosis, and cryptococcosis, produce granulomatous disease that is very similar to tuberculosis.

Another relatively common granulomatous disease is sarcoidosis, a disease of unknown cause characterized by widespread noncaseous granulomas. It produces a mild to moderately debilitating illness often involving lungs and lymph nodes as well as many other organs. It is more common in young adult women, in blacks, and in southern United States. Most patients are asymptomatic or have a mild illness that disappears in a few years. A few die from progressive granulomatous involvement of the lungs or complications of the lesions.

Foreign body granulomas are less stereotyped than the "tuberculoid" or "sarcoid" granulomas described above. They result from indigestible "foreign" material being surrounded by epithelioid cells and giant cells. Common causes are suture material, splinters, talc, mineral oil inhaled into the lung, crystalline cholesterol deposits derived from blood or bile, and large microorganisms such as helminths. The "foreign" body is usually quite evident within the granuloma.

The term granuloma has been used in different ways. The best use is for the characteristic histologic appearance, which suggests that it would be profitable to look for a specific cause. Round lesions seen

GRANULOMATOUS INFLAMMATION		4-4
causes	**lesions**	**manifestations**
Tuberculosis Fungal infections Foreign bodies Sarcoidosis	Focal collections of plump macrophages and giant cells Often multiple foci Caseous necrosis with some causes	Nonspecific, may be none Positive tests for causative organisms Tissue destruction which may affect organ function

on chest x-rays are often termed granulomas because most of these are due to old healed tuberculosis or fungal infection.

Exudates and Transudates

Exudates should be distinguished from transudates. A *transudate* is a collection of fluid in tissue or in a body space due to increased hydrostatic or decreased osmotic pressure in the vascular system without loss of protein into the tissue. Thus transudates are watery with low protein content. *Exudates* are the result of increased osmotic pressure in the tissue due to high protein content and are caused by inflammation or obstruction of lymphatic flow. Thus a swelling with cloudy or protein rich fluid is caused by inflammation or lymphatic obstruction, whereas a swelling with thin watery fluid might be caused by heart failure with its increased venous pressure or by depleted serum proteins. Exudates tend to be more localized than transudates because most inflammations are localized whereas the effects of increased hydrostatic pressure or depleted serum proteins are usually generalized.

Serous exudate contains fluid as well as small amounts of protein and often implies a lesser degree of damage. For example, the fluid content of blisters that follow skin burns is serous exudate.

A *fibrinous exudate* is an exudate composed of large amounts of fibrinogen from the blood that is polymerized to form fibrin. For example, in bacterial pneumonia fibrinous exudate forms a mesh that helps trap the bacteria; on a skin wound, dried fibrinous exudate forms a scab.

Purulent exudate (also called *pus*) is an exudate that is loaded with live and dead leukocytes, mostly neutrophils. An inflammatory reaction with much purulent exudate is called *suppurative inflammation*. A localized collection of pus is an *abscess*. When pus fills a body cavity such as the pleural cavity, the term *empyema* is used.

Gross Inflammatory Lesions

Lesions with relatively specific gross appearance include abscess, cellulitis, and ulcer. An *abscess* is a localized, usually spherical lesion containing liquified dead tissue and neutrophils (purulent exudate) (Figure 4–9). Pyogenic bacteria are the most typical cause of abscesses because they liberate chemotactic factors and proliferate to produce an exuberant acute inflammatory reaction. The host is induced to destroy and liquify its own tissue to limit the spread of the offending agent. Abscesses are typically caused by bacteria of the skin (staphylococci), oral cavity (streptococci including pneumococci, anaerobic bacteria), and lower intestinal tract (coliform bacteria and anaerobic bacteria). The bacteria, which enter the tissue and proliferate due to obstruction of ducts and glands, tissue injury, or foreign bodies, are opportunists. Examples of abscesses include the *boil* or *furuncle* usually due to an obstructed skin appendage or foreign body, a *paronychia* due to purulent infection around a fingernail, and pimples of acne due to greasy secretions with obstruction and infection of sebaceous glands associated with onset of sexual maturity. Abscesses also occur in areas where there is change from one tissue type to another

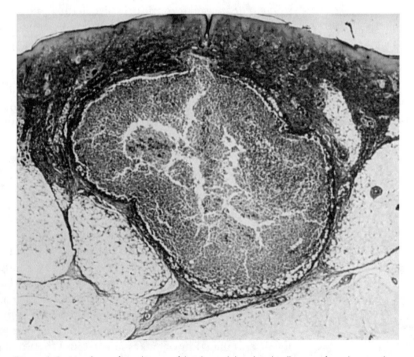

Figure 4–9. Histology of an abscess of the skin with localized collection of purulent exudate.

such as around the nares, teeth, and anus. The combination of foreign material, necrotic tissue, and bacteria trapped in wounds or in operative incisions is particularly likely to produce an abscess. In more serious breakdowns of the body defense mechanisms, such as perforation of the intestines, large areas of necrosis, and infarcts in organs open to the bacterial environment, such as lung, intestine, or legs, anaerobic organisms of intestinal, oral, or soil origin often cause abscesses.

The typical small abscess is red, hot, swollen, and quite painful. When the abscess reaches a "head," the center is liquified and fluctuant and the edge is beginning to wall off. Puncture of the abscess causes an outpouring of pus, relief of pain, and more rapid healing. If punctured before this stage, the abscess may be spread. Larger abscesses are more irregular and may spread in tissue spaces and cause extensive damage. If the host wins, an abscess will be walled off and replaced by fibrous tissue after drainage or resolution (resorption) of the purulent exudate. If uncontained, an abscess may enlarge, spread, and kill the host. For example, acute appendicitis with abscess formation can lead to death; early appendectomy prevents such an outcome.

Cellulitis refers to a spreading acute inflammatory process. This type of inflammation is commonly seen with streptococcal bacterial infections and is due to the body's inability to confine the organism. Cellulitis is seen in the skin and subcutaneous tissue and is characterized by nonlocalized edema and redness.

An *ulcer* is a locally excavated area of skin or mucous membrane secondary to an injury and the subsequent inflammation. Ulcers are commonly seen in the stomach and duodenum secondary to local injury by acid from the stomach. Bedsores, resulting from pressure atrophy, are another example of ulcers.

REPAIR

Regeneration

The body's two basic methods of repair following tissue destruction are *regeneration* and *fibrous connective tissue repair* (scarring or fibrosis). Regeneration is replacement of the destroyed tissue by cells similar to those previously present, i.e., the parenchymal cells of the organ are regenerated. For example, the epidermal surface of a cut is replaced by epidermis, fractured bone is united by bone, or scattered dead liver cells are replaced by new liver cells. In fibrous connective tissue repair, tissue previously present is replaced by fibrous tissue (scar). For example, the dermal edges of a cut are united by scar, a bone fracture that is not properly united is healed by scar tissue, extensively damaged liver may be replaced by fibrous tissue. Many tissue injuries heal in part by regeneration and in part by fibrosis.

Regeneration is the most desirable form of repair, because normal function is often restored. As a prerequisite to regeneration, cells next to those that have died must be able to multiply. For example, neurons and cardiac muscle fibers cannot undergo cell division in adults; therefore, these cells cannot regenerate. Tissues that are continuously replacing their cells under normal circumstances also have great capacity for regeneration. Examples of such tissues include the epidermis, the mucosal lining of the intestinal tract, and bone marrow. Bone marrow can replace itself when only a few cells survive an injury. Epidermis and intestinal mucosa can repair defects up to several centimeters in diameter through the process of regeneration (Figure 4–10). Most of the tissues of the body normally undergo cell replacement at a slow rate and are intermediate in their ability to regenerate. Regeneration can usually occur in parenchymal organs if the architectural framework is

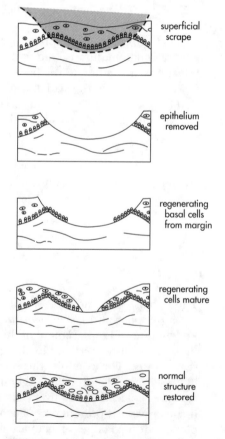

superficial scrape

epithelium removed

regenerating basal cells from margin

regenerating cells mature

normal structure restored

Figure 4–10. Complete regeneration of lost surface epithelium.

not destroyed. Tissues particularly noted for their regenerative capacity include liver, renal tubules, and bone. More complex structures, such as lung and renal glomeruli, do not regenerate.

Regeneration is particularly important when there has been widespread-damage to a vital organ. When there is generalized hypoxia, renal tubular cells, hepatocytes, and neurons are most susceptible to necrosis because of their high metabolic requirements. Typical causes of generalized hypoxia include shock, cardiac arrest followed by successful resuscitation, and carbon monoxide poisoning. Renal and hepatic function is likely to be restored because the few surviving cells can regenerate and restore normal structure. Brain function cannot be restored when neurons die because they cannot regenerate. Bone marrow is an organ that may be wiped out by drug therapy for cancer and other causes; it has tremendous capacity to regenerate from only a few cells and, in some cases, may be restored by cells from another individual by bone marrow transplantation.

Fibrous Connective Tissue Repair (Scarring or Fibrosis)

Fibrosis can occur in any tissue and produces the same result regardless of site, namely the formation of a dense, tough mass of collagen called a *scar*. Unlike regeneration, replacement by fibrous tissue does not restore the original function. The purpose of fibrosis is to provide a strong bridge between normal tissue and the damaged area.

The process of fibrous repair is also called *organization* and consists of a granulation tissue stage and a scar formation stage. *Granulation tissue* consists of capillaries and fibroblasts. The process, which begins when the injury has been stabilized, is initiated by the ingrowth of new capillaries and fibroblasts into the injured area. The capillaries bring blood to provide the nutrition for the repair process. Capillaries also carry away liquid remains of dead tissue and particulate material removed by macrophages. The removal process is called *resolution*. The fibroblasts proliferate rapidly and then initiate the stage of scar formation by laying down collagen. Initially, there are small amounts of loose collagen within the mass of capillaries and fibroblasts. With time, more collagen is formed and the number of capillaries and fibroblasts decreases. The final stage, which takes weeks to months, involves shrinking and condensation of the fibrous scar (Figure 4–11).

Wound Repair

The process of repair of wounds is artificially separated into repair by primary union and secondary union, depending on whether the wound edges are placed together or left separated. The best example

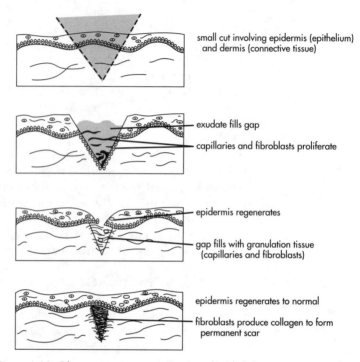

small cut involving epidermis (epithelium) and dermis (connective tissue)

exudate fills gap

capillaries and fibroblasts proliferate

epidermis regenerates

gap fills with granulation tissue (capillaries and fibroblasts)

epidermis regenerates to normal

fibroblasts produce collagen to form permanent scar

Figure 4–11. Fibrous connective tissue repair and epithelial regeneration in a skin cut.

of repair by primary union is that which follows a clean surgical incision of the skin in which there is minimal tissue damage and the edges of the wound are closely approximated by tape or sutures. In this example, the narrow space between the two wound edges fills with a small amount of serum, which quickly dries and clots forming a scab. Within 1 to 2 days, the narrow zone of acute inflammation at the wound edges has lessened and new capillaries begin to bridge the gap between the wound edges. By this time, the epithelium has already grown across the surface of this gap. Within a few more days, fibroblasts grow across the subepithelial portions of the wound gap and begin to deposit collagen, the collagen eventually contracts, pulling the wound edges together and giving them strength. Although this incision may appear well healed by about 2 weeks, it may take a month or more for the strength of the scar tissue to equal that of the original tissue.

Repair by secondary union utilizes the same basic process as primary union, except that there is greater injury with consequent greater tissue damage and more inflammation to resolve (Figure 4–12). To fill the void left by tissue damage, there is a tremendous proliferation of capillaries and fibroblasts, which actually start growing after the injury is just a few days old and acute inflammation may still be

unsutured cut

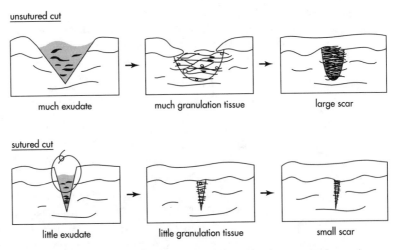

much exudate   much granulation tissue   large scar

sutured cut

little exudate   little granulation tissue   small scar

Figure 4–12. Repair of an unsutured and sutured skin cut leading to secondary and primary union, respectively.

intense. After a week or more, the wound will be filled with this tissue, composed largely of capillaries, fibroblasts, and variable numbers of residual acute inflammatory cells (neutrophils) with some chronic inflammatory cells (lymphocytes). This tissue is friable and red with oozing blood and is called *granulation tissue*. It is what is seen when one picks a scab off a skin wound. Granulation tissue eventually is replaced as more and more collagen is deposited by fibroblasts. Fibroblasts and collagen have inherent contractile properties, which aid in shrinking a wound and drawing the edges together. Fibroblast proliferation and collagen synthesis by fibroblasts are both stimulated by pro-inflammatory cytokines such as TNF and IL-1. It may take a long time for a wound that heals by secondary union to achieve strength approximating that of the normal tissue. If a skin wound is very large, the epithelium may never completely bridge the wound, and skin may need to be grafted to the wound site from another area of the body. Transplanted skin usually grows quite readily in such a situation, because the underlying granulation tissue is so rich in capillaries. One of the greatest impediments to healing and repair of a wound is the amount of dead tissue and foreign material (dirt, bacteria, shrapnel, etc.) present. It might take the body's inflammatory cells many months to phagocytize a large amount of dead tissue and foreign material, and the presence of bacteria in a wound may produce necrotic tissue and inflammatory cells as fast as they are removed. For this reason, the medical care of a large wound should always include thorough cleaning and *debridement* (removal of foreign material and necrotic tissue).

Inflammation and subsequent repair of tissue is a very dynamic process that is influenced by numerous modifying factors. The following factors may detract from the body's ability to most effectively deal with an injury:

1. Virulence of the infective organisms; for example, staphylococcus is more capable of destroying tissue than alpha streptococcus.
2. Advancing age; elderly people heal more slowly than younger people for various reasons.
3. Poor nutrition; protein and vitamin C are needed to produce collagen.
4. Diabetes; small blood vessels are abnormal in diabetics and consequently they do not deliver materials to the tissues optimally.
5. Steroid therapy; steroids inhibit the inflammatory response by preventing vascular permeability, hindering cellular digestion of debris, and blocking antigen–antibody reactions. Steroids can be very useful in those situations where inhibition of inflammation is desired; for example, steroids are used to slow the destructive inflammation of rheumatoid arthritis.

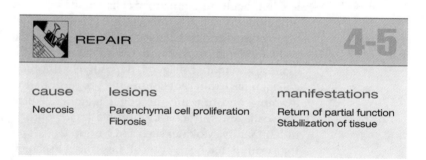

REPAIR		4-5
cause	lesions	manifestations
Necrosis	Parenchymal cell proliferation	Return of partial function
	Fibrosis	Stabilization of tissue

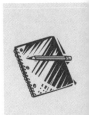

Review Questions

1. How does the duration of an injury affect the interrelationship between injury, inflammation, and repair?

2. What are the major causes, lesions, and manifestations of necrosis, inflammation, and repair?

3. What functional and histologic changes indicate cell death?

4. What is the difference between cell necrosis and apoptosis?

5. How do the various types of necrosis, atrophy, and accumulations differ in appearance and cause?

6. What distinguishes metastatic from dystrophic calcification?

7. How do acute inflammation, chronic inflammation, and granulomatous inflammation differ in cause, histologic appearance, and manifestations?

8. What is the sequence of events in a typical acute inflammatory reaction and how does this relate to the local and systemic signs and laboratory findings?

9. How do chemical mediators, including cytokines, control the acute inflammatory response?

10. How do serous, fibrinous, and purulent exudates differ in composition and gross appearance?

11. How do abscesses, cellulitis, and ulcers differ in gross appearance and location within the body?

12. What is the usual cause of an abscess? What type of inflammatory cell is most characteristic of an abscess?

13. What determines whether repair will be by regeneration or fibrous connective tissue repair? What is the sequence of each and how do the outcomes differ?

14. What is the difference in sequence and outcomes of repair of an open versus a closed (sutured) wound?

15. What conditions inhibit wound healing?

16. What do the following terms mean?
Allergy
Amyloid
Anaphylatoxins
Anoxia
Autoimmune reaction
Chemotaxis
Debridement
Edema
Embolus
Empyema
Exudate
Fatty metamorphosis
Gangrene
Granulation tissue
Hyalin
Hyperemia
Hypoxia
Infarct
Ischemia
Karyolysis
Karyorrhexis
Organization
Phagocytosis
Pus
Pyknosis
Pyogenic
Resolution
Suppuration
Thrombus
Transudate

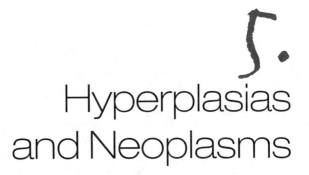

Hyperplasias and Neoplasms

REVIEW OF STRUCTURE AND FUNCTION
Classification of Tissues and Cells • Physiologic Replacement
• Cell Differentiation

BASIC DEFINITIONS

SIGNIFICANCE OF HYPERPLASIAS
AND NEOPLASMS

CLASSIFICATION OF NEOPLASMS
Benign Neoplasms • Malignant Neoplasms • Epithelial
• Mesenchymal • Other

MORPHOLOGIC FEATURES
Hyperplasias and Hypertrophies
Benign Neoplasms
Malignant Neoplasms

LIFE HISTORY AND SPREAD OF CANCER

GRADING AND STAGING

REVIEW QUESTIONS

REVIEW OF STRUCTURE AND FUNCTION

The cells of the body are derived from one cell, the fertilized ovum. During embryonic development successive cell divisions lead to more and more specialized cell types and the less differentiated embryonic cells disappear. The cells of the developed organism can be divided into germ cells (normally confined to the gonads) and somatic cells. Somatic cells are classified under four major categories: epithelial cells, connective tissue cells, muscle cells, and nervous tissue cells.

Epithelial cells are generally those that arise from the embryonic ectoderm and endoderm to form the lining of body spaces and surfaces and the various glands. Surface lining cells are of squamous, transitional, or columnar types. Stratified squamous epithelium forms a tough protective barrier, often with a layer of keratin on the surface. Stratified squamous epithelium lines the skin, mouth, pharynx, larynx, esophagus, and anus. Transitional epithelium is also multilayered but lacks the surface layer of keratin. Transitional epithelium is confined to the urinary tract including renal pelvis, ureter, bladder, and urethra. Columnar epithelium is usually composed of one layer of tall cells, which often are mucus secreting. The surface columnar epithelium is often in continuity with underlying glands; its pathologic reactions are similar to those of glandular epithelium, hence, it is often referred to as glandular epithelium. Columnar epithelium lines the nose, trachea, bronchi, stomach, small intestine, colon, and many of the ducts leading to glands such as the bile ducts and breast ducts.

Epithelial cells comprising the various epithelial organs may be arranged as glands (acini), tubules, or cords. Glandular organs include breast, salivary glands, thyroid, and pancreas. The kidney is an example of an organ composed predominantly of tubules. The liver, adrenal, and pituitary are arranged in cords or sheets, with blood sinusoids between the sheets of cells.

Connective tissue cells, which are mostly derived from mesoderm, are recognized by their lack of close approximation with other cells and by the substances they produce. Fibroblasts produce and are associated with collagen, chondrocytes with cartilage, osteocytes with bone, and endothelial cells with blood vessels. White blood cells are recognized by their round appearance and distinctive nuclei.

Muscle cells are also derived from mesoderm but resemble epithelial cells in their close approximation to each other. They differ from epithelium by their elongated fiber-like structure and abundant contractile cytoplasm.

Nervous tissue cells are derived from ectoderm and include neurons and their supporting cells. Neurons have very long processes (axons), which carry electrical impulses. The supporting cells in the brain and spinal cord are glial cells (astrocytes and oligodendroglia). Supporting cells in peripheral nerves are Schwann cells.

The tendency of cells to undergo hyperplasia and neoplasia is roughly related to their involvement in physiologic replacement. Surface epithelial cells undergo continuous replacement, and this process of replacement can be accelerated by mild injury. Glandular epithelial cells are more stable but can proliferate following injury. Connective tissue cells also have great capacity to proliferate. Blood cells are replaced continuously. Fixed connective tissue cells are replaced more slowly except when stimulated by injury. Heart muscle cells cannot be replaced, and skeletal muscle cells have very limited replacement capacity. Smooth muscle cells, especially those in small blood vessels, can proliferate. Of the nervous tissue cells, only the neurons are incapable of replacing themselves following injury.

The proliferative capacity of cells relates to the process of differentiation. Differentiation is the process of maturation from a nonspecific cell type to a specialized cell. For example, the stem cell in the bone marrow is a poorly differentiated cell whose main function is to divide and produce daughter cells. The daughter cell passes through several intermediate stages of differentiation until it becomes a mature, differentiated white or red blood cell. The stages of differentiation are also well illustrated in the epidermis—the basal cells are poorly differentiated and concerned primarily with cell division; the surface cells are differentiated with formation of keratin to protect the surface.

BASIC DEFINITIONS

Hyperplasias and neoplasms are both characterized by proliferation of cells that increase tissue mass. They differ on the basis of cause and growth potential.

Hyperplasias are exaggerated responses to various stimuli or presumed stimuli (a nonexaggerated response to injury is called repair). Hyperplasia may recede if the stimulus is removed, provided permanent structural changes have not occurred. Hyperplasia typically involves tissues that undergo physiologic replacement but may involve stable tissues.

Neoplasms are growths that proliferate with varying degrees of independence from normal cellular control mechanisms. Neoplasms are presumed to arise by mutation or altered genetic control, they behave as if they were an independent parasitic organism struggling to overwhelm the host. Neoplasms may arise from embryonic cells, germinal cells, or mature somatic cells. Like hyperplasias, the majority of neoplasms arise from cells that undergo physiologic replacement. Therefore, hyperplasias and neoplasias cannot be distinguished on the basis of cell type alone.

Hyperplasias may be caused by a wide variety of stimuli, such as a remote response to inflammation (e.g., lymph node hyperplasia, bone marrow hyperplasia), hormone excess or hormone deficiency (e.g., thyroid goiter), chronic irritation (e.g., skin callus), or unknown factors (e.g., hyperplasia of the prostate gland in elderly men). Hypertrophy should be distinguished from hyperplasia; both frequently occur together. *Hypertrophy* refers to an increase in cell size, whereas *hyperplasia* refers to increase in cell numbers (Figure 5–1). The term *hypertrophy* is best applied to muscles, as the muscle fiber (cell) enlarges as a response to increased work load rather than undergoing hyperplasia.

Most neoplasms represent an overgrowth of a single cell type; however, neoplasms of germ cells and embryonic cells may contain more than one cell type. A germ cell neoplasm that produces tissue representing more than one of the three germ cell layers (ectoderm, mesoderm, endoderm) is called a *teratoma*. Neoplasms thought to be derived from embryonic cells are termed *embryonal.*

Neoplasms are classified on the basis of the cell type they resemble and from which they presumably arise. Almost all cell types in the body can undergo neoplasia, but some do so much more frequently than others. The growth potential for each type of neoplasm is best determined by analysis of patients who have had similar neoplasms.

Most neoplasms can be classified as benign or malignant (a few are intermediate). *Benign neoplasms* are generally localized, single masses of cells that remain localized at their site of origin and limited in their growth (although some become very large). *Malignant neoplasms* are defined by their potential to invade and metastasize at some point in their life history. *Invasion* refers to direct extension of neoplastic cells into surrounding tissue without regard to tissue boundaries. *Metastasis* means transplantation of cells to a new site. The neoplastic cells must be transported through vascular channels or body spaces and must grow at the new site. Metastasis is the single most

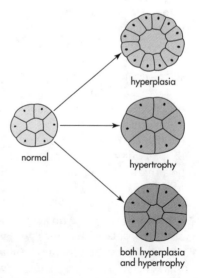

Figure 5–1. Hyperplasia and hyper-trophy of a gland.

important feature of malignant neoplasms, although some types can kill by local invasion alone. The term *cancer* is a synonym for *malignant neoplasm*. The term *tumor* classically meant swelling or mass, but now is more commonly used as a synonym for neoplasm.

SIGNIFICANCE OF HYPERPLASIAS AND NEOPLASMS

Hyperplasias and neoplasms commonly produce masses that are discovered by direct vision, palpation, radiographic imaging, or by presumption from the effects of the mass on organ function. Once discovered, the nature of a mass must be determined to be inflammation, hyperplasia, or neoplasia because the treatment for these processes is radically different. Subclassification within each category allows for even more rational treatment based on past experience with similar lesions.

With inflammation and hyperplasia, therapy focuses on the causative stimulus. With some forms of hyperplasia, the potential development of cancer is also a concern. With a benign neoplasm, therapeutic concern is limited to accurate diagnosis and removal of the lesion. With a malignant neoplasm, therapy is based on an estimate of the possibility for complete destruction of the neoplasm. Curative therapy is the attempt to remove all of the cancer, whether by surgical operation, radiation, or administration of drugs. Palliative therapy, whether by operative removal, radiation, or by administration of drugs, attempts to control the effects of the cancer rather than to cure it. Overall, about 50 percent of patients with malignant neoplasms die of the cancer (this does not include skin cancers).

An example will illustrate the differences in approach to hyperplasias, benign neoplasms, and malignant neoplasms. A woman discovers a lump in her breast. The mass is removed by excisional biopsy. If the pathologist classifies the lesion as a benign neoplasm, nothing further need be done and the patient is cured. If the lesion is a malignant neoplasm and judged to be potentially curable, some combination of surgical and radiation therapy will be used to remove or kill all of the cancer cells. If the neoplasm has spread beyond the breast and regional lymph nodes, palliative therapy may be used. If the pathologist diagnoses the breast lump as hyperplasia, the situation is more complex. It is unlikely that the stimulus can be removed (presumed to be the patient's own hormonal variations). If the pathologist judges the hyperplasia to be a potential site of malignancy (precancerous), the surgeon is faced with the choice of whether to remove the breast(s) to prevent cancer or to see the patient at regular intervals to detect the development of a cancer in its early stage. If the

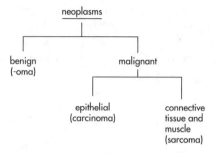

Figure 5–2. Major categories and suffixes for neoplasms.

pathologist judges the lesion to be simple hyperplasia, it is still likely that further lumps will develop, because hyperplasia, unlike neoplasia, tends to be multifocal or diffuse. When another lump develops, the same diagnostic procedure must be repeated.

CLASSIFICATION OF NEOPLASMS

Most neoplasms are named by the cell or tissue they resemble plus a suffix or word indicating neoplasm. For a benign neoplasm, the suffix -*oma* is added after the name of the tissue, for example, *fibroma*. For a malignant neoplasm, either the term *carcinoma* or *sarcoma* is added to the name of the tissue. If the malignant neoplasm is from epithelium, *carcinoma* is used; if from nonepithelial tissue, *sarcoma* is used (Figure 5–2). A few additional types of neoplasm of nonepithelial or ambiguous origin are named separately. Benign neoplasms, which follow standard nomenclature, are listed in Table 5–1.

TABLE 5–1. NAMES OF BENIGN NEOPLASMS

Cell or Tissue of Origin	Name
Squamous epithelium	Squamous papilloma
Glandular or surface columnar epithelium	Adenoma
Fibrous tissue	Fibroma
Adipose tissue	Lipoma
Cartilage	Chondroma
Bone	Osteoma
Blood vessels	Hemangioma
Smooth muscle	Leiomyoma
Nerve sheath	Neurilemoma

Unfortunately there are several glaring exceptions to this naming system. A *hematoma* is a collection of blood, not a neoplasm. A *lymphoma* is a malignant neoplasm of lymph node cells (there is no benign counterpart). A *melanoma* is a malignant neoplasm of melanocytes (the benign counterpart is called a *nevus*). *Glioma* is used to refer to all neoplasms of the supporting cells of the brain (glial cells). Gliomas represents an example of neoplasms that are ambiguous in terms of the usual classification. They are benign in that they usually do not metastasize and malignant in that most kill the patient. Biologically they represent a spectrum from slow growth to rapid growth.

The naming system for the most common types of malignant neoplasms is given in Table 5–2. Two exceptions worth noting include the common use of *hepatoma* to mean liver-cell carcinoma and *hypernephroma* to mean renal tubular cell carcinoma.

TABLE 5–2. NAMES OF MALIGNANT NEOPLASMS

Cell or Tissue of Origin	Name
Epithelium	
Site not specified	Carcinoma
Squamous epithelium of skin	Squamous cell carcinoma of skin
Basal cells of epithelium of skin	Basal cell carcinoma (unique to skin)
Colonic mucosa	Adenocarcinoma of colon
Breast glands	Adenocarcinoma of breast
Bronchial epithelium of lung	Bronchogenic carcinoma
Prostatic glands	Adenocarcinoma of prostate
Bladder mucosa	Transitional cell carcinoma of bladder
Endometrium	Adenocarcinoma of endometrium
Cervix	Squamous cell carcinoma of cervix
Stomach mucosa	Adenocarcinoma of stomach
Pancreatic ducts	Adenocarcinoma of pancreas
Connective tissue and muscle	
Site not specified	Sarcoma
Lymphoid tissue	Malignant lymphoma
Bone marrow	Leukemia
Plasma cells in bone marrow	Multiple myeloma
Cartilage	Chondrosarcoma
Bone	Osteosarcoma
Fibrous tissue	Fibrosarcoma
Smooth muscle	Leiomyosarcoma
Other	
Site not specified	Malignant neoplasm
Glial cells	Glioma
Melanocytes	Malignant melanoma
Germ cells	Teratocarcinoma

MORPHOLOGIC FEATURES

Hyperplasias and Hypertrophies

Hyperplasias represent a very diverse group of conditions about which it is difficult to generalize. Diffuse organ hyperplasias are characterized by an increase in the normal cellular elements of the organ. Common examples include lymph node hyperplasia with increased lymphocytes and macrophages in response to an inflammatory condition, physiologic breast hyperplasia with increased number and size of glands in response to pregnancy, nodular goiter (enlarged thyroid) with enlarged thyroid acini in response to prolonged iodine deficiency, and hyperplasia of the prostate with enlarged glands and fibromuscular stroma in response to uncertain stimuli in elderly men. These types of hyperplasia are grossly diffuse (they lack the discreteness of neoplasms) and, histologically, some cells appear normal but may be somewhat distorted in their arrangement and increased in density. Sometimes degeneration and fibrosis within a hyperplastic organ produces a nodularity that may diagnostically require differentiation from cancer.

Hyperplasias of epithelial surface cells are particularly important as sites of cancer development in some organs. Surface hyperplasias produce slightly raised lesions due to piling up of cells. Where they can be visualized grossly (skin, oral cavity, respiratory tract, cervix), these lesions appear more opaque than surrounding surface. In mucous membranes, opaque white lesions are called *leukoplakias*. Surface hyperplasias are easily confused grossly with inflammation or early neoplastic lesions. Microscopically, the hyperplastic nature will be evident, but the pathologist will need to judge whether it is a simple innocuous hyperplasia or whether it is premalignant hyperplasia. A premalignant lesion is one in which there is an increased likelihood of cancer as compared to adjacent normal tissue. If premalignant, the relative potential for malignancy must be estimated, based on analysis of similar lesions in other patients. As a general rule, this judgment will be based on the atypical appearance of the cells (atypia) in the hyperplastic surface epithelium. This atypical change includes increased size and staining of the nucleus, irregular shape of the nucleus, and decreased amount and maturity of the cytoplasm.

A change closely associated with hyperplasia is metaplasia. *Metaplasia* is a change from one type of tissue to another. Most commonly this involves change from columnar epithelium to stratified squamous epithelium (*squamous metaplasia*). In addition, the metaplastic tissue is often hyperplastic because both occur together in response to mild injury.

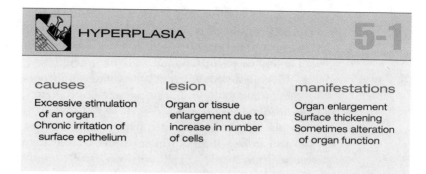

HYPERPLASIA   **5-1**

causes	lesion	manifestations
Excessive stimulation of an organ Chronic irritation of surface epithelium	Organ or tissue enlargement due to increase in number of cells	Organ enlargement Surface thickening Sometimes alteration of organ function

Hypertrophy is organ enlargement at the gross level and increased cell size at the microscopic level. It is usually a diffuse process. The best examples of hypertrophy are those of muscle such as the enlarged skeletal muscles of weight lifters, the enlarged cardiac muscle that occurs with high blood pressure, and the enlarged uterine smooth muscle in pregnancy.

Benign Neoplasms

Benign neoplasms are relatively easy to recognize grossly and microscopically, because they produce a single mass that is discrete from surrounding tissue. When originating on a body surface, benign neoplasms extend outwardly, producing a polyp (Figure 5–3). A *polyp* is

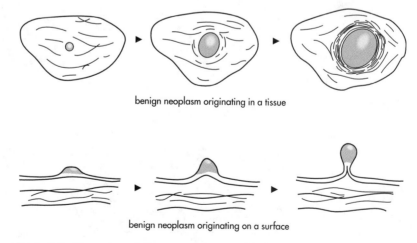

benign neoplasm originating in a tissue

benign neoplasm originating on a surface

Figure 5–3. Comparison of a benign neoplasm in solid tissue such as breast with a benign neoplasm developing in an organ with mucosal surface such as the colon. The breast neoplasm is encapsulated; the colon neoplasm is polypoid.

any abnormal protrusion from a mucosal surface. Polypoid growth is characteristic of benign neoplasms on surfaces; however, polypoid growth sometimes occurs with other types of lesions, such as inflammations, hyperplasias, and malignant neoplasms.

Benign neoplasms that originate within solid organs or connective tissue usually compress tissue around them to form a fibrous rim (capsule) (Figures 5–3, 5–5A). Because of the fibrous rim, benign tumors are easily separated from surrounding tissue during removal. This can be a distinguishing feature from malignant neoplasms. Histologically, benign neoplasms very closely resemble their cells of origin. Minimal to moderate degrees of cellular atypia are encountered with various types of benign neoplasms. The normal architectural arrangement of tissue or organ is lost within the neoplasm. The most important criteria are the discreteness of the lesion and the uniform, relatively mature appearance of the cells.

Malignant Neoplasms

Early lesions are hardest to diagnose but are most important. Diagnostic differentiation from premalignant surface hyperplasia may be difficult. Two criteria are required for the diagnosis of a malignant neoplasm—establishing that the cells are neoplastic and demonstrating invasion. The cells are judged to be neoplastic by microscopic criteria. Proof would require genetic study which is impractical or impossible. Microscopic criteria for identification of malignant cells include uniformity of cell population, formation of a mass with

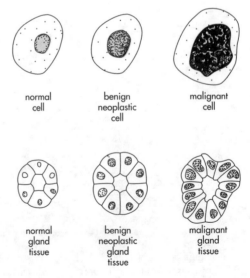

Figure 5–4. Comparison of cells and glands from normal tissue, benign neoplasm, and malignant neoplasm.

replacement of the normal components of the organ, and, to a variable extent, the degree of cellular atypia. Atypical hyperplasias may have similar degrees of atypia to some neoplasms, but they fail to form a mass or replace normal landmarks. Very severe atypia is nearly diagnostic of cancer, but many cancers have a relatively mild degree of atypia, which is not diagnostic in itself (Figure 5–4).

Invasion and metastasis are the principal criteria used to distinguish benign and malignant neoplasms. Metastasis is the most definitive criterion but is not a desirable means of diagnosing cancer because it occurs late in the evolution of a malignant neoplasm. Proof of metastasis requires biopsy to demonstrate that the apparent metastatic lesion contains neoplastic cells rather than inflammatory cells, because infections can also "metastasize."

Local invasiveness is a more commonly used criterion for cancer than is metastasis (Figure 5–5B). As mentioned earlier, invasion is characterized by infiltration of cancer cells with poor respect for tissue

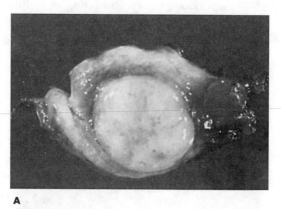

A

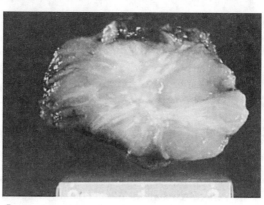

B

Figure 5–5. Excisional biopsy specimens of breast neoplasms. A. Spherical, encapsulated benign neoplasm (fibroadenoma). B. Invasive, crab-like streaks of a breast cancer (adenocarcinoma).

NEOPLASIA		5-2
causes	**lesions**	**manifestations**
Genetic change in clone of cells Promoting factors	Mass of abnormal cells Invasion and metastasis if malignant	Mass interfering with function Secondary effects such as infection and anemia

boundaries. Invasiveness is recognized grossly by irregularity of tumor tissue margins, failure of the tumor to separate from surrounding tissue during removal, and, when advanced, direct spread beyond the organ of origin.

Additional features that are helpful but not entirely specific in separating malignant from benign neoplasms include hardness (many malignant neoplasms provoke proliferation of fibrous tissue with scarring), necrosis (soft yellow areas resulting from the cancer outgrowing its blood supply), ulceration (necrotic tissue of surface cancers sloughs, leaving an ulcer defect), and multilobulation (uncommon in benign neoplasms). Malignant neoplasms are usually larger than benign neoplasms, but this is a very unreliable generalization. Both benign and malignant neoplasms are usually solitary in their origin; however, skin cancers and a few benign neoplasms are characteristically multiple (nevi, leiomyomas of the uterus, neurofibromas, and sometimes adenomas of the colon).

LIFE HISTORY AND SPREAD OF CANCER

Cancers have a long life history, most of which occurs before there is any lesion that can be called a cancer. We know of the early events through experimentation and inference rather than through direct observations of each type of cancer that occurs in humans.

Genetic alteration is the basis for development of cancer, but, of all the mutations that occur in cells, very few lead to cancer. Further, most cells with cancer potential do not express that potential. A cell must undergo an alteration or series of alterations called *initiation* to acquire the autonomous growth potential referred to as cancer. Agents that so alter cells are called *carcinogens*. Carcinogens may be physical, chemical, or biologic agents. Once a carcinogen has genetically altered a cell, a second, nongenotoxic agent called a *promoter* may act to further the expression of the cancer in that cell and its progeny.

Some carcinogens act as both initiators and promoters but many others serve only one function or the other. The mechanism of action of the carcinogen is direct or indirect at the level of the cell's deoxyribonucleic acid (DNA), that comprises *oncogenes.* Oncogenes are special genes that, when stimulated, code for growth-enhancing products (growth factors) that can contribute to neoplasia under the right circumstances. Cells also contain tumor suppressor genes (e.g., p53) that normally keep the oncogenes in check. However, when there is a mutation in a suppressor gene, it no longer functions as a control on an oncogene. The net result is replication of DNA and consequent cell division outside of the normal control mechanisms. Thus, the development of cancer is an extremely complex process that entails multiple variables. A "cure for cancer" takes on new meaning when the complexities of the developmental events are appreciated.

Transformation is the process by which normal cells acquire cancer potential. The cancer cells must proliferate rapidly enough to maintain and expand the size of their population. Further, they must either influence the surrounding tissue from which they originated to supply their nutritional and metabolic needs, or they must adapt themselves nutritionally and metabolically. Antagonism between the body and these aberrant cells is continuous. If the body gains the upper hand, the aberrant population may disappear. If the aberrant cells gain the upper hand, they can become established.

These colonies of aberrant cells are not necessarily neoplasms. If they have permanently and irreversibly established themselves as an expanding population in the body, then they are considered neoplasms. If they are not firmly established and there remains a potential for their spontaneous disappearance (regression), they are said to be preneoplastic. If the preneoplastic states are clinically discoverable, surgical removal of the aberrant cell populations can be undertaken before a cancer actually develops. Unfortunately, it is not possible to detect preneoplastic phases for most types of neoplasms. There are a few cancer types where preneoplastic tissue may manifest itself in a detectable manner. Squamous epithelium may go through a slow series of changes, including simple epithelial hyperplasia, atypical hyperplasia (often called *dysplasia*), and finally carcinoma in situ. With *carcinoma in situ,* the transformed cells are confined to the epithelial layer and have not yet manifested themselves as frank neoplastic cells by invading the surrounding tissue (Figure 5–6). The in situ stage can be microscopically detected in the uterine cervix, oral cavity, and larynx. Cancer can be prevented by removal of either the dysplastic lesion or the in situ lesion.

There are a number of lesions from which cancers arise in noticeable frequency that are not in themselves definable as carcinoma in situ. These predisposing lesions are definable by statistical association with the development of cancer. Examples are a hyperplastic lesion of

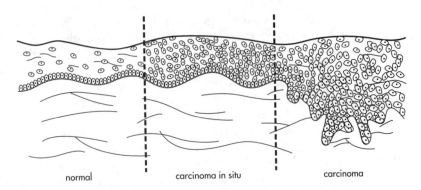

normal   carcinoma in situ   carcinoma

Figure 5–6. Invasion of the basement membrane differentiates carcinoma in situ.

the gums due to ill-fitting dentures or atypical hyperplasia and squamous metaplasia of bronchi in a chronic smoker. In some sites, particularly epithelial surfaces, chronic inflammation may be predisposing
for the development of neoplasms.

Local invasion is a critical step in the development of overt cancer. For epithelial cancers (carcinomas), this is the point where malignant cells break through the basement membrane that separates
epithelium from connective tissue. Once this break occurs, the cancer
can grow and spread to destroy tissue, produce a mass, and further
spread via the vascular system and body passageways. Local growth may
be slow or rapid. Some cancers kill mainly by local destruction. Examples include blockage of ureters by local spread of carcinoma of the
cervix, obstruction of the common bile duct by carcinoma of the pancreas, and obstruction of the esophagus by esophageal carcinoma.

Regional and distant spread through lymphatics is an important
step in the life history of most carcinomas. Sarcomas less commonly
spread by this route. Lymph nodes can filter out the cancer cells for a
while, but eventually the cancer cells spread beyond the nodes and to
the bloodstream for wide dissemination. Absence of lymph node
involvement is a favorable stage for surgical cure. Some patients with
regional spread (involved lymph nodes) can also be cured. Those with
distant spread less commonly survive. Sarcomas usually spread directly
in the bloodstream and are filtered out first in the lungs, where they
may grow and produce metastatic nodules. The spread of breast carcinoma is illustrated in (Figure 5–7).

GRADING AND STAGING

The terms *grade* and *stage* refer to the histologic differentiation and
degree of spread of cancers, respectively. *Differentiation* refers to the

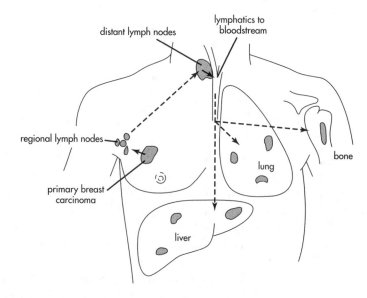

Figure 5–7. Typical pattern of metastasis from a breast cancer. For carcinomas, metastasis via lymphatics usually precedes metastasis via the blood.

degree of resemblance of the cancer to its tissue of origin. Thus, cancers are commonly graded as well-differentiated, moderately differentiated, poorly differentiated, or undifferentiated. Poorly differentiated neoplasms exhibit more cellular atypia and less structural similarity to the tissue of origin than do well-differentiated neoplasms. Numerical systems are used for grading of some cancers.

Staging reflects the degree of local invasion and regional and distant metastasis. Rules for staging have been established for each of the common cancer types. These rules for staging involve evaluation for in situ change, localization to the organ of origin, direct spread beyond the organ, lymph node metastasis, and distant metastasis. Both grading and staging are used to predict likelihood of cure (*prognosis*), but staging usually is the better predictor.

Review Questions

1. What is the difference in pathogenesis of hyperplasias and neoplasms? What is the significance of this difference? How does hypertrophy differ from hyperplasia?

2. How do hyperplasias, benign neoplasms, and malignant neoplasms differ in behavior, morphology, and treatment?

3. How does the appearance of hyperplasias and neoplasms differ from inflammation?

4. What conventions are used to name the various types of benign and malignant neoplasms? What are the exceptions to these conventions?

5. Which organs or tissues commonly undergo hyperplasia? Which organs characteristically undergo hypertrophy rather than hyperplasia?

6. What is the significance of surface epithelial hyperplasia?

7. What criteria are used to diagnose cancer?

8. What are the temporal relationships among mutation, transformation, premalignant lesions, in situ cancer, local invasion, metastasis, and death?

9. How do carcinomas and sarcomas differ in their spread?

10. What do *grading* and *staging* refer to and why are they used?

11. What do the following terms mean?
    Carcinogen
    Carcinoma in situ
    Differentiation
    Dysplasia
    Initiation
    Metaplasia
    Polyp
    Predisposing condition
    Promotion
    Squamous metaplasia
    Tumor

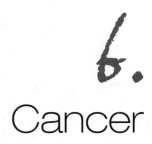

Cancer

FREQUENCY AND SIGNIFICANCE

ETIOLOGY

LOCAL AND SYSTEMIC MANIFESTATIONS
  Mass
  Pain
  Obstruction
  Hemorrhage
  Pathologic Fracture
  Infection
  Anemia
  Cachexia
  Hormone Production

DIAGNOSIS

NATURAL HISTORY

TREATMENT

REVIEW QUESTIONS

Chapter 5 covered the basic concepts of cell proliferative disorders, separating hyperplasias from neoplasms and benign from malignant neoplasms. The emphasis in this chapter is on malignant neoplasms (cancers)—their frequency and significance, etiology, manifestations, natural history, and treatment. This chapter is an overview; much more will be said about specific cancers in Chapters 8 through 25.

FREQUENCY AND SIGNIFICANCE

Cancer is often fatal and ranks as the second leading cause of death in the United States. However, the term *cancer* encompasses a large number of specific types of malignant neoplasms that must be considered individually, because their behavior, their treatment, and probably their causes vary considerably. The prognosis of a cancer depends upon the natural history of that type of cancer, the extent of spread at the time of discovery, and efficacy of existing therapy for that particular type of cancer. In general, the incidence of malignant tumors is about twice the mortality rate. Stated differently, the overall survival rate of cancer is approximately 50 percent. There is a great variability in the behavior of different cancers. Some types, such as carcinoma of the pancreas, almost always kill the patient, whereas others, such as skin carcinoma, rarely kill the patient.

Three important variables relating to cancer frequency and significance are site of development, sex, and age. Cancers developing from epithelium (carcinomas) outnumber cancers from nonepithelial cells (sarcomas, leukemias, and lymphomas) by 6 to 1. The most common cancers of humans are actually basal and squamous cell carcinomas of the skin, comprising about 40 percent of all cancers and 99 percent of all skin cancers. Despite their frequency, they are very seldom fatal because they are readily visualized, grow slowly, metastasize only rarely, and can be completely excised. In contrast, malignant melanoma comprises only 1 percent of all skin malignancies but is fatal in about 20 percent of patients. Thus, a large proportion of the mortality associated with cancers of the skin is accounted for by the least common type. In addition to being the most common cancers, basal and squamous cell carcinomas are the only common cancers that are frequently treated in a physician's office and thus escape hospital statistics. Thus, these two common skin cancers are often omitted from overall collections of cancer statistics.

Aside from skin cancers, carcinomas of the lung, colon, breast, prostate, and uterus are the most common types. The five most common types in males and females are given in Tables 6–1 and 6–2.

Lung cancer is responsible for over one-third of cancer deaths in males and nearly one-fifth of cancer deaths in females. Treatment is relatively ineffective (13 percent 5-year survival), but prevention of most cases (by cessation of smoking) is possible. Treatment of colon cancer (surgical removal) cures more than 50 percent of patients, and, although we know that a dietary factor is the likely cause, we have no practical way of preventing its occurrence at the present time. Breast and uterine cancers are often detected early and are quite accessible to surgical and radiation therapy, but their high frequency still accounts for a large number of cancer deaths. Prostate cancer is a dis-

TABLE 6–1. FREQUENCY AND SURVIVAL OF COMMON CANCERS IN MALES

	Relative Incidence (%)	Cancer Deaths (%)	Relative 5-Year Survival (%)
Lung	19	34	13
Prostate	22	12	72
Colon	14	11	54
Bladder	10	5	77
Leukemias/Lymphomas	7	8	33–74
	72	70	

ease of elderly men, so its impact is lessened by the fact that these patients are likely to die of other causes. Leukemias and lymphomas have variable survival rates, depending on the specific type. Aggressive radiation and chemotherapy of leukemias and lymphomas consume a disproportionate share of medical resources and are associated with more complications than those cancers treated by surgical therapy alone.

In general, cancer is much more common in older persons; this is particularly true for carcinomas. Of the ten most common carcinomas, most have a peak frequency in the seventies (Table 6–3). Cancers of the breast and female genital tract tend to occur in midlife. Cancer of the lung also presents somewhat earlier than carcinomas in general, with the peak number of new cases occurring in the sixties. Of the many other less common types of cancer, most have a characteristic age incidence. Although cancer is much less frequent in younger

TABLE 6–2. FREQUENCY AND SURVIVAL OF COMMON CANCERS IN FEMALES

	Relative Incidence (%)	Cancer Deaths (%)	Relative 5-Year Survival Rate (%)
Breast	28	18	76
Colon	16	13	54
Cervix/Endometrium	10	4	68/86
Lung	11	21	13
Leukemias/Lymphomas	6	6	33–74
	71	62	

TABLE 6–3. AGE PEAK OF COMMON CARCINOMAS

Site	Peak Age
Cervix	40s and 50s
Breast	40s and 50s
Endometrium	50s
Ovary	50s to 70s
Lung	60s
Bladder	70s
Colon	70s
Pancreas	70s
Stomach	70s
Prostate	70s

people, some types occur predominantly in the young (Table 6–4). All of the common cancers of young people listed in this table are non-epithelial, except for adenocarcinoma of the thyroid, a carcinoma most common in young adult women.

ETIOLOGY

Cancers arise in a variety of circumstances, which suggests that more than one factor is involved in the development of any neoplasm. Experimental studies suggest that cancers go through progressive

TABLE 6–4. CANCER TYPES CHARACTERISTICALLY OCCURRING IN PERSONS UNDER AGE 30

0–10 years
  Acute lymphocytic leukemia
  Neuroblastoma
  Wilm's tumor of kidney
  Retinoblastoma
  Medulloblastoma of cerebellum
10–20 years
  Osteogenic sarcoma
20–30 years
  Hodgkin's disease
  Adenocarcinoma of thyroid
  Testicular cancers

changes before becoming clinically evident. Some even become more aggressive after being temporarily inhibited by cancer therapy. As indicated in Chapter 5, neoplasms are usually considered to originate from a single, genetically altered cell (initiation). This cell, in turn, divides to form a discrete population of altered cells (a clone). Further alterations may occur (promotion) and give rise to new clones. Agents causing transformation of mutant cells into cancer may differ from those causing the initial mutation. If the new clone has a higher rate of cell division than the old clone, the new will outgrow the old. As a general rule, the more a cell deviates in character from analogous normal cells (i.e., the more poorly differentiated it becomes), the more rapidly it grows. The more poorly differentiated cells are usually more invasive and more likely to metastasize.

Prevention of cancer will be dependent upon discovery of, and mechanism of action of oncogenes, tumor suppressor genes, and initiating agents that cause the original genetic change or the circumstances that cause malignant transformation of mutated cells. At the present time, three initiating factors can be identified—chemical carcinogens, radiation, and oncogenic viruses. Their roles as carcinogens will be briefly discussed.

The recognition of a high incidence of scrotal skin cancer in London chimney sweeps led to the discovery that repeated occupational exposure to coal tar was carcinogenic. Later, through experimentation, methylcholanthrene was identified as a specific polycyclic hydrocarbon that could cause cancer. Since then, a large number of man-made compounds have been discovered that are potentially carcinogenic. Chemical carcinogens also occur in nature. One of the most potent carcinogens, known as aflatoxin, is a product of fungi that contaminates peanuts, corn, and other human and animal foods.

The mechanism of chemical carcinogenesis is complex. Generally, carcinogens must be metabolized by cells to an active metabolite, which, in turn, interacts with deoxyribonucleic acid (DNA), ribonucleic acid (RNA), or cell proteins. The interaction with DNA is potentially mutagenic. However, the cell has an enzyme system that actively repairs DNA defects such as those caused by carcinogens. It may be that the establishment of a carcinogenic effect depends on failure to repair DNA. The appearance of tumors takes months to years after exposure to a carcinogen (latent period). What happens in this intervening time is not well known. The latent period can be reduced by increasing the frequency of exposure and size of the dose of carcinogen. Other factors modifying the effects of chemical carcinogens include age, sex, diet, genetic factors, and immune deficiencies. Certain chemicals that do not cause cancer when given alone (promoters), enhance the chance of neoplastic conversion when applied to tissues after exposure to carcinogens.

There are many examples of human cancer associated with recognizable exposure to carcinogenic chemicals. Many of the examples involve occupational chemical exposure, resulting in increased incidence of a specific cancer in a definable population. Compounds implicated include certain dyes, vinyl chloride, alkylating agents, and asbestos. Hormones may increase the incidence of certain neoplasms by mechanisms that are not understood. For example, administration of diethylstilbesterol to pregnant women has been found to correlate with increased incidence of an otherwise rare vaginal adenocarcinoma in their female offspring. Based on present knowledge, the cancer-inducing chemical agent(s) affecting the largest number of people is/are contained in cigarette smoke. Smokers have a 10- to 50-fold greater chance of developing bronchogenic carcinoma than non-smokers, and the risk can be significantly correlated with the number of packs smoked per day multiplied by the number of years an individual has smoked (pack-years). Squamous cell carcinomas of the oral region, larynx, and esophagus and transitional cell carcinomas of the urinary bladder are also significantly associated with cigarette smoking.

Ultraviolet radiation, x-radiation, and gamma radiation are all carcinogenic, with the effect dependent on dose, duration, and the portion of the body exposed. As with chemical carcinogens, a latent period of years to decades intervenes between exposure and the appearance of neoplasms. Just how radiation initiates cancer is not known, although we do know that radiation produces localized breaks in DNA strands.

Examples of radiation-induced cancer include thyroid carcinoma in children, a neoplasm that was rarely encountered before the advent of therapeutic radiation. Now 75 percent of children with this cancer have a history of radiation of the neck for conditions that are no longer treated in this manner. Survivors of the Hiroshima and Nagasaki atomic blasts who were exposed to whole body gamma radiation have an increased incidence of leukemias and thyroid carcinomas. Radiologists not uncommonly developed skin cancers before the benefits of protective shielding were realized. People having extended exposure to the sun (farmers, mariners, and sunbathers) experience a high incidence of basal or squamous cell skin carcinomas due largely to the ultraviolet component of sunlight.

Both RNA- and DNA-containing viruses have oncogenic (tumor-producing) potential. In the DNA groups, members of the papova, herpes, pox, and adenovirus groups have been found to produce tumors in animals. Tumor-producing RNA viruses are called oncornaviruses (onco + RNA) or retroviruses. In cells infected by DNA oncogenic viruses, the viral genome is incorporated in host cell genome and is expressed with it. This insertion of viral genome occurs in only a few cells of an infected population. In cells infected by RNA oncogenic viruses, the virus carries an enzyme, reverse transcriptase, that makes a copy of DNA complementary to the virus' RNA, and this DNA becomes inserted into the host genome.

Viral causation of neoplasms has been demonstrated in numerous animal cancers, but few strong cases of demonstrable viral oncogenesis in humans can be found. Papovaviruses cause squamous papillomas in humans including the common wart (verruca vulgaris), venereal warts (condyloma acuminata), and laryngeal papillomas. Several viruses have been associated with malignant neoplasms in humans, but the exact role of the virus in causing these cancers has not been established and most people with these viruses do not get cancer. Epstein-Barr virus, the cause of infectious mononucleosis, has been associated with Burkitt's lymphoma, a neoplasm most prevalent in Africa, and with undifferentiated nasopharyngeal carcinoma. Specific strains of human papilloma virus play an important role in the etiology of carcinoma of the uterine cervix. Hepatitis B virus has been associated with hepatocarcinoma.

The interactions between chemical carcinogens, radiation, and viruses on one hand, and oncogenes and tumor suppressor genes on the other hand are the subject of intensive and fascinating research.

LOCAL AND SYSTEMIC MANIFESTATIONS

Local manifestations include mass, pain, obstruction, hemorrhage, pathologic fracture, and infection. Systemic manifestations include infection, anemia, cachexia, and hormone production. Any one of these manifestations is present in a minority of patients with cancer; in fact, many cancers are asymptomatic until late in their course.

Mass

If a cancer becomes very large or is situated in a location that is readily visible or palpable, it may be first noted as a mass. Otherwise, one or more of the complications listed below may become evident before a mass is noted.

Pain

Cancer produces pain by local destruction of tissue, with invasion of nerves, by obstructing hollow organs such as the intestine, and by causing inflammation, which, in turn, is associated with pain. In advanced cases, surgical interruption of nerve tracts is sometimes needed to relieve the discomfort. Many cancers are nonpainful.

Obstruction

Body passageways may be obstructed by tumors growing within their lumens or by external compression by a mass. Symptoms depend on the passages involved. Examples of internal obstruction include the obstruction of a bronchus by lung cancer or bowel obstruction by colonic carcinoma. An example of external obstruction is the blockage of the common bile duct by a carcinoma of the pancreas.

Hemorrhage

Cancers on internal or external surfaces may ulcerate and bleed, leading to either acute or chronic blood loss. Inapparent blood in feces (occult blood) may be detected by a simple chemical test.

Pathologic Fracture

Primary bone cancer or metastatic cancers may invade and locally destroy bone, weakening it so that fracture may occur with minimal injury. Cancers of lung, breast, and prostate are especially likely to metastasize to bone. Multiple myeloma, a neoplastic proliferation of plasma cells, is a primary cancer of bone marrow that commonly destroys adjacent bone. A third mechanism by which a neoplasm can cause pathologic fracture is by induction of osteoporosis. Osteoporosis may be caused by inactivity or by rare tumors secreting high levels of corticosteroids or ACTH.

Infection

Infection is a common and often disastrous complication of neoplasia. A variety of overlapping mechanisms produce infections in patients with cancer. At the local level, erosion or ulceration of tumors of epithelial surfaces allows entry of microorganisms. Impaired host responses to infection can arise from a number of causes. Leukopenia may result from extensive replacement of bone marrow in leukemias and lymphomas or in other metastatic cancers. In leukemias and lymphomas, the circulating neoplastic leukocytes are deficient in phagocytic activity. Inadequate nutrition and other factors in the terminally debilitated cancer patient may be associated with a decline in the general capacities of the immune system. Chemotherapy of cancer has a side effect of suppressing the bone marrow's production of leukocytes. Because lymphocyte quantity and quality are often deficient in neoplastic disease, cell-mediated immunity may be particularly impaired. Immune deficiency is manifested by unusual causal agents of infections, such as fungi, protozoa, and viruses, and bacteria that are ordinarily not pathogens.

Anemia

Anemia is one of the most frequent manifestations of malignant neoplasms. Major mechanisms include decreased erythropoiesis resulting from the effects of chemotherapeutic drugs or radiation on bone marrow, bone marrow replacement by neoplastic cells, and blood loss caused by ulceration of the cancer.

Cachexia

Cachexia is the generalized wasting that occurs in the terminal cancer patient. It is probably caused by a combination of anorexia (loss of appetite), nutritional problems, and demands of the rapidly growing neoplasm.

Hormone Production

A few neoplasms secrete hormones that lead to effects associated with excess hormone. Benign neoplasms, particularly those of the endocrine glands, are most commonly involved (see Chapter 25 for specific examples). Sometimes, malignant endocrine gland neoplasms or other neoplasms such as small cell carcinoma of the lung produce hormones in sufficient quantity to cause clinical effects.

DIAGNOSIS

The diagnosis of cancer is based on investigation of the cause of a patient's symptoms or on screening. The diagnosis is confirmed by biopsy, or sometimes by blood smear or cytology. The astute physician will recognize that a patient's symptoms may be due to cancer and will do the appropriate physical examination or order appropriate laboratory tests, radiologic procedures, and endoscopic examinations. Before carrying out irreversible treatment procedures that always entail some risk, a final biopsy report should be in hand, because noncancerous lesions often mimic cancer clinically.

Case finding for cancer is often done, especially in the elderly, when the patient is seen for some other disease. Asymptomatic cancer of the breast or prostate may be detected by palpation, and the skin can be inspected for malignant melanoma and carcinoma. The most common routine screening tests for cancer are cytology of the uterine cervix, testing feces for occult blood, mammography, and chest x-ray. The screening procedures produce a lot of false-positive results that require follow-up tests and biopsies.

NATURAL HISTORY

Each malignant neoplasm possesses its own expected behavior pattern. For example, it is known from past experience that a given malignant neoplasm will likely metastasize to certain organs and will likely take the life of a patient within a certain length of time. Thus, we speak in terms of 5- or 10-year survival for neoplasms, meaning that a certain percentage of patients with that particular neoplasm will still be alive (with or without disease) 5 or 10 years after initial diagnosis. This prognostication of tumor behavior is far from exact. One person with a malignant metastatic neoplasm may die within months of diagnosis, whereas another patient with the same type of neoplasm may live for several years.

Infection is the most common cause of death in cancer patients. Commonly, as the terminally ill patient with a malignant neoplasm becomes more and more immobilized and bedridden, the lungs fail to remove secretions, allowing bacteria to proliferate and cause pneumonia. Infections of the genitourinary tract are also common in terminally ill patients. Whatever the initial site of the infection, many patients eventually develop bacteremia, with spread of organisms to other organs. The predisposing factors for terminal infections are the previously mentioned immune and white cell deficiencies, immobilization, obstruction of body passageways, and general debilitation manifested by cachexia.

Cachexia itself seems to be the cause of death in many cancer patients. Cachexia may be the result of loss of appetite or of a mass obstructing the gastrointestinal tract in some instances. In other instances, there is no logical explanation for cachexia. In some cases, the increased metabolic needs of a neoplasm can explain cachexia, but at other times, patients with very little neoplastic mass become cachectic.

Metabolic and endocrine effects of neoplasm and hemorrhage are occasional causes of death of cancer patients. Often, a single immediate cause of death in a patient with terminal cancer is not identifiable.

TREATMENT

The basic modality of cancer treatment is surgical removal. Even in those cases where total removal of a malignant neoplasm cannot be accomplished, some tumor tissue must be biopsied to establish a tissue (histologic) diagnosis. If a tissue diagnosis is not established for a given cancer, then treatment such as chemotherapy or radiation therapy would be based on less than optimum knowledge of the type of tumor present; sometimes, the diagnosis of cancer may be erroneous. The amount of the cancer removed at operation depends upon its accessibility to surgical removal and its amenability to other modes of therapy. For example, a surgeon may remove very little of a cerebellar medulloblastoma because surgical exposure of the tumor is difficult and there is a risk of destroying adjacent brain structures. In addition, the surgeon knows that this type of cancer responds readily to radiation therapy. Conversely, when a cancer is discovered in the large bowel, total removal is anticipated because the tumor is usually accessible to the surgeon in its entirety. In the latter example, even if metastasis has already occurred, removal of the primary tumor may prevent bowel obstruction.

Radiation therapy is employed in the treatment of localized neoplastic masses that are not surgically accessible (inoperable) or in situations where surgery would be impractical or deleterious to the patient. Radiation therapy is also used following surgery to treat residual neoplasm. Another use of radiation therapy is in the treatment of lymph nodes in the expected metastatic pathway of a particular type of neoplasm. For example, carcinoma of the medial aspect of the breast would be expected to metastasize via the internal mammary lymphatic channels; consequently, these lymph node channels are often irradiated prophylactically following mastectomy. Radiation therapy is generally most effective with tumors composed of rapidly dividing cells. Only a limited number of cancer types can be cured by radiation. For many types of cancers, radiation therapy is palliative; that is, it temporarily abates the progress of a cancer without curing it.

Chemotherapy employs a wide variety of powerful metabolic inhibitors and other cell-killing chemicals that are often used in various combinations for treatment of different cancers. The rationale behind the use of all chemotherapeutic agents is that they will kill or inhibit the growth of neoplastic cells to a greater degree than that of the body's normal cells. However, in some instances not enough differential response exists, and consequently, it is understandable that serious side effects from chemotherapy can occur, most of which are based on the deleterious effects on rapidly metabolizing normal body tissues such as bone marrow. Chemotherapy has been most successful for certain types of leukemias and lymphomas and for choriocarcinoma in females, resulting in cures.

Hormonal therapy may cause significant regression of some cancers of the breast and prostate gland and prolong life. The response may be induced by administering hormone or by removing hormone-producing organs such as testes, ovaries, adrenal glands, or pituitary gland. Breast cancers that have estrogen receptors on their cell surfaces (about two-thirds) often regress when estrogen levels are lowered by oophorectomy or adrenalectomy. Similarly, some prostate cancers regress when testosterone levels are lowered by castration or by administration of an opposing hormone, estrogen. Hormonal therapy is most used as palliative therapy for metastatic cancer.

Review Questions

1. What are the most common carcinomas? How do they differ in frequency, sex ratios, and survival rate?

2. Which carcinomas occur predominantly in the middle aged? in the elderly?

3. Which cancers occur predominantly in each of the first three decades of life?

4. What types of agents have been implicated in the development of cancers?

5. What are six local manifestations of cancer? How does cancer cause these manifestations?

6. What is the pathogenesis of the three major systemic manifestations of cancer?

7. What are the forms of cancer therapy? What are the advantages and disadvantages of each?

7.

Genetic and Developmental Diseases

REVIEW OF STRUCTURE AND FUNCTION
Chromosomal Duplication and Fertilization • Genetic Inheritance • Embryonic Development • Fetal Development • Perinatal Period • Infancy • Childhood • Adolescence

DEFINITIONS

FREQUENCY AND SIGNIFICANCE OF DEVELOPMENTAL ABNORMALITIES
Monogenetic (Single-Gene) Diseases
Polygenetic (Multigene) Disorders
Chromosomal Diseases
Embryonic Anomalies
Fetal Diseases
Perinatal Diseases
Diseases of Infancy
Diseases of Childhood and Adolescence

SYMPTOMS, SIGNS, AND TESTS
Genetic Diseases
Chromosomal Diseases
Embryonic Anomalies
Fetal Diseases

EXAMPLES OF SPECIFIC DISEASES
Genetic Diseases
Diabetes Mellitus • Gout • Sickle-Cell Anemia • Hemophilia • Phenylketonuria • Muscular Dystrophy • Cystic Fibrosis

Chromosomal Diseases

Down's Syndrome • Klinefelter's Syndrome • Turner's Syndrome • Fragile X-Syndrome

Embryonic Anomalies

Tetralogy of Fallot • Agenesis of One Kidney • Meckel's Diverticulum • Meningomyeiocele

Fetal Diseases

Erythroblastosis Fetalis • Congenital Syphilis • Fetal Alcohol Syndrome

REVIEW QUESTIONS

REVIEW OF STRUCTURE AND FUNCTION

The development of a mature individual takes approximately 18 years and can be divided into the following stages: fertilization, embryonic period, fetal period, perinatal period, infancy, childhood, and adolescence.

Fertilization involves the uniting of a sperm and ovum, with each contributing 23 chromosomes to the newly created human organism. These chromosomes contain all of the genetic information needed to control the succeeding stages of development. Because many human diseases result from abnormalities in the genetic makeup as a result of events occurring before fertilization, the events occurring before fertilization will be briefly reviewed.

All of the cells of a normal mature individual have 46 chromosomes. These chromosomes may duplicate themselves and divide to form two daughter cells each with 46 chromosomes. This process is called *mitosis* and can occur in most of the cells in the body (Figure 7–1). The germ cells that develop into sperm and ova undergo a different type of cell division called *meiosis*. In meiosis, only one chromosome from each pair is passed on to each gamete (sperm or ovum) (Figure 7–1). Thus, each gamete has only 23 chromosomes.

Because each pair of chromosomes is unique with an orderly arrangement of its subunits (genes), abnormalities of separation of the chromosome pairs or breakage of chromosomes during meiosis will be reflected in the chromosomal makeup of a new individual at the time of fertilization. Abnormalities in chromosome number result from nondisjunction, a process in which two chromosomes go to one gamete and none to another (Figure 7–2). When such gametes result in fertilization, the zygote formed has three homologous chromosomes (trisomy) or only one (monosomy). Abnormalities in chromosome structure result from breakage of chromosomes during the process of cell division. Resulting fragments may pass to the wrong

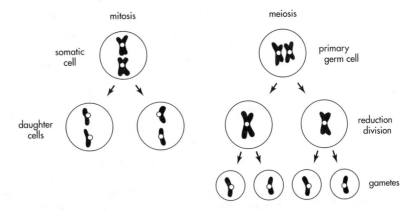

Figure 7–1. Comparison of mitosis in somatic cells with meiosis in germ cells. A homologous pair of chromosomes that have already duplicated but are still connected by a centromere are illustrated at the top. In mitosis, the centromere is duplicated and each daughter cell receives one of each of the duplicated chromosomes from each pair. In meiosis, the paired chromosomes align opposite each other and are separated at the first (reduction) division. The second division sends only one chromosome duplicate from the original pair to each gamete.

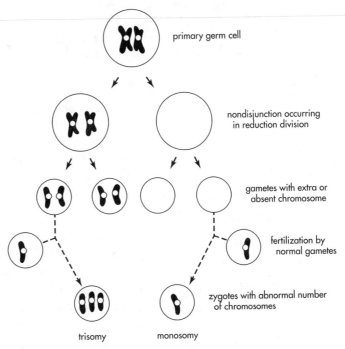

Figure 7–2. The results of nondisjunction at reduction division of meiosis.

daughter cells, resulting in duplication or deletion of parts of a chromosome, or fragments may exchange places with fragments from nonhomologous chromosomes, resulting in translocations (Figure 7–3). Occasionally, nondisjunction, duplication, deletion, or translocation occur in the first or second cell division after fertilization, resulting in an individual with cells of differing chromosomal makeup. This is called *mosaicism.* Because of the vast amount of genetic information carried by each chromosome, the new organism may be severely affected by abnormalities in chromosomes.

Chromosomes are made of deoxyribonucleic acid (DNA) molecules arranged into specific sequences. These sequences define the subunits of a chromosome known as *genes.* One or more genes are responsible for determining a genetic trait. An abnormality in a gene may result in the genetic trait being expressed in an abnormal way. Each individual harbors a few abnormal genes that may cause disease and many genes that cause nonharmful traits such as red hair. There are two ways an individual can acquire an abnormal gene. When a gene is altered chemically, it is called a *mutation.* When a mutation occurs during meiosis, the resulting sperm or ovum can pass the abnormal gene to the new individual. This abnormal gene will be present in all the cells of the new individual and will be passed to subsequent generations by the germ cells. Thus, abnormal genes can arise by mutation of germ cells or by passage from previous generations. It should also be noted that mutations can occur in nongerm cells (somatic cells), but the effects are limited because of the limited number of new cells resulting from any given somatic cell. As we have

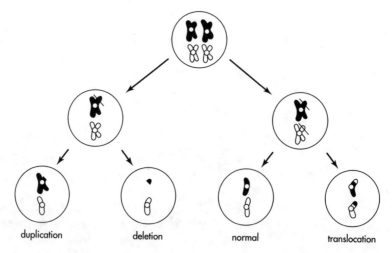

duplication   deletion   normal   translocation

Figure 7–3. Illustration of how breaks in chromosomes can result in duplication, deletion, and translocation.

noted in previous chapters, neoplasms can result from mutations in somatic cells.

Not all abnormal genes produce an abnormal genetic trait. Each genetic trait is influenced by two genes, one on each of the paired chromosomes. One of the genes of a pair may be dominant over the other, that is, it will determine the genetic trait that the individual expresses. There is one exception to this rule; males have some unpaired genes on the sex chromosomes (X and Y).

A recessive gene will be expressed only if it is paired with another recessive gene. Thus, recessive genes for abnormal traits can only be expressed if both genes are abnormal or if they are located on the X chromosome of a male, where there is no second gene for the trait.

Sometimes abnormal dominant genes or pairs of abnormal recessive genes fail to cause expression of the abnormal trait. This is called *nonpenetrance*. If the abnormal trait is expressed to a variable extent in different individuals, it is called *variable expressivity*. To complicate matters even further, the expression of some genetic traits is dependent on multiple factors such as other genes and environmental factors including time. It is difficult to determine the genetic makeup (genotype) of an individual except for completely expressed dominant traits that become evident early in life. The term *phenotype* refers to those traits that are manifest by form or function. Most of the abnormal genes in the population are not manifest. Abnormal genes are only discovered by inference, by establishing which family members have the disease and deducing which ones carried the abnormal genes.

Embryonic development occurs in the first 8 weeks after fertilization. This developmental sequence, which transforms a single fertilized ovum to an individual with body structure and organs, may be influenced by abnormal genes or by environmental factors such as nutrition, infection, chemicals, and radiation exposure.

Fetal development occurs from the eighth week after fertilization to birth. The fetal period is primarily one of growth and maturation of organs and tissues and results in an individual who can survive and grow without the direct support of a maternal blood supply. The lungs, kidneys, and liver require the longest time to reach this stage.

The perinatal period is defined as the period from 2 weeks before birth to 4 weeks after birth. The major events of this period are survival from the trauma of birth and adjustment to external life. The lungs and vascular system must adjust to breathing and rerouting of oxygenated blood. Kidney and liver function increase at this time to meet new demands.

The period of infancy is defined as 1 month to 1 year of age. Major events during this period include growth, development of motor and intellectual functions, and development of immunologic defense against foreign substances.

The period of childhood covers the period from infancy to puberty and is primarily one of growth and refinement of motor and intellectual functions.

Adolescence is the final developmental period before the process of aging begins. Sexual maturation is the major physical event that distinguishes this period.

DEFINITIONS

Abnormalities of development may be due to altered genetic structure or environmental effects or a combination of the two. The interaction of genetic and environmental factors is complex, and for a given disease may not be well understood. We will use the term developmental abnormality in a broad sense to refer to diseases that affect normal maturation.

A genetic disease is an established disease caused by an abnormal gene. Simply having an abnormal gene is not a disease. Although abnormal genes are acquired at the time of fertilization, most genetic diseases do not develop until some time after birth if they develop at all. Single-gene defects encompass the classic genetic diseases in which the abnormal gene may be traced through family trees. Multiple-gene or complex gene defects involve more than one abnormal gene and sometimes environmental factors for their expression. Inheritance patterns are not clear-cut, but there is some tendency for the disease to occur in families. Diabetes mellitus is an example of a complex genetic disease.

Chromosomal diseases are also genetic in nature but will be treated separately in this text because they differ considerably from other genetic diseases. Chromosomal abnormalities are defined by visible misplacement of, or damage to, chromosomes. Chromosomes can be visualized by a process known as *karyotyping*. This involves culture of cells, inducing the cells to divide, arresting the dividing cells during mitosis, and squashing and staining the cells so that the chromosomes can be seen under a microscope (Figure 7–4). Sex chromosome numbers can be evaluated by a simpler test known as a *buccal smear* (a scraping of epithelial cells from inside the mouth). X-chromatin bodies (Barr bodies) can be seen on the periphery of cell nuclei with ordinary stains when more than one X chromosome is present (Figure 7–5). Thus, Barr bodies are absent in normal males. The Y chromosome (F body) can be seen using a fluorescent staining technique. Chromosomal diseases often result in abnormalities so severe as to preclude reproduction and further passage of the abnormality.

Abnormalities developing between the time of fertilization and birth are divided into two types, based on whether they are initiated

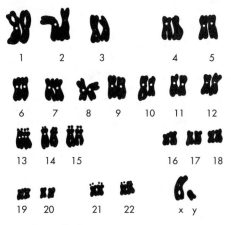

Figure 7–4. A normal male karyotype.

during the embryonic period (first 8 weeks) or the fetal period (the final 32 weeks to birth). Changes occurring in the embryonic period produce gross malformations of body or organ structure and are referred to as *embryonic* or *congenital anomalies.* Diseases of the fetal period are less common and are more similar to diseases of later life in that they produce destructive lesions.

Congenital means present at birth. Embryonic anomalies and fetal diseases are present at birth but may go undetected until adult life (e.g., two ureters on one side). Genetic and chromosomal diseases may also be congenital; however, many genetic diseases are not manifest until sometime after birth and therefore are not congenital. Familial diseases are diseases in which several family members have the same disease. Familial diseases are not necessarily genetic in origin (e.g.,

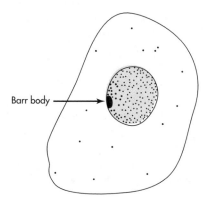

Figure 7–5. Squamous epithelial cell from a female with a Barr body at the nuclear membrane.

common colds tend to be familial but not genetic). We generally tend to think of genetic diseases when we talk of familial disease because of genes being passed from generation to generation. However, many individuals with genetic diseases do not have a family history of the disease because of the recessive nature of many of these diseases or because the disease is caused by a new germ cell mutation. Also, some embryonic anomalies are caused by abnormal genes and may be familial (e.g., polycystic kidneys, cleft lip and palate). In the latter situation, the disease can be classified as both congenital and familial. Most genetic diseases are not congenital. Although the abnormal gene may be present, the disease usually does not develop by the time of birth and may never develop.

FREQUENCY AND SIGNIFICANCE OF DEVELOPMENTAL ABNORMALITIES

Monogenetic (Single-Gene) Diseases

These diseases are inherited by one of four mechanisms: autosomal recessive, autosomal dominant, sex-linked recessive, sex-linked dominant. Autosomal diseases are much more common than sex-linked diseases, and recessive diseases are much more common than dominant diseases. Many of the thousands of types of genetic diseases are incompletely penetrant (not all persons with the appropriate genes will have the disease) and many are variably expressed (not all persons will have the disease to the same severity). Most genetic diseases are uncommon or rare; yet, when taken in aggregate, most families will be influenced by some type of multifactorial genetic disease and may have members with single-gene diseases. Dominant genes are easily recognized when completely penetrant, because the presence of the disease identifies those individuals with the gene, and the line of inheritance can be followed through each generation (Figure 7–6).

Recessive disorders usually appear sporadically. When they occur, about one-fourth of siblings are involved (both parents are carriers, so the chance of a child getting both abnormal genes is $\frac{1}{2} \times \frac{1}{2}$). The family history for others with the disease will usually be negative unless the recessive gene has a very high frequency in the population or there was marriage among related individuals (Figure 7–7).

Sex-linked recessive disorders will appear in every other generation. Females with the abnormal gene on the X chromosome will not have the disease, because they have an opposing normal gene on the other X chromosome; males with the gene will have the disease, because the Y chromosome has no gene to oppose the abnormal one on the X chromosome (Figure 7–8).

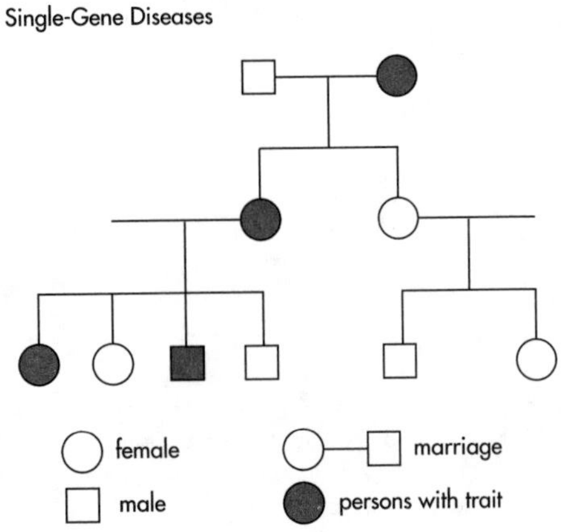

Single-Gene Diseases

Figure 7–6. Family tree for a dominantly inherited trait. The abnormality appears in the parent of each involved individual unless it arises by mutation or is nonpenetrant.

Recessive disorders are very difficult to control, because the abnormal genes can be perpetuated through many generations before two carriers mate. Many dominant diseases will arise as the result of mutations and, if severe, will disappear as involved individuals fail to reproduce. Factors favoring the perpetuation of dominant diseases include late onset, mild disease, nonpenetrance, and variable expressivity.

Polygenetic (Multigene) Disorders

These disorders are difficult to define, because inheritance patterns are not clear and because similar disorders may be caused by nongenetic mechanisms. Diabetes mellitus is a good example. Diabetes

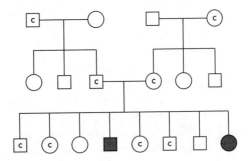

Figure 7–7. Family tree for a recessively inherited trait. The trait appears in one-fourth of offspring when both parents carry the recessive gene. The trait is often absent in previous generations, although carriers (represented by the letter c) are likely to have been present but undetected.

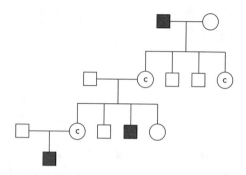

Figure 7–8. Family tree for a sex-linked recessive trait. The trait only appears in males. Uncles or grandfathers are likely to be affected. The abnormal gene may be passed through carrier females for generations.

tends to occur in families but not in a predictable manner. Some cases of diabetes are due to destruction of the pancreas, a nongenetic cause. Some congenital anomalies, such as cleft lip and congenital heart disease, are established as genetic by a definite tendency to occur in families without other explanation for the familial tendency. In addition to the multigene disorders that are reasonably well established as genetic, there is a much broader category of multifactorial disease that may have abnormal genes as one of the factors. Such multifactorial diseases probably include many cases of atherosclerotic heart disease, hypertension, and cancer.

Chromosomal Diseases

Most diseases of autosomal chromosomes are so severe as to be incompatible with embryonic development. These account for one-third of the spontaneous abortions that occur during the first third of pregnancy. The other two-thirds of early spontaneous abortions are of unknown cause. Of the types of chromosomal diseases compatible with survival to birth, Down's syndrome (trisomy 21 or "mongolism" as it used to be called) is most common. Other autosomal chromosomal disorders compatible with survival to birth usually produce severely deformed infants who die within a few months. Abnormalities of sex chromosome number produce relatively mild abnormalities that often are not detected until puberty, when secondary sex characteristics are found to be abnormal.

The overall frequency of genetic disease is difficult to establish because of delayed onset of some types and the variable effects of environmental factors. An estimate of the frequency of genetic disease in children is given in Table 7–1.

TABLE 7–1. INCIDENCE OF GENETIC DISEASES AS PERCENT OF LIVE BIRTHS	
Genetic Disease	Incidence (%)
Chromosomal abnormalities	0.4
Single-gene defects	2.0
Multigene disorders	2.6
Total	5.0

(Data from The National Health Education Committee, The Killers and Cripplers—Facts on Major Diseases in the U.S. Today. New York: D. McKay, 1976, p. 127.)

Embryonic Anomalies

Approximately 2 percent of newborns are said to have significant congenital anomalies. The causes of these anomalies can be roughly estimated as follows: 65 percent unknown, 20 percent genetic, 5 percent chromosomal, and 10 percent environmental. The genetic causes can be classified as monogenetic (abnormal gene or pair of genes), polygenetic (effects of several genes), or multifactorial (combined effect of genes and environmental factors). The chromosomal causes have been discussed previously. Of the environmental causes, radiation is quite capable of causing anomalies but care with diagnostic and therapeutic use of radiation makes this a rare cause. Rubella virus is an important cause of congenital anomalies, but its effects have been reduced by vaccination. Maternal metabolic disorders, such as iodine deficiency and diabetes, can cause anomalies. Drugs, environmental chemicals, and alcohol account for about half of the known nongenetic causes of developmental defects. Thalidomide is a drug that produced many babies with short arms before its effects were discovered. Other drugs, such as anticonvulsants, are less predictable in their effects and more important for maternal health. The effects of environmental chemicals has received much attention, but the effects are difficult to evaluate unless there is a dramatic increase in the frequency of anomalies above the background level. Alcohol abuse is a preventable cause of growth and mental retardation in infants.

Among the various types of anomalies, congenital heart defects are common and most important. Many can be successfully repaired surgically. Abnormalities of the kidney and urinary tract are also quite common; they are often hidden, in which case they are discovered later in life or at autopsy. The gastrointestinal tract harbors many different anomalies, many of which are treatable. Anomalies of the central nervous system are often serious and nonrepairable. Approximately 15 percent of embryonic anomalies are multiple, involving several organs.

Fetal Diseases

Although there is overlap with embryonic anomalies, fetal diseases are less frequent than other types of developmental disorders. The most important is erythroblastosis fetalis, which is caused by the mother producing antibodies to the fetus' red blood cells. This disease is a concern whenever the mother has Rh negative red blood cells and the fetus has Rh positive red blood cells. All women should be tested for their Rh status during their first pregnancy, because erythroblastosis fetalis can be prevented or controlled (see below). Syphilis in the fetus is uncommon, but it can be completely prevented if the mother is treated before the middle of pregnancy. Therefore, all pregnant women should be tested for syphilis early in pregnancy to prevent congenital syphilis. Fetal rubella can also be prevented by ensuring that the mother is immunized prior to becoming pregnant. Infectious agents such as HIV, cytomegalovirus, herpes virus, and toxoplasma usually produce their effects during fetal development. Alcohol and other drugs are important causes of damage to the fetus.

Perinatal Diseases

Prematurity and cerebral palsy are two major categories of disease caused during the perinatal period. Approximately 10 percent of babies are born prematurely, as indicated by subnormal birth weight. Major problems resulting from prematurity include brain damage and development of hyaline membrane disease due to immaturity of the lungs. If there is no brain damage and the infant survives, a normal life may be expected. Brain damage in the late fetal or perinatal period often results in cerebral palsy, a condition characterized by abnormal muscular coordination with or without mental retardation.

Diseases of Infancy

Major problems of infancy that relate specifically to this developmental stage include infections due to lack of previous experience with infectious agents and nutritional problems. Antibodies acquired from the mother tend to protect the infant for about 6 months, after this the infant must experience the infection or be immunized in order to develop antibodies against infectious agents. A common nutritional problem is the failure to get enough iron. Babies fed on milk and fruit, without sources of iron such as cereals, will develop iron-deficiency anemia beginning around 6 months of age, when iron stores acquired from the mother are used up. Iron-deficient babies perform less well on standarized tests of development compared to iron-sufficient peers.

Diseases of Childhood and Adolescence

Diseases of these periods rarely relate to developmental problems. They differ from diseases of older age groups only in relative frequency. Accidents and infections are more common, whereas degenerations and neoplasms (except for a few types) are uncommon.

SYMPTOMS, SIGNS, AND TESTS

Genetic Diseases

Each specific disease has its own highly individual manifestations, which vary in time of onset and nature of the lesions. Some genetic diseases are present at birth (congenital), but most appear later. Some genetic diseases present as inflammations, degenerations, or growth disturbances. For example, cystic fibrosis presents with pancreatitis and pneumonia, Friedreich's ataxia presents with degeneration of nerve cells, and retinoblastoma presents as a malignant neoplasm of the eye in children. A large number of genetic disorders produce specific recognizable biochemical defects. These are called inborn errors of metabolism and therefore may be also classified as metabolic diseases.

Biochemical defects can be subdivided into defects in structural protein and defects in enzymes. An example of structural protein defect is sickle-cell anemia, in which the hemoglobin of red blood cells is defective, resulting in premature death of red blood cells. Enzyme defects are subdivided on the basis of the type of substance affected into disorders of carbohydrate, protein, lipid, and mineral metabolism. An example of an inborn error of carbohydrate metabolism is glycogen storage disease, in which glucose can be converted into glycogen for storage, but one of the enzymes needed to convert the glycogen back to glucose is missing. This results in excessive storage of glycogen and enlargement of organs in which glycogen is stored. Biochemical tests are available for some inborn errors of metabolism, but many are diagnosed mainly by clinical findings. A few genetic diseases can be diagnosed before birth by testing of the amniotic fluid (Figure 7–9). Several biochemical diseases, including sickle-cell anemia, phenylketonuria, galactosemic, and hypothyroidism, are routinely tested for at birth, using a small blood sample obtained from the head, and early treatment can prevent long-term disability.

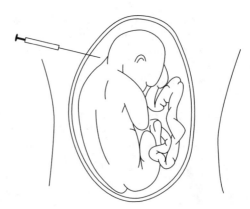

Figure 7–9. Amniocentesis to obtain fluid and cells for the detection of some genetic, chromosomal, and fetal diseases.

Chromosomal Diseases

These diseases are suspected and often diagnosed by physical examination. Karyotyping should be used to substantiate the diagnosis. Karyotyping is performed only at large referral centers, but is essential for accurate diagnosis and counseling.

Embryonic Anomalies

These gross anomalies are detected by physical examination, radiologic procedures, or exploratory surgery.

Fetal Diseases

The method of diagnosis depends on the nature of the disease. Infections are diagnosed by culture or measurement of antibodies (e.g., serology for syphilis). Immunologic diseases are diagnosed by measuring antigen and antibodies (e.g., Rh factor in fetal and maternal red blood cells). Hydrocephalus, polycystic kidneys, and severe bone disease can be detected by ultrasound.

EXAMPLES OF SPECIFIC DISEASES

Genetic Diseases

Relatively common and important examples of genetic diseases include sickle-cell anemia, hemophilia, phenylketonuria, muscular dystrophy, diabetes mellitus, gout, and cystic fibrosis.

The gene for sickle-cell anemia causes a structural defect in the hemoglobin molecule. When two such genes are present (homozygous), the blood cells of such individuals often are sickle-shaped. Under stressful circumstances, such as a respiratory infection, the red cells are destroyed, producing severe anemia (so-called sickle-cell crisis). Over a period of years the disease is fatal, more rapidly in colder climates. This is a recessive disorder prevalent among blacks. Heterozygotes can be identified because their red blood cells show a slight tendency to sickle.

The two types of hemophilia (classic hemophilia and Christmas disease) are similar, sex-linked disorders. Hemophilia is an example of a rare genetic disease (2 per 100,000 persons) that commands a large amount of medical care in the treatment of severe bleeding and long-term prevention of bleeding. A specific enzyme in the blood-clotting mechanism (factor VIII or factor IX) is deficient, leading to spontaneous bleeding into joints or uncontrollable bleeding when cut. The missing factor can be replaced on a temporary basis, but at great expense.

Phenylketonuria is caused by an absence of phenylalanine hydroxylase, which results in accumulation of phenylketones. Over a period of months, brain damage results. Diagnosis can be made by testing newborns for phenylketones in the blood and is mandatory in all 50 states. This is an example of screening to detect a rare disease.

The most common type of muscular dystrophy (Duchenne) occurs in males because it is a sex-linked recessive disorder. Skeletal muscles degenerate over a period of years, leading to death in childhood. The genetic defect results in an abnormality in a muscle protein called *dystrophin*. Diagnosis of muscular dystrophy requires expertise in differentiation from other genetic and acquired musculoskeletal disorders.

Cystic fibrosis is an autosomal recessive disorder characterized by thick secretions that lead to obstruction of body passageways. The pancreas is particularly affected, because blockage of ducts leads to decreased delivery of pancreatic enzymes to the intestine and thus to poor digestion of food and marked weight loss. In the lungs, the obstruction of bronchi predisposes to bouts of pneumonia caused by the trapped bacteria. Prevention of pneumonia may prolong life to adulthood. Analysis of chloride secretion in sweat provides a diagnostic test (sweat chloride test). The defect is in the secretory cell's chloride ion channels (see also Chapter 12).

Diabetes mellitus is probably the most important genetic disease, because it is common (2 percent of the population), requires treatment (diet and drugs), and has many complications. It is discussed in Chapter 25.

Gout is about one-tenth as common as diabetes (2 per 1000 persons). It is due to an unknown biochemical defect that causes over-

<table>
<tr><td colspan="3">GENETIC DISEASES   7-1</td></tr>
</table>

cause	lesion	manifestations
Inherited or mutation Sometimes other promoting factors	Specific to each disease Many are metabolic	Specific to each disease May be familial

production of uric acid. Uric acid is a normal breakdown product of purines (used to build DNA) and is excreted by the kidney. When the blood level of uric acid is high, crystals sometimes form in joints, leading to the acute inflammation of gout. If untreated, deposits of urate crystals build up over a period of years in cartilage of the joints and the ear. These deposits are called tophi. Acute and chronic changes in joints are referred to as acute and chronic gout, respectively. For some reason, gout affects men, not women, and is a disease of older men. Three types of drug treatment are available: allopurinol inhibits the body's production of uric acid, probenecid promotes excretion of uric acid by the kidneys (and thereby may promote formation of uric acid stones in the kidney), and colchicine inhibits the acute inflammatory reaction in joints to relieve pain temporarily.

The genes that cause sickle-cell disease, phenylketonuria, and Duchenne's muscular dystrophy have been identified using DNA techniques, resulting in improved testing for carriers and prenatal diagnosis, and providing hope for advances in treatment. Techniques in DNA analysis are being applied to many other diseases, including cystic fibrosis.

Chromosomal Diseases

The most common types of chromosomal disorders include increases (trisomy) or decreases (monosomy) in the normal complement of autosomes or in the sex chromosomes, combining of chromatin material, or damage to, deletion, or duplication of parts of one or more arms of the involved chromosome. Examples include Down syndrome, Klinefelter syndrome, Turner syndrome, and the fragile X syndrome.

Down syndrome (trisomy 21) occurs in 1 of every 1000 newborns and is the most common genetic cause of mental retardation. It is a chromosomal disorder associated with mental deficiency and other minor common dysmorphic characteristics. With appropriate surgical and medical treatment of anatomic (cardiac septal defects), physiologic (anemia), and neoplastic (leukemia) disorders, as well as the provision of adequate educational, vocational, and social opportu-

CHROMOSOMAL ABNORMALITIES 7-2

cause	lesion	manifestations
Defective or missing chromosomes	Gross changes in body structure or sex characteristics	Observable changes in body structure Abnormal chromosomes Mental retardation

nities, the life expectancy and quality of life for persons with Down syndrome have markedly improved.

Klinefelter syndrome occurs in males with one Y and two X chromosomes. It is usually not diagnosed until puberty, when lack of male sexual development, breast enlargement, and chubby appearance may be detected. One in every 1000 males is affected.

Turner syndrome occurs in females with only one X chromosome who fail to show normal female secondary sex development at puberty. They are short in stature with a broad neck. The condition is less common than Klinefelter's syndrome.

Fragile X-syndrome produces mild to moderate mental retardation and is the most common genetic cause of mental retardation in males. A fragile site on an X chromosome is transmitted from generation to generation and can become more unstable with each successive generation. Males have a characteristic phenotype with long facies and enlarged ears in addition to mental retardation. Females show variable degrees of retardation. The diagnosis is made by DNA analysis of the fragile site. Unlike most chromosomal diseases, this condition is familial with a sex-linked recessive pattern of inheritance.

Embryonic Anomalies

Tetralogy of Fallot, agenesis of one kidney, Meckel's diverticulum, and meningomyelocele are representative examples from the four most commonly involved organs.

Tetralogy of Fallot is one of the more common serious anomalies of the heart in which a defect between the two chambers of the heart and misplacement of the aorta allow blood to flow from the right side of the heart to the left side without being oxygenated by the lungs. The infants are often cyanotic (blue) from lack of oxygen in their red blood cells and have a loud heart murmur. The defects can be repaired in some cases.

One kidney may be small (hypoplastic) or missing (agenesis). This only presents a problem if the other kidney becomes diseased and needs to be removed. Otherwise this anomaly may go undetected.

EMBRYONIC ANOMALIES

7-3

causes	lesions	manifestations
Genetic	Abnormalities of size,	Grossly observable
Chromosomal	location, or structure	changes
Environmental	Missing or extra parts	Organ malfunction
Radiation		
Drugs		
Toxic chemicals		
Infection		
Maternal metabolic		
disease		
Unknown		

Meckel's diverticulum is an outpouching of the distal small intestine and is a remnant of an embryonic connection between the intestine and yolk sac. It occurs in 2 percent of the population and is usually harmless.

Meningomyelocele is an outpouching (-*cele*) of meninges (covering of spinal cord) and spinal cord (-*myelo-*) through a defect in the bony structure of lumbar vertebrae. The brainstem often has an associated defect, with the brain being pushed into the foramen magnum (hole at base of skull). Compression of the brainstem may block the flow of cerebrospinal fluid, resulting in hydrocephalus (enlargement of brain and head due to increased fluid in the ventricles of the brain). Surgical repair of the meningomyelocele will prevent secondary infection of the protruding mass but will neither correct the damage done to nerves nor the hydrocephalus.

Fetal Diseases

Examples include erythroblastosis fetalis and congenital infections.

Erythroblastosis fetalis occurs when maternal antibodies destroy fetal red blood cells. In the latter part of pregnancy or at the time of delivery, some Rh+ fetal red blood cells leak across the placenta and enter the maternal circulation. The mother forms antibodies to the Rh factor. This rarely causes any problem with the first pregnancy. With a second or later pregnancy involving an Rh positive fetus, maternal serum antibodies may cross the placenta and destroy the fetal red blood cells. This is called *erythroblastosis fetalis*. The severity varies greatly. The fetus may go into heart failure because of the anemia produced by destruction of red blood cells and be stillborn, or the problem may not develop until after birth, when massive destruction of blood cells may produce jaundice. The bilirubin pigment responsible for the jaundice is a breakdown product of red blood cells. Bilirubin in high concentration can produce brain damage and mental retardation. It is now possible to limit maternal antibody production caused by leakage of fetal red cells at the time of delivery. Gamma globulin containing Rh positive antibodies is given to the mother just after delivery. These antibodies tie up the Rh positive antigen on the fetal cells that have leaked into the maternal circulation, thus preventing the mother's immune system from recognizing them as foreign and producing antibodies to them. If this procedure is followed for each pregnancy involving an Rh negative mother and Rh positive fetus, the incidence of erythroblastosis is reduced.

Syphilis is a disease that may go unrecognized, especially in females, where the primary lesion is hidden in the vagina. The spirochetes (organisms causing syphilis) may circulate in the blood for months without being noticed. During the second half of pregnancy, the spirochetes are capable of crossing the placenta and causing syphilis in the fetus. The severity of the disease in the fetus varies greatly; it may cause death of the fetus and stillbirth or may only be discovered years later as mental retardation or deformity of bones. The disease can be prevented by giving the mother penicillin during the first half of pregnancy. Maternal syphilis is easily diagnosed by testing for antibodies to the spirochetes (serology). For this reason, a serologic test for syphilis is recommended at the time of the first prenatal visit.

Congenital syphilis is rare in the United States because we understand the disease and know how to treat it. Toxoplasmosis and cytomegalovirus infections can be transmitted transplacentally and can cause acute illnesses or destructive brain lesions. Herpes simplex infection can be transmitted during birth and produce a generalized fatal infection.

Heavy alcohol intake, especially during early pregnancy, produces the *fetal alcohol syndrome,* which is characterized by growth retardation, abnormal facial appearance, septal defects in the heart, and mental retardation due to malformation of the brain.

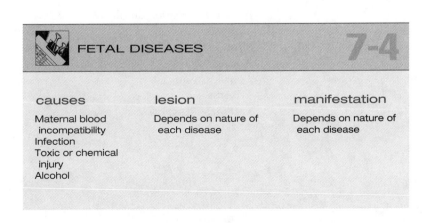

FETAL DISEASES   **7-4**

causes	lesion	manifestation
Maternal blood incompatibility Infection Toxic or chemical injury Alcohol	Depends on nature of each disease	Depends on nature of each disease

Review Questions

1. What are the causes of genetic diseases, chromosomal abnormalities, and congenital anomalies? At what stage of development do these diseases become manifest?

2. What is the value of karyotyping?

3. What are the differences among congenital diseases, familial diseases, and genetic diseases?

4. What are the differences in inheritance patterns among multigene genetic disease, variably expressed inherited disease, and the four types of single-gene inheritance?

5. Approximately what percentage of births are associated with single-gene abnormalities, recognized multigene abnormalities, chromosomal abnormalities, and embryonic anomalies? What is the relative frequency of the various inheritance patterns for single-gene abnormalities? What organs are most frequently involved by embryonic anomalies?

6. What types of diseases are common in the perinatal period, in infancy, and in childhood?

7. How are genetic diseases, chromosomal abnormalities, and embryonic congenital anomalies likely to differ in their appearance? Illustrate these differences by citing specific diseases.

8. What do the following terms mean?
   Deletion
   Duplication
   Inborn error of metabolism
   Monosomy
   Mosaicism
   Nonpenetrant
   Translocation
   Trisomy
   Variable expressivity

MAJOR ORGAN-RELATED DISEASES

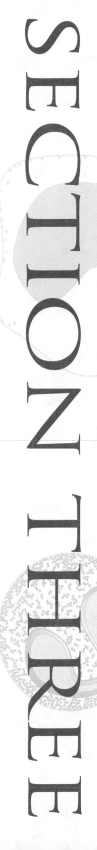

The purpose of this section is to survey the diseases of humans as they cause problems in the various organs. Most diseases present with a problem that can be associated with an organ; most laypersons can tell you the organ that is causing their problem. To deal with these problems, it is necessary to know which are most likely, how they can be diagnosed, and the specific features of the possible diagnoses. With the exception of Chapter 22 (Mental Illness), each chapter is organized for your convenience according to the following format:

- *Review of Structure and Function*
- *Most Frequent and Serious Problems*
- *Symptoms, Signs, and Tests*
- *Specific Diseases*
    Genetic/Developmental Diseases
    Inflammatory/Degenerative Diseases
    Hyperplastic/Neoplastic Diseases
- *Organ Failure*

Degenerative diseases is used here as a nonspecific classification to include all acquired non-neoplastic conditions that are presumably the result of exogenous or endogenous injuries.

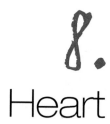

8.
Heart

REVIEW OF STRUCTURE AND FUNCTION
Great Vessels • Chambers • Valves • Blood Flow • Coronary Arteries • Conduction System

MOST FREQUENT AND SERIOUS PROBLEMS
Atherosclerotic Heart Disease • Hypertensive Heart Disease • Valvular Heart Disease • Congenital Heart Disease

SYMPTOMS, SIGNS, AND TESTS
Pain • Angina Pectoris • Congestive Heart Failure • Murmurs • Electrocardiogram • Echocardiogram • Enzymes • Chest X-ray • Cardiac Catheterization • Blood Pressure

SPECIFIC DISEASES
Genetic/Developmental Diseases
Atrial Septal Defect
Ventricular Septal Defect
Tetralogy of Fallot
Coarctation of Aorta
Inflammatory/Degenerative Diseases
Coronary Artery Atherosclerosis
(Arteriosclerotic Heart Disease)
Rheumatic Heart Disease
Infective Endocarditis
Hypertensive Heart Disease
Cor Pulmonale
Hyperplastic/Neoplastic Diseases

ORGAN FAILURE
Cardiogenic Shock • Congestive Heart Failure

REVIEW QUESTIONS

REVIEW OF STRUCTURE AND FUNCTION

The heart functions as two pumps working synchronously to move blood to all sites in the body (Figures 8–1 and 8–2). The right side of the heart receives poorly oxygenated blood from the vena cava and pumps it under relatively low pressure to the lungs where it is oxygenated. The left side of the heart receives the well-oxygenated blood from the pulmonary veins and pumps it at high pressure to all areas of the body. The right heart is less muscular than the left heart due to the lower pressure on the right side and minimal pulmonary vascular resistance. The muscles of each side of the heart are capable of undergoing hypertrophy to pump blood at higher pressure under disease conditions, such as when blood has to be pumped through a narrowed valve. Within each side of the heart, there is a receiving chamber (atrium) and a major pumping chamber (ventricle). Delicate fibrous valves open and close efficiently with a quick snap in response to pressure changes, producing the normal heart sounds. Valves control the inflow of blood in the ventricle and prevent back flow. If the valves fail to close completely, some blood will be pumped by the ventricle back into the atrium during contraction (systole), or blood will flow back into the ventricle from the major artery during relaxation (diastole). In either case, the ventricle would have to pump the blood more than once, with resultant loss of efficiency of the heart. If the valves fail to open completely, more pressure is needed to force the blood through the narrowed valves. To some extent, the heart can gain this needed increase in force by hypertrophy of its muscles. Atrial muscle enlarges when the atrioventricular valves (tricuspid or mitral)

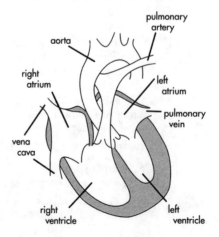

Figure 8–1.   Great vessels and chambers of the heart.

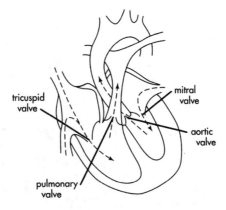

Figure 8–2. Blood flow and valves of the heart.

are narrowed and fail to open completely, and ventricular muscle enlarges when the pulmonary or aortic valves are narrowed and fail to open completely.

Cardiac muscle must have a generous supply of oxygenated blood to provide the fuel for its high energy needs. Blood is supplied to the muscle via two medium-sized arteries, the right and left coronary arteries, which have their origin from the aorta immediately above the aortic valve (Figure 8–3). In addition to the rich blood supply, an electrical pulse is needed to initiate each rhythmical contraction of the heart. This pulse is generated spontaneously within a pacemaker focus called the sinoatrial node and is conducted to the ventricles by the arterioventricular node and specialized bundles (Figure 8–4). The pulse may be disturbed by disease in the area of the node, by metabolic

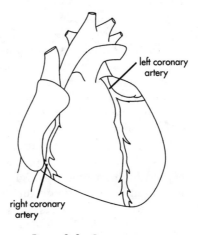

Figure 8–3. Coronary arteries.

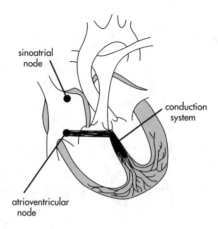

sinoatrial
node

conduction
system

atrioventricular
node

Figure 8–4. Conduction system.

changes in the blood, such as changes in serum potassium level, and by a number of drugs.

MOST FREQUENT AND SERIOUS PROBLEMS

Major diseases of the heart result from ischemic injury to cardiac muscle, damaged heart valves, and increased work load for the pumps produced by altered blood flow or high blood pressure in pulmonary or systemic vascular circuits.

Compromise of the blood supply to the heart (ischemia) caused by narrowing of the main coronary arteries from atherosclerosis is by far the most common cause of death in the United States and thus is the most common cause of cardiac deaths (Figure 8–5). Atherosclerosis leads to cardiac muscle dysfunction through myocardial infarction and/or abnormal heart rhythms (arrhythmias). Coronary atherosclerosis not only is common as a cause of death, it is also common as a cause of disability, which may last for weeks to years prior to death. The major forms of disability are angina pectoris and heart failure.

Hypertensive heart disease, the second most common heart problem, is underestimated in the mortality figures, because it often occurs in conjunction with coronary atherosclerotic heart disease. Hypertensive heart disease is not a primary disease of the heart, but rather it is caused by high blood pressure in the systemic arteries causing an increased work load for the heart. Congenital heart disease and rheumatic endocarditis are less common, but are particularly important as causes of valve deformity. Many types of congenital heart disease also produce abnormalities in the pathway of blood flow leading

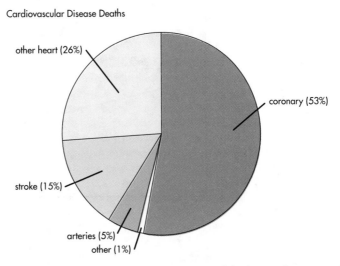

Cardiovascular Disease Deaths

other heart (26%)

coronary (53%)

stroke (15%)

arteries (5%)

other (1%)

Figure 8–5. Cardiovascular diseases, percent as cause of death. (Data from National Institutes of Health, 1990.)

to poor oxygenation of blood and increased work load on the heart. Chronic lung disease can cause hypertension in the pulmonary arteries and lead to heart failure. Heart failure secondary to lung disease is called *cor pulmonale*. The frequency of cor pulmonale as a cause of death is not known, because these patients are usually recorded as having died from lung disease.

Most persons succumbing to congenital heart disease die in the first year of life (Figure 8–6). Those that survive have less severe anomalies or undergo surgical correction of their defect and have variable survival times extending to old age. Rheumatic and hypertensive heart diseases have a prolonged course, so that most deaths occur in older people. Atherosclerotic heart disease has a shorter course, and the mortality rate rises rapidly after age 30 and continues to increase at all older age levels (Figure 8–6).

Sudden death resulting from heart disease is most often associated with one of several complications of coronary atherosclerosis but may also be associated with other types of heart disease. Sudden death due to a "heart attack" generally is the result of ventricular fibrillation, probably due to a sudden episode of myocardial ischemia. Ventricular fibrillation is an uncoordinated, ineffective, weak contraction of ventricular muscle due to spontaneous generation of impulses within the muscle rather than coordinated electrical stimulation through the conduction system. Overdosage with certain cardiac drugs may also produce ventricular fibrillation. Rupture of the heart is not common but does produce sudden death, because the pericardial sac fills with

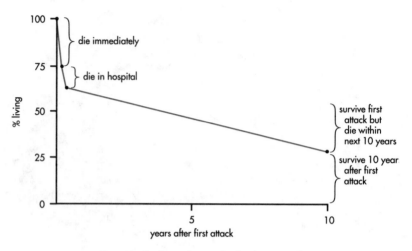

Figure 8–6. Survival time after first heart attack.

blood and prevents adequate pumping of blood out of the heart. Rupture may be due to the softening of a large myocardial infarct or trauma (car accident, stabbing, gunshot wound). Marked narrowing of the aortic valve (aortic stenosis) also is associated with sudden death. Many deaths are due to congestive heart failure (pump failure), irrespective of underlying cause, when the heart cannot pump blood out efficiently. The resulting congestion in the lungs prevents oxygenation of the blood. Primary failure of the heart muscle (*cardiomyopathy*) also results in congestive failure and is a reason for heart transplant, especially in younger patients.

SYMPTOMS, SIGNS, AND TESTS

Sudden severe pain is a symptom of many but not all myocardial infarcts. The pain of myocardial infarction is persistent and may be a squeezing chest pain or may be pain referred to the shoulder, arm, neck, or jaw. The term *angina pectoris* refers to transient chest pain brought on by exercise or emotional stress and relieved by rest or vasodilator drugs. Angina pectoris is due to transient hypoxia to the heart with spasm of atherosclerotic coronary arteries. Congestive heart failure is a cluster of symptoms, signs, and laboratory measurements that indicates inadequate pumping of the heart relative to the demands of the peripheral tissues. The resultant buildup of pressure in the pulmonary or systemic veins leads to venous distention and edema.

Important aspects of physical examination, which relate to possible heart disease, include listening for murmurs, estimating heart size, measuring blood pressure, and checking for signs of heart failure. Heart murmurs are abnormal sounds of the heart usually heard with the aid of a stethoscope. The process of listening through a stethoscope is called *auscultation*. Murmurs are caused by abnormal flow of blood through the heart valves or major vessels. A heart murmur may be functionally unimportant or may indicate serious underlying disease.

Arterial blood pressure is usually referred to simply as the *blood pressure* and is measured using a sphygmomanometer. A sphygmomanometer is a cuff with an attached pressure gauge that can be applied to an extremity and inflated above arterial pressure. By listening over an artery distal to the cuff, one can hear the pulse when the pressure drops below the systolic pressure. The pulse sound disappears when the blood pressure drops below the diastolic pressure.

Venous blood pressure, which is used as an indicator of congestive heart failure, is estimated on physical examination by the degree of distention of neck veins and, when necessary, is measured accurately through a catheter placed intravenously. The manifestations of heart failure are discussed at the end of this chapter in the section on Organ Failure.

Procedures and laboratory tests used in the evaluation of heart disease include chest x-ray, electrocardiogram (ECG), echocardiogram, serum enzyme levels, and cardiac catheterization. Chest x-ray is used to evaluate the size and shape of the heart. Enlargement of the heart usually reflects muscle hypertrophy or dilatation of the chambers.

Electrocardiography is carried out by the placement of a series of electrodes at various standard locations on the body surface. From electrical activity at these sites, the electrical activity of the heart can be inferred. ECG is most often used in the diagnosis of myocardial infarcts, either recent or old. Results may be normal, nonspecific, or relatively specific and usually require interpretation by an experienced physician. ECG is also used to define rhythm disturbances (arrythmias) and to monitor the course of a disease or the effect of therapy. An ECG taken after exercise is used to detect evidence of ischemia due to atherosclerotic narrowing of the coronary arteries.

Echocardiography provides an image of the heart based on ultrasound waves which are reflected at tissue interphases. This allows for assessment of size and function of various aspects of the heart and also depicts abnormal structures.

Enzymes released from dying muscle can be measured in the blood and are helpful in determining if and when an acute myocardial infarct has occurred. Creatinine phosphokinase (CK), aspartate aminotransferase (AST), and lactic dehydrogenase (LDH) have peak elevations at different times following onset of a myocardial infarct

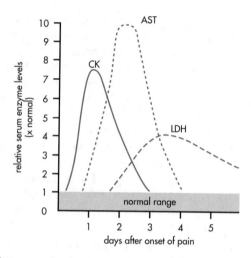

Figure 8–7. Patterns of serum enzyme elevations following a myocardial infarct.

(Figure 8–7). Cardiac troponins and myoglobin may also be useful markers for early diagnosis of myocardial injury.

Cardiac catheterization is used for more extensive evaluation of serious cardiac problems. Catheters are tubes that can be threaded into the vessels and heart to measure pressure and to allow injection of radiopaque dyes. X-rays taken following injection of radiopaque dyes into the vascular system are called *angiograms.* Abnormalities in the rate and route of blood flow in various parts of the heart and great vessels can be detected through cardiac catheterization. The angiograms taken during catheterization reveal the anatomy of the heart chambers and blood vessels. Radiopaque dyes can even be injected directly into the coronary arteries to outline atherosclerotic plaques. Newer, non-invasive techniques for evaluating heart disease include echocardiography, which utilizes ultrasound to define anatomic structures, and radioisotope techniques, which are used to evaluate the rate of flow in the ventricles and coronary arteries.

SPECIFIC DISEASES

Genetic/Developmental Diseases

Developmental abnormalities of the heart are almost all embryonic anomalies, which collectively are called *congenital heart disease.* Of all the organs, the heart and great vessels are the most common sites of congenital defects, and the defects are likely to have serious conse-

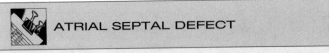

cause	lesion	manifestations
Embryonic anomaly	Hole in the septum between right and left atria	Murmur Heart failure (late)

ATRIAL SEPTAL DEFECT

8-1

quences. Early diagnosis and surgical correction of the defect alter the life expectancy in many cases. Ventricular septal defects account for 30 percent of congenital heart diseases. The variety of other types each comprise less than 10 percent. A few classic types are briefly presented below to illustrate the variety of blood flow disturbances of congenital disease of the heart and great vessels.

Atrial Septal Defect

During the fetal period, there is a hole (called *foramen ovale*) in the septum between the right and left atria that usually closes shortly after birth. If this septal defect remains open and is large (Figure 8–8), blood may flow from the left atrium to the right atrium causing increased work load on the right side of the heart.

Ventricular Septal Defect

A hole in the interventricular septum (Figure 8–9) is more serious than an atrial septal defect, because there is a greater pressure difference between the two ventricles than between the two atria. Some

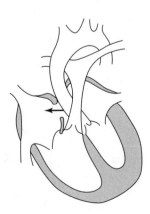

Figure 8–8. Atrial septal defect.

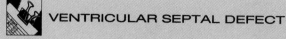

cause	lesion	manifestations
Embryonic anomaly	Hole in the septum between right and left ventricles	Murmur Heart failure

blood flows from the left ventricle (high pressure) to the right ventricle (low pressure), forcing both ventricles to pump the same blood more than once. Over a number of years, the added work load will lead to left and/or right heart failure.

Tetralogy of Fallot

This is the most common cause of cyanotic congenital heart disease. *Cyanosis* refers to the blue color of the skin caused by poor oxygenation of blood. In cyanotic heart disease, the poor oxygenation is caused by shunting of blood from the right heart to the systemic circulation, so that some blood fails to reach the lung to receive oxygen. The four changes of tetralogy (Figure 8–10) are (1) shift in position of the aorta so that both ventricles empty into the aorta, (2) a stenosis (narrowing) of the pulmonary outflow tract, (3) a ventricular septal defect allowing the blood that cannot get through the pulmonary valve to pass into the systemic circulation, and (4) right ventricular hypertrophy caused by the increased force required of the right ventricle. Because only a fraction of the blood will be oxygenated, the

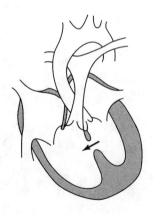

Figure 8–9. Ventricular septal defect.

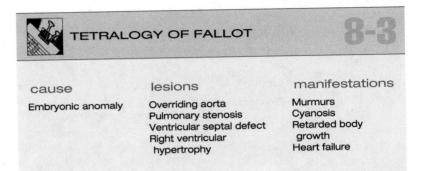

TETRALOGY OF FALLOT   **8-3**

cause	lesions	manifestations

Embryonic anomaly	Overriding aorta
	Pulmonary stenosis
	Ventricular septal defect
	Right ventricular
	  hypertrophy
		Murmurs
		Cyanosis
		Retarded body
		  growth
		Heart failure

child usually will be cyanotic. Life expectancy is variable, depending on the severity of the defects. Surgical correction of the abnormalities may allow prolonged survival.

Coarctation of Aorta

Coarctation is a narrow fibrous constriction in the descending thoracic aorta (Figure 8–11). Proximal to the coarctation the blood pressure is usually elevated, and distal to the coarctation it is decreased. Diminution of the femoral artery pulse in a child may lead one to suspect the presence of this defect, and a marked difference in blood pressure in the arm versus the leg strengthens the suspicion. Surgical correction usually is curative if the disease is diagnosed early. The disease may easily go undetected, however, and, if so, the high blood

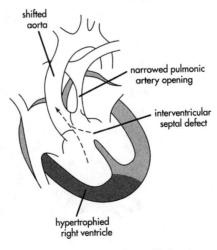

shifted aorta

narrowed pulmonic artery opening

interventricular septal defect

hypertrophied right ventricle

Figure 8–10. Tetralogy of Fallot.

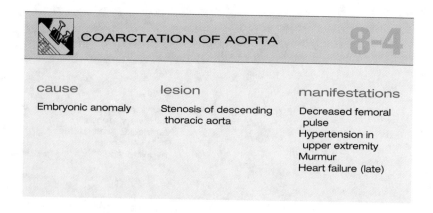

COARCTATION OF AORTA   8-4

cause	lesion	manifestations
Embryonic anomaly	Stenosis of descending thoracic aorta	Decreased femoral pulse Hypertension in upper extremity Murmur Heart failure (late)

pressure proximal to the coarctation eventually leads to left ventricular hypertrophy and heart failure.

Inflammatory/Degenerative Diseases

Degenerative and inflammatory diseases of the heart are the most important group of diseases in the United States. They are of diverse causes, but the outcome is similar in that they cripple this vital organ. Hypertensive heart disease is not really a primary heart disease but is discussed here because of its importance and similarity to other heart disease. See Chapter 9 for further discussion of hypertension.

Coronary Artery Atherosclerosis (Arteriosclerotic Heart Disease)

The intimal plaques that build up with age in the right and left coronary arteries produce the most significant disease in the United States.

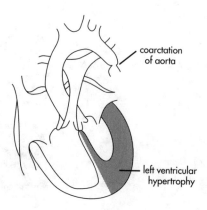

Figure 8–11. Coarctation of aorta.

The etiology and epidemiology of atherosclerosis are discussed in Chapter 9.

We are concerned here with how these small plaques may kill or cripple an individual. Simplistically, we can say that the plaques narrow the lumens of the coronary arteries, thus reducing blood flow to heart muscle and to the conduction system of the heart (Figure 8–12). In practice, the correlation between the number and size of plaques and significant damage to the heart is not so simple, because the patterns of circulation vary considerably depending on anastomoses (connections) between right and left coronary arteries. For example, a single strategically placed plaque may kill one person at a young age, whereas on rare occasions another person may gradually develop complete occlusion of both coronary arteries and survive to old age. Increased vascularization of the myocardium due to development of anastomoses occurs with recovery from a myocardial infarct and with aging.

Symptoms of inadequate blood flow in the coronary arteries may be acute, chronic, or both. In either case, the coronary arteries have one or more areas of significant narrowing by atherosclerotic plaque.

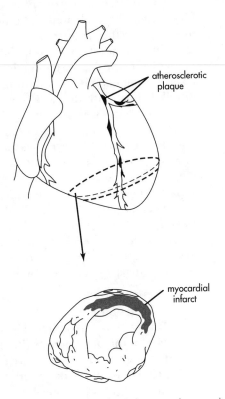

atherosclerotic plaque

myocardial infarct

Figure 8–12. Coronary artery atherosclerosis and myocardial infarct.

An area of marginally adequate blood flow may suddenly become inadequate when there is an increased need for oxygen by the myocardium due to exercise or emotional stress or when the artery is blocked due to thrombosis (formation of blood clot), vasoconstriction (spasm), or a dissection of blood into the plaque (plaque hemorrhage) with resultant pushing of the plaque into the lumen of the coronary artery. The roles of thrombosis in coronary artery obstruction has been debated; currently, it is thought to be an important factor in many cases even though it is not always present at autopsy in fatal cases.

The results of sudden insufficiency of coronary artery blood flow are arrhythmia, infarct, or both. Persons who die suddenly of "heart attacks" have an arrhythmia with a failure of the electrical impulse that times the pump; persons who survive the attack usually develop a myocardial infarct. Arrhythmias are usually reversible, so emergency resuscitation is practical; infarcts can heal.

Chronic insufficiency of coronary artery blood flow causes pain accentuated by exertion (angina pectoris) because of the relative ischemia produced by the increased need of the myocardium for oxygen. Vasodilator drugs usually relieve the pain.

The degree of coronary artery obstruction by atherosclerotic plaque may be evaluated directly and indirectly. Radiopaque dyes injected into the coronary arteries to produce arteriograms are used to evaluate areas of obstruction; however, they are not always accurate in predicting the degree of functional obstruction. Electrocardiograms taken during exercise may demonstrate electrical changes associated with ischemia. With the development of techniques for bypassing the coronary arteries with vein grafts, the evaluation of the degree of coronary atherosclerosis has become more important. Current evidence, however, suggests that bypass is most useful with severe angina and in some patients in the early stage of infarction. It should be noted that the viewing of collapsed atherosclerotic arteries at autopsy is not a very accurate measure of their functional state during life.

When an area of myocardium dies, the lesion is called a *myocardial infarct* and the process is called *myocardial infarction*. The major site of involvement is the left ventricle, although some infarcts extend into the right ventricle. Once an area of muscle is killed by lack of oxygen, the following sequence of changes occurs:

1. For 12 to 18 hours, the heart appears normal both grossly and microscopically.
2. During days 1 to 5, there is progressive softening and disintegration of the dead muscle fibers and an inflammatory reaction at the edge of the necrotic area.
3. Healing begins at day 5 with the ingrowth of fibroblasts and capillaries (granulation tissue), which replace the dead muscle and form collagen.

4. By 2 weeks, sufficient collagen has been laid down to give new strength to the softened area, and the collagen continues to accumulate and contract for weeks to months. The end result is a dense tough scar not unlike that which can occur in the skin following a cut.

Complications can develop at any stage of the process of myocardial infarction. Arrhythmias, such as ventricular fibrillation, may occur. Ventricular fibrillation produces sudden death except in some cases where medical care is immediately available. Artificial maintenance of heart contraction and breathing (cardiopulmonary resuscitation) may be successful. Another possible complication is heart failure due to loss of function of a large area of myocardium. Heart failure may cause venous congestion in the lungs with seepage of fluid into the pulmonary air spaces (pulmonary edema). When more severe, there may be an inability to maintain the arterial blood pressure (cardiogenic shock). Heart failure in the first few days after a myocardial infarct is more common in persons whose heart has been weakened by previous myocardial infarcts.

Following a myocardial infarct, the area of damage may extend due to further inadequacy of the blood supply. A major reason for requiring bed rest is to prevent intolerable demand on the heart through exercise. Extension of the infarct may tip the patient into heart failure or cause a fatal arrhythmia. If sufficient muscle is lost, by single or multiple infarcts, the remaining muscle hypertrophies in response to the increased demand placed on it. Thus, myocardial infarcts are one cause of cardiac enlargement. Myocardial hypertrophy is a reflection of the heart's inadequacy to function normally, and eventually this will be expressed by heart failure. Hypertrophy is a late complication of myocardial infarct, because it requires time to develop.

Three less common complications of large infarcts are rupture, ventricular aneurysm, and endocardial thrombus formation. Myocardial rupture occurs when blood dissects through necrotic myocardium into the pericardial space with resultant compression of the heart and sudden death. Rupture occurs at the time of maximum softening (about 5 to 7 days) of a large infarct. Aneurysms are sac-like outpouchings of the heart or vessels. A ventricular aneurysm is an outward bulging of the scar of a large, healed left ventricular infarct. The aneurysm tends to make the left ventricle an ineffective pump because the blood is not effectively moved out of the aneurysm. Mural thrombosis is the formation of a thrombus over the inner endocardial wall of an infarct. Sometimes material breaks loose from a mural thrombus, producing free-floating material in the systemic arterial circulation (arterial emboli) that can lodge at distant sites producing infarcts. Brain, intestines, and extremities are most commonly affected. For example, a patient recovering from a myocardial infarct may suddenly

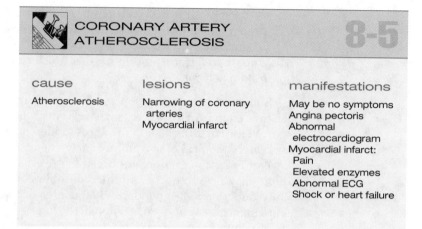

CORONARY ARTERY ATHEROSCLEROSIS 8-5

cause	lesions	manifestations

Atherosclerosis	Narrowing of coronary arteries
	Myocardial infarct
		May be no symptoms
		Angina pectoris
		Abnormal electrocardiogram
		Myocardial infarct:
		  Pain
		  Elevated enzymes
		  Abnormal ECG
		  Shock or heart failure

develop a stroke because thrombotic material has embolized from the heart to cerebral vessels causing an infarct of the brain. Because myocardial infarcts may be caused by coronary artery thromboses and they may also result in mural thrombosis, pharmaceutical agents that lyse thrombi are often prescribed.

Symptoms and signs of myocardial infarcts are quite variable. Most patients have no symptoms prior to their first myocardial infarct, although a few may experience angina pectoris. Angina pectoris is more frequent in persons who have had one or more previous myocardial infarcts and have a marginally adequate blood supply to the heart. Although pain is the major symptom of myocardial infarction, infarcts may be asymptomatic and heal without the patient being aware of them. Thus, some patients may first present with heart failure due to advanced disease.

Rheumatic Heart Disease

Rheumatic fever is a hypersensitivity disorder occurring in a small percentage of persons following a streptococcal infection, usually pharyngitis. Apparently, the protein of group A hemolytic streptococci is similar to the proteins in the heart and other connective tissues of these susceptible individuals, so that the antibodies that develop against the streptococci, not only attack the bacteria but also the host tissue (especially the heart and joints). The inflammatory reaction produced by this hypersensitivity is usually mild or asymptomatic but may produce a full-blown illness called *rheumatic fever* characterized by myocarditis and arthritis. The illness is not usually serious in the acute stages and may gradually resolve without apparent residual effects. The sequelae of one or more episodes of rheumatic fever cause inflammation of the heart valves (valvulitis) rather than the myocardium and lead to scarring and deformity of the valves (Figure 8–13).

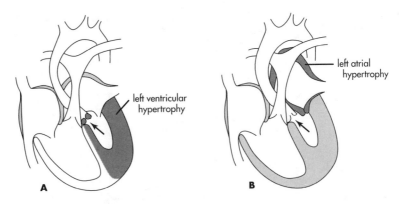

Figure 8–13. A. Aortic stenosis. B. Mitral stenosis.

At variable times following a known or presumed acute illness, chronic damage to heart valves may become evident. The functional valve damage is produced by narrowing of valve opening (stenosis) and/or failure of the valve to close completely (valvular insufficiency). Fibrosis of the mitral valve, the valve most commonly involved, usually leads to left heart failure. The left heart failure is due either to backup of blood into the lungs caused by stenosis or to regurgitation of blood back through the insufficient valve. Stenosis and insufficiency of the aortic valve, the other commonly affected valve, cause left ventricular hypertrophy and eventually heart failure. Surgical replacement of damaged valves may prolong life.

In addition to heart failure, the valves may become secondarily infected, producing infective endocarditis (discussion follows). Thus, rheumatic fever itself is less serious than its potential sequelae, rheumatic valvulitis and infective endocarditis. The pathogenesis of rheumatic heart disease is summarized in Table 8-1.

To prevent the long chain of events of rheumatic heart disease, pharyngitis caused by group A hemolytic streptococci should be treated with antibiotics to minimize the development of antibodies to

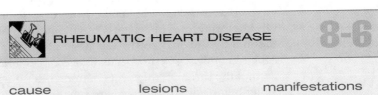

RHEUMATIC HEART DISEASE 8-6

cause	lesions	manifestations
Hypersensitivity reaction to antigen of group A hemolytic streptococci	Diffuse myocarditis (early) Fibrous thickening of heart valves (late)	Fever, arthritis, cardiac abnormalities (early) Murmur, heart failure (late)

TABLE 8–1. PATHOGENESIS OF RHEUMATIC HEART DISEASE

Sequence of Steps	Causes	Lesions	Manifestations
Ordinary strep throat	Throat infection due to group A streptococcus	Pharyngitis	Sore throat
Rheumatic fever	Antibodies to group A streptococcus cross-react with human tissues	Carditis, arthritis	Fever, joint pains, murmurs, may be no symptoms
Recurrent rheumatic carditis	Further throat infections with group A streptococci	Recurrent carditis	Usually none
Latent rheumatic valvulitis	Long latent period (years), presumed continuation of previous injury	Scarring of heart valves	Murmurs, heart failure (late)
Rheumatic valvulitis complicated by subacute bacterial endocarditis	Transient bacteremia with organisms normally present in mouth (usually alpha hemolytic streptococci)	Infective endocarditis	Fever, leukocytosis, bacteremia, emboli, heart failure

the streptococcal antigen. Accurate diagnosis of group A hemolytic streptococci by culture and prolonged treatment (10 days) is effective in preventing rheumatic fever.

Infective Endocarditis

Infective endocarditis, in contrast to rheumatic valvulitis, is caused by organisms living on the heart valves and producing an inflammatory reaction. Bacteria are the most common cause, hence the name *bacterial endocarditis*. Most cases occur on previously damaged valves, most often caused by rheumatic heart disease but also by congenital valve deformities. The bacteria often enter the bloodstream through the mouth and stick to the damaged valve to initiate the infection. Alpha hemolytic streptococcus (*Streptococcus viridans*), a normal resident of the throat, is the most common offending organism. Because alpha hemolytic streptococci are very weak pathogens, they produce a smoldering infection on the heart valve (subacute bacterial endocarditis), which gradually destroys the valve and leads to death either by heart failure or by damage from emboli dislodged from the valve. In contrast, when a more virulent organism such as *Staphylococcus aureus* lodges on a heart valve, an acute infection (acute bacterial endocarditis) ensues, and organisms dislodged from the valve travel to other organs producing multiple abscesses and rapid death.

Many cases of infective endocarditis can be prevented by preventing rheumatic fever, because rheumatic valvulitis is the most common predisposing factor to the development of infective endocarditis. Those persons who already have damaged heart valves can be protected from the bacteremia resulting from manipulative procedures, such as dental extractions, by antibiotics. Once developed, early diagnosis of infective endocarditis may result in treatment that will reduce the amount of damage, but overall the disease is very serious.

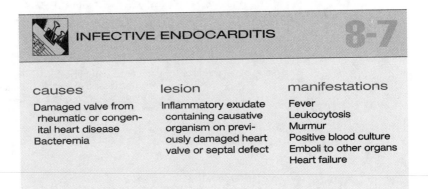

INFECTIVE ENDOCARDITIS   8-7

causes	lesion	manifestations
Damaged valve from rheumatic or congenital heart disease Bacteremia	Inflammatory exudate containing causative organism on previously damaged heart valve or septal defect	Fever Leukocytosis Murmur Positive blood culture Emboli to other organs Heart failure

Hypertensive Heart Disease

High blood pressure (hypertension) will lead to an increased work load on the heart, which leads to cardiac hypertrophy and eventually heart failure (Figure 8–14). Hypertension also accelerates the development

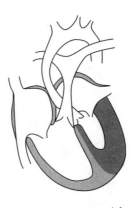

Figure 8–14. Effect of systemic hypertension—left ventricular hypertrophy.

of atherosclerotic plaques, so it is often combined with coronary atherosclerotic heart disease. Hypertension within the systemic arterial blood circuit is quite common and increases in frequency with age. It is usually of unknown cause, hence the name *idiopathic* or *essential hypertension*. However, every patient should be medically evaluated for causes that are curable, such as coarctation of aorta, narrowing of renal artery, which leads to increased release of hormones causing hypertension, or tumors of the adrenal gland, which secrete hormones that elevate blood pressure.

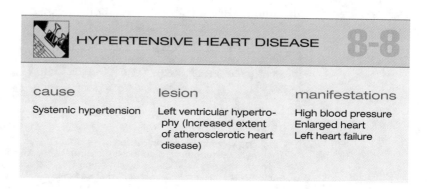

HYPERTENSIVE HEART DISEASE 8-8

cause	lesion	manifestations
Systemic hypertension	Left ventricular hypertrophy (Increased extent of atherosclerotic heart disease)	High blood pressure Enlarged heart Left heart failure

Cor Pulmonale

Hypertension can also occur in the pulmonary arterial system due to long-standing diffuse pulmonary disease or failure of the left heart. Pulmonary hypertension with right heart failure caused by chronic lung disease is called *cor pulmonale*. Pulmonary hypertension leads to right ventricular hypertrophy and eventually to right heart failure (Figure 8–15).

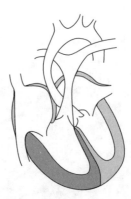

Figure 8–15. Effect of pulmonary hypertension—right ventricular hypertrophy.

Hyperplastic/Neoplastic Diseases

Hypertrophy has already been discussed. All neoplasms of heart, whether benign, malignant, or metastatic, are rare.

ORGAN FAILURE

Inadequacy of cardiac pumping action may take two forms—cardiogenic shock and congestive heart failure. Shock is inadequate perfusion of tissues with oxygen due to low blood pressure. Congestion is distention of veins due to increased pressure within the veins. Shock, whether due to heart damage or other conditions such as blood loss, is a serious acute condition. If blood pressure is not restored quickly, the patient will die. Congestion, on the other hand, usually develops gradually and is less life threatening.

Cardiogenic shock is usually the result of extensive myocardial infarction and rapidly leads to death in the majority of patients. Drugs given to constrict the vascular bed and improve the force of contraction of the heart are sometimes effective in controlling the shock.

Congestive heart failure means the inability of the heart to pump enough blood to meet the demands of peripheral tissue. When this occurs, there is increased pressure in the pulmonary or systemic veins, or both, resulting in "backing up" of blood with consequent transudation of fluid into the pulmonary alveoli and tissues supplied by the systemic circulation. Congestive heart failure, like cardiogenic shock, is most commonly a sequela of myocardial infarcts but also occurs in the later stages of other forms of heart disease.

Congestive heart failure is divided into left and right heart failure, although both commonly occur together. Left heart failure involves increased venous pressure from the left side of the heart into the lungs and is usually manifest by shortness of breath (dyspnea) due to transudation of fluid into pulmonary alveoli (pulmonary edema). Right heart failure causes enlargement of the liver and spleen (hepatosplenomegaly) due to congestion; edema, particularly noticeable in the ankles because of their dependent position; and distention of neck veins due to increased venous pressure (Figure 8–16). Left heart failure may lead to right heart failure because increased pressure is transmitted through the pulmonary circuit to the right heart.

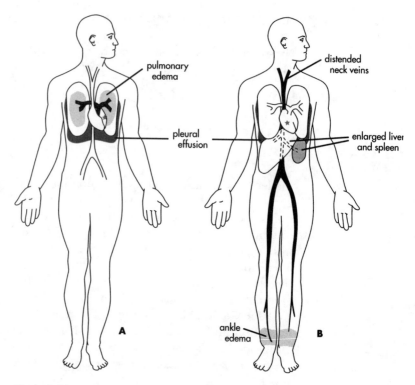

Figure 8–16. A. Left-sided congestive heart failure. B. Right-sided congestive heart failure.

Severe chronic heart disease is often expressed as congestive heart failure. The severity and duration of heart failure varies. At its worst, it leads to death. In its mild forms, it may be controllable for many years with rest and drugs, such as digitalis, which improve myocardial contractal force, and diuretics, which promote renal excretion of edema fluid.

Review Questions

1. What are the major causes of heart disease? What is the relative frequency of each type?
2. What is the pathogenesis of three causes of sudden death from heart disease?
3. How are each of the following tests or procedures helpful in evaluation of a patient with heart disease?
   - Blood pressure
   - Electrocardiogram
   - Serum enzyme levels
   - Chest x-ray
   - Cardiac catheterization
4. What are the causes, lesions, and major manifestations of each of the specific heart diseases discussed in the chapter?
5. What are the steps involved in the evolution of a myocardial infarct?
6. What is the pathogenesis of the various complications of myocardial infarcts?
7. What is the pathogenesis of each stage of rheumatic heart disease and its complications?
8. Which two types of heart disease predispose to infective endocarditis? What are the consequences of infective endocarditis?
9. How is hypertension related to atherosclerosis?
10. How do cardiogenic shock and congestive heart failure differ in terms of acuteness, seriousness, cause, and manifestations?
11. What do the following terms mean?
    - Ventricular fibrillation
    - Cardiac arrhythmia
    - Angina pectoris
    - Heart murmur
    - Myocardial infarct
    - Ventricular aneurysm
    - Mural thrombosis
    - Rheumatic fever
    - Rheumatic valvulitis
    - Cardiogenic shock
    - Congestive heart failure

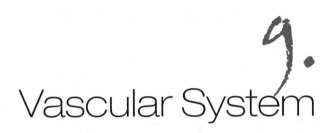

Vascular System

REVIEW OF STRUCTURE AND FUNCTION
Blood Vascular System • Arteries • Veins • Capillaries • Sinusoids • Lymphatic Vascular System

MOST FREQUENT AND SERIOUS PROBLEMS
Atherosclerosis • Thrombi and Emboli • Varicosities • Hypertension

SYMPTOMS, SIGNS, AND TESTS
Infarcts • Ischemic Atrophy • Angiography • Hypertension • Elevated Venous Pressure • Funduscopic Examination

SPECIFIC DISEASES
Genetic/Developmental Diseases
  Angiomas
Inflammatory/Degenerative Diseases
  Atherosclerosis
  Hypertension
  Vasculitis
  Functional Vascular Disease
  Thrombophlebitis
  Varicose Veins
Hyperplastic/Neoplastic Diseases

ORGAN FAILURE
Shock • Congestion • Edema • Elephantiasis

REVIEW QUESTIONS

REVIEW OF STRUCTURE AND FUNCTION

The vascular system actually comprises two systems—the blood vascular system and the lymphatic vascular system. The blood vascular system is a continuous-flow system transporting blood to and from the heart via arteries, capillaries, and veins. Because the blood does not directly surround tissue cells, the vascular system must allow for exchange of gases, nutrients, and metabolic wastes across its walls. This exchange takes place primarily in the smallest component of the blood vascular system, the capillaries and small venules where blood flow is slowest and where the walls are the thinnest.

The arteries and veins have three concentric layers—intima, media, and adventitia (Figure 9–1). The intima is lined by broad flat endothelial cells with an underlying basement membrane and a few connective tissue cells for support. The endothelial cells in the smaller vessels control the exchange between blood and tissue. The media is composed of elastic tissue and smooth muscle. Either sympathetic stimulation or circulating adrenergic hormones can produce contraction of the muscle layer, which decreases the caliber of vessels. Cholinergic hormones and, in some vessels, parasympathetic stimulation cause vasodilation. The adventitia is composed of supporting connective tissue cells.

The arterial side of the vascular system has intraluminal pressures of about 100 mm Hg throughout most of its length. In accordance with this high pressure, arteries are thick-walled muscular structures. Major determinants of pressure are the amount of blood flowing through the vessels and the resistance of the vessels to this flow. Therefore, either an increased amount of blood or decreased vessel caliber due to contraction will elevate the blood pressure. Normally, pressure is controlled mainly by the degree of dilatation or constriction of arteries and arterioles (very small arteries). The amount of blood flow is a function of the rate of contraction of the heart and the volume of blood pumped with each contraction.

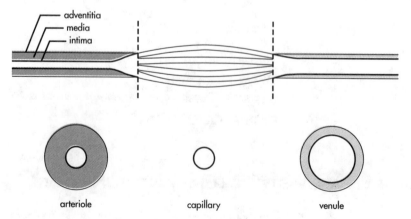

Figure 9–1. Comparison of arterioles, capillaries, and venules.

The venous side of the vascular system has a mean pressure of less than 30 mm Hg. Accordingly, veins have thinner muscular walls than arteries and larger lumens to carry blood at a slower rate under less pressure. The function of veins is to return blood to the heart from the tissue capillary beds. The force that pushes blood in the veins back to the heart is the pressure that is left after the passage of blood through arteries, arterioles, and capillaries. This force is only adequate to return blood to the heart when the body is in a horizontal position. Unless compensated for, blood in the head and upper parts of the body would gravitate to the abdomen and lower extremities in a person standing upright. Among the compensatory mechanisms to prevent this are venomotor reflexes that constrict the lower body veins, the massaging action of skeletal muscles, and action of respiratory movements on the great veins in the chest. In addition, veins contain valves, which aid in the vertical flow of blood against gravity.

Obstruction of blood flow in veins by such mechanisms as compression, thrombosis, or heart failure elevates venous and capillary blood pressures, causing accumulation of blood in these highly distensible structures. Distention of veins and capillaries due to increased venous pressure is called *congestion.* Continued congestion results in leakage of fluids through capillary endothelium into tissues. This accumulation of fluid is called *edema,* and it results in a disturbance of tissue–capillary exchange of oxygen, nutrients, and metabolites.

The portal vein is an exceptional vein that collects blood from most of the intestinal tract and spleen and carries it to the liver, where nutrients and metabolic products are removed before it is returned to the heart via the hepatic vein.

The capillaries are small vessels that connect arteries and veins and are essentially composed of an intimal layer. Capillaries comprise by far the largest volume of the vascular system, although most are in a state of collapse at any given time. Capillaries are extremely adaptable in being able to open in response to increased blood flow needs and in being able to proliferate to help repair an injured area. Capillary flow is controlled by contraction or relaxation of small arteries (arterioles) and possibly by small veins (venules).

In some organs, such as liver, spleen, adrenal gland, and pituitary gland, the capillaries take the form of sinusoids. Sinusoids are dilated capillaries that are more continuously open to blood flow than ordinary capillaries. Sinusoids are associated with specialized functions, such as filtering out particulate matter, including damaged blood cells in the liver and spleen, and hormone regulation in the adrenal and pituitary glands. The most structurally complex capillaries are found in the renal glomerulus, where filtration of waste products into the urine is the specialized function.

The lymph vascular system (lymphatic system) is unique in that it has no vessels flowing into the system. Lymphatic vessels originate as blind-ended, thin-walled channels that extend to lymph nodes and beyond, becoming larger, and eventually emptying into the thoracic duct. The thoracic duct flows into the superior vena cava, thus emptying lymph into the venous blood. To a lesser extent, lymphatic vessels may empty into other veins. Lymphatic vessels function as a low-pressure drainage system, much like the tiles draining a farmer's field, as they return some of the excess tissue fluid back into the venous system. Also, lymphocytes may reenter the circulation from tissue via this route.

MOST FREQUENT AND SERIOUS PROBLEMS

Atherosclerosis is a disease characterized by lipid, calcium, and fibrous deposits in the intima of large- and medium-sized arteries and is by far the most significant disease in the United States in terms of death and morbidity. We have already described its effects on the heart, which account for the most common cause of death. The arteries to the brain are the second most important site of atherosclerosis. Cerebral infarcts resulting from atherosclerosis of cerebral vessels are the third most common cause of death in the United States. Atherosclerosis of the arteries of the legs and of the main artery to the intestines (superior mesenteric artery) less commonly leads to arterial obstruction and infarction, but when it occurs, the effects are quite serious.

The formation of thrombi (blood clots formed within vessels) in the deep veins of the legs is a relatively common and sometimes serious problem that occurs particularly in bedridden patients. The most important complication of thrombi occurs when they break away from the vessel wall to form emboli. The emboli are then carried through the veins to the right side of the heart, where they are pumped into the branches of the pulmonary arteries, producing obstruction of blood flow to portions of the lungs.

Varicosities are permanently dilated venous channels. They most commonly occur in the legs (varicose veins) and about the anus (hemorrhoids). Varicose veins may cause discomfort, disfigurement, edema, ulceration of the lower extremities, and predispose to the formation of thrombi. Hemorrhoids may be asymptomatic or may cause itching, pain on defecation, bright red bleeding, or sudden severe pain if thrombosis occurs.

High blood pressure (hypertension) is one of the most important conditions for the health care team to understand, because its recognition and treatment can prevent or delay complications for a large number of people. Most cases of hypertension are idiopathic (called *essential hypertension*). The effects of hypertension have a latent period of many years and take the form of accelerated atherosclerosis leading to myocardial and cerebral infarcts, heart failure, cerebral hemorrhage, and occasionally renal failure.

SYMPTOMS, SIGNS, AND TESTS

The manifestations of arterial obstruction due to atherosclerosis, inflammation, thrombosis, embolism, or external compression are either infarcts or more gradual loss of tissue due to insufficient blood supply (ischemic atrophy). Either infarcts or ischemic atrophy will result in loss of function in the organs supplied by the affected vessel. Pain may also occur.

The integrity of arteries can be directly evaluated by arteriography, a procedure in which radiopaque dye is injected into arteries and successive x-ray films are taken to show the caliber of the vessels and distribution of blood flow. For example, a cerebral angiogram, made by injecting radiopaque dye into the carotid artery, may demonstrate an aneurysm of the circle of Willis or displacement of cerebral vessels by a tumor. Commonly, a carotid angiogram will demonstrate atherosclerotic narrowing or occlusion of the carotid artery, a significant predisposing factor to strokes (Figure 9–2).

Functional disease of arteries caused by high or low blood pressure has entirely different symptoms than arterial occlusion. High blood pressure (hypertension) is usually asymptomatic, but it may be manifested by headaches and dizziness. Low blood pressure (hypotension), if severe, will be manifested by symptoms of shock, which include faintness, cold skin due to vasoconstriction, and reduced blood flow to the brain and the kidneys.

The functional status of the arterial system is usually evaluated by measuring the arterial blood pressure with a sphygmomanometer and by determining the fullness of the pulse using a finger placed over a pulsating artery.

The status of the venous system can be estimated by inspection or measured using specialized instruments. Distention of neck veins when the patient is in an upright position is an obvious sign of increased pressure in the venous system. More subtle increases can be measured by inserting a pressure gauge into an arm vein. Thrombosis of deep leg veins causes cyanotic congestion, edema, and sometimes pain. Ultrasound techniques measuring the Doppler effect provide a sophisticated method of evaluating venous flow at deep sites, including deep vein thrombosis of the legs. Incompetent valves in superficial leg veins lead to distended, tortuous, protruding, rope-like varicosities that are

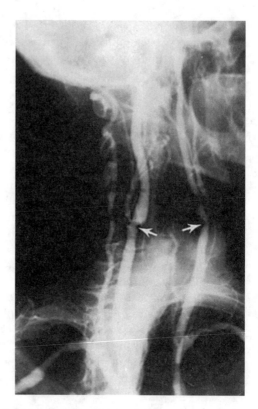

Figure 9–2. An arteriogram of a carotid artery with areas of narrowing (*arrows*).

obvious on inspection. Likewise, hemorrhoidal and esophageal varicosities are evaluated by inspection of the anus and by endoscopy, respectively.

Generalized disease of small vessels, such as occurs with hypertension and diabetes mellitus, may be manifested by decreased visual acuity, and can be evaluated by looking at the eyegrounds (back of the eye) with an ophthalmoscope (funduscopic examination). Small vessels are easily seen here, because they lie immediately beneath the highly translucent retina.

SPECIFIC DISEASES

Genetic/Developmental Diseases

Congenital variations in the vascular system are common but rarely cause problems except for congenital heart diseases and anomalies of the great vessels.

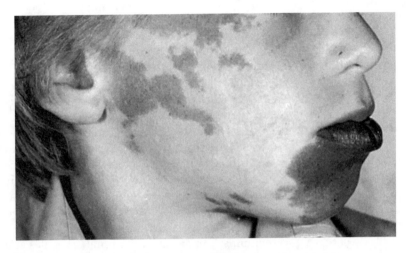

Figure 9–3. Hemangiomas of the face (port wine stains).

Angiomas

Hemangiomas are local proliferations of capillaries that may be present at birth. They are common in the skin, where they vary from small red dots to large cosmetically distracting "port wine stains" (Figure 9–3). Because the dilated vessels fill with blood, they are red to blue and blanch under the pressure of a finger as the blood is pushed out of them. Hemangiomas of the skin rarely cause any problem, but they are occasionally removed for cosmetic reasons. Lymphangiomas, dilated masses of lymphatics, are much less common. When they occur in the neck of an infant (cystic hygroma), they may be frightening in appearance, but they usually regress with age. Hemangiomas and lymphangiomas may be considered as congenital anomalies when their growth is commensurate with that of the patient's body. If their

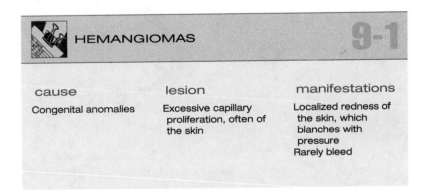

HEMANGIOMAS 9-1

cause	lesion	manifestations
Congenital anomalies	Excessive capillary proliferation, often of the skin	Localized redness of the skin, which blanches with pressure Rarely bleed

growth is disproportionately great, they are considered to be neoplasms of vessels.

Inflammatory/Degenerative Diseases

Atherosclerosis and hypertension will be discussed first and in more detail than the other conditions. The term *atherosclerosis* should be distinguished from the term *arteriosclerosis*. *Arteriosclerosis* means hardening of the arteries and is the general term used to include thickening of the intima and media of small arterioles (arteriolosclerosis or arteriolarsclerosis), calcification of the media of large arteries (medial sclerosis), and plaque formation in the intima of large arteries (atherosclerosis) (Figure 9–4). Arteriolosclerosis occurs in response to increased blood pressure and thus is associated with hypertension. It is seen most commonly in the renal arterioles and may contribute to decreased renal function. In fact, decreased blood flow to the kidney is known to cause hypertension, so arteriolosclerosis may be contributing to a vicious cycle of events.

Medical calcification occurs in the medium-sized to large arteries of the thyroid, genital tract, and extremities with aging and is not considered to be a cause of significant disease.

Atherosclerosis

Atherosclerosis is a degenerative condition, with prevalence and severity increasing with advancing age. The basic lesion of atherosclerosis is a fibrofatty deposit in the intima of blood vessels, particularly in the major muscular arteries (Figure 9–5). This deposit is called an *atheroma*

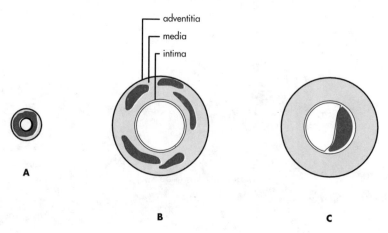

adventitia
media
intima

A

B

C

Figure 9–4. Types of arteriosclerosis: A. Arteriolosclerosis. B. Medial calcification. C. Atherosclerosis.

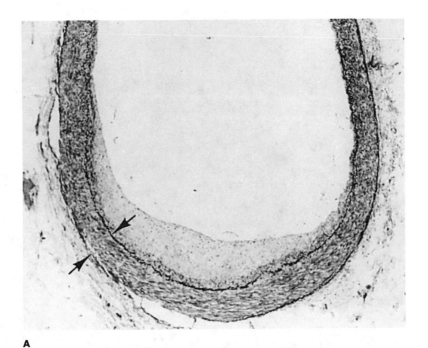

A

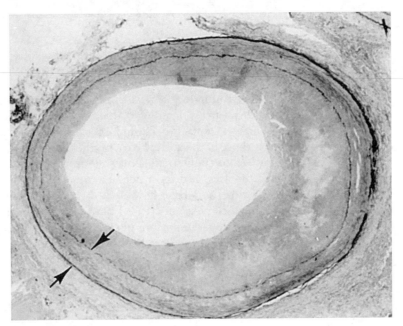

B

Figure 9–5. Progressive stages of narrowing of the lumen of coronary artery by atherosclerotic plaque (A, B, C). The internal and external elastic lamina define the media of the artery (*arrows*). In A, the early intimal thickening at the bottom of the photograph is contrasted with the normal intima. In B the plaque is mostly fibrous tissue, with patchy areas of lipid deposit (*lighter areas*).   *(Continued)*

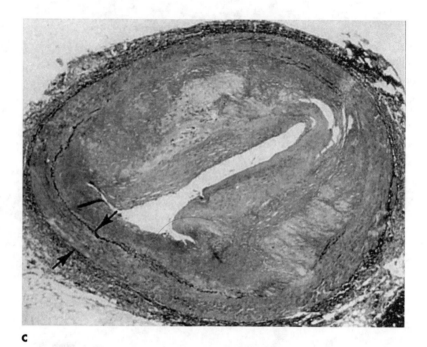

c

Figure 9–5. *Continued.* As seen in B, the plaque is mostly fibrous tissue, with patchy areas of lipid deposit (*lighter areas*).

or, more commonly, a *plaque*, and its continued growth will eventually occlude an artery, leading to an infarct in the territorial distribution of that artery. Deposits occur in large- and medium-sized arteries, particularly those of the aorta, heart, brain, kidneys, legs, and intestines. The early lesions (fatty streaks) may be found in children dying from unrelated diseases, and most persons over the age of 30 will have grossly visible atherosclerotic lesions in their larger arteries. Complications of atherosclerosis (decreased blood flow, thrombosis, or embolism) begin to appear in persons in their thirties and increase with each year of age thereafter. The increase in frequency of complications in women is usually delayed until after menopause, presumably due to a protective effect of female hormones. The low-pressure pulmonary arteries are not usually involved.

An atherosclerotic lesion starts with the accumulation of smooth muscle cells and macrophages in the vessel intima. Lipid accumulates in these cells giving them a foamy appearance histologically and grossly imparting a yellow color to the plaque. These small fatty plaques occur in all populations. In populations with a high prevalence of atherosclerotic vascular disease, the plaques gradually enlarge over years and become progressively more fibrous (sclerotic). The sclerosis presumably occurs in response to the low-grade degeneration and necrosis of cells in the lesion. A white-yellow, shaggy, crusted appearance to the developing fibrous plaque is due to crystallization of the cholesterol that is accumulating in the plaque and to dystrophic calcification.

Eventually, atherosclerotic plaques may cause harm in one of several ways. The lumen of the blood vessel may be obstructed to produce ischemia distally. Ulceration of the surface of the plaque invites thrombus formation there, which may in turn lead to occlusion or embolization. The plaque may produce damage to the vessel wall so that it balloons under pressure to form an aneurysm, a complication most often found in the abdominal aorta (Figure 9–6) and iliac arteries.

Atherosclerosis in the coronary arteries tends to produce occlusion, superimposed thrombosis, or sometimes ulceration with hemor-

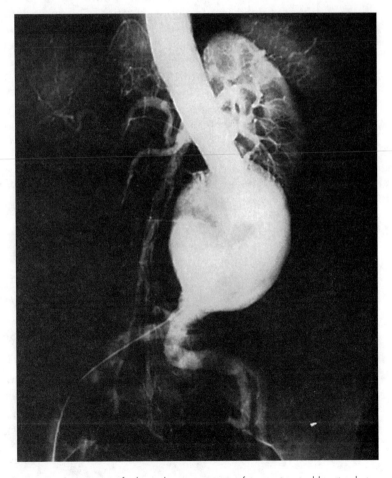

Figure 9–6. Arteriogram of atherosclerotic aneurysm of aorta at typical location between the renal and iliac arteries. Note the catheter in the right iliac artery that was used to inject the radiopaque dye.

rhage into a plaque. Plaques in the carotid arteries tend to produce occlusion (see Figure 9–2). Atherosclerosis of the abdominal aorta, the most common site for atherosclerosis, is usually asymptomatic even when extensive (Figure 9–7). Complications of aortic athero-sclerosis occur if a tributary is blocked by plaque, if embolization occurs from the surface of the plaque, or if the aorta bulges to form an aneurysm. Atherosclerosis in the arteries of the lower extremity may cause an infarct of the foot (gangrene) (Figure 9–8) or produce more gradual ischemic changes in the leg. The latter are associated with ischemic atrophy of muscle and pain that is aggravated by walk-ing and relieved by rest (*intermittent claudication*).

It is not understood at present what initiates and perpetuates the atherosclerotic process. The more prevalent theories propose initial damage followed by lipid infiltration of the intima, possibly aug-mented by platelet aggregation and microclotting. Smooth muscle cells with phagocytic properties, called *myointimal cells*, and macro-phages phagocytose the lipoprotein, cholesterol, and other lipid to form the early atherosclerotic lesion. Collagenous and elastic connec-tive tissue is formed in response to the lipid and contributes to the bulk of the developing lesion. Lipid deposition is clearly the factor that perpetuates the evolution of the lesion. But what causes the lipid depo-sition? Much attention has been paid to the role of injury to the endothelial surface as an initiating factor. This would explain the loca-

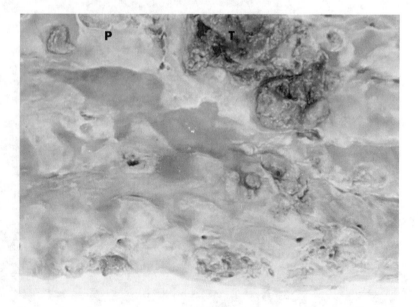

Figure 9–7. Atherosclerosis of the aorta. Note plaques (P) and fibrin thrombi (T) on the sur-face of plaques.

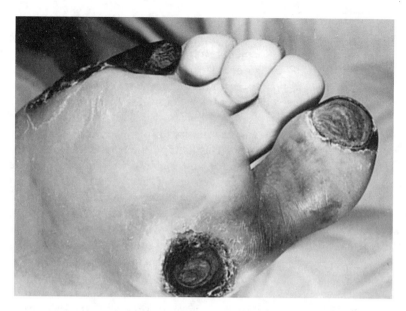

Figure 9–8. Infarcts of the great and small toes (gangrene) resulting from atherosclerosis.

tion of plaques near bifurcations of arteries where the pressure of the arterial stream might cause injury and the increased frequency of plaques in hypertensive patients where the injury might be more severe. Another interesting observation is that the myointimal cells can be derived from one clone of proliferating cells, suggesting that they might be tiny hyperplasias or even neoplasias. In summary, serum lipid abnormalities promote the development of atherosclerosis, but local factors, which are poorly understood, are necessary for plaque development. The complexity and graded severity of both serum and local factors makes isolation of specific causes difficult.

All people have some degree of atherosclerosis, yet one individual may die of a myocardial infarct from an atherosclerotic, occluded coronary artery at the age of 35, whereas another individual may die of cancer at the age of 90 with only mild atherosclerosis. The recognition of this variation in individual susceptibility has led to the elucidation of risk factors, those conditions that when present will render an individual more susceptible to atherosclerosis. The major risk factors are:

1. *Hyperlipidemia.* Increased dietary intake and familial elevations of serum lipids, are predisposing factors to atherosclerosis. Serum cholesterol values over 200 mg/dL are generally considered to carry an increased risk, although this figure is relative and risk can only be crudely estimated in any individual by taking all risk factors into consideration. Further, serum cholesterol levels

represent the total of several forms of cholesterol in the serum and some forms are more strongly associated with the development of atherosclerosis than others. Lipoproteins, the major carriers of cholesterol in the serum, have been classified on the basis of their density and electrophoretic migration. High serum levels of low-density lipoproteins (LDL) are associated with more severe atherosclerosis, whereas high-density lipoproteins (HDL) are somewhat protective. Hyperlipoproteinemic states have been classified on the basis of serum levels of lipoproteins, cholesterol, and triglycerides. The classification of hyperlipidemias is not very exact, except perhaps for some familial types that carry a high risk for atherosclerosis at an early age.

2. *Hypertension.* The greater the hypertension, the greater the risk of atherosclerosis. The reason is not known, but it may be related to trauma to the arterial intima, as veins very seldom develop significant atherosclerosis. On the other hand, when a vein is transplanted to a position where it carries arterial blood, it may develop atherosclerosis very rapidly. Thus, atherosclerosis may develop in veins that are utilized as coronary artery bypass grafts.

3. *Cigarette smoking.* The death rate from coronary atherosclerosis in heavy smokers may double that of nonsmokers.

4. *Diabetes.* Diabetics have more atherosclerosis on the average than nondiabetics, but in spite of this many diabetics, especially those with later onset of the disease, live a normal lifespan. Atherosclerosis tends to be more severe in insulin-dependent diabetes of long duration.

The minor (other) risk factors are:

5. *Age.* In general, the older a person, the more atherosclerosis present.

6. *Sex.* Men have a much higher incidence of serious atherosclerosis. In women, the frequency of atherosclerosis increases after menopause and approaches that of men in the elderly.

7. *Family.* Some families have a much higher incidence of atherosclerosis and resulting diseases than other families. In some instances, this may be related to a common diet, but in other cases, there is a clear genetic influence such as familial hypercholesterolemia.

8. *Activity level.* Reasonable exercise reduces lipid levels and the amount of atherosclerosis.

9. *Obesity.* People with obesity and/or high caloric intake of carbohydrates and lipids have a greater incidence of atherosclerosis.

10. *Stress.* Emotional stress is often blamed for an increased incidence of atherosclerotic coronary disease, but this is not well substantiated.

Of all these risk factors, the major treatable ones are hypertension, smoking, and hyperlipoproteinemias. Several pharmaceutical agents are now available that can reduce serum lipid levels. Treatment of atherosclerosis involves taking care of complications as they arise and preventing further ones from developing. An enormous portion of our health care resources is utilized in managing myocardial infarcts and angina pectoris, inserting coronary artery bypass grafts, caring for stroke victims, removing plaques from carotid arteries, bypassing occlusions and aneurysms of the aorta and leg arteries with grafts, and amputating gangrenous legs.

Surgical therapy for atherosclerosis has become very important and dramatic over the last several decades. Abdominal aortic aneurysms are bypassed by using a tube of biologically inert material. Ultrasound techniques allow diagnosis and measurement of asymptomatic aneurysms so that they can be treated after they reach a critical size and before they fatally rupture. Operations for carotid and coronary artery atherosclerosis are reserved for symptomatic patients, and then only after careful evaluation of potential risks and benefits. Carotid artery plaques, which occur at the bifurcation of internal and external carotid arteries and reduce cerebral blood flow, are removed by opening the artery and shelling out the plaque, a process called *endarterectomy*. Atherosclerotic lesions in coronary arteries may be bypassed using a portion of the patient's own vein (usually saphenous) or mammary artery carefully stitched into the ascending aorta proximally and into the coronary artery distal to the occlusion. Techniques have been developed to insert balloon catheters into coronary arteries that can be expanded to break and crush plaques without subjecting the patient to an operation.

In recent years, more attention to preventing or delaying the development of atherosclerosis has produced some hopeful results. Preventive measures focus on reducing risk factors. Early diagnosis and treatment of hypertension clearly has a beneficial effect. Cessation of smoking, even by those who have smoked for many years, reduces the frequency of atherosclerotic complications. Smoking appears to exert its effects both by affecting the development of plaques and by causing vasopasms, which increase the likelihood of complications. Dietary preventative measures attempt to reduce serum cholesterol in individuals at high risk and in the population as a whole by altering eating patterns. In an individual, serum cholesterol can be lowered by dietary manipulation, but the effect is limited by genetic factors and the outcome depends on a combination of risk factors. In the United States there has been some drop in the incidence of heart disease and this has been attributed to reduced cholesterol intake, but cause and effect are hard to prove. Some populations in the world have very little atherosclerosis. When people from these populations emigrate to high-risk areas, they develop atherosclerosis. This provides a very

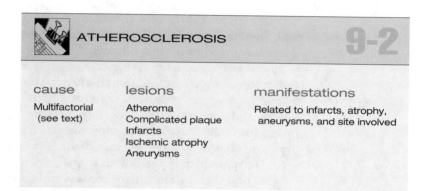

cause	lesions	manifestations
Multifactorial (see text)	Atheroma Complicated plaque Infarcts Ischemic atrophy Aneurysms	Related to infarcts, atrophy, aneurysms, and site involved

compelling argument for attempts to prevent atherosclerosis among high-risk populations.

Hypertension

Hypertension means high blood pressure. The upper limits of normal blood pressure are generally considered to be 90 mm Hg diastolic and 140 mm Hg systolic. As thus defined, over 50 million persons in the United States have hypertension. Transient hypertension, such as is caused by anxiety or physical activity needs to be distinguished from hypertensive disease in which there is sustained hypertension leading to gradual development of cardiovascular lesions. The systolic pressure is created by the force of the heart's contraction as it expels blood into the aorta. Large arteries expand to dampen the force of the pulse. Loss of the ability to expand, as occurs in the aorta with atherosclerosis, produces systolic hypertension. Thus, elderly persons with atherosclerosis tend to have high systolic blood pressure. Systolic hypertension also may be produced by increased cardiac output, such as occurs with exercise, hyperthyroidism, or fever. The diastolic pressure represents the minimum pressure within arteries between heart contractions and is created by arterial relaxation, as during cardiac diastole. Injury from prolonged hypertension correlates best with the diastolic pressure, because eventually the small, rigid peripheral arteries and arterioles will not allow adequate tissue delivery of blood during diastole. However, over the age of 50 increasing systolic pressure appears to correlate better with complications overall.

Essential hypertension refers to primary or idiopathic hypertensive disease. It is the most common form, accounting for over 90 percent of persons with hypertensive disease. *Secondary hypertension* refers to hypertensive disease in which a cause is evident.

Although an exact cause of essential hypertension cannot be identified, it is clearly a multifactorial disease involving both genetic and environmental factors. The genetic factor is suggested by the tendency for essential hypertension to be familial and by the high prevalence among American blacks. The genetic factor probably involves multiple genes and does not produce clear lines of inheritance. Among the many possible environmental factors, a high salt diet has been identified as a factor by animal experiments and by some epidemiologic studies. Psychologic stimuli appear to aggravate hypertension in some individuals. It is possible that many cases of essential hypertension are perpetuated by the hypertensive effects on the kidney vessels, which results in increased renin secretion, which, in turn, sustains the hypertension. This mechanism is described below.

Causes of secondary hypertension include renal disease, endocrine disorders, brain disorders, coarctation of the aorta, arteriovenous fistulas, and toxemia of pregnancy. Three types of renal disorders that produce hypertension are (1) chronic destructive renal disease, such as chronic glomerulonephritis, chronic pyelonephritis, or polycystic kidneys; (2) acute renal disease, such as glomerulonephritis; and (3) narrowing of the main renal artery due to atherosclerosis or smooth muscle hypertrophy. Chronic destructive renal disease is the most common cause of secondary hypertension. Partial occlusion of the renal artery is diagnosed by arteriograms and is often surgically treatable. Unilateral renal artery stenosis causes the affected kidney to secrete increased amounts of renin, an enzyme that activates angiotensin. Angiotensin causes hypertension by contracting small arteries as well as by causing release of aldosterone, which, in turn, aggravates the hypertension because of its salt-retaining effects. Renin may also be important as a cause of hypertension in acute or chronic renal parenchymal disease, although it is less commonly found in elevated levels in the blood under these circumstances.

Endocrine causes of hypertension usually relate to increased secretion of adrenal hormones. Corticosteroids and aldosterone from the adrenal cortex cause salt retention and often lead to hypertension. Epinephrine and norepinephrine are produced by a rare neoplasm of the adrenal medulla called a *pheochromocytoma* and cause hypertension by constricting blood vessels. Endocrine causes of hypertension are often treatable by removal of a benign neoplasm or hyperplastic gland.

Increased intracranial pressure is often associated with hypertension. Coarctation of the aorta produces hypertension proximal to the coarctation by obstruction of the aorta and is treatable by surgical removal of the coarcted segment. Arteriovenous fistulas are connections between arteries and veins that cause more rapid drainage of blood from arteries, producing a low diastolic pressure and a greater cardiac output leading to systolic hypertension. Toxemia of pregnancy is a cause of hypertension in pregnant women. Toxemia of pregnancy is discussed in Chapter 17.

Hypertension takes years to produce its damaging effects. The basic lesion consists of thickening and rigidity of small arteries and arterioles due to the prolonged increase in pressure, especially in the kidney. Hypertrophy of the left ventricle due to the increased pumping force required of the heart is an almost invariable finding. Acceleration of the development of atherosclerosis also occurs commonly in hypertensive patients. Most hypertensive patients die from heart disease due to heart failure. This is the result of the increased work imposed on the left ventricle as well as the damage to the myocardium from the concomitant coronary artery atherosclerosis. The second most common cause of death in hypertensives is from strokes as a result of bleeding from the damaged small arteries in the brain.

Small arteries are best visualized clinically in the retina, where they show thickening and focal narrowing. In fact, the degree of arteriolar involvement can be assessed by ophthalmoscopic examination of the retina. Retinal hemorrhages may lead to blindness. The renal involvement is occasionally severe enough to produce renal failure. At autopsy, the damage to arterioles can be seen microscopically in the kidneys. Rarely, the course of hypertensive disease may become accelerated, with severe renal and retinal vascular disease and very high blood pressure, often in the range of 300/150 mm Hg or more, and manifested by severe headaches and convulsions. This is termed *malignant hypertension* and leads to rapid death within months if not controlled. Severe thickening of arteries and arterioles with obliteration of the lumens are seen in patients who die of malignant hypertension (Figure 9–9).

Most hypertensive disease is asymptomatic; thus, it must be diagnosed by screening. When symptoms develop, they are usually complications of the lesions described above. Heart lesions produce myocardial infarcts or heart failure; brain lesions produce strokes, headaches, and sometimes dizziness or light-headedness; retinal lesions produce blind spots; and renal lesions produce proteinuria. Severe epistaxis (nose bleeds), hemoptysis (coughing up blood), and metrorrhagia (uterine bleeding at an abnormal time) may occur due to the effects of hypertension on small vessels.

Prognosis depends on many factors, such as the levels of blood pressure, variability in the natural course of the disease, occurrence with other potentiating disease, such as atherosclerosis, presence of a treatable cause, stage at time of diagnosis, ability to alter environmental factors, such as stress and diet, and effectiveness of drug therapy in reducing the blood pressure. Untreated hypertensive disease might be expected to run a course of 20 years or so, with the first 15 years being asymptomatic. Although it is difficult to measure the effects of treatment in a predominantly elderly group of patients, there is no

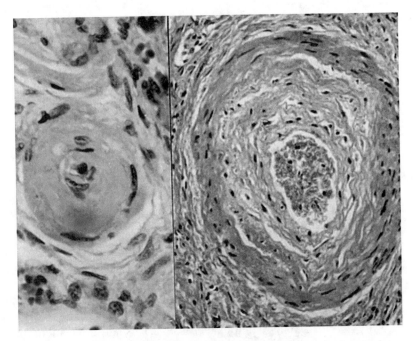

Figure 9–9. Changes in arteriole (*left*) and small artery (*right*) associated with severe hypertension. The arteriole is hyalinized, with obliteration of the lumen. The small artery is greatly thickened by concentric layers of connective tissue and smooth muscle. The narrowed lumen contains red blood cells.

doubt that treatment adds years to the life of an average hypertensive patient.

The strategy of approach to hypertensive disease is threefold: (1) make the diagnosis early through screening, (2) undergo thorough medical investigation to discover the 5 to 10 percent who have secondary hypertension that may be curable, and (3) reduce the blood pressure through environmental manipulation and drug therapy. The environmental manipulation refers to proper diet and exercise as well as attaining psychologic well-being. Numerous drugs are used to treat hypertension. Among the more common classes are diuretics, which decrease the vascular volume; beta-adrenergic agents, which decrease the heart rate and cardiac output; calcium channel blockers, which dilate peripheral blood vessels; and angiotension-converting enzyme (ACE) inhibitors and angiotension II blockers, which inhibit natural body chemicals that elevate blood pressure. Drug therapy requires that the patient be under continuous medical surveillance. As mentioned in Chapter 2, carrying out these strategies accounts for hypertension being the most common chronic disease in terms of visits to family physicians.

HYPERTENSION   9-3

causes	lesions	manifestations
Unknown (most)	Arteriolosclerosis	Elevated blood pressure
Chronic renal disease	Left ventricular	Complications related to
Acute	hypertrophy	myocardial infarct, heart
glomerulonephritis	Accelerated	failure, cerebral
Renal artery stenosis	atherosclerosis	hemorrhage, cerebral
Pheochromocytoma		infarct, renal failure
Corticosteroids		
Coarctation of aorta		
Toxemia of pregnancy		

Vasculitis

There are several uncommon, relatively low-grade and sporadic, non-infectious inflammatory diseases that affect arteries and sometimes veins. Their exact causes are usually not evident, but in most instances they are probably autoimmune in nature. Vasculitis produces significant diagnostic problems, because its variable distribution produces unpredictable and often serious effects. Collections of acute and/or chronic inflammatory cells are found in the walls of and scattered around the vessels.

The most common type of vasculitis is systemic lupus erythematosus, which is noted for a butterfly-shaped rash over the cheeks, effusions (collections of watery fluid) in joints and other body cavities such as the pericardial sac and pleural space. Muscle weakness may occur, and eventual involvement of the kidney vessels may lead to renal failure. Serum antibodies to cell nuclei provide the antinuclear antibody test.

 VASCULITIS   9-4

cause	lesion	manifestations
Usually immunologically mediated	Collection of inflammatory cells in the walls of small- and medium-sized vessels	Infarcts in the areas supplied by affected vessel
		Renal failure
		Muscle weakness

Polyarteritis nodosa is another type of vasculitis that consists of nodular inflammatory thickenings of medium-sized arteries, particularly those of the kidneys, intestines, and skeletal muscles. Inflammation of these arteries (Figure 9–10) may lead to luminal occlusion, resulting in small- to medium-sized infarcts in many organs.

Functional Vascular Disease

Various disease states exist in which arterioles and venules constrict secondarily to local influences such as precipitation of intraluminal proteins, chemicals applied to the adventitia, or disturbance of autonomic function. One of these states is called Raynaud's phenomenon. In this condition, the small vessels of the extremities (usually hands) constrict markedly, leaving the extremity cold and blue. Raynaud's phenomenon occurs with some collagen–vascular diseases, such as lupus erythematosus, but at other times the reason for its occurrence is unknown.

Thrombophlebitis

Literally, thrombophlebitis means thrombosis in an inflamed vein. The term *phlebothrombosis* may be more appropriate, because the veins are not usually inflamed. Thrombophlebitis occurs most frequently in the deep veins of the legs or pelvis, where thrombosis is the important finding. Thrombophlebitis may also occur in arm veins as a complication of intravenous catheters that are left in place for several days. Sluggish and turbulent blood flow is probably more important in causing thrombosis than is inflammation. If the thrombi are dislodged from the vein wall, they will become emboli and will be carried to the lung (Figure 9–11), where they may produce varying pulmonary symptoms and sometimes death.

Pulmonary emboli are common in hospitalized patients, particularly following surgical operations and childbirth, presumably because lack of exercise causes stasis of blood in leg veins and blood platelet concentration is increased. The prevention of thrombi in leg veins is

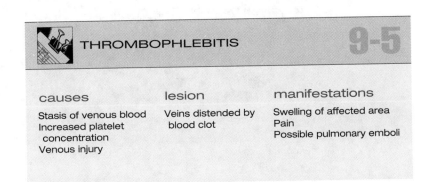

THROMBOPHLEBITIS   9-5

causes	lesion	manifestations
Stasis of venous blood Increased platelet concentration Venous injury	Veins distended by blood clot	Swelling of affected area Pain Possible pulmonary emboli

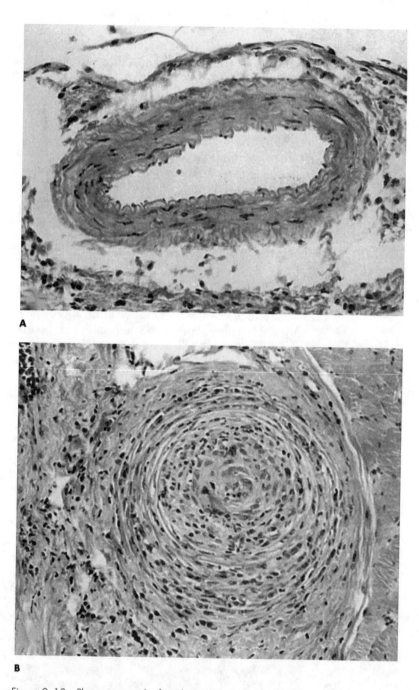

Figure 9–10. Photomicrograph of medium-sized artery. A. Normal. B. Vasculitis with infiltration of inflammatory cells and obliteration of vascular lumen.

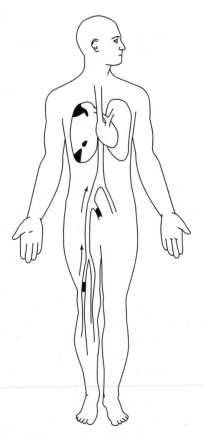

Figure 9–11. Thrombi in leg and pelvic veins leading to pulmonary embolism and infarcts. *Arrows* indicate direction of blood flow.

the reason for early ambulation following operation or childbirth. Most venous thrombi and even pulmonary emboli are undiagnosed; this is known because they are found frequently at autopsy when they were clinically unsuspected. Local symptoms of thrombophlebitis may include leg pain and tenderness, but these symptoms are unreliable diagnostic indicators. Accurate diagnosis depends upon techniques involving injection of radiopaque dyes or use of ultrasound to detect venous occlusions. Treatment consists of anticoagulant drugs and may involve surgical ligation of the veins to the legs to prevent pulmonary emboli. With time, the thrombi are either dissolved or replaced by scar.

Varicose Veins
Varicose veins are dilated tortuous veins. Three important sites of involvement are legs, anus, and lower esophagus. Esophageal varices are caused by increased pressure in the portal vein, usually due to cirrhosis of the liver, and may readily bleed, with a fatal outcome. Hem-

VARICOSE VEINS		**9-6**

causes	lesion	manifestations
Chronically increased venous pressure Incompetent valves in legs	Dilated tortuous veins including esophageal varices hemorrhoids varicose leg veins	Edema Visibility of veins Hemorrhage

orrhoids are enlarged veins of the lower rectum and anus, usually without definable cause, although they are common following childbirth due to external pressure and consequent venous distention from pregnancy. Esophageal varices and hemorrhoids are discussed in Chapters 14 and 15.

Varicose veins of the lower extremities commonly involve the greater saphenous vein, a superficial vein just beneath the skin surface of the medial side of the leg. Normally, valves in the leg veins aid in the return of blood upward to the heart by preventing backflow once the blood has been forced upward by muscular activity. Varicose veins have incompetent valves, so hydrostatic pressure is transmitted through the entire course of the vein. The increased internal pressure leads to dilated, tortuous, and visible veins, and standing for long periods of time may further lead to edema, and eventually, ulceration of the skin from the pressure of the edema fluid. Because there are many alternate venous routes for blood to return to the heart, these superficial varicosities can be removed by a surgeon when symptoms indicate the need.

Hyperplastic/Neoplastic Diseases

Except for hemangiomas, discussed earlier, benign and malignant tumors of vessels are rare.

ORGAN FAILURE

Failure of the cardiovascular system to maintain adequate blood pressure is called *shock*, and it is clinically manifest by decreased blood pressure, increased heart rate, decreased urine output, and altered states of consciousness. The two important determinants of arterial blood pressure are the amount of blood pumped by the heart and the resistance of arteries, which is determined by muscular and elastic tension in their walls, as well as by the amount of blood in the vascular system. The types of shock relate to failure of these functions (Table 9–1). Cardiogenic shock, which was discussed in the previous chapter, results when the heart cannot pump enough blood under sufficient arterial pressure to maintain oxygenation of tissues. Hemorrhagic shock results when bleeding leads to an insufficient amount of blood in the vascular system to maintain arterial pressure. Neurogenic shock results when small vessels dilate resulting in an insufficient amount of blood for the remainder of the vascular system. Syncope (fainting) is most often due to neurogenic shock and often occurs in response to emotional situations.

In neurogenic shock, pooling of blood in the lower body results in brain ischemia. After approximately 10 seconds of ischemia, neurons cease to function properly and the person loses consciousness. Syncope is relieved by lowering the position of the head so that less pressure is needed to get blood to the head. In the more severe forms of shock (cardiogenic, hemorrhagic), the kidney, along with the brain, is a sensitive indicator of the severity of the shock. Urine output will be low if the kidney has been damaged by the decreased circulation of blood. Hemorrhagic shock may be treated by expanding the vascular compartment with plasma or whole blood. Severe shock is often treated with drugs (pressor agents) that contract small vessels, thereby increasing the resistance of arteries and elevating the blood pressure.

Failure of the systemic and pulmonary venous systems to return blood to the heart results in congestion and edema due to the increased hydrostatic pressure in venules and capillaries. Failure of the portal venous system has an additional effect, namely, the creation of anastomotic channels between the lower-pressure portal system and the systemic venous system. These anastomoses occur at many sites in the abdomen, but most importantly in the submucosa of the distal esophagus, where the dilated venous channels are prone to rupture and produce fatal bleeding into the gastrointestinal tract. Failure of the systemic and pulmonary venous systems most commonly results

TABLE 9–1. TYPES AND CAUSES OF SHOCK

Type	Cause
Cardiogenic	Inadequate pumping by the heart
Hemorrhagic	Loss of blood
Neurogenic	Inappropriate dilation of small vessels, resulting in pooling of blood

from right and left heart failure, respectively. Failure of the portral venous system most commonly results from cirrhosis of the liver, because the fibrous scarring in the liver acts as an external compressor of the portal veins.

Failure of the capillaries to regulate fluid exchange between blood and tissue results in edema. Three factors determine the ability of capillaries and venules to control fluid exchange: (1) the hydrostatic pressure transmitted from the venules, (2) the osmotic pressure determined by the amount of solutes (particularly protein) in blood and tissue fluid, and (3) the integrity of endothelial cells. As previously mentioned, a generalized increase in hydrostatic pressure leading to edema is a result of heart failure. Altered osmotic pressure leading to edema may result from decreased serum proteins or increased electrolyte (salt) content of tissues. Decreased serum proteins result from a variety of disease conditions, including poor absorption of dietary protein due to malabsorption, chronic liver disease with low production of albumin, and injury to renal glomeruli with loss of protein. Increased salt retention in the tissues occurs from increased dietary intake or decreased renal excretion of salt. Disruption of capillary endothelial cell integrity or function leading to edema is usually a localized accompaniment of the inflammatory reaction caused in part by the release of vasodilatory substances such as histamine.

Edema that is generalized throughout the body and associated with accumulation of fluid in the chest cavity (hydrothorax) and abdominal cavity (ascites) is called *anasarca*. Anasarca is particularly likely when serum proteins are very low or when low serum protein level is associated with salt retention and heart failure. The edema fluid produced by increased hydrostatic pressure in the blood or decreased osmotic pressure in the blood has a low protein content and is called a *transudate*. The edema fluid associated with endothelial injury, as occurs with inflammation, has a high protein content due to the leaky endothelium and thus is an *exudate*.

Failure of the lymphatic system may result from permanent and extensive obstruction to the many lymphatic channels of a particular region of the body. The result is a chronic edema due to failure to drain excess tissue fluid. This type of chronic lymphatic edema, called *elephantiasis*, produces marked enlargement of the affected region, which has a firm doughy consistency. Chronic lymphedema may be secondary to obstruction of lymph nodes by cancer or to surgical removal of lymph nodes with resultant backup of lymphatic fluid, a possible complication of radical mastectomy in which axillary lymph nodes are removed. In the tropics, elephantiasis is caused by a helminthic worm infection called *filariasis*. The worms cause fibrosis and blockage of lymphatic vessels.

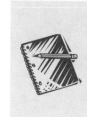

Review Questions

1. What organs are most frequently affected by atherosclerosis?
2. How are each of the following tests utilized in the diagnosis of vascular disease?
   Angiography
   Antinuclear antibody test
   Funduscopic examination
   Sphygmomanometry
   Ultrasound
   Venous pressure measurement
3. What are the causes, lesions, and major manifestations of each of the specific vascular diseases discussed in this chapter?
4. What are the three different types of arteriosclerosis and which type is the most significant? Why?
5. What are the steps in the development of atherosclerosis?
6. What are four ways in which atherosclerotic deposits can cause complications?
7. What are the major risk factors in atherosclerosis?
8. What are the major sites of atherosclerosis and the potential manifestations of involvement in each of these sites?
9. How does essential hypertension differ from secondary hypertension in terms of cause and treatment?
10. What are the major effects of hypertension?
11. How does malignant hypertension differ from benign hypertension in terms of lesions and manifestations?
12. What is the relationship between hypertension and atherosclerosis?
13. What are the most common sites of involvement of each of the common types of vasculitis?
14. How do the manifestations and complications of varicose veins differ from those of thrombophlebitis?
15. What do fainting and hemorrhage have in common?
16. How do venous and arterial failure differ in terms of causal mechanisms, manifestations, and complications?

17. What are the major mechanisms causing localized and/or generalized edema?

18. What do the following terms mean?
    Thrombus
    Embolus
    Cystic hygroma
    Arteriosclerosis
    Arteriolosclerosis
    Medial sclerosis
    Atherosclerosis
    Intermittent claudication
    Aneurysm
    Raynaud's phenomenon
    Phlebothrombosis
    Pulmonary emboli
    Esophageal varices
    Hemorrhoids
    Hemorrhagic shock
    Syncope
    Hydrostatic pressure
    Osmotic pressure
    Anasarca
    Elephantiasis

10.

Hematopoietic System

REVIEW OF STRUCTURE AND FUNCTION
Blood Cells • Lymphoid Tissue • Mononuclear Phagocytic System • Bone Marrow • Production and Destruction of Red Blood Cells

MOST FREQUENT AND SERIOUS PROBLEMS
Anemia • Leukocytosis • Leukemia, Lymphoma, and Multiple Myeloma

SYMPTOMS, SIGNS, AND TESTS
Lymphadenopathy, Splenomegaly, Hepatomegaly • Petechiae • Hematocrit • Hemoglobin • Red Blood Cell Count • Mean Corpuscular Volume • Mean Corpuscular Hemoglobin Concentration • White Blood Cell Count • White Blood Cell Differential Count • Platelet Count • Reticulocyte Count • Bone Marrow Examination • Lymph Node Biopsy

SPECIFIC DISEASES
Genetic/Developmental Diseases
Inflammatory/Degenerative Diseases
   Anemias in General
   Blood-Loss Anemias
   Hemolytic Anemias
   Anemias with Decreased Red Blood Cell Production
   Disorders of White Blood Cells
   Disorders of Platelets
   Infections
Hyperplastic/Neoplastic Diseases
   Polycythemia
   Leukemias
   Lymphomas
   Multiple Myeloma

ORGAN FAILURE

REVIEW QUESTIONS

REVIEW OF STRUCTURE AND FUNCTION

The major functional components of the hematopoietic system are blood, bone marrow, lymphoid tissues, mononuclear phagocytic system, and immune system. Unlike other systems, these components are located within several organs and have overlapping functions. The major organs where these functional components reside are bone marrow, blood vessels, spleen, lymph nodes, and thymus. We will concentrate on the blood and its cellular components and the bone marrow with brief mention of lymphoid tissues and the mononuclear phagocytic system. The immune system is covered in Chapter 27.

The blood consists of plasma and cells. The plasma alone will clot due to the conversion of fibrinogen to fibrin. If the fibrin is removed, the remaining fluid is called *serum*. The cells include red blood cells, which will fall to the bottom of a tube of blood upon standing, and the platelets and white blood cells, which will form a thin white layer between the serum and red blood cells called the *buffy coat*.

The cells of the hematopoietic system are produced at one site (bone marrow) and live their mature lives at other sites (blood, lymphoid, and mononuclear phagocytic tissues). In the bone marrow, common precursor cells produce offsprings that mature along any one of several pathways to produce erythrocytes, platelets, granulocytes, lymphocytes, and monocytes.

Mature erythrocytes live their 120-day life span in the blood carrying out the highly specialized function of oxygen transport; when senile they are removed in the spleen and other mononuclear phagocytic tissues and their chemical constituents are returned to the body pool.

Red blood cells (erythrocytes) are specialized cells that have no nucleus and whose hemoglobin-filled cytoplasm is shaped like a biconcave disk. The principal function of red blood cells is oxygen transport. The amount of oxygen that can be transported by the blood is determined by the number of red cells in circulation and the amount of hemoglobin in them.

Millions of old red blood cells are removed from the circulation each hour by mononuclear phagocytes in the spleen, liver, and, to a lesser extent, other sites. The most important product of the breakdown process is the iron portion of the hemoglobin molecule, which must be stored by the mononuclear phagocytic system for later production of new red blood cells. Proteins from the degraded red cells (and white cells) are returned to the body's protein pool. The major product of red blood cell breakdown, which requires excretion, is bilirubin. Bilirubin is derived from the noniron-containing portion of the heme molecule. Bilirubin is carried by the blood to the liver, conjugated by liver cells, and excreted into the intestine through the bile duct. Serum bilirubin levels may rise if there is increased breakdown of red blood cells, if the liver is diseased, or if the bile duct is obstructed.

Platelets are actually fragments of a bone marrow cell, the megakaryocyte. The megakaryocyte remains in the bone marrow but its cytoplasmic fragments enter the blood where they are ready to participate in the blood clotting system when needed. Platelets are short lived and must be replaced continuously. The role of platelets is discussed in Chapter 11.

Granulocytes also live their short lives (half a day for neutrophils) in the blood where they are ever ready to participate in an inflammatory reaction; they are removed in the same manner as red blood cells.

After leaving the bone marrow, lymphocytes undergo further maturation. Some differentiate in the thymus to become T lymphocytes and become involved in cell-mediated immunity. Others differentiate in other lymphoid tissues to become B lymphocytes that are capable of further transforming into plasma cells for antibody production. Non-B, non-T lymphocytes have still other functions (see Chapter 27 for details).

Monocytes are the most widespread of the bone marrow derived cells. Some circulate in the blood ready to participate in an inflammatory reaction; others reside in tissues, particularly the sinusoids of liver, spleen, lymph nodes, and bone marrow, but also in practically every tissue of the body. In tissues they are referred to by many names: macrophages, histiocytes, reticuloendothelial cells, and Kupffer cells (in liver). Tissue macrophages as a whole, which carry out the scavenger function of removing debris including foreign materials and the body's own dead cells, are referred to as the *mononuclear phagocytic system* (previously called the *reticuloendothelial system*). Macrophages also play a major role in cellular immune responses.

The bone marrow consists of specialized connective tissue through which flows many capillaries. Filling the tissue are immature forms of the various blood cells to intermediate forms to mature forms (Figure 10–1). Red blood cell intermediate forms are called rubricytes or normoblasts up until the time that the nucleus is extruded to form a red blood cell. Immature red blood cells retain basophilic material in their cytoplasm and are called reticulocytes. An increase in reticulocytes in the blood is an indication of early release from the bone marrow and thus suggests accelerated red blood cell production. Red cells proliferate in clusters recognized by the small, round, dense nucleus of normoblasts in the cluster. Granulocytes mature from myeloblast to myelocyte to mature granulocytes. The band, or stab, neutrophil occurs at a stage just before the lobes of the nucleus become separated by a thin strand. When found in increased numbers in the blood (more than 6 percent), band neutrophils indicate increased production and early release of neutrophils from the bone marrow. The characteristic

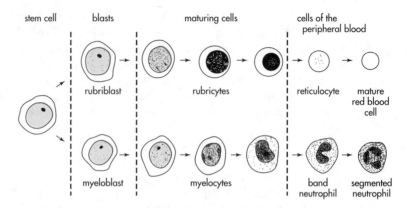

Figure 10–1. Maturation sequence of red blood cells and polymorphonuclear leukocytes.

neutrophilic, basophilic, or eosinophilic granules are acquired in the later stages of myelocyte differentiation. Granulocytic cells are spread diffusely throughout the bone marrow; their normal concentration is about four times that of red blood precursor cells. Monocytes develop from monoblasts and are mixed in with the granulocytes.

The bone marrow serves as a storage site for blood cells, which can be released when needed. The bone marrow can increase its production of blood cells in response to increased demand. Under normal circumstances erythrocytes live 120 days and neutrophils a half day. Erythropoietin is a hormone, released from the kidney, that stimulates erythropoiesis. When there are too few erythrocytes in circulation, more hormone is released to accelerate production of new cells. The production of neutrophils is thought to be mediated by a hormonal substance released from damaged tissue. Mechanisms that control production of other bone marrow elements are poorly understood.

MOST FREQUENT AND SERIOUS PROBLEMS

Overall, the most common clinical problem relating to the hematopoietic system is anemia. Anemia is a decrease in the circulating red blood cell mass. Thus, it is a finding rather than a disease per se. It may be due to decreased production of red blood cells or to increased destruction or loss of red blood cells. The most common types of anemia are: (1) iron-deficiency anemia resulting from dietary deficiency, (2) iron-deficiency anemia resulting from chronic bleeding from the uterus or gastrointestinal tract, (3) anemia associated with various chronic diseases, and (4) vitamin B_{12}–deficiency anemia (pernicious anemia) and folic acid-deficiency anemia. Anemia may be serious in

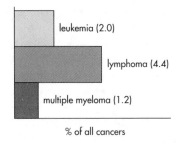

leukemia (2.0)

lymphoma (4.4)

multiple myeloma (1.2)

% of all cancers

Figure 10–2. Relative frequency of primary hematopoietic cancer.

itself if severe; otherwise, it is often a clue to the discovery and treatment of its underlying cause.

Most disorders of white blood cells are secondary effects of other diseases rather than primary in the hematopoietic system. For example, most infections are associated with an increased need for white blood cells and thus cause leukocytosis. If the infection is severe or prolonged, myeloid and/or lymphoid hyperplasia results.

Primary cancers of the hematopoietic system comprise leukemias, lymphomas, and multiple myeloma. These cancers of white blood cells and their derivatives account for 6 percent of all cancers and most of the deaths from primary disease of the hematopoietic system (Figure 10–2).

SYMPTOMS, SIGNS, AND TESTS

Most symptoms of hematopoietic system disease are nonspecific; they can be caused by diseases of other systems. The symptoms of anemia vary from no symptoms to heart failure. Heart failure occurs when there is an insufficient amount of blood to pump and, thus, insufficient oxygenation of the tissues of the body. Nonspecific symptoms of anemia include headache, easy fatigability, loss of appetite, heartburn, shortness of breath, edema of the ankles, and numbness and tingling sensations.

Physical examination may detect enlargement of lymph nodes (lymphadenopathy), spleen (splenomegaly), and liver (hepatomegaly), which can be due to a wide variety of hematopoietic and non-hematopoietic diseases. The occurrence of tiny hemorrhages in the skin (petechiae) is an important finding that suggests a decrease in the number of circulating platelets. Other types of hemorrhage, such as nosebleeds or ecchymoses (large areas of hemorrhage into the skin), may be associated with decreased platelet count or they may be associated with a coagulation disorder (discussed in Chapter 11). Pallor of the skin is found with severe anemia but is an unreliable sign for mild anemia.

Laboratory tests for hematopoietic disease include analysis of blood cells, biopsy of lymph nodes or bone marrow, and special tests for specific diseases. Analysis of blood cells is used for screening and diagnostic purposes. The most commonly used tests in this category are the hematocrit, hemoglobin, red blood cell count, white blood cell count, white blood cell differential count, red blood cell morphology, platelet count, and reticulocyte count.

The hematocrit, hemoglobin, red blood cell count, and blood smear are used to indicate the presence or absence of anemia, and to characterize it as microcytic, normocytic, or macrocytic and as normochromic or hypochromic. Anemia is defined as a decrease in circulating red cell mass as measured by a low hematocrit, hemoglobin, or red blood cell count. Hematocrit is the volume of the red blood cells as compared with other blood elements. When blood is centrifuged, the red cells form the sediment. The percentage of the blood occupied by the red blood cells is the hematocrit. The hemoglobin is a measurement of the amount of hemoglobin in grams per deciliter (g/dL). The red blood cell count, performed by counting the cells in a small chamber, is the number of red blood cells per cubic millimeter of blood.

The size and hemoglobin concentration of red blood cells can be visualized directly by placing a blood smear under a microscope or may be calculated from the hematocrit, hemoglobin, and red blood cell count. The blood smear is a useful, rapid means of classifying red blood cells as macrocytic, normocytic–normochromic, or microcytic–hypochromic (Figure 10–3). Other changes in red blood cell morphology may also be present and may give more specific clues to the cause of the anemia. The mean corpuscular volume (MCV), or mean red blood cell size, is calculated by dividing the hematocrit by the red blood cell count. The mean corpuscular hemoglobin concentration (MCHC) is calculated by dividing the hemoglobin by the

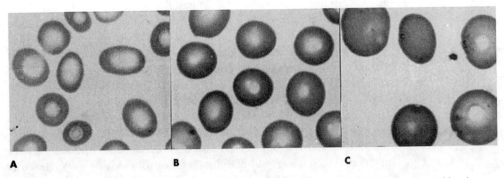

A B C

Figure 10–3. Classification of red blood cells by size and hemoglobin content as visualized on a blood smear. A. Hypochromic, microcytic red blood cells. B. Normochromic, normocytic red blood cells. C. Macrocytic red blood cells.

TABLE 10–1. MEASUREMENTS OF RED BLOOD CELLS

Test	Normal Values	Name of Low Value	Name of High Value
Hematocrit	Male: 40–54% Female: 37–49%	Anemia	Polycythemia
Hemoglobin	Male: 14.1–18.0 g/dL Female: 12.3–16.2 g/dL	Anemia	Polycythemia
Red blood cell count	Male: 4.7–6.1 million/mm³ Female: 4.2–5.6 million/mm³	Anemia	Polycythemia
MCV	82–97 cu μ	Microcytosis (microcytic anemia)	Macrocytosis (macrocytic anemia)
MCHC	32–36 g/dL	Hypochromia (hypochromic anemia)	Hyperchromia (rarely occurs)

hematocrit. Table 10–1 gives the normal values for measurements of red blood cells and interpretations of high and low values.

The white blood cell count and differential white blood cell count are used to evaluate white blood cells. The white blood cell count involves the counting of cells in a chamber and calculating the number of cells per cubic millimeter. The differential count involves identifying consecutive white blood cells on a smear and calculating the percentage of each type present. Absolute counts can be calculated from the percentages of each cell type and the total count. Absolute counts are of more value than the relative percentages, because the numbers of specific types of leukocytes may vary independently of each other. Table 10–2 gives the normal values and names applied to increases and decreases.

Platelets are evaluated by the platelet count, expressed as thousands per cubic millimeter. Normal values are between 150,000 and 400,000 per cubic millimeter. A platelet decrease is called *thrombocytopenia* and an increase *thrombocytosis.*

The reticulocyte count is a measure of the percentage of immature red blood cells in circulation. Values greater than 2 percent are referred to as *reticulocytosis* and indicate an increased rate of production and release of new red blood cells.

Biopsy of the bone marrow is performed by boring a needle into the iliac crest, vertebra, or sternum to obtain bone marrow tissue. The tissue can be smeared on a slide and stained or embedded in paraffin and sectioned. Bone marrow examination is used in the diagnosis of hematopoietic cancers and selected other hematopoietic diseases. Lymph node biopsy is most often used to evaluate the presence or

		TABLE 10–2. MEASUREMENTS OF WHITE BLOOD CELLS (WBCs)	

Test	Normal Values	Name of High Value	Name of Low Value
WBC count	4,300–11,600/mm³	Leukocytosis	Leukopenia
WBC differential count			
Neutrophils	42–81%	Granulocytosis or neutrophilic leukocytosis	Granulocytopenia or neutropenia
Lymphocytes	10–47%	Lymphocytosis	Lymphopenia
Monocytes	0–10%	Monocytosis	Not applicable
Eosinophils	0–7%	Eosinophilia	Not applicable
Basophils	0–1%	Basophilia	Not applicable

absence of cancer, but it is also used to diagnose rare types of chronic infections.

Examples of special hematology tests include *hemoglobin electrophoresis* to evaluate genetic abnormalities in the hemoglobin molecule, *sickle-cell preparation* to induce the sickle-shaped red blood cells associated with sickle-cell anemia, *red cell fragility test* to detect spherical red blood cells (spherocytes), which burst when exposed to hypotonic solutions. Iron concentrations may be measured in serum. Diseases that are the result of antibodies against red or white cells are evaluated by special immunohematology procedures.

SPECIFIC DISEASES

Genetic/Developmental Diseases

There are several important hereditary defects that cause anemia including sickle-cell disease, thalassemia, hereditary spherocytosis, and glucose-6-phosphatase deficiency. For clarity, they will be discussed in the following section with the other types of anemia. The much rarer genetic defects of white blood cells, which lead to death in childhood from repeated infections, are discussed in Chapter 26.

Inflammatory/Degenerative Diseases

This section deals with anemias, disorders of white blood cells, disorders of platelets, and certain inflammatory disorders that characteristically affect the mononuclear phagocytic and lymphoid tissues.

Many of these conditions are indirect results of injury, inflammation, and repair. Others, included in this section for convenience, are better classified as genetic disorders, metabolic disorders, or both.

Anemias in General

Anemia may be a finding in many diseases, including primary diseases of red blood cells and diseases that secondarily involve the hematopoietic system. A pathogenetic classification is given in Table 10–3. Anemia may be due either to removal of red blood cells at a rate that exceeds the replacement capacity of the bone marrow (blood-loss anemias and hemolytic anemias) or to decreased production of red blood cells by the bone marrow. Blood-loss anemia involves loss of blood from the vascular system, either externally to the body or internally. Hemolytic anemia involves destruction of red blood cells within the vascular or mononuclear phagocytic systems. When the mononuclear phagocytic system (particularly the spleen) removes red blood cells before their normal lifespan is up, it is called *extravascular hemolysis*. If the red blood cells are actually destroyed in the bloodstream, it is called *intravascular hemolysis*.

A laboratory-oriented approach to the classification of anemia is based on common laboratory findings that help separate the most frequently encountered types of anemia in an efficient manner. Evaluation of red blood cell size and hemoglobin concentration gives three major categories of anemia. Microcytic hypochromic anemia occurs with iron

---

TABLE 10–3. CLASSIFICATION OF ANEMIA

Blood-loss anemias
   Acute blood-loss anemia
   Chronic blood-loss anemia
Hemolytic anemias
   Sickle-cell anemia
   Thalassemia
   Hereditary spherocytosis
   Glucose-6-phosphate dehydrogenase deficiency
   Immune hemolytic anemia
   Hypersplenism
   Microangiopathic hemolytic anemia
Anemias with decreased red blood cell production
   Deficiency anemia
     Iron deficiency
     Vitamin B_{12}–deficiency (pernicious anemia)
     Folic acid deficiency
   Anemia of chronic disease
   Myelophthisic anemia
   Aplastic anemia

deficiency, with some cases of anemia of chronic disease, and with a few other rare diseases. Macrocytic (normochromic) anemia is usually due to vitamin B_{12} or folic acid deficiency. Normocytic normochromic anemia is a feature of most other types of anemia. The reticulocyte count helps separate anemias of decreased production (normal or low reticulocyte count) from those of increased destruction or loss (elevated reticulocyte count). The laboratory approach to classification must be applied with care, for there are some ambiguities. For example, chronic blood loss is not associated with an elevated reticulocyte count, because the mechanism by which chronic blood loss produces anemia is iron deficiency. Thus, chronic blood-loss anemia is both a blood-loss anemia and a decreased-production anemia. Another example is thalassemia. In thalassemia, there is both decreased production of red blood cells because of the deficient hemoglobin production and increased extravascular hemolysis because the resulting cells are defective and consequently more subject to removal.

The classification of anemia is obviously very important, because incorrect interpretation may result in failure to diagnose the underlying disease or apply the proper treatment. We suggest that you consider each type of anemia in terms of its pathogenetic mechanism, laboratory classification, and the context in which it is likely to occur.

Blood-Loss Anemias

Acute blood loss will produce anemia within a few hours because of hemodilation, a process that allows replacement of blood serum before the bone marrow can replace lost cells. The red blood cells remaining in the anemic blood will be normochromic and normocytic. Within a few days, an elevated reticulocyte count will herald the stepped-up production and release of new cells from the bone mar-

---

BLOOD-LOSS ANEMIA 10-1

causes	lesions	manifestations
Acute bleeding	Hyperplasia of bone marrow (compensatory)	Normochromic normocytic anemia Reticulocytosis
Chronic bleeding	Decreased iron stores	Hypochromic microcytic anemia Decreased serum iron

row. The bone marrow is capable of replacing a large amount of lost blood. For example, a blood donor who gives one pint of blood suffers no ill effects. Blood lost need not be replaced unless the amount is such that hemodynamic effects, such as shock, occur.

Chronic blood loss is the slow loss of small amounts of blood over a period of time. The most common causes are excessive menstrual bleeding and bleeding from the gastrointestinal tract. The bone marrow has plenty of capacity to replace this type of blood loss. Anemia occurs late in the course of chronic blood loss due to failure to recycle the iron from the lost red blood cells. Thus, chronic blood-loss anemia is a subcategory of iron-deficiency anemia. Chronic blood loss is discovered by taking a menstrual history or checking the feces for blood (occult fecal blood test). Other forms of chronic blood loss are usually obvious from the patient's history.

Hemolytic Anemias

In hemolytic anemias, red blood cells are prematurely removed from the bloodstream (extravascular hemolysis) or destroyed within the bloodstream (intravascular hemolysis). Extravascular hemolysis is more common. Hemolysis may be caused by the bone marrow producing defective red blood cells that are destined to a short life or by events that affect normal cells after they are released from the bone marrow.

In hemolytic anemia, there is an increased production of bilirubin as macrophages degrade the dead red blood cells. The transportation of this pigment to the liver for excretion is often manifest by an elevation of serum bilirubin and by mild jaundice. The bone marrow, which is stimulated by the anemia to produce more erythrocytes, becomes hyperplastic and releases more immature erythrocytes than normal, causing a reticulocytosis. With intravascular hemolysis, there also will be free hemoglobin in the blood and urine and a decrease in serum haptoglobin, a serum protein that binds free hemoglobin. Patients with hemolytic anemia do not become depleted of iron because iron from the destroyed cells reenters the body's iron pool. In fact, increased absorption of iron and transfusion therapy often leads to hemosiderosis (excessive iron deposition) in these patients.

The mechanisms of hemolytic anemia include hereditary defects in red blood cells that decrease their lifespan, antibodies to red blood cells that cause their destruction or premature removal by the mononuclear phagocytic system, premature removal of red blood cells by the spleen due to chronic passive congestion (*hypersplenism*), and mechanical injury to red blood cells by rough surfaces in the bloodstream (*microangiopathic hemolytic anemia*). Important diseases that illustrate these mechanisms will be discussed.

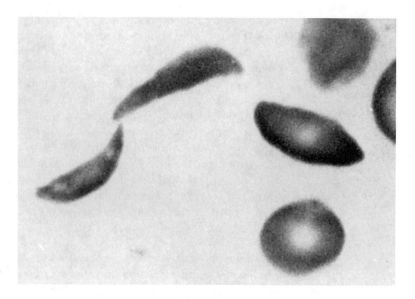

Figure 10–4. Sickled red blood cells.

Sickle-cell anemia is one of several genetic abnormalities of hemoglobin structure due to an altered sequence of amino acids in the globin molecule. The diseases produced by these genetic defects are called *hemoglobinopathies,* and the abnormal hemoglobin is designed by a letter or name of a place where it was first described. Sickle-cell anemia occurs in persons with two genes for hemoglobin S (the homozygous state). Persons with one hemoglobin S gene (the heterozygous state) are said to carry the sickle trait and can be identified by a positive sickle-cell preparation test (Figure 10–4), but do not have anemia. Identification of the trait is quite useful for purposes of genetic counseling. Hemoglobin S is a genetic abnormality predominantly of blacks; about 10 percent are heterozygous carriers and about 1 percent are homozygous persons with the disease. The abnormal hemoglobin results in some red blood cells becoming sickle shaped under situations of low oxygen tension. The sickle cells are not only more susceptible to rupture and premature death, but they also tend to sludge and obstruct small blood vessels. Vascular obstructions are particularly common in the spleen and bone, where they produce multiple small infarcts over a period of years. Patients with sickle-cell anemia often live reasonably well with their anemia except during periods of so-called crisis, when more cells become sickled, leading to abdominal and bone pain from small infarcts and jaundice from the increased breakdown of red blood cells. Leg ulcers are a common complication of long-standing disease. Most patients with sickle-cell anemia die by age 30 to 40.

SICKLE-CELL ANEMIA 10-2

cause	lesions	manifestations
Recessive genetic abnormality for hemoglobin S	Sickled red cells Vascular occlusions with infarcts Hyperplasia of bone marrow	Crises of anemia and pain from thrombosis Sickled red cells Hemoglobin S Occurs in blacks

Thalassemia is a genetic defect affecting the rate of synthesis of normal hemoglobin (hemoglobin A) due to a deficient production of alpha or beta globin. There is a compensatory increase in a type of hemoglobin found in the fetus (hemoglobin F) or in a type of hemoglobin found normally in small amounts (hemoglobin A2). Thalassemia is most common in Mediterranean countries and some parts of Africa and Southeast Asia. Thalassemia-major occurs in homozygous individuals with severe anemia developing in infancy and leads to death in childhood or adolescence. There is a decrease in production of red blood cells because of increased destruction of immature red blood cells in the bone marrow.

THALASSEMIA 10-3

cause	lesion	manifestations
Genetic defect of hemoglobin synthesis	Severe anemia due to decreased production and increased destruction of red blood cells	Anemia Hemoglobin F Occurs in persons of Mediterranean, African, or Southeast Asian descent

Hereditary spherocytosis is a genetic defect of the red blood cell membrane with an autosomal dominant inheritance pattern. The abnormal red blood cells are spherical rather than the normal flat, biconcave disks. As they filter through the spleen, they are more easily removed than normal cells. The anemia is usually mild and often not discovered until adulthood. The spleen is enlarged because it traps the abnormal red blood cells. Removal of the spleen usually is curative. This is an example of a dominant disease that is perpetuated because its relative mild nature and prolonged course allows persons with the disease to reach maturity and reproduce.

HEREDITARY SPHEROCYTOSIS 10-4

cause	lesions	manifestations
Dominant genetic defect	Spherocytic red blood cells Splenomegaly Bone marrow hyperplasia	Spherocytes Increased red-blood-cell fragility Splenomegaly

Glucose-6-phosphate dehydrogenase deficiency is a genetic enzyme defect that only becomes manifest when red blood cells are exposed to certain oxidant drugs such as antimalarial drugs, sulfas, nitrofurantoin, aspirin, and other analgesics. These patients have a mutant enzyme that becomes deficient in older red blood cells, allowing oxidants to damage the cell membrane and produce hemolysis. Discontinuance of the drug and normal replacement by young red blood cells end the hemolytic episode. The genetic abnormality is sex-linked and is present in 10 percent of blacks. Males are much more prone to develop anemia because most affected females are heterozygous carriers. The disease can be prevented by screening high-risk individuals (black males) for the defect and then avoiding exposure to oxidant drugs.

GLUCOSE-6-PHOSPHATE DEHYDROGENASE DEFICIENCY 10-5

cause	lesion	manifestations
Sex-linked recessive genetic defect	None except biochemical abnormality	None unless certain drugs given Enzyme deficiency Occurs in blacks

Immune hemolytic anemia may be associated with antibodies that activate complement and lyse the red blood cell in the bloodstream or with antibodies that facilitate removal of the red cell by the spleen. Transfusion of blood with a major incompatibility between the donor's and recipient's ABO systems and severe cases of erythroblastosis fetalis are examples of causes of intravascular hemolysis. Certain drugs may induce antibodies to red blood cells and thus cause immune hemolytic anemia. In many cases of immune hemolytic anemia, the source of the antigen is the patient's own red cell antigens; thus, the anemia is classified as autoimmune hemolytic anemia. The Coombs' test measures the presence of antibodies attached to the surface of red blood cells and therefore is the test used to detect immune hemolytic anemias.

Hypersplenism is most commonly caused by chronic passive congestion of the spleen, a condition where the venous pressure is increased due to obstruction of the portal venous system, usually due to cirrhosis of the liver. The venous congestion causes the spleen to remove more blood cells than normal, thus producing a type of extravascular hemolytic anemia. The condition is suspected in a patient with cirrhosis and enlarged spleen and who often has leukopenia and thrombocytopenia along with anemia.

Microangiopathic hemolytic anemia is caused by rough surfaces in the bloodstream as sometimes produced by prosthetic heart valves, rough atherosclerotic plaques, and disseminated intravascular thrombosis. The blood smear will show the fractured cells, called schiztocytes or helmet cells.

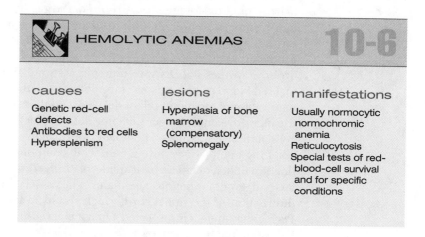

HEMOLYTIC ANEMIAS   10-6

causes	lesions	manifestations
Genetic red-cell defects	Hyperplasia of bone marrow (compensatory)	Usually normocytic normochromic anemia
Antibodies to red cells	Splenomegaly	Reticulocytosis
Hypersplenism		Special tests of red-blood-cell survival and for specific conditions

Anemias with Decreased Red Blood Cell Production

The bone marrow may fail to put out enough red blood cells if it has an inadequate supply of nutrients to produce red blood cells, if its function is suppressed by the presence of chronic disease, or if the bone marrow tissue is insufficient in amount. The blood smear is quite helpful in initial screening because deficiency of iron produces a microcytic, hypochromic anemia and deficiency of either vitamin B_{12} or folic acid produces a macrocytic anemia. Most other types of anemias are normocytic and normochromic.

Iron-deficiency anemia is a common type of anemia. It may be due to loss of iron or inadequate intake of iron. Loss of iron most commonly results from chronic blood loss, as has been discussed. Inadequate intake of iron occurs in infants fed on a milk and fruit diet without meat or supplemental iron; in women during the menstrual years (a combination of inadequate intake and increased loss); during pregnancy, when iron must be provided to the fetus; and in chronic intestinal diseases associated with malabsorption of iron. In iron-deficiency anemia, the cells produced are smaller and paler than normal because there is less hemoglobin per cell (microcytic hypochromic anemia). The anemia is often mild and unrecognized by the patient. Because iron stores are depleted, the serum iron is decreased and the proteins that bind iron in the serum are increased (elevated serum iron-binding capacity). Administration of iron causes an elevation of the reticulocyte count in a few days and increases in hemoglobin after about 10 days.

Vitamin B_{12}–deficiency anemia is caused by failure to absorb vitamin B_{12} from the intestinal tract and not from deficiency of the diet. Dietary vitamin B_{12} (extrinsic factor) must combine with a protein produced in the gastric mucosa (intrinsic factor) and be carried to the distal small intestine before it can be absorbed and carried to the bone marrow or body storage sites. Atrophy of the gastric mucosa, occurring mostly in persons over 60, with resultant insufficiency of intrinsic factor, is the most common cause of vitamin B_{12}–deficiency. The disease produced is called *pernicious anemia*. Vitamin B_{12}–deficiency causes disordered synthesis of DNA, resulting in accumulation of large, abnormal red blood cell precursors (megaloblasts) in the bone marrow. The maturation of red blood cells is delayed, and the red cells released into the bloodstream are larger than normal (macrocytic). The macrocytic cells have a tendency to hemolyze more than normal cells, so the resulting anemia may have a hemolytic component as well as a production deficiency. The basic defect also affects other blood cells to a lesser degree. Pernicious anemia may be associated with permanent destruction of the spinal cord, which results in loss of coordination. Pernicious anemia is suspected when a macrocytic anemia with megaloblasts in the bone marrow is found, and it is confirmed by low serum levels of vitamin B_{12}. The Schilling test, which measures the degree of absorption of vitamin B_{12} from the intestine, is also a useful diagnostic test. Injections of vitamin B_{12} cure the anemia and are continued at regular intervals to prevent recurrence of the disease.

Folic acid deficiency also results in impaired DNA synthesis and produces a macrocytic anemia similar to pernicious anemia, except that the spinal cord degeneration does not occur. Folic acid deficiency results from inadequate diet such as is common in alcoholics, from increased need such as occurs in pregnancy, and from chronic intestinal diseases that produce malabsorption. Folic acid levels in the serum are used to distinguish folic acid deficiency from vitamin B_{12}–deficiency.

Anemia of chronic disease is an anemia of unknown cause that is diagnosed in patients with chronic disease after exclusion of other causes. It is the most common type of anemia and is unresponsive to therapy. Associated diseases include long-standing infections, cancer, chronic inflammatory diseases, such as rheumatoid arthritis, and chronic renal disease. Ten to 15 percent of hospitalized patients may exhibit this type of anemia. The cost of differentiating this untreatable type of anemia from other treatable forms is considerable. Differentiation from mild iron-deficiency anemia is a particular problem because both may be borderline microcytic with borderline serum iron levels and both may be present at the same time. The pathogenesis of the anemia is unclear, although there is suppression of red blood cell reproduction, reluctance of mononuclear phagocytic cells to release stored iron for production of new cells, and a mildly shortened red blood cell survival time. Diagnosis rests on a history of chronic disease in addition to laboratory studies that show normocytic, normochromic (or sometimes mildly microcytic, hypochromic) red blood cells, normal to slightly low serum iron and serum ferritin levels, and normal serum iron-binding capacity (elevated in iron deficiency). Also, in contrast to iron-deficiency anemia, mononuclear phagocytic cells in the bone marrow contain abundant iron.

Myelophthisic anemia refers to anemia caused by replacement of the bone marrow by diseased tissue such as cancer or fibrous tissue. Cancer is the most common cause. Leukemias, lymphomas, multiple myeloma, and metastatic carcinoma from lung, breast, or prostate can replace the bone marrow so that normal blood cells are produced in subnormal numbers. In addition to the anemia, there will be leukopenia and thrombocytopenia. Replacement of the bone marrow by fibrous tissue is called *myelofibrosis*. It may be the result of irradiation or drugs or of unknown cause. To compensate for bone marrow destruction, hematopoietic cells may take up residence in other sites, such as spleen, liver, and lymph nodes, a process called *myeloid metaplasia* or *extramedullary hematopoiesis*.

Aplastic anemia is an atrophy of the bone marrow, usually of unknown cause, but sometimes caused by chemical poisons such as benzene, drugs such as anticancer agents and chloramphenacol, and by radiation. As in myelophthisic anemia, all blood cell elements may be reduced. Bone marrow biopsy is useful in distinguishing myelophthisic anemia from aplastic anemia, the former displaying the disease replacing the bone marrow and the latter displaying only a hypocellular bone marrow.

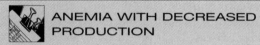

causes	lesion	manifestations
Iron deficiency	Usually abnormal bone	Microcytic
Vitamin B₁₂ deficiency	marrow	hypochromic anemia
Folic acid deficiency		(iron deficiency)
Chronic disease		Macrocytic anemia
Bone marrow		(vitamin B₁₂ or folic
replacement		acid deficiency)
Bone marrow atrophy		Normochromic ane-
Thalassemia		mia (bone marrow
		replacement)
		Normal or low reticu-
		locyte count

Disorders of White Blood Cells

Degenerative and inflammatory disorders involving white blood cells are almost always secondary to disease of some other system. Granulocytosis is characteristic of acute inflammation; lymphocytosis and monocytosis occur with some chronic inflammations; and eosinophilia is characteristic of parasitic infections and some types of allergy. Neutropenia and lymphopenia occasionally occur with some types of infections. White blood cell count may be decreased (leukopenia) by excessive removal with hypersplenism or insufficient production in association with myelophthisic or aplastic anemia.

Disorders of Platelets

Thrombocytopenia is more common and more significant than thrombocytosis. Mechanisms of thrombocytopenia include increased platelet destruction and decreased platelet production. Causes of increased destruction include antibodies to platelets, increased utilization of platelets such as occurs in some blood coagulation disorders, and hypersplenism. Occasionally, treatment with any of a variety of drugs may be associated with the development of antibodies to platelets. Causes of decreased production of platelets include myelophthisic and aplastic anemia.

Idiopathic thrombocytopenic purpura (ITP) refers to thrombocytopenia without evident cause and is believed to be due to antibodies to platelets in most instances. It occurs as a short-lived disorder in children following infections. It also occurs in adults, especially young women, without a precipitating episode and with a prolonged course. In chronic cases, removal of the spleen often results in remission, because the spleen can no longer remove the antibody-coated platelets. Corticosteroid drugs may cause a temporary rise in platelets.

Regardless of cause, a markedly depressed platelet count will be associated with bleeding from small blood vessels to produce petechiae. Thrombocytosis is associated with a few uncommon diseases and usually produces no ill effects.

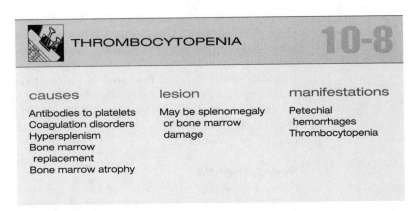

THROMBOCYTOPENIA   10-8

causes	lesion	manifestations

Antibodies to platelets
Coagulation disorders
Hypersplenism
Bone marrow
  replacement
Bone marrow atrophy
	May be splenomegaly
	  or bone marrow
	  damage
		Petechial
		  hemorrhages
		Thrombocytopenia

Infections

As mentioned previously, infections frequently cause a secondary hyperplasia of myeloid, lymphoid, and mononuclear phagocytic tissues. A few types of infections, mostly chronic types, have their major effects in the hematopoietic system. Malaria is caused by small protozoa that live in red blood cells and cause episodes of red cell destruction manifested by fever and anemia. Infectious mononucleosis is caused by a virus that produces enlargement of lymphoid tissue, including lymph nodes, pharyngeal lymphoid tissue, and spleen. The disease runs a prolonged course, producing weakness, sore throat, and lymphadenopathy. Atypical reactive lymphocytes in the blood and a positive mono spot test for antibodies to the virus are the means of diagnosis.

Granulomatous diseases such as tuberculosis and systemic fungal infections have a strong tendency to localize in organs with much mononuclear phagocytic tissue, including lymph nodes, spleen, liver, and bone marrow. Sarcoidosis is an idiopathic granulomatous disease that also produces widespread granulomatous lesions in the mononuclear phagocytic tissues.

Hyperplastic/Neoplastic Diseases

The diseases called *leukemias* are white blood cell cancers characterized by extensive bone marrow replacement with neoplastic white blood cells. The condition *leukemia* is an elevated blood cell count due to leukemic cells, and is usually, but not always, present in patients with leukemia (the disease). Leukemias can be either granulocytic or lymphocytic. *Lymphomas* are also white blood cell cancers and are characterized by involvement of sites peripheral to the bone marrow, often with production of mass lesions (as opposed to diffuse involvement of bone marrow and leukemia), and are mostly of lymphocytic origin. *Multiple myeloma* is a cancer of plasma cells, usually arising in the bone marrow without producing leukemia. The effects of multiple myeloma are due to cancerous replacement of bone marrow and production of abnormal immunoglobulins that are deposited in other organs. Without treatment hematopoietic malignancies are uniformly fatal. Establishment of the curative potential of various drug regimens and/or radiation therapy and the introduction of bone marrow transplantation have made the classification of these diseases based on cell type much more important. Only a general outline of this complicated subject will be presented.

Polycythemia

Polycythemia is an increase in red blood cells due to persistent overproduction. It is a form of hyperplasia that may be primary (of unknown cause) or secondary. Primary polycythemia is called *polycythemia vera*. Secondary polycythemia is mediated by erythropoietin. The causes of excess erythropoietin production include (1) hypoxia due to chronic lung disease, cyanotic heart disease, or living at a high altitude and (2) excess production of erythropoietin by any one of several rare neoplasms.

Secondary polycythemia due to hypoxia is necessary to sustain oxygenation of tissue. Polycythemia leads to difficulty by increasing the viscosity of the blood, which may lead to thrombosis and hemorrhage. Polycythemia vera is much less common than secondary polycythemia and appears to be a primary proliferative disease of bone marrow. White blood cells and platelets may also be increased, and the disease may lead to myelofibrosis, and, in rare cases, leukemia develops.

POLYCYTHEMIA   10-9

causes	lesion	manifestations
Unknown	Hyperplasia of bone	Thromboses and
Chronic hypoxia	marrow	bleeding
Rare neoplasms		Polycythemia
secreting		
erythropoietin		

Leukemias

Leukemias comprise several types of malignant neoplasms of white blood cells that originate and spread diffusely in the bone marrow and usually produce high white blood cell counts. Leukemic cells often diffusely infiltrate other organs, such as spleen, liver, and lymph nodes.

Leukemias are usually classified by the type of white cell involved and the chronicity of the disease. The degree of differentiation of the leukemic cells relates closely to the likely duration; thus, acute leukemias have poorly differentiated cells and a rapid course, whereas chronic leukemias have well-differentiated cells and a slow course. Most leukemias involve either lymphocytes or granulocytes (mostly neutrophils). Monocytic leukemia is less common. Acute lymphocytic leukemia is the most common type of childhood leukemia and is rapidly fatal unless treated very aggressively with multiagent chemotherapy. Successful therapy may lead to long-term survival and cure. Chronic lymphocytic leukemia is a much different disease; it occurs in the elderly and runs a prolonged, indolent course with many patients dying from other causes before the leukemia has time to kill the patient. Both acute and chronic granulocytic (myelogenous) leukemia occur predominantly in adults and are less likely to be cured than leukemia in children.

Acute leukemias are composed of more primitive or less well-differentiated cell types; chronic leukemias are composed mainly of mature cells with some primitive blast forms. Acute leukemias have an abrupt onset with bleeding due to thrombocytopenia, anemia, fatigue, fever, and weight loss. The white blood count may be normal or elevated. In chronic leukemia, the symptoms, although similar, appear gradually and by the time they develop the white blood count may be very high and organs, such as spleen, liver, and lymph nodes, enlarged by leukemic infiltrates. Diagnosis is made by examination of the blood smear and bone marrow, and patients are often referred to major centers for treatment.

LEUKEMIAS 10-10

cause	lesions	manifestations
Unknown	Bone marrow replacement by neoplastic cells Leukemic cells in blood Organ infiltrates	Weakness Anemia Bleeding Infections Leukemic cells in blood and bone marrow

Lymphomas

Lymphomas comprise several types of malignant neoplasms of lymphocytes and histiocytes that originate in lymphoid tissues outside of the bone marrow, most often in lymph nodes. Lymphomas usually produce mass lesions, in contrast with leukemias in which disease is concentrated within the bone marrow. Further, lymphomas usually do not spill malignant cells into the bloodstream, i.e., they are aleukemic.

The classification of lymphomas is based on cell type and is very complex. Major categories include Hodgkin's disease and non-Hodgkin's lymphoma. Hodgkin's disease is characterized by a large, malignant cell with a multilobed nucleus containing prominent nucleoli that is known as a *Reed-Sternberg cell*. Unlike most malignancies, Hodgkin's disease contains many benign cells including lymphocytes, histiocytes, neutrophils, eosinophils, and fibroblasts; these additional cells are used for subclassification and their presence or absence relates to prognosis. Non-Hodgkin's lymphomas are classified on the basis of cell size (small vs large), immunologic markers (T cell, B cell, or neither), histologic pattern (follicular vs diffuse), and details of cell structure.

The ultimate purpose of trying to subclassify disease is to better estimate prognosis and provide optimal therapy; considerable progress has been made with regard to lymphomas. The survival from Hodgkin's disease, once considered to be zero, is greatly improved for all types with aggressive radiation therapy and/or chemotherapy, and survival is now expected in many patients with the less malignant types of disease. Follicular lymphomas have a long median survival without therapy but are not cured by chemotherapy. In contrast, diffuse large cell lymphoma can be cured or life greatly prolonged by aggressive chemotherapy; but has a short survival without therapy.

Diagnosis and classification of a lymphoma is made by biopsy; patients are often referred to major centers for therapy.

LYMPHOMAS   **10-11**

cause	lesion	manifestations
Unknown	Neoplastic masses in lymph nodes or other organs	Lymphadenopathy or other mass Lymphoma by biopsy

Multiple Myeloma

Multiple myeloma is a malignant neoplasm of plasma cells. For unknown reasons, it arises in the bone marrow and grows to replace bone marrow with localized destruction of surrounding bone. Another characteristic feature is the production of immunoglobulins, which can be detected in the blood and urine. Multiple myeloma is a disease of the middle-aged and elderly that presents with anemia, infection, multifocal destructive bone lesions, and sometimes renal failure from immunoglobulin precipitates in renal tubules. Although chemotherapy has prolonged survival, the ultimate prognosis is poor.

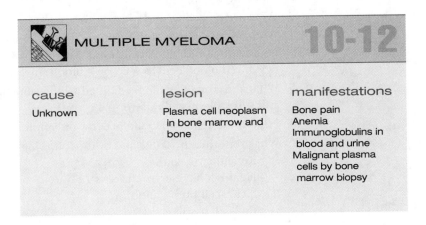

MULTIPLE MYELOMA		10-12
cause	**lesion**	**manifestations**
Unknown	Plasma cell neoplasm in bone marrow and bone	Bone pain Anemia Immunoglobulins in blood and urine Malignant plasma cells by bone marrow biopsy

ORGAN FAILURE

Bone marrow failure has been discussed above as myelophthisic anemia and aplastic anemia, conditions associated with replacement or atrophy of the bone marrow. The results of bone marrow failure are anemia, leukopenia, and thrombocytopenia. These effects, in turn, lead to increased likelihood of infection and bleeding. Failure of the lymphoid system is associated with immune deficiency (discussed in Chapter 26). Failure of the mononuclear phagocytic system is not clearly defined.

Review Questions

1. What are the most common types of anemias and cancers of the hematopoietic system?
2. What are the manifestations of anemia?
3. What are petechiae and what do they suggest?
4. What are the names of the abnormalities defined by hematocrit, hemoglobin, red blood cell count, MCV, MCHC, and morphology of red blood cells as seen on a blood smear?
5. What abnormalities can be defined by the white blood cell count and white blood cell differential count?
6. What is the value of a bone marrow or lymph node biopsy?
7. What abnormality is detected by the following tests?
   Reticulocyte count
   Hemoglobin electrophoresis
   Sickle-cell preparation
   Red-cell fragility test
   Serum iron
   Coomb's test
   Mono spot test
8. What are the causes, lesions, and major manifestations of each of the diseases or groups of diseases discussed in this chapter?
9. What are the major categories of anemia as classified by pathogenesis and by laboratory findings?
10. What are the major causes of leukocytosis, leukopenia, and thrombocytopenia?
11. What are the major differences between leukemias and lymphomas?
12. What are the causes and effects of bone marrow failure?

13. What do the following terms mean?
    Reticuloendothelial system
    Mononuclear phagocytic system
    Intravascular hemolysis
    Extravascular hemolysis
    Pernicious anemia
    Myelophthisic anemia
    Aplastic anemia
    Reed–Sternberg cell
    Multiple myeloma

11.

Bleeding and Clotting Disorders

REVIEW OF STRUCTURE AND FUNCTION
Role of Vessels • Role of Platelets • Plasma Coagulation

MOST FREQUENT AND SERIOUS PROBLEMS
Trauma • Vascular Disease • Platelet Disorders • Coagulation Disorders • Thrombotic Disorders

SYMPTOMS, SIGNS, AND TESTS
Type of Bleeding • Family History • Platelet Count • Bleeding Time • Activated Partial Thromboplastin Time • Prothrombin Time • Fibrinogen Assay • Fibrin Degradation Products

SPECIFIC DISEASES
Disorders Characterized by Hemorrhage
  Vascular Disorders
  Platelet Disorders
  Coagulation Disorders
Disorders Characterized by Thrombosis
  Vascular Disorders
  Platelet Disorders
  Coagulation Disorders

REVIEW QUESTIONS

Bleeding and clotting disorders are treated in this separate chapter because they involve both the vascular and hematopoietic systems and their classification does not fit into the scheme used for other chapters.

This chapter was coauthored by John Olson, M.D.

REVIEW OF STRUCTURE AND FUNCTION

Hemostasis is the process that prevents excessive bleeding following injury. The mechanisms of hemostasis involve a complex interaction of blood vessels, platelets, and chemical coagulation factors in plasma. Hemostasis is highly regulated by numerous activating and inhibiting mechanisms that allow the process to proceed rapidly but not excessively under normal conditions.

Blood vessels confine blood and allow it to circulate. The endothelial cells lining blood vessels normally prevent the activation of blood platelets and plasma coagulation factors, but when the endothelium is removed or injured, platelets and the coagulation mechanism are activated to prevent leakage of blood from the injured vessel. The activating mechanisms will be discussed. Blood vessels undergo spastic contraction in response to injury, thus aiding hemostasis by decreasing the blood flow to the injured area. Spasm of the smooth muscle of small arteries (arterioles) can occlude the vascular lumen and stop bleeding from an injured vessel in a few minutes. Shunting of blood to non-injured vessels provides collateral circulation for healing of the injured vessels. Spasm in medium and larger arteries may aid in hemostasis by decreasing blood flow but is often not sufficient to stop bleeding.

Platelets are cytoplasmic fragments of megakaryocytes. Normally 150,000 to 400,000 platelets per microliter circulate in the blood with a lifespan of 8 to 10 days each. If they are not needed for hemostasis, they are removed by the mononuclear phagocytic system as they become senescent.

The major functions of platelets at the site of an injury are to physically obstruct blood flow, to release chemicals that further the hemostatic process, and to facilitate clot retraction in the healing phase. Platelets will stick to any surface other than normal endothelium—a process called *adhesion*. Endothelial cells produce a potent inhibitor of these functions called *prostacyclin*, which is thought to prevent platelet activation under normal conditions. Minor injury to the endothelial layer with exposure of underlying extracellular connective tissue components will activate platelets and coagulation factors. Adhesion is accompanied by *aggregation* of platelets to each other to form a *platelet plug*. In small vessels, the plug itself may be sufficient to effect hemostasis. Aggregation is potentiated by collagen (exposed by the endothelial injury), by epinephrine (released from adrenal glands during stress and from the platelets themselves), by arachidonic acid (from platelets and other cells in the injured areas), and by thrombin (an enzyme in the coagulation mechanism).

Chemicals released from platelet granules as they adhere and aggregate facilitate all three components of the hemostatic mechanism and are essential to the coagulation mechanism. Vasoactive amines cause vascular smooth muscle contraction. Epinephrine and arachidonic acid accelerate aggregation of additional platelets. Components of the platelet surface are a necessary ingredient of the plasma coagulation mechanism. The role of platelets in the repair process will be discussed later.

The process of converting plasma from a liquid to a solid is called *blood coagulation* or *blood clotting*. The solidification step in this process involves the conversion of fibrinogen, a large, soluble plasma protein produced by the liver, to form fibrin monomer. Fibrin monomer polymerizes to form fibrin, a stringy, strong, insoluble protein. As noted in Chapter 4, fibrinogen may leak into tissues during inflammation and coagulate to form a fibrinous exudate. When the process occurs in a blood vessel the product is called a *thrombus*. Thrombi can contain fibrin with entrapped red blood cells and platelets (Figure 11–1).

Thrombosis, the process of thrombus formation, is a complex process involving tissue, platelet, and plasma protein coagulation

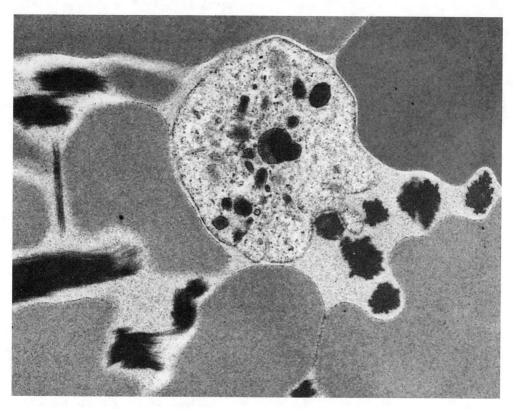

Figure 11–1. Fibrin fibers with an entrapped platelet and portions of several red blood cells (*larger dark bodies*).

factors. The formation of fibrin occurs through a series of enzymatic steps often referred to as the coagulation cascade because the product of each step catalyzes the next step, and often preceding steps so that the reaction can accelerate rapidly. The reaction can be slowed or stopped by inhibitors of the reaction. Factors involved in the reaction have been designated by Roman numerals, which are used interchangeably with their names. Some knowledge of this highly complex scheme is needed to understand and diagnose bleeding and clotting disorders.

The complex process of blood coagulation is presented in an abbreviated form (Figure 11–2). As mentioned, the mechanism is designed to achieve the goal of converting fibrinogen to a stable fibrin clot and thereby converting the blood from a liquid to a solid. The conversion of fibrinogen to fibrin is dependent upon two active enzymes. The first is the enzyme thrombin that converts fibrinogen to fibrin monomer. The fibrin monomer then polymerizes and is reacted upon by a second enzyme called fibrin stabilizing factor (Factor XIII). Factor XIII converts the polymer of fibrin monomer to a stable fibrin clot. These active enzymes and the others of the coagulation mechanism are derived from inactive precursors. In the case of Factor XIII, the inactive precursor is converted to the active enzyme by thrombin. Thrombin also is derived from an inactive precursor called prothrombin (Factor II). The conversion of prothrombin to thrombin is dependent upon the active form of Factor X. Factor X with the cofactor, Factor V, in the presence of calcium ions and phospholipids

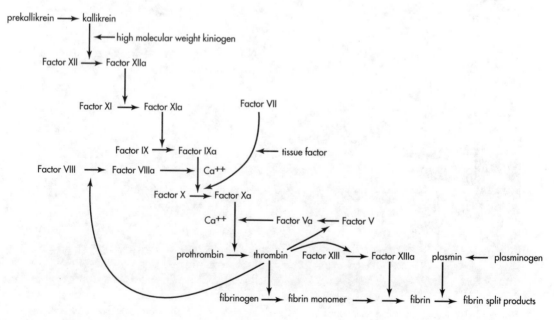

Figure 11–2. Chemical reactions of blood coagulation and fibrinolysis.

convert prothrombin to thrombin. The cofactor, Factor V, also circulates in an inactive form and is activated by thrombin.

Factor X can be converted to its active form, Factor Xa, by two distinct mechanisms. In the first mechanism (traditionally called the extrinsic pathway), tissue juices, which contain tissue factor, combine with plasma Factor VII. This complex of tissue factor and Factor VII, in the presence of calcium ions, converts Factor X to Factor Xa. In the second mechanism (traditionally called the intrinsic pathway), Factor X can be converted to Factor Xa by the activated form of plasma Factor IX. Plasma Factor IX also requires a cofactor (Factor VIIIa) and calcium ions to facilitate its activity. Factor VIII is also converted to its active form, Factor VIIIa, by thrombin. Factor IX is converted to Factor IXa by Factor XIa and Factor XI is converted to Factor XIa by the active form of Factor XII.

Factor XII along with prekallikrein and high molecular weight kininogen are part of a complex system called the contact activation system. Contact activating factors are of interest because their absence greatly prolongs the clotting time of blood in the test tube. These contact factors are of interest in explaining abnormal laboratory tests but of little consequence in the hemostatic mechanism in the patient, as patients who lack them do not bleed. The mechanism by which contact activation is initiated in vivo is unknown, however, exposure of charged molecules such as collagen may be important.

It is apparent that once a clot has formed, it is necessary to have a mechanism for the appropriate removal of the clot in the repair process. This removal is accomplished by the fibrinolytic system. The active enzyme plasmin is formed from plasminogen in the presence of a variety of activators. Tissue-derived plasminogen activator and urokinase appear to be the physiologic activators. Streptokinase, an enzyme derived from the bacteria streptococcus, is also used as a therapeutic agent to activate plasminogen. Plasmin acts upon fibrin to break down the insoluble fibrin clot into soluble fragments called fibrin-split products. Some large thrombi are not completely lysed, in which case they are replaced by granulation tissue and become scar tissue. A thrombus converted to scar tissue is called an *organized thrombus*.

Hemostasis is needed to prevent bleeding, but unregulated intravascular activation of hemostasis is not otherwise desirable. Several inhibitors of the coagulation mechanism have been identified to protect against the devastating consequences of unchecked coagulation. The most prominent of these inhibitors is named antithrombin III. Antithrombin III binds to and inactivates thrombin and the other activated enzymes in the coagulation mechanism. If the active enzymes were generated at a slow rate, or if free active enzymes were found in the circulation in small quantities, antithrombin could bind to and inactivate them. In addition, another inhibitor called protein C, when activated in the presence of its cofactor (protein S), can inactivate the active form of Factor V and Factor VIII. These three molecules plus many others then are capable of slowing or stopping the coagulation process. Finally, the endothelium produces prostacyclin, which is a potent inhibitor of platelet function.

MOST FREQUENT AND SERIOUS PROBLEMS

Everyone experiences bleeding due to physical injury (trauma). Most of the time traumatic hemorrhage is controlled by the normal hemostatic mechanisms. Along with maintenance of an airway, control of bleeding is the major consideration in accident victims. Pressure on bleeding vessels can be used as an emergency measure, but access to medical facilities where the lost blood volume can be replaced and surgical control of internal bleeding can save many lives.

Bleeding may occur with many vascular diseases, but those that cause sudden rupture of a large artery are most life threatening. For example, fatal hemorrhage may occur from a ruptured aortic or cerebral aneurysm or from a bleeding peptic ulcer. Trauma and surgical operations increase the likelihood of significant hemorrhage in patients with preexisting vascular disease.

Spontaneous bleeding may be anticipated when the platelet count drops below 10,000 per microliter or when platelets are defective. Typical causes of thrombocytopenia (platelet deficiency) include bone marrow failure where production is deficient and peripheral destruction of platelets as seen with idiopathic thrombocytopenic purpura where antibodies cause premature removal of platelets. Patients with temporary platelet deficiency, such as might be caused by cancer chemotherapy, can be treated with platelet transfusions.

Hereditary coagulation disorders, such as hemophilia, are rare, but people with these disorders require considerable medical care over many years. Acquired coagulation disorders are typically associated with other diseases, with drugs, or are induced by anticoagulation therapy.

Thrombosis is usually secondary to some other condition. Deep vein thrombosis and pulmonary embolism are quite common and may occur in persons who are minimally ill such as after childbirth or an operation. Disseminated intravascular coagulation usually occurs in patients with significant underlying disease.

SYMPTOMS, SIGNS, AND TESTS

A patient with a tendency to bleed, whether known by a history of bleeding or by abnormal laboratory tests, is said to have a *hemorrhagic diathesis.*

Bleeding from decreased or deficient platelets causes bleeding from small vessels in the skin and internal surfaces such as nose, gastrointestinal tract, and urinary tract in the form of *petechiae* (small hemorrhages in the skin) (Figure 11–3), nose bleeds, hematuria (blood in the urine), and occult fecal blood (positive test for blood in the stool). Tissue bleeding, such as occurs with coagulation deficiencies, tends to occur at one site at a time with minor trauma and produces a localized collection of blood (*hematoma*). Typical sites are joints (Figure 11–4), soft-tissues, and brain.

A history of previous bleeding, such as after circumcision or tooth extraction, and a family history of bleeding may provide the clues to diagnosis of a hereditary coagulation defect. Such a history is particularly important in patients scheduled for an operation because the history may call attention to a problem when screening tests for bleeding disorders are normal.

Laboratory tests for bleeding disorders are used to determine the specific pathogenesis of the problem (vascular, platelet, or coagulation disorder), to monitor the process of the problem or the effect of therapy, and to preoperatively screen patients who are at high risk. Some of the more common tests will be discussed here.

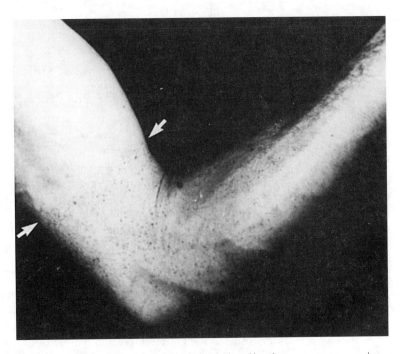

Figure 11–3. Petechial hemorrhage (*black dots*) induced by placing a tourniquet on the arm (*at the site of the arrow*) in a patient with platelet deficiency.

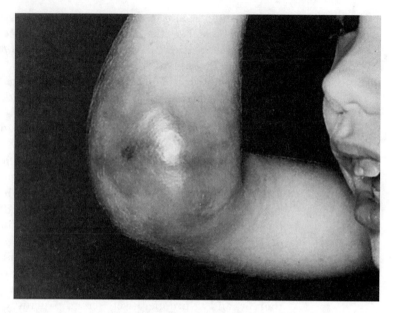

Figure 11–4. Hematoma in the elbow joint of a child with hemophilia.

The *platelet count* is simple and informative. It is performed on most hospitalized patients as a part of a complete blood count. Although the normal platelet count is 150,000 to 400,000 per microliter, spontaneous hemorrhage due to thrombocytopenia is rare if the count exceeds 10,000 per microliter. Abnormalities in platelet function will not be identified by this test.

Bleeding time is the time needed for bleeding to stop after a small skin incision at a standard venous pressure (obtained by putting a tourniquet on the arm). Normal hemostatic mechanisms stop the bleeding in 6 to 9 minutes. Bleeding will be prolonged with a low platelet count, with abnormalities of platelet function, and with diseases affecting small vessels. If the platelet count is normal and bleeding time prolonged, other special tests may be needed to distinguish between abnormal platelets and vascular disease.

The *activated partial thromboplastin time* tests for deficiencies in the coagulation mechanism except for Factor VII. A sample of the patient's blood is drawn into a container containing citrate. The citrate binds calcium, an essential ingredient in clotting, so that the sample can be taken to the laboratory without clotting. At the start of the test three ingredients are added: calcium, a surface contact material, such as finely ground glass, to activate the contact system, and phospholipid as a substitute for platelets. Normally fibrin will solidify the plasma in this test in about 30 seconds. The test is sensitive to defects in the intrinsic pathway, such as hemophilia, and less sensitive to prothrombin and fibrinogen deficiencies. Specific tests are available to test for each of the factors that might be deficient.

The *prothrombin time* is a more sensitive measure of prothrombin and fibrinogen deficiency, but also reflects adequacy of Factors V, VII, and X. Factor VII activates Factor X when tissue factor and calcium are added to the citrated plasma (see Figure 11–1). Normally fibrin forms in about 12 seconds in this test. The prothrombin time is quite sensitive to prothrombin, Factor VII, Factor V, and Factor X deficiencies and less sensitive to fibrinogen deficiency. The *fibrinogen assay* can be used to measure fibrinogen levels.

Measurement of *fibrin degradation products* reflects fibrinolysis in vivo (the amount of fibrin or fibrinogen being split by plasmin). The test is particularly useful in the diagnosis of disseminated intravascular coagulation, which will be discussed later.

SPECIFIC DISEASES

Disorders Characterized by Hemorrhage

Vascular Disorders

The most common vascular causes of hemorrhage are trauma and diseases that erode blood vessels. In these situations, the cause and effect are usually obvious and bleeding is controlled by normal hemostatic process or mechanically by the patient or physician. One should be aware that patients on anticoagulant therapy may bleed excessively from minor or major trauma. Some forms of vasculitis may be associated with petechial hemorrhage. They need to be distinguished from platelet disorders using the appropriate tests.

Bleeding from vascular disruption may be life threatening. Immediate consideration should be given to stop the bleeding and to replace the blood volume. If the bleeding site is accessible, pressure, suture, or a tourniquet can be employed. If the bleeding is internal, access to a hospital is critical. If sufficient blood is lost, plasma or a plasma expander should be given during and after transport to a hospital. Replacement of red blood cells usually is not needed because the patient has a considerable reserve capacity, but blood volume must be replaced immediately to prevent shock.

Platelet Disorders

Decreased numbers of platelets leads to petechial hemorrhages, hematuria, and gastrointestinal hemorrhage. The cause is either decreased production or increased destruction of platelets. Production problems are usually due to extensive bone marrow disease as was discussed in Chapter 10. A bone marrow examination will confirm decreased megakaryocytes; whereas, with increased platelet destruction megakaryocytes will be normal or increased.

There are three major mechanisms of increased platelet destruction. Antibodies to platelets, as occurs in idiopathic thrombocytopenic purpura (Chapter 10), cause their premature removal by the spleen. Diseases of the spleen can cause excessive removal of normal platelets as well as other blood cells—a condition called *hypersplenism.* Finally, disseminated intravascular coagulation can use up platelets faster than the bone marrow can produce new ones.

Disorders of platelet function may be hereditary or acquired. Hereditary disorders are rare but interesting as they help us understand platelet function. Patients with *von Willebrand's disease,* an autosomal dominant disease, lack a plasma factor (von Willebrand factor) that facilitates platelet adhesion. They also have a deficiency of Factor VIII (hemophiliac factor), so they may have abnormal tests for platelet function (bleeding time) and coagulation function (activated partial thromboplastin time). It is important to identify these patients because they may not manifest significant bleeding problems until operated upon. Other hereditary platelet disorders include a deficiency of platelet receptors for von Willebrand factor, a deficiency of platelet aggregation and clot retraction, and deficiency of the release of platelet components.

Acquired disorders of platelet function include renal failure and aspirin therapy. In severe renal failure (uremia), waste products accumulate in the blood that may interfere with the platelet's ability to support coagulation. A platelet exposed to aspirin will no longer be able to release its storage granules. This, obviously, does not usually cause a problem, as millions of people consume aspirin. Aspirin may potentiate an existing bleeding tendency, however. Other drugs also affect platelet function.

Coagulation Disorders

Coagulation disorders may be hereditary or acquired. Hereditary disorders are nature's experiments that have greatly enhanced our understanding of the role of the various coagulation factors.

Hemophilia is the most common of the hereditary coagulation disorders, and both forms are sex-linked. Hemophilia A or classic hemophilia is a deficiency of Factor VIII and occurs in about 1 of 5000 males (females are rarely affected) and about 20 percent appear as new mutants (negative family history). This was a prevalent disease among European royalty. Hemophilia B or Christmas disease is a deficiency of Factor IX and is about one-tenth as common as hemophilia A and somewhat less severe. Persons with hemophilia bleed into joints, muscle, and soft tissues and can bleed excessively from minor operations such as circumcision or tooth extraction. The diagnosis is based on the history of bleeding, screening tests that indicate a coagulation factor defect (normal bleeding time, platelets, and prothrombin time; prolonged activated partial thromboplastin time), and specific tests for Factors VIII and IX. Hemophiliacs suffer lifelong bleeding problems and typically become crippled by bleeding into joints, leading to degenerative arthritis. Factor VIII and IX are available commercially for lifelong replacement and emergency therapy, but are costly and can transmit other diseases (hepatitis and acquired immune deficiency syndrome).

Other hereditary coagulation disorders are autosomally transmitted, much rarer, usually less severe, and lack specific treatment. Fresh-frozen plasma may be used to provide the missing factor in emergencies or prior to an operation.

Acquired causes of bleeding due to coagulation factor deficiency are caused by inadequate production of coagulation factors, excessive destruction of coagulation factors, or drugs that inhibit coagulation. Acquired coagulation disorders, especially platelet function defects, are much more common than inherited ones. All of the plasma factors are proteins produced in the liver (except for von Willebrand factor, which is a product of endothelial cells). Severe acute or chronic liver disease may be associated with bleeding because of deficiency of one or more of these factors. Some of the factors require vitamin K for their synthesis in the liver. Vitamin K is a fat-soluble vitamin produced by bacteria in the intestines, so reduction of the bacteria with antibiotics or malabsorption of fats can lead to a hemorrhagic diathesis due to vitamin K deficiency. Although the main source of vitamin K is diet, newborns, who lack intestinal flora, are given vitamin K parenterally to prevent *hemorrhagic disease of the newborn.*

Coagulation factors may be consumed rapidly by excessive coagulation, thus paradoxically superimposing a hemorrhagic diathesis on top of a coagulation process. This has led to the term *consumption coagulopathy,* which, in its most severe form, may become disseminated intravascular coagulation (discussion follows). Another form of destruction of coagulation factors occurs when antibodies to exogenous Factor VIII or Factor IX develop in hemophilia A or B, respectively.

Warfarin (one of several coumarin drugs) and heparin are used to prevent thrombosis, so they cause a hemorrhagic diathesis at therapeutic levels and active bleeding at toxic levels. Warfarin inhibits vitamin K utilization by liver cells, thus inhibiting production of some coagulation factors. Warfarin takes several days to act and its effect is long-acting. Activity is measured by the prothrombin time and counteracted by vitamin K.

The inhibition of thrombin by antithrombin III is greatly accelerated by heparin. It also inhibits Factors XI, IX, and X, so the activated partial thromboplastin time can be used to monitor the degree of anti-coagulation. Heparin is used for acute therapy in hospitals (it has to be given by injection). Its half-life is only about 90 minutes although newer heparin-like drugs have much longer half-lives. Protamine is used to treat an overdose of heparin. Warfarin is more appropriate for long-term therapy and can be taken orally.

Disorders Characterized by Thrombosis

Vascular Disorders

Vascular changes that lead to thrombosis include acute and chronic injuries to vessel walls (including the endocardium) and turbulent blood flow. The most important of these conditions, including thrombi in leg veins, thrombi on atherosclerotic plaques, mural thrombi over a myocardial infarct, and atrial thrombi, are discussed in Chapters 8 and 9. Any vascular injury or site of turbulence can lead to thrombosis.

Platelet Disorders

Excessive platelets (thrombocytosis) is uncommon but can lead to thrombosis. When the platelet counts exceed 1,000,000 per microliter, there may be an increased likelihood of thrombosis or, paradoxically, bleeding. Causes include idiopathic thrombocythemia, bone marrow hyperplasia secondary to loss or destruction of red blood cells, cancer, splenectomy, and inflammatory diseases. More common is the transient increase in platelets that follows trauma, operations, and childbirth, which, along with venous stasis caused by bed rest, has been incriminated as a predisposing cause of deep leg vein thromboses and subsequent pulmonary embolism.

Coagulation Disorders

Disseminated intravascular coagulation is a clinical syndrome caused by coagulation within the bloodstream. Multiple small thrombi may plug many small vessels throughout the body; however, bleeding often predominates due to consumption of coagulation factors and platelets. Coagulation tests reveal many defects and fibrin degradation products are elevated. Disseminated intravascular coagulation (DIC) is caused by release of tissue thromboplastin, activation of the contact system, or by excessive thrombolysis. It is usually associated with serious underlying disease such as massive trauma, shock, septicemia, or cancer, but it also can occur as a complication of pregnancy due to tissue factors entering the maternal bloodstream from the placenta. DIC is often a terminal event; however, if there is reason to believe that the underlying cause can be treated, anticoagulation therapy may buy time for treatment of underlying cause of the coagulopathy.

Rare hereditary deficiencies of antithrombin III, protein C, or protein S cause spontaneous thrombosis due to lack of these inhibitors of coagulation. Spontaneous thrombosis may also be associated with a common (5 percent of the population) inherited mutation in the factor V molecule, preventing its activation by protein C. As with platelets, coagulation factors are increased after trauma, operations, and childbirth, thus contributing to the tendency to form thrombi under these conditions.

As mentioned earlier, heparin and vitamin K antagonists are used to prevent thrombosis. Long-term therapy with aspirin to prevent thrombosis in coronary and cerebral arteries is based on the known effects of aspirin on platelet function; however, the long-term effects of such therapy require more study. Attempts are also made to dissolve existing thrombi by using enzymes that convert plasminogen to plasmin such as tissue plasminogen activator, streptokinase, and urokinase. Catheters have been used to inject these enzymes into recently plugged coronary and pulmonary arteries.

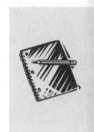

Review Questions

1. Thrombi, hematomas, and fibrinous exudates all contain fibrin. How do they differ?

2. What are the roles of vessels, platelets, and plasma coagulation factors in hemostasis?

3. How are bleeding disorders classified? What types are most common? Most life threatening?

4. What signs of hemorrhage would distinguish a patient with hemophilia from one with platelet deficiency?

5. What is the significance of an abnormal value for each of the following tests?
   Platelet count
   Bleeding time
   Activated partial thromboplastin time
   Prothrombin time
   Fibrin degradation products

6. What is the mechanism and possible treatment for bleeding in each of the following conditions?
   Trauma
   Vasculitis
   Idiopathic thrombocytopenic purpura
   Thrombocytopenia due to hypersplenism
   Hemophilia A
   Hemophilia B
   Severe liver disease
   Hemorrhagic disease of the newborn
   Disseminated intravascular coagulation
   Coumadin therapy
   Heparin therapy

7. How does atherosclerosis predispose to arterial thrombosis?

8. How does a major surgical operation predispose to venous thrombosis?

9. What are the causes, pathogenesis, and prognosis for intravascular thrombosis?

10. What treatments are used to prevent or dissolve thrombi?

11. What do the following terms mean?
    Hemostasis
    Fibrinolysis
    Organized thrombus
    Hemorrhagic diathesis
    Petechiae

12.
Lung

REVIEW OF STRUCTURE AND FUNCTION
Ventilation, Diffusion, and Perfusion • Acini and Alveoli • Trachea and Bronchi • Respiratory Tract Defense Mechanisms

MOST FREQUENT AND SERIOUS PROBLEMS
Pneumonia Chronic • Chronic Bronchitis and Emphysema • Asthma • Cancer

SYMPTOMS, SIGNS, AND TESTS
Dyspnea • Orthopnea • Narcosis • Wheezing • Cough • Hemoptysis • Tachypnea • Cyanosis • Consolidation • Rales • Arterial Gases • Ventilatory Capacity • Chest X-ray • Bronchoscopy • Pleural Aspiration

SPECIFIC DISEASES

Genetic/Developmental Diseases
Respiratory Distress Syndrome of the Newborn (Hyaline Membrane Disease)
Cystic Fibrosis

Inflammatory/Degenerative Diseases

Infections
Lobar Pneumonia
Bronchopneumonia
Abscess
Interstitial Pneumonia
Tuberculosis
Fungal Diseases
Atelectasis
Chronic Obstructive Pulmonary Disease

Asthma
Bronchiectasis
Chronic Bronchitis
Emphysema
Acute Noninfectious Interstitial Disease
Chronic Noninfectious Interstitial Disease
Vascular Conditions

Hyperplastic/Neoplastic Diseases
Bronchogenic Carcinoma
Bronchoalveolar Carcinoma
Bronchial Carcinoid

Metastatic Cancer
Other Lung Tumors

ORGAN FAILURE
Acute Airway Obstruction • Malfunction of Respiratory Control •
Chronic Obstructive and Restrictive Disease • Muscular Disease

REVIEW QUESTIONS

REVIEW OF STRUCTURE AND FUNCTION

The main function of the lungs is to transfer oxygen from the atmosphere to the blood and carbon dioxide from the blood to the atmosphere. The lungs also serve as a filter of air and blood, and, like the kidney and liver, they are involved in the detoxification and excretion of certain toxins and normal metabolites. The term *pulmonary* means "of the lungs."

To carry out its main function, air must be moved from the atmosphere to the terminal units of the lung, a process called *ventilation*, and gas must pass across tissue from air to blood and blood to air, a process called *gas exchange* or *diffusion*. Pathologic processes interfering with ventilation are referred to as *obstructive* and those that decrease lung volume as *restrictive*.

The functional units for gas exchange are thin-walled, wide-mouthed sacs called *alveoli*. A cluster of alveoli with their associated respiratory bronchioles form an *acinus* (Figure 12–1). Alveolar walls consist of capillaries, a scant amount of connective tissue, and epithelial lining cells called Type I and Type II pneumocytes. Type I pneumocytes have very thin cytoplasm, much like an endothelial cell, and comprise most of the inner lining of the alveolus. Type II pneumocytes secrete surfactant, a phospholipid that lowers surface tension, and proliferate when the lining is injured. Monocytes emigrate from the

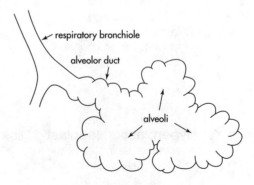

respiratory bronchiole

alveolor duct

alveoli

Figure 12–1. Portion of a pulmonary acinus.

capillaries to the alveolar surface or lumen where they are known as alveolar macrophages and play their usual roles as scavengers of foreign particles. The capillaries bulge into the alveolus. The endothelium and epithelium share basement membranes in areas, providing a very short distance for gases to move across tissue. *Perfusion* refers to blood flow through the pulmonary capillary bed.

The ventilatory pathway is tree-like with the trachea as a trunk and branching bronchi as limbs. Bronchi occupy only a small fraction of the lung space compared with the alveoli (Figure 12–2). Movement of air in the tracheobronchial tree is brought about by muscular movement of the thorax and diaphragm and elastic recoil of the lungs. The bronchial muscle controls the size of the bronchi and thus the resistance to air flow.

Although the skin, mouth, and intestines are more exposed to gross environmental contamination, the lung is more vulnerable because the lining of the distal air sacs is designed for gas exchange, not protection. Proximal to the acinus, the bronchi and trachea are lined by columnar epithelial cells with cilia that propel solid material upward. This is aided by mucus secreted by surface goblet cells and mucosal mucous glands. When excessive material accumulates in the bronchi, the cough reflex helps expel it. Excessive particulate material in alveoli is countered by increased numbers of alveolar macrophages.

MOST FREQUENT AND SERIOUS PROBLEMS

The lung is the site of a wide variety of inflammatory and destructive diseases as well as being the most common primary site of lethal cancer. The majority of deaths from disease of the lung can be attributed to cigarette smoking, the major cause of emphysema and bronchogenic carcinoma.

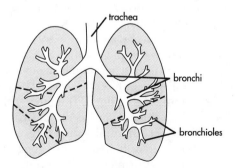

Figure 12–2. Gross anatomy of the trachea and lungs. Lobes are separated by dashed lines.

Pneumonia means an inflammation of the lungs with consolidation and is most often used to describe infections of the lung. The term *pneumonitis* is used in a less specific sense to indicate inflammation. Bacterial pneumonias commonly occur terminally in debilitated persons dying from other causes. Antibiotics have greatly reduced the effects of primary bacterial pneumonias. Viral and mycoplasmal pneumonias are fairly common but rarely cause death.

Chronic bronchitis and emphysema cause a great deal of disability from chronic lung disease. Most cases are associated with smoking. *Pneumoconioses* are diseases of the lung caused by deposition and reaction to inhaled particles such as silica, asbestos, or cane fibers. They occur in miners and others exposed to particulate matter, and may cause destructive pulmonary fibrosis.

Asthma is a common nondestructive lung disease that has its greatest effect on children and young adults. It requires considerable medical attention; acute episodes may be severe enough to require emergency treatment.

In the United States, lung cancer causes over one-third of cancer deaths in men. In women, the frequency of lung cancer has increased rapidly and now causes more deaths than breast cancer.

SYMPTOMS, SIGNS, AND TESTS

Difficulty with breathing is called *dyspnea*, and lack of breathing is called *apnea*. *Orthopnea* refers to difficulty in breathing while reclining. A person who is not getting enough oxygen will attempt to breathe faster and may often become frightened. A person not getting rid of enough carbon dioxide will be somnolent (carbon dioxide narcosis) and may even be unaware of danger. Partial obstruction of major airways will produce noisy breathing such as wheezing.

Cough is due to irritation of bronchi or accumulation of fluid. Fluid coughed up from the lungs is *sputum. Hemoptysis*, the coughing of blood, suggests serious destructive disease such as cancer or tuberculosis.

Physical examination involves observation of the rate and type of breathing. Rapid breathing, *tachypnea*, occurs in response to increased oxygen need whether it be from lung disease or increased general body needs such as fever. *Cyanosis* is blue skin due to inadequate oxygen saturation of the blood. Difficulty with inhaling suggests bronchospasm, as in asthma, whereas difficulty in exhaling is typical of emphysema. *Percussion*, thumping on a finger placed against the chest, may reveal dull or low-pitched sounds suggestive of underlying pulmonary consolidation or pleural effusion. Listening to the chest with a *stethoscope*, a cupped diaphragm that, when placed on the chest wall, transmits sounds from the lung to the examiner's ear via air-filled tubes, may be even more revealing. Bubbly sounds, called *rales*, are created by turbulent air–fluid mixtures and indicate transudate or exudate in the lung as might be caused by heart failure or pneumonia. Diminished normal breath sounds suggest consolidation or pleural effusion.

The ultimate measure of pulmonary function is the oxygen and carbon dioxide content of arterial blood. These tests along with measurement of the capacity to move air in and out of the lung (ventilation) allow assessment of the severity of chronic lung disease. With ventilation defects, the capacity to move air in and out will be decreased and lungs will not empty as much as normal. With diffusion or perfusion defects, blood gases will be abnormal with relatively normal ventilation. Low blood oxygen is *hypoxemia* and high blood carbon dioxide is *hypercapnia*.

The chest roentgenogram (x-ray) is the major diagnostic tool used to look for lung lesions. Once a lesion is found, it is often necessary to determine whether it is inflammatory or neoplastic. If inflammatory, is it due to infection or other cause? If neoplastic, is it primary or metastatic? To make these determinations, samples of lung need to be obtained for culture, cytologic evaluation, or histologic evaluation. Sputum can be used for culture and cytology. Biopsy of trachea, bronchi, and lung can be done at bronchoscopy (endoscopic examination of the trachea and bronchi). Fluid or tissue obtained from the pleural cavity or pleura with a needle can be used for culture, cytology, or histology. If these techniques fail, open lung biopsy may be necessary to establish the nature of the lung disease.

SPECIFIC DISEASES

Genetic/Developmental Diseases

Congenital anomalies of the lung, which are rare, include hypoplastic lobes, lobes with a separate blood supply, and multiple cysts. At birth, pulmonary function suddenly becomes critical, so it is not surprising to find a serious disease, hyaline membrane disease, occurring at this time. Cystic fibrosis is a genetic disease that has more delayed effects.

Respiratory Distress Syndrome of the Newborn (Hyaline Membrane Disease)

The importance of pulmonary alveolar surfactant is nowhere more evident than at birth. If sufficient surfactant is present, the alveoli will inflate and allow diffusion of gases, otherwise they will collapse, a

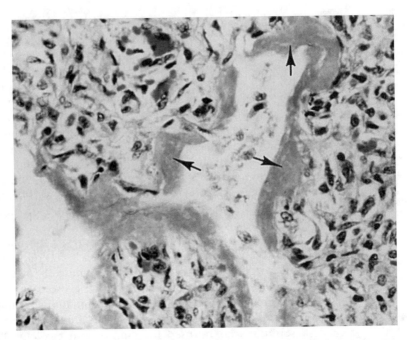

Figure 12–3. Microscopic view of hyaline membranes (*arrows*) in pulmonary alveoli.

condition called *atelectasis*. Surfactant is excreted into the amniotic fluid in utero where it can be measured in samples obtained by amniocentesis. Such samples are useful in determining when elective premature delivery is safe for the fetus. If surfactant is deficient, a proteinaceous precipitate rich in fibrin builds up in dilated bronchioles and alveolar ducts (Figure 12–3). This eosinophilic membrane, although now known to be a nonspecific manifestation to epithelial injury, accounts for the name hyaline membrane disease. Oxygen therapy, which is essential in this situation, also causes injury to the lining cells leading to more hyaline membrane formation. Improved ventilation techniques and awareness of oxygen toxicity have low-

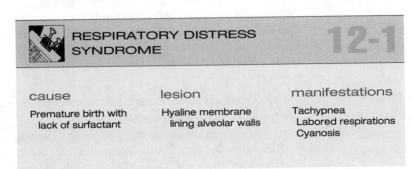

RESPIRATORY DISTRESS SYNDROME   12-1

cause	lesion	manifestations
Premature birth with lack of surfactant	Hyaline membrane lining alveolar walls	Tachypnea Labored respirations Cyanosis

ered the age and birth weight at which prematurely born infants can survive. Untreated infants with respiratory distress syndrome live 1 or 2 days. With treatment, they may survive long enough for the lungs to mature and recover to normal. Prolonged survival, however, may be associated with permanent lung damage in some infants and may unmask other complications of prematurity such as necrotizing enterocolitis. Prematurity is the most common underlying cause of neonatal mortality and hyaline membrane disease is the usual finding at autopsy.

Cystic Fibrosis

This autosomal recessive disease occurs in about 1 of every 2000 whites with an estimated carrier rate of 1 in 20. It is rare in blacks and orientals. It is discussed here because most patients die of lung disease, and attention to medical care of the lung disease has raised the average life expectancy from childhood to adulthood. Cystic fibrosis is caused by mutation of a gene on chromosome 7, the gene product being a protein that compromises the chloride channel of secretory cells, resulting in plugging of various ducts and body passageways with thick mucus. Treatment consists of clearance of secretions and control of lung infections.

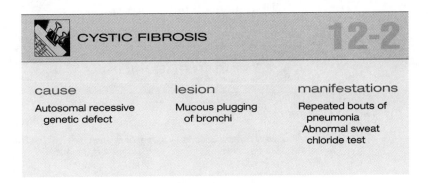

CYSTIC FIBROSIS		12-2
cause	lesion	manifestations
Autosomal recessive genetic defect	Mucous plugging of bronchi	Repeated bouts of pneumonia Abnormal sweat chloride test

Inflammatory/Degenerative Diseases

For this discussion we will group the diseases into four categories: infections, chronic obstructive pulmonary diseases, acute and chronic noninfectious interstitial diseases, and vascular diseases.

Infections

Bacteria are the principal causes of lobar pneumonia, bronchopneumonia, and abscesses. Tuberculosis is an entirely different type of bacterial infection. Several fungi cause pulmonary lesions similar to tuberculosis, whereas others act more like opportunistic bacteria. Viruses and mycoplasma produce an interstitial pneumonia. We have chosen to treat tuberculosis in some detail here, rather than in Chapter 26.

Lobar Pneumonia

Lobar pneumonia involves an area of lung (often a single lobe, hence the name) in a diffuse manner and is caused by *Streptococcus pneumoniae* (pneumococcus) in most cases. It used to be the most common form of pneumonia and involved relatively healthy as well as debilitated people. Most strains of the organism are very susceptible to antibiotics such as penicillin, and the disease responds dramatically to treatment. However, a few resistant strains have emerged, justifying the development of vaccines. The bacteria and resulting exudate spread through the pores in alveolar walls in a wave-like fashion, incapacitating the involved areas. This classic bacterial inflammatory disease can be diagnosed by the finding of respiratory distress, fever, leukocytosis, lobar density on chest x-ray (Figures 12–4 and 12–5A), many gram-positive diplococci on Gram's stain smear of sputum (coughed up from the lungs), and culture of *S. pneumoniae*. The organism itself is always around as an inconstant and variable component of the normal throat flora. There is great variability in the pathogenicity of various strains of pneumococci.

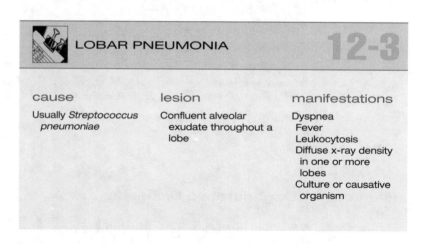

LOBAR PNEUMONIA   **12-3**

cause	lesion	manifestations
Usually *Streptococcus pneumoniae*	Confluent alveolar exudate throughout a lobe	Dyspnea Fever Leukocytosis Diffuse x-ray density in one or more lobes Culture or causative organism

Bronchopneumonia

In contrast to lobar pneumonia, bronchopneumonia has a patchy distribution throughout the lungs, with multiple foci of infection occurring at sites where clumps of bacteria and debris lodge in bronchi (Figure 12–5B). The essential causative factor is obstruction of small bronchi by mucus or aspirated gastric contents, so that bacteria that

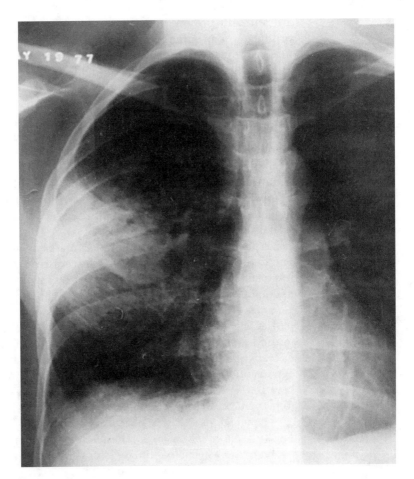

Figure 12–4. Lobar penumonia by chest x-ray. Note radiodensity in right middle lobe caused by inflammatory exudate filling the alveoli.

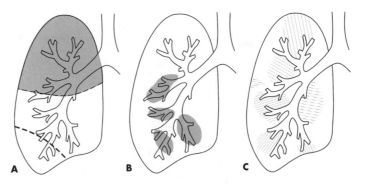

A   **B**   **C**

Figure 12–5. Comparison of lobar (A), broncho- (B), and interstitial (C), pneumonia. Note lobar, bronchial, and patchy distributions.

are normally present in small numbers are trapped and multiply to produce foci of infection in the lung. Various types of bacteria and other nonbacterial organisms may be involved. The lesion consists of inflammatory exudate filling bronchi and alveoli. The extent and location depends on the underlying cause and source of causative organisms. If lung lesions, such as an obstructing cancer, viral bronchitis, or chronic lung disease of various types, are the predisposing cause, the bacteria causing the pneumonia are likely to be normal residents of the upper respiratory tract that were not removed normally. In debilitated patients and those with abdominal infections, gram-negative intestinal organisms, including anaerobic bacteria, are commonly the cause. Circulating bacteria in septic patients may seed the lung and cause multifocal pneumonia.

Bronchopneumonia is more difficult to diagnose and treat than lobar pneumonia, because multiple organisms may be involved, the pneumonia may be masked by underlying disease, and x-ray changes are less distinctive. Bronchopneumonia is a very significant cause of death in debilitated and bedridden patients with chronic diseases.

Aspiration pneumonia is a subtype of bronchopneumonia in which particulate material carrying bacteria gets into the lungs and gravitates to the lower, more dependent lobes. This occurs most often in postoperative and debilitated persons and is enhanced by lack of full expansion of the lungs. The postoperative patient wants neither to breath deeply nor to cough because it hurts, but both are important to prevent bronchopneumonia.

Legionnaire's disease is a bacterial pneumonia due to inhalation of *Legionella pneumophilia,* an organism that lives in water storage tanks and cooling systems. The confluent areas of pneumonia may be extensive enough to be fatal if not treated in time.

Pneumonia is one of the commonest causes of death in immunosuppressed patients. Immunosuppression is a consequence of protec-

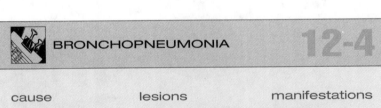

BRONCHOPNEUMONIA		12-4
cause	**lesions**	**manifestations**
Obstruction of small bronchi with subsequent bacterial invasion	Patchy distribution of alveolar inflammatory exudate Exudate in bronchi	Dyspnea Fever Leukocytosis Patchy x-ray appearance

tion of organ transplant recipients from transplant rejection and of chemo- and radiation therapy for cancer. The organisms, which are usually harmless to persons with normal defense mechanisms, include protozoa (*Pneumocystis carinii*), viruses (cytomegalovirus), fungi (aspergillus, mucor, cryptococcus), and bacteria (staphylococcus, gram-negative bacteria).

Abscess

Lung abscesses are localized areas of suppuration, which may develop as a complication of bacterial pneumonia. They may result from aspiration of a foreign body, obstruction of a bronchus by neoplasm, infection in an infarct, or from sepsis. Massive bacterial infection of the pleural cavity with outpouring of purulent exudate is called, *empyema*. This serious condition usually results from underlying lung infection.

Interstitial Pneumonia

When the inflammatory reaction involves the walls of alveoli with relatively little exudation and relatively few polymorphonuclear leukocytes, the reaction is called *interstitial pneumonia* or *pneumonitis*. It is distributed throughout all lobes but tends to be more central than peripheral (Figure 12–5C).

Interstitial pneumonias due to infection usually are associated with an upper respiratory infection and vary from mild and unnoticed by the patient to severe with cough, fever, and malaise. The term primary atypical pneumonia has been applied to acute infectious interstitial pneumonias. The most commonly identified agent (most often the agent is unidentified) is *Mycoplasma pneumoniae*, a bacteria-like organism. Viral causes include influenza A and B, respiratory syncytial virus, and rhinoviruses. The course of mycoplasmal pneumonia may be shortened by antibiotic therapy. Antibiotics may also be useful to treat bacterial complications of viral pneumonia.

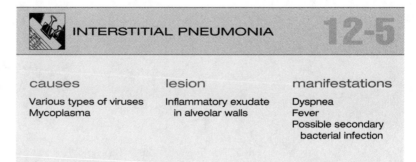

INTERSTITIAL PNEUMONIA   **12-5**

causes	lesion	manifestations
Various types of viruses Mycoplasma	Inflammatory exudate in alveolar walls	Dyspnea Fever Possible secondary bacterial infection

Tuberculosis

Although the disease is under control in the United States, it still occurs, often unexpectedly. Tuberculosis is the most significant lung disease in many areas of the world. The initial or primary lesion is usually asymptomatic. Later, usually years later, secondary lesions develop in some individuals, and these lesions gradually destroy the lung, often with the diseased individual being unaware of the severity of the illness. Such persons spread organisms into the environment and to other individuals.

Tuberculosis is caused by the bacterium *Mycobacterium tuberculosis* and some related atypical strains. The organism is spread from person to person by coughing. A cluster of organisms lodge at the periphery of the lung to set up a focal granulomatous reaction. A few organisms spread through lymphatic vessels to hilar lymph nodes, setting up another granulomatous focus. These foci usually undergo necrosis (caseous type), and they heal by fibrosis and calcification. They may remain indolent for years as small calcified nodules and are then known as the *primary*, or *Ghon complex* (Figure 12–6A). If this primary infection is severe enough, a few organisms may be carried through the bloodstream, seeding the infection in other organs or new sites in the lung. These foci may lie dormant for months to years and then spring up as isolated tuberculous lesions in organs such as kidney, fallopian tubes, bone, or brain. Occasionally, especially in children, the spread from the lungs will be massive, with multiple small foci (miliary lesions) developing in many organs. Meningeal involvement usually leads to fatal outcome (tuberculous meningitis).

Much more common than the spread to other organs is the development of new lung lesions either through breakdown of the primary lesion or by way of reinfection from another individual. These secondary lung infections are different in terms of localization, amount of

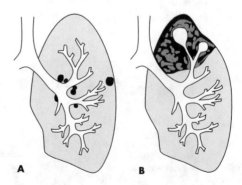

Figure 12–6. A. Ghon complex with solitary peripheral primary granuloma and secondary granulomas in hilar lymph nodes. B. Advanced pulmonary tuberculosis with cavities (connecting to bronchi), granulomas, and scarring of lung and pleura.

tissue destruction, and site in the lungs. Because of previous exposure, lymphocytes now recognize the tubercle bacilli as foreign, resulting in a more rapid reaction and greater amount of necrosis. The disease is usually found in the apices (top) of the lungs, because the organisms presumably grow better with the higher oxygen concentrations found in the upper lobes of the lung. The necrosis may involve the bronchial walls. This allows tissue to be sloughed out through the bronchi, leaving a cavity in the area of necrosis (Figure 12–6B). This sloughed tissue may be coughed, thereby spreading the disease to other persons.

Healing by scar formation destroys the involved portion of lung. The balance between destruction and healing may go on for years. In days gone by, rest was the only treatment, and hospitals were filled with incapacitated infective persons. These patients were usually cachectic and appeared to be "consumed" by their disease, consequently, the term *consumption* became synonymous with *tuberculosis*. Presently, antituberculous drugs control the progression of disease in many persons, and many are able to have parts of their lungs removed, while the drugs prevent recurrence of the disease. Through massive screening efforts, the number of persons with tuberculosis has been greatly reduced, and advanced cavitary disease is rare.

There are two methods of screening, each with its advantages. Skin testing measures hypersensitivity—whether a person's lymphocytes have encountered tubercle bacilli before. Hypersensitive persons may be checked for active disease by a chest x-ray. Skin testing is best for large-scale screening of children, because it is less expensive and when positive tests are found they are more significant than in adults. The reason they are more significant is because children have had less time to acquire an innocuous primary infection, and contacts are more likely to be traceable. Chest x-rays are more definitive than skin tests in finding significant lesions and are less likely to uncover falsely positive cases. For example, an irregular apical lesion in an asymptomatic

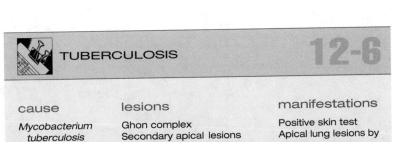

TUBERCULOSIS   12-6

cause	lesions	manifestations
Mycobacterium tuberculosis	Ghon complex Secondary apical lesions with granulomas, cavities, and fibrosis	Positive skin test Apical lung lesions by x-ray Coughing Dyspnea Cachexia if advanced

adult is very suspicious for tuberculosis. The definitive diagnosis is made by culture of sputum or concentrated gastric contents (the coughed-up lung material is normally swallowed). It takes several weeks for the organism to grow in culture. Patients with positive cultures are those who are infectious.

After decades of progress in combating tuberculosis, its incidence is on the rise again and the atypical strains of mycobacterium are becoming more common.

Fungal Diseases

Two primary fungal infections produce diseases much like tuberculosis. Histoplasmosis, which occurs predominantly in midwestern United States, and coccidioidomycosis, which occurs in southwestern United States, are noteworthy. Like tuberculosis, they are usually asymptomatic diseases but may disseminate throughout the lung to cause serious acute illnesses manifested by dyspnea, fever, and incapacitation. Organisms are inhaled after becoming airborne in dust or in dried bird droppings. The lung lesions are granulomatous inflammations but usually do not cavitate as does tuberculosis. Other fungi, such as candida, aspergillus, and mucor, are opportunistic pathogens that may produce pneumonia.

Atelectasis

This means collapse of lung and is not a disease but rather a finding. There are two causative mechanisms (Figure 12–7): (1) external pressure on the lung, such as fluid in the pleural space or poor expansion

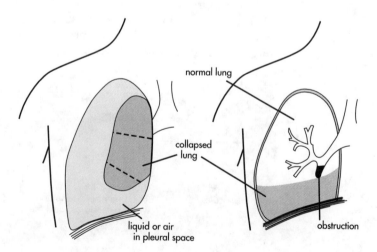

Figure 12–7. Atelectasis produced by external compression (A) and by bronchial obstruction (B).

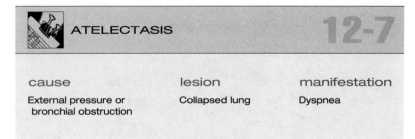

ATELECTASIS   **12-7**

cause	lesion	manifestation
External pressure or bronchial obstruction	Collapsed lung	Dyspnea

of the chest following surgical operation or (2) complete obstruction of a bronchus with reabsorption of the air in alveoli distal to the obstruction. In contrast to complete obstruction, partial bronchial obstruction usually produces an expanded segment of lung, because air gets in past the obstruction more easily than it gets out (ball-valve effect).

Chronic Obstructive Pulmonary Disease (COPD)

This term and the acronym refer collectively to diseases characterized by chronic partial obstruction of airways and inadequate ventilation. COPD is more often used to indicate chronic bronchitis and/or emphysema, which have a similar etiology, than asthma and bronchiectasis, which are different diseases. Asthma may be a lifelong disease, but tends to be more severe in children and young adults. Bronchiectasis is really a complication of previous disease rather than a disease in itself. Chronic bronchitis and emphysema will be discussed together because they are overlapping conditions usually due to heavy cigarette smoking.

Asthma

Asthma is labored breathing due to spasm of bronchioles. It is characterized by episodic attacks characterized by forced inhalation and exhalation due to bronchospasm and excess mucous. The patient appears short of breath, produces wheezing sounds, and may be frightened. Bronchodilating drugs may relieve the symptoms or the patient may seek emergency medical help. The patient appears normal between episodes. There is little permanent damage to the lung unless the disease is complicated by repeated bacterial infections. The bronchial muscle may become hypertrophied and there is hyperplasia of mucous glands in the bronchi associated with increased mucous secretion. During recovery from an attack, coughing leads to expectoration of large amounts of mucus.

The cause of asthma is complex, involving external allergens or irritants, increased reactivity of the bronchi, and inflammation. Some patients have obvious external allergens as the cause, such as those

ASTHMA		12-8
causes	**lesions**	**manifestations**
Allergens	Bronchial spasm	Wheezing
Irritants	leading to bronchial	Dyspnea
Infection	hypertrophy	
	Increased mucus	

who become asthmatic during the hay fever season. Avoidance of rag-weed pollen and/or desensitization may prevent the asthmatic attacks. Other agents that should be evaluated by history and/or skin testing include house dust, animal dander, foods, aspirin, chemicals and molds. In many cases, a specific allergen or irritant cannot be identified; therefore, prevention and treatment are directed at reducing the reactivity of the bronchial muscles and mucous glands. Respiratory tract infections, such as the common cold, typically trigger nonallergic types of asthma. Cold, stress, and exercise may also trigger an asthmatic attack. A severe prolonged attack is called *status asthmaticus* and occasionally is fatal. Most patients can be controlled by avoiding precipitating factors, desensitization of those with atopic allergies (see Chapter 27 for more detail), and administration of bronchodilating agents and corticosteroids. This common disease requires considerable medical attention and may require monitoring of drug levels in patients receiving maintenance bronchodilators.

Bronchiectasis

Bronchiectasis is a dilatation of a bronchus or group of bronchi due to chronic inflammation (Figure 12–8). Classically, it occurs in lower lobes or the right middle lobe following childhood infections complicated by pneumonia. The prevention of bacterial complications of childhood viral pneumonias and the success of measles vaccine have greatly reduced the incidence of this condition. Bronchiectasis can occur with a variety of chronic pulmonary diseases such as cystic fibrosis, tuberculosis, cancer, and obstruction of a bronchus by aspirated foreign body. It is often manifested by copious production of thick, foul-smelling sputum. Diagnosis is made by computerized tomography or bronchogram (a roentgenogram of the lung after infusion of radiopaque dye into the bronchial tree). When the disease is isolated to one lobe, surgical removal of the diseased lobe ends the continuing inflammatory and destructive process.

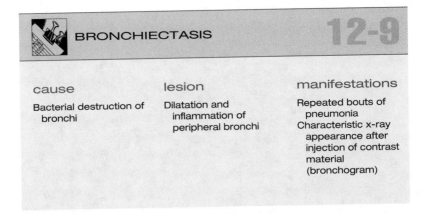

BRONCHIECTASIS   12-9

cause	lesion	manifestations
Bacterial destruction of bronchi	Dilatation and inflammation of peripheral bronchi	Repeated bouts of pneumonia Characteristic x-ray appearance after injection of contrast material (bronchogram)

Chronic bronchitis has been arbitrarily defined to be a clinical term meaning persistent cough with sputum production for at least 3 months in at least 2 consecutive years. Thus chronic bronchitis is a disorder invented because of its high specificity (about 90 percent) for heavy smokers. *Emphysema* is defined as permanent enlargement of acinar air spaces due to destruction of their walls (Figure 12–9). Thus emphysema is an anatomic abnormality that is usually observed at autopsy. Chronic bronchitis and emphysema are not really diagnoses, but rather nonspecific reactions to injury made more specific by a common cause (smoking). No wonder the acronym COPD has become popular! With these definitional problems out of the way, let us try to describe these conditions.

Chronic Bronchitis

Chronic bronchitis is correlated histologically with hyperplastic bronchial mucous glands and goblet cells. Some degree of obstruction may occur in small bronchioles due to mucus and mild inflammatory

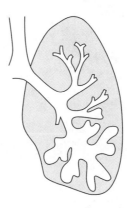

Figure 12–8. Dilated lower lobe bronchi of bronchiectasis.

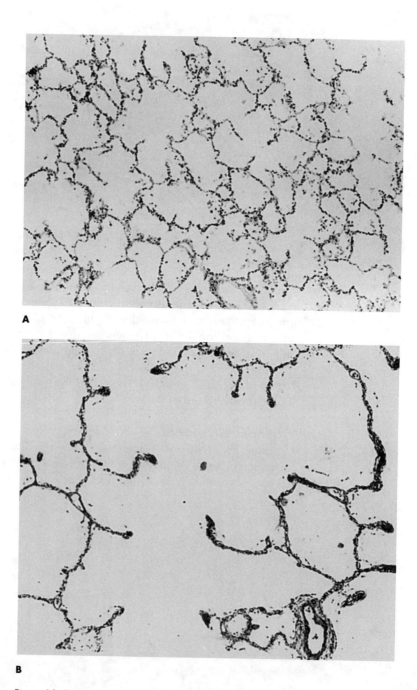

Figure 12–9. Normal lung (A) and emphysema (B) taken at the same magnification. Note that the alveoli are larger and fewer in number in emphysema.

changes, but changes at autopsy are not striking. Chronic bronchitis is a reversible condition, as the symptoms and, presumably, the underlying lesions go away when smoking is stopped. Patients with chronic bronchitis tend to have frequent respiratory infections. In the late stages, they have hypoxia and hypercapnea associated physiologically with resistance to air flow in bronchioles.

Emphysema

Smokers gradually develop more and more emphysema so that there is a great overlap in those with chronic bronchitis and those with emphysema. In emphysema, the ventilation problem is mainly due to trapping of air so that oxygen poor, carbon dioxide rich air is not exchanged effectively with fresh air. This occurs because the walls of alveoli have been destroyed leaving large air spaces with little elastic recoil to force air out. The total size of the lungs increases, often with an expanded fixed chest wall (*barrel chest*) and depressed diaphragm. The lungs are more radiolucent on chest roentgenograms due to the increased air/tissue ratio. Retention of carbon dioxide stimulates the respiratory center to increase the rate of breathing. Eventually, the respiratory center becomes refractory to high carbon dioxide levels and low blood oxygen becomes the stimulus for breathing. At this end stage of the disease, oxygen therapy may kill a patient due to removal of the stimulus for breathing (low oxygen). Some patients with emphysema develop pulmonary hypertension leading to right heart failure (cor pulmonale). They are also more susceptible to pneumonia.

Several types of emphysema have been identified that likely have different causes. In centriacinar emphysema, the common type found in smokers, the respiratory bronchioles in the center of an acinus are dilated and the alveoli at the periphery of the acinus are spared. The upper lobes tend to be more affected. In advanced stages grossly dilated blebs occur. Panacinar emphysema involves all of the alveoli and tends to be more severe in the lower lobes of the lung. This type of emphysema is of interest because it occurs in homozygous alpha-1-antitrypsin deficiency. Alpha-1-antitrypsin inactivates proteases (including elastase). Without the counter activity, elastase, activated by inflammation, can destroy elastic tissue in alveolar walls leading to emphysema. In patients with the deficiency, the rate of destruction is greatly enhanced by smoking. The evidence suggests that smoking produces injury that attracts neutrophils, and neutrophils release elastase that destroys elastic tissue in alveolar walls. The process occurs slowly and locally in respiratory bronchioles in smokers with normal alpha-1-antitrypsin deficiency, but is rapid and generalized in those with the deficiency. Other forms of emphysema include paraseptal emphysema that occurs in the outer part of the acinus, particularly in subpleural areas. This form may be the cause of spontaneous

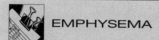

causes	lesion	manifestations

Smoking
Alpha-1-antitrypsin
  deficiency
Fibrosing lung diseases
	Rupture of alveolar
	  walls with
	  coalescence
	  of alveoli
		Dyspnea with
		  continuous
		  shortness of breath
		Barrel chest

pneumothorax in young adults. Rupture of a bleb forces air into the pleural space, collapsing the lung, and leading to sudden dyspnea. If the lobe does not seal spontaneously, a tube may be placed in the pleural space to siphon off air until healing occurs. Irregular emphysema occurs with various chronic destructive diseases of the lung in association with scarring.

Acute Noninfectious Interstitial Disease

Diffuse acute and chronic injuries to alveolar walls by inhaled fumes and small particulate matter or by hypoxemia and blood-borne toxins generally cause restrictive pulmonary disease with inadequate perfusion of oxygen leading to dyspnea, tachypnea, and, when severe, cyanosis. The airway is not obstructed.

Acute alveolar injuries, which have been given many names depending on cause, are collectively referred to as *adult respiratory distress syndrome* or *diffuse alveolar damage*. The damage to pneumocytes produces edema and inflammatory cell infiltrate that enlarge the alveolar walls. Exudate into alveoli is scant compared to the purulent exudate of bacterial pneumonia. Fibrinous exudate and necrotic lining cells may form hyaline membranes in the alveoli.

Causes of diffuse alveolar damage include shock (sometimes called shock lung), oxygen toxicity, nitrogen dioxide, hypersensitivity reaction to volatile chemicals, and drugs. The outcome may be death, recovery, or progression to chronic interstitial lung disease.

Chronic Noninfectious Interstitial Disease

Chronic diffuse interstitial disease may be due to the same agents that cause acute interstitial disease. The most common known causes are pneumoconioses and sarcoidosis. Fibrosis of the alveolar walls leads to restrictive disease of variable severity. Complications include pulmonary hypertension leading to cor pulmonale and increased susceptibility to infection.

Pneumoconiosis refers collectively to environmentally induced pulmonary fibrosis resulting from inhalation of particulate matter. *Anthracosis* is carbon accumulation in the lungs and its draining lymph nodes. It is more severe in city dwellers, factory workers, and coal miners. Anthracosis is generally harmless because carbon by itself elicits very little fibrous reaction. On the other hand, coal miners may develop progressive fibrosis after many years in the mines. This is probably due to the fact that coal miners inhale silica as well as carbon, although the role of silica versus carbon versus infection in producing coal miners' pneumoconiosis is debated. *Silicosis* is caused by inhalation of crystalline forms of silica and occurs in miners and fabricators of silica products such as glass cutters, sand blasters, pottery workers, and foundry workers. Very small crystalline particles of silica are potent inducers of fibrosis. *Asbestosis*, a condition caused by the inhalation of fibrous silicates, is associated with pulmonary fibrosis, bronchogenic carcinoma, and mesothelioma of the pleura (a malignant neoplasm of pleural lining cells). The effects of asbestosis are somewhat unpredictable as many people harbor the fibers without obvious deleterious effect. Because asbestos has been so widely used as an insulating and fireproofing product, it will be decades before its effects subside. *Berylliosis* appears to be a hypersensitivity reaction (it occurs in only a fraction of exposed persons) and may produce acute diffuse injury or a chronic granulomatous reaction. Beryllium is a metal used in alloys because of its strength and heat resistance.

Sarcoidosis is a generalized noncaseating granulomatous disease of unknown cause and with varying clinical manifestations associated with involvement of various organs. In some individuals, pulmonary fibrosis is the dominant process and these patients have a worse prognosis than others with predominantly lymph node disease. Sarcoidosis is most common in young adults and is more common in women,

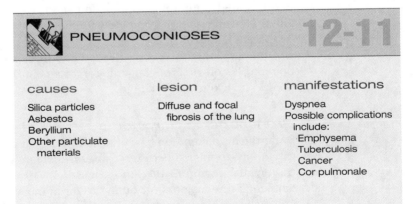

PNEUMOCONIOSES 12-11

causes	lesion	manifestations
Silica particles	Diffuse and focal	Dyspnea
Asbestos	fibrosis of the lung	Possible complications
Beryllium		include:
Other particulate		Emphysema
materials		Tuberculosis
		Cancer
		Cor pulmonale

blacks, and residents of southern United States. Immunologically, delayed hypersensitivity reactions are decreased or absent and antibody-mediated reactions are normal or enhanced.

Diffuse idiopathic pulmonary fibrosis occurs when no cause is found for progressive diffuse alveolar injury. The course is unpredictable but often fatal in months to a few years.

Vascular Conditions

Pulmonary congestion results from left heart failure with increased venous pressure in the pulmonary veins. When severe or prolonged, fluid passes through the alveolar walls into alveoli, producing pulmonary edema, and into the pleural space, producing *pleural effusion.* Both of these complications impair breathing. Right heart failure due to lung disease (cor pulmonale) may be caused by acute or chronic lung diseases that result in increased pulmonary blood pressure. For example, acute cor pulmonale may result from pulmonary emboli, and chronic cor pulmonale is associated with emphysema and fibrotic lung lesions. In both of these conditions, blood can only be forced into and through the lungs by increased right heart pressure.

Pulmonary embolism results from thrombi in the leg or pelvic veins being carried to the right heart and into the pulmonary arteries (discussed in Chapter 9). Pulmonary emboli are sometimes apparent clinically but are much more often found at autopsy. Sometimes they play a role in causing death, but when small, they usually resolve without producing significant injury. Occasionally they cause infarcts.

Hyperplastic/Neoplastic Diseases

Cancer of the lung is one of the three most common nonskin cancers in the United States (along with colon and breast) and is the leading killer. The lung is also a leading site for metastatic cancer. Benign lung neoplasms are rare.

Primary lung cancers are divided into three types based on location and histology: bronchogenic carcinoma, bronchoalveolar carcinoma, and bronchial carcinoid.

Bronchogenic Carcinoma

By far the most common type of primary lung cancer is bronchogenic carcinoma, so named because it arises from large bronchi in the central or hilar region of the lung (Figures 12–10, 12–11, and 12–12). Smoking is the major contributing factor in most cases. Asbestos and radioactive ores are also factors in exposed individuals. The total exposure to cigarettes is estimated in terms of pack-years (the number of

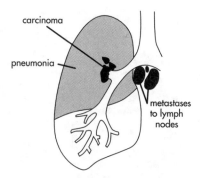

Figure 12–10. Bronchogenic carcinoma, arising in the right upper lobe bronchus with obstruction leading to pneumonia and metastasis to hilar lymph nodes producing a mediastinal mass.

packs of cigarettes smoked per day times the number of years smoked). The number of pack-years correlates with the likelihood of developing lung cancer. Although more lung cancers occur in men, the relative frequency in women is rising.

Bronchogenic carcinomas are subclassified histologically into squamous cell carcinoma (most common), adenocarcinoma, large

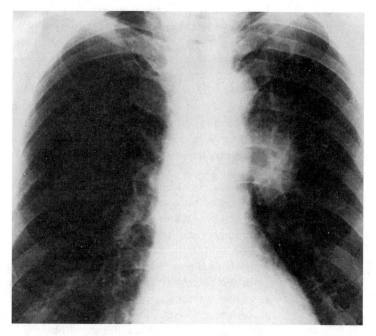

Figure 12–11. Bronchogenic carcinoma of the hilus of left lung by chest x-ray.

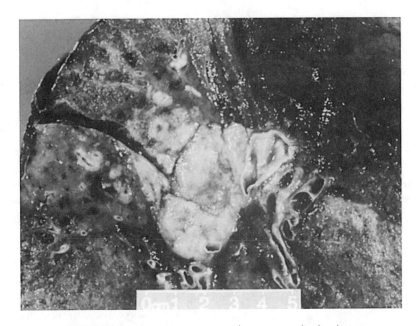

Figure 12–12. Bronchogenic carcinoma with pneumonia distal to the tumor.

cell undifferentiated carcinoma, and small cell undifferentiated carcinoma (oat cell carcinoma). The first three subtypes are treated similarly. If there is no apparent spread by the time of diagnosis (30 percent), a surgical cure is possible by removing the lesion; otherwise, palliative therapy is indicated. Small cell carcinoma, which is identified by small cells that look like lymphocytes and contain neuroendocrine granules, almost always has spread beyond the point of surgical cure by the time it becomes manifest. Radiation and chemotherapy prolong life but do not effect a cure. Some small-cell carcinomas become manifest due to hormone production.

The behavior of bronchogenic carcinomas is variable. About 20 percent are localized at the time of diagnosis, and the overall cure rate is about 12 percent. Bronchogenic carcinomas spread in many directions, including local invasion of the lung, pleura, and mediastinum and metastasis to lymph nodes of the lung and neck. Hoarseness may result from involvement of the recurrent laryngeal nerve. Lung cancer may also metastasize through the bloodstream to many organs. Metastasis to the brain and bone is notorious for producing clinical problems, whereas liver metastasis is frequently evident in advanced stages. Symptoms may include shortness of breath, weight loss, pneumonia secondary to bronchial obstruction, or coughing of blood (hemoptysis). The diagnosis may be suggested by x-ray but is usually made by sputum cytology and biopsy.

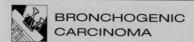

BRONCHOGENIC CARCINOMA   12-12

causes	lesion	manifestations
Unknown	Masses of squamous,	Dyspnea
Smoking	glandular, or	Weight loss
Asbestosis	undifferentiated cells,	Pneumonia
	usually arising from a	Hemoptysis
	bronchus	X-ray appearance

Bronchoalveolar Carcinoma

Adenocarcinomas that arise in the periphery of the lung, spread in alveoli, and are not related to smoking are called bronchoalveolar carcinomas. They are uncommon but have up to a 50 percent cure rate with resection. This small group of tumors must be differentiated from more peripherally located bronchogenic carcinomas and metastatic adenocarcinomas.

Bronchial Carcinoid

Carcinoid tumors are low-grade carcinomas that arise from neuroendocrine cells. This rare variety of lung cancer arises in the hilar region, has very characteristic clusters of neuroendocrine cells, and spreads very slowly. Most have not spread to lymph nodes by the time of diagnosis and, even if they have, progression may occur over many years.

Metastatic Cancer

The lung is a common site of metastatic cancer spread by the bloodstream. Clumps of tumor cells are carried through the bloodstream to the periphery of the lungs, and some grow to produce spherical tumor nodules. Because sarcomas preferentially spread via the bloodstream, the lung is a characteristic site of sarcoma metastases. Many advanced carcinomas also spread to the lung.

Other Lung Tumors

Benign neoplasms of the lung are rare. Most benign nodules in the lung are old healed granulomas from a primary tuberculous or fungal infection. Many patients with benign lung nodules undergo excisional biopsies, however, because the x-ray appearance of the nodules often resembles carcinoma. Occasional carcinomas arise in the periphery of the lung; these are adenocarcinomas and produce a single large mass, in contrast to the multiple nodules of metastatic carcinoma.

ORGAN FAILURE

Death is associated with failure of pulmonary, cardiac, or brain function. Failure of any one of these organs causes the others to fail. Pulmonary causes of death may be acute and chronic. Acute obstruction of the trachea and major bronchi may cause rapid death. Obstruction may be external (strangulation) or internal (aspiration of a large foreign body, massive hemorrhage). Acute restrictive disease may be caused by pulmonary edema or pneumonia. Inadequate expansion of the lung may be caused by pneumothorax, hydrothorax, multiple rib fractures, or muscular paralysis.

Chronic lung disease causes death by producing slowly worsening hypoxia, by cor pulmonale, or by superimposed pneumonia. Lung cancer may cause death by diverse mechanisms including infection, obstruction, and cachexia.

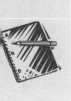

Review Questions

1. How do obstructive and restrictive pulmonary disease differ in terms of location, causes, and manifestations?
2. Why is the impact of lung disease so great? Can anything be done about it?
3. How are lung diseases detected and diagnosed?
4. What are the causes, lesions, and major manifestations of each of the specific diseases listed in this chapter?
5. What is the cause and significance of respiratory distress syndrome of the newborn?
6. What are the similarities and differences among lobar, broncho-, and interstitial pneumonia?
7. Why is pulmonary tuberculosis such an important disease? How do primary and secondary forms differ?
8. What are the two mechanisms of atelectasis?

9. What do the terms chronic obstructive pulmonary disease, chronic bronchitis, and emphysema mean?
10. How does emphysema differ from chronic noninfectious interstitial disease in terms of lesions, cause, and physiologic effect?
11. What is asthma?
12. Why is bronchogenic carcinoma the most important cancer in the United States today?
13. By what mechanisms does lung disease cause death?
14. What do the following terms mean?

> Ventilation
> Perfusion
> Pneumonia
> Dyspnea
> Orthopnea
> Hemoptysis
> Tachypnea
> Rales
> Hypercapnia
> Hyaline membrane
> Legionnaire's disease
> Emphysema
> Mycoplasma
> Ghon complex
> Adult respiratory distress syndrome
> Pneumoconiosis
> Anthracosis
> Silicosis
> Asbestosis
> Berylliosis
> Sarcoidosis

13.

Oral Region, Upper Respiratory Tract, and Ear

REVIEW OF STRUCTURE AND FUNCTION
Mouth • Salivary Glands • Nose • Pharynx • Larynx • Ear

MOST FREQUENT AND SERIOUS PROBLEMS
Dental Caries • Periodontal Disease • Upper Respiratory Infection •
Sinusitis • Allergic Rhinitis • Otitis Media • Carcinoma

SYMPTOMS, SIGNS, AND TESTS
Dental Screening • Pain • Loss of Hearing • Direct Examination •
X-rays • Throat Culture • Audiometry

SPECIFIC DISEASES
Genetic/Developmental Diseases
Cleft Lip and Cleft Palate
Inflammatory/Degenerative Diseases

Dental Caries
Periodontal Disease
Acute Necrotizing Ulcerative
   Gingivitis (Vincent's Infection,
   Trench Mouth)
Herpes Stomatitis (Cold Sores)
Aphthous Stomatitis
   (Canker Sores)

Upper Respiratory Infection
   (URI)
Sinusitis
Allergic Rhinitis (Hay Fever)
Otitis Media
Meniere's Syndrome
Presbycusis
Otosclerosis

Hyperplastic/Neoplastic Diseases
Squamous Cell Carcinoma
Salivary Gland Tumors
ORGAN FAILURE
Loss of Mastication • Swallowing Detects • Airway Obstruction •
Deafness

REVIEW QUESTIONS

REVIEW OF STRUCTURE AND FUNCTION

The structure and function of these organs are generally known to most persons, and their importance is exemplified by the number of specialists involved in health care of diseases of these organs (dentists—including many subspecialists; otolaryngologists, otologists, plastic surgeons, speech pathologists). The oral cavity, including teeth, tongue, and walls of the mouth, serves in the mastication and swallowing of food, as a phonetic box for speech, and as a secondary pathway for breathing. The salivary glands (parotid, submandibular, lingual, and minor salivary glands of the oral mucosa) provide moisture to soften and, of lesser importance, to add carbohydrate-digesting enzymes to the food.

The nose is a passageway for breathing and also partially filters air. Its upper portion contains the sense organ for smell. The pharynx serves as a passageway for air, provides the musculature for swallowing, and contains the openings of the eustachian tubes, which serve as pressure outlets for the middle ears. The pharynx also contains abundant lymphoid tissue, which aids in the recognition of antigens such as foreign materials and microorganisms. The larynx is a major air passage to the lungs and contains the vocal cords.

The ear detects sound and also contains in its inner portion the vestibular apparatus, which is a sensory organ for body equilibrium.

MOST FREQUENT AND SERIOUS PROBLEMS

Diseases of these organs account for an enormous proportion of health care problems. The most common include dental caries, periodontal disease, and upper respiratory infections. Other common diseases include sinusitis, allergic rhinitis, otitis media, and deafness. Of the relatively few potentially fatal conditions, carcinoma of the mouth, pharynx, and larynx are most common.

SYMPTOMS, SIGNS, AND TESTS

Dental caries is either asymptomatic or causes pain. Symptoms of periodontal disease include loose teeth and bleeding gums. Most instances of dental caries and periodontal disease are detected by screening (routine dental examination). The propensity of the nasal mucosa to secrete mucoid exudate in response to mild stimuli is well known to all sufferers of hay fever and the common cold. Pain is the principal symptom of sinusitis, pharyngitis, and otitis media. Loss of hearing occurs with many types of ear diseases. Bleeding from the mouth may signal periodontal disease, an ulcerating neoplasm, or may often be the first manifestation of a systemic bleeding disorder.

Most diseases of the organs under consideration are evaluated by direct vision with or without the aid of specialized instruments such as mirrors, laryngoscopes, and otoscopes. X-rays are particularly helpful in detection of disease in teeth and nasal sinuses. Function tests for hearing employ audiometers. The most important laboratory test is the throat culture for beta hemolytic streptococci, because treatment of streptococcal pharyngitis prevents rheumatic fever (see Chapter 8 for further discussion). Other laboratory tests are of value under a limited number of circumstances.

SPECIFIC DISEASES

Genetic/Developmental Diseases

Various rare types of abnormalities occur in the oral and ear structures that may be either isolated or occur in conjunction with defects of other organs. Cleft lip and cleft palate are two of the more common abnormalities of this area. Various forms and degrees of improper dental development may occur. The most common is *malocclusion* (improper contact between upper and lower teeth). Bizarre abnormalities of facial structure may occur in children with severe mental retardation; fortunately, most of these are rare.

Cleft Lip and Cleft Palate
Cleft lip, a defect on either side of the midline of the upper lip (Figure 13–1), occurs with or without cleft palate, a defect in the roof

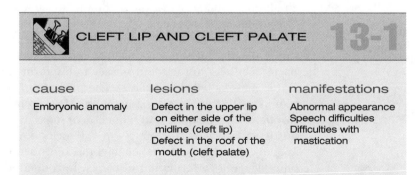

CLEFT LIP AND CLEFT PALATE 13-1		
cause	lesions	manifestations
Embryonic anomaly	Defect in the upper lip on either side of the midline (cleft lip) Defect in the roof of the mouth (cleft palate)	Abnormal appearance Speech difficulties Difficulties with mastication

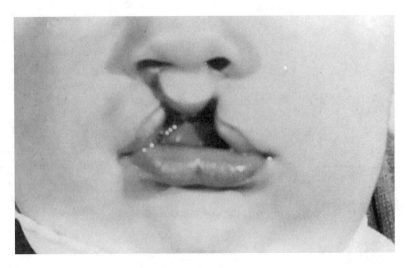

Figure 13–1. Cleft lip.

of the mouth connecting with the nasal cavity (Figure 13–2). These failures of late embryonic development usually can be corrected surgically to improve voice, mastication, and cosmetic appearance.

Inflammatory/Degenerative Diseases

Most health problems of the oral region, upper respiratory tract, and ear are acute or chronic infections. The most significant inflammatory diseases of these regions will be discussed followed by several less frequent but significant degenerative conditions of the ear.

Dental Caries

Caries is a microbial disease of the calcified portion of the teeth (enamel and dentin) characterized by demineralization. Caries is the disease that produces cavities in teeth. Disease activity is greatest in childhood so that caries is the predominant cause of tooth loss in persons under 35 years of age.

The cause of caries is complex, although bacteria are essential factors and a diet high in carbohydrate content is a contributing factor. Bacteria adhere to the tooth surface in the form of a tenacious nonvisible mass called *dental plaque*. The plaque can be made visible by staining with the red dye basic fuchsin. Daily removal of the plaque through tooth cleaning and reduction of sugar in the diet reduce the incidence of caries. Introduction of fluoride ion into the hydroxyapatite crystal of the dental enamel markedly decreases the susceptibility of teeth to formation of caries. Introduction of fluoride into

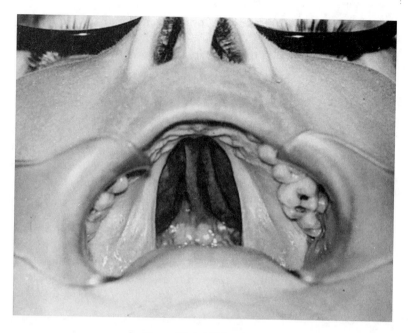

Figure 13–2. Cleft palate.

drinking water and tooth paste has reduced the incidence of caries by more than 75 percent over the past 40 years. Caries may erode into the central connective tissue core of a tooth (dental pulp), producing infection and necrosis of the pulp. Complications of pulpitis include tooth loss, periapical abscess, periapical granuloma, and periapical cyst. Abscess is the most acute and destructive complication. A periapical granuloma is not really a granuloma but rather a low-grade inflammation with abundant granulation tissue. Periapical cysts form

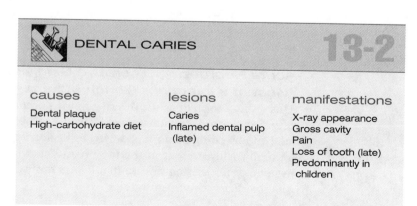

DENTAL CARIES   13-2

causes	lesions	manifestations
Dental plaque	Caries	X-ray appearance
High-carbohydrate diet	Inflamed dental pulp	Gross cavity
	(late)	Pain
		Loss of tooth (late)
		Predominantly in
		children

from islands of odontogenic epithelium that are trapped in a periapical granuloma and proliferate to form a squamous-lined cyst. Root canal therapy can prevent tooth loss due to pulpitis.

Periodontal Disease

Periodontal disease refers to a usually painless chronic low-grade inflammation of the supporting tissues of teeth. It is a disease of adults that increases in prevalence with age and is the major cause of tooth loss in adults. As with caries, dental plaque is the major etiologic factor. Accumulation of plaque on the tooth between tooth and gingiva produces a low-grade inflammation of the gingiva, which may be recognized by direct inspection as changes in color, texture, and amount of gingival tissue. Daily removal of plaque from between the teeth and gingiva with dental floss and brushing is the major means of preventing and reducing periodontal disease. If allowed to progress, the low-grade inflammation extends to the underlying alveolar bone and connective tissue, thus loosening the teeth and causing them to be extruded. Most adults have some degree of periodontal disease, but its severity varies greatly.

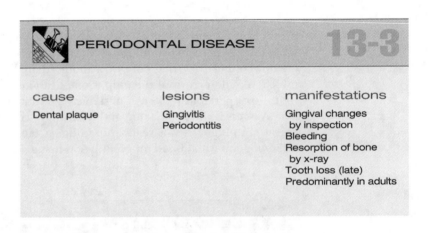

PERIODONTAL DISEASE 13-3

cause	lesions	manifestations
Dental plaque	Gingivitis Periodontitis	Gingival changes by inspection Bleeding Resorption of bone by x-ray Tooth loss (late) Predominantly in adults

Acute Necrotizing Ulcerative Gingivitis (Vincent's Infection, Trench Mouth)

This distinct form of acute, severe gingivitis occurs predominantly in young adults and is characterized by halitosis (bad breath) and ulcerated and bleeding gums. It is caused by fusiform and spirochetal bacteria, normally present in the mouth and associated with poor oral hygiene or underlying disease that lowers host resistance. Treatment is peroxide rinses and antibiotics.

Herpes Stomatitis (Cold Sores)

Herpes simplex type I is a very prevalent virus of humans. Following primary infection, herpes has the ability to lie dormant in nervous tissue until activated by stress, trauma, or immunosuppression. Its favorite site is the mucocutaneous border of the lips, gums, and hard palate, where it produces blisters followed by ulcerating and crusting inflammatory lesions when activated by sunburn or the fever of a common cold (Figure 13–3). The lesion will recur at intervals throughout life. Genital herpes is caused by a different virus (type II).

Aphthous Stomatitis (Canker Sores)

Aphthous means spot, *stoma* means mouth, so aphthous stomatitis is a painful inflammatory spot in the mouth. These are very discrete, shallow, painful ulcers within the mouth that gradually heal in 7 to 10 days (Figure 13–4). The lesions are similar to herpes stomatitis in that they are activated periodically, but differ from herpes in their discrete appearance and occur on nonkeratinized areas of the oral mucosa. The causative agent is unknown.

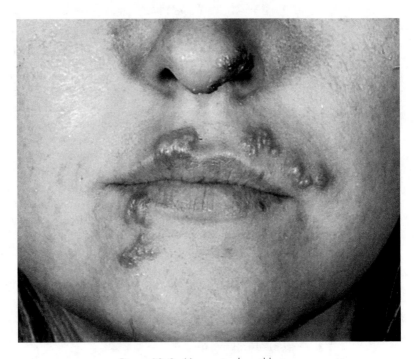

Figure 13–3. Herpes simplex cold sores.

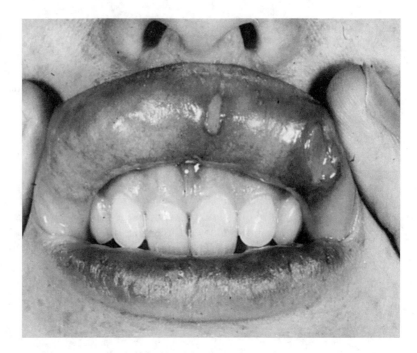

Figure 13–4. Aphthous stomatitis (canker sore).

Upper Respiratory Infection (URI)

This term encompasses a wide spectrum of illnesses in terms of sites, causative organisms, and severity. Inflammation of nasal sinuses, lung, and conjunctiva are commonly associated with upper respiratory infections. Terms based on site include *rhinitis* (nose), *pharyngitis, tonsillitis,* and *laryngitis.* Terms based on cause include viral sore throat and streptococcal sore throat. Nonspecific terms include *common cold, sore throat, flu,* and *coryza. Coryza* is a descriptive term meaning profuse nasal discharge. Most upper respiratory infections are caused by viruses of various types that are not ordinarily identified. Rhinoviruses are the most common cause. A few cases are caused by group A beta hemolytic streptococci. It needs to be emphasized that the amount of redness and exudate in the throat and the white blood count are not reliable in distinguishing viral from bacterial upper respiratory infections. Both may be mild or severe, both may be associated with elevated white blood counts. Throat culture will detect beta hemolytic streptococcus and the numbers (many versus few) present will help distinguish persons with strep throat from persons who are merely carriers of the organisms.

Upper respiratory infections are the most significant cause of work loss in adults, but complications are more common in children and in

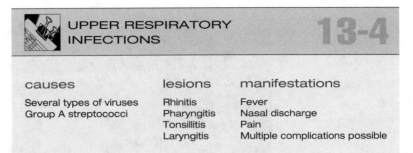

causes	lesions	manifestations
Several types of viruses	Rhinitis	Fever
Group A streptococci	Pharyngitis	Nasal discharge
	Tonsillitis	Pain
	Laryngitis	Multiple complications possible

the elderly. In children, the abundant lymphoid tissue of the naso-pharynx (adenoids) and pharyngeal tonsils enlarge in response to upper respiratory infections. Commonly, the enlargement of the adenoids surrounding openings of the eustachian tubes blocks these openings and predisposes to middle ear infection (otitis media). Repeated bouts of otitis media may be cause for removal of the adenoids. Enlarged tonsils may partially obstruct breathing and sometimes are removed for this reason. Pneumonia is a frequent complication of upper respiratory infections in both children and the elderly. Epidemics of upper respiratory infections increase the death rate of the elderly. Sometimes, upper respiratory infections predominantly involve the larynx, producing edema, partial obstruction, and difficult inspiration. In children, this produces a condition known as *croup*, a laryngeal spasm characterized by a loud, high-pitched, inspiratory sound, which is frightening to the patient because of inability to breathe and to bystanders because of the labored respiration. Usually the edema can be reduced with great relief. In adults, laryngitis is manifest by a rough quality to the voice (hoarseness).

Two other uncommon but serious respiratory infections are whooping cough and *Haemophilus influenzae* infection. These will be discussed in the chapter on infectious diseases (Chapter 26).

Sinusitis

Infection in the paranasal sinuses is a cause of pain and headache in some individuals. Obstruction of the opening to sinus cavities leads to fluid accumulation and infection (Figure 13–5). Treatment that reduces the inflammatory swelling in the lining epithelium of the sinus and its opening may allow the exudate to drain and the infection to be brought under control. Sometimes the sinus opening must be surgically enlarged to allow drainage. Chronic infections with continuous drainage into the pharynx (postnasal drip) may lead to pulmonary infections. Sinusitis is the most common chronic medical condition overall.

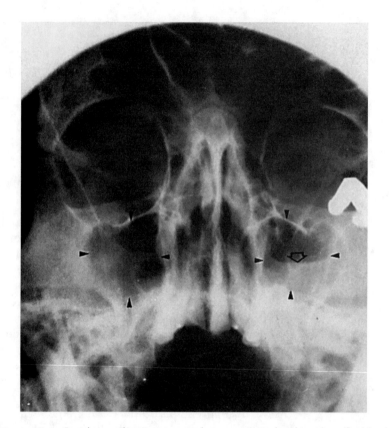

Figure 13–5. Facial x-ray showing paranasal sinuses (*arrow heads*) and air/fluid level (*open arrow*) in patient's left sinus due to chronic sinusitis and obstruction of the opening to the sinus.

Allergic Rhinitis (Hay Fever)

Hay fever is an outpouring of watery exudate from the nose due to mild inflammation, which is in turn caused by exposure to antigenic substances in the environment. Ragweed pollen is the most important seasonal allergen, although various other pollens may be the cause in some individuals. House dust and dander from pets are important causes of chronic allergic rhinitis. In some individuals, the boggy, swollen nasal mucosa may form polyps, which obstruct breathing and require surgical removal. Allergic rhinitis is also covered in Chapter 27 as an immunologic condition.

Otitis Media

Otitis media is inflammation of the middle ear. It is most common in young children as a sequela of upper respiratory infections. Pharyngeal edema causes obstruction of the eustachian tube, with resultant

OTITIS MEDIA   13-5

causes	lesion	manifestations
Obstruction of eustachian tube Bacteria Viruses	Inflammation of the middle ear	Pain Swollen, red eardrum Multiple complications possible

spread of infection through the eustachian tube to the middle ear. In most instances, the otitis media is presumed to be caused by bacteria, although culture is usually not performed because of the inaccessible location of the middle ear behind the eardrum. Antibiotic therapy usually is curative, although some children are subject to repeated episodes of otitis media. Otitis media is suspected in a child who may be irritable and who can often localize the pain to one ear. Inspection through an otoscope reveals a swollen, inflamed eardrum (Figure 13–6). Complications of otitis media include rupture of the eardrum, with drainage of pus and mastoiditis due to spread of the infection to surrounding mastoid bone. The development of mastoiditis is particularly serious, because it may lead to permanent hearing loss or spread of infection into the brain. Chronic low-grade otitis media may lead to the formation of a mass of keratinized tissue called a *cholesteatoma.*

Meniere's Syndrome
Meniere's syndrome is a degenerative disease in which the vestibular apparatus becomes dilated with fluid. The symptoms of Meniere's syndrome are *tinnitus* (ringing in the ears), deafness, and episodic *vertigo* (illusion of movement).

Presbycusis
Hearing loss accompanying increasing age is called *presbycusis* and may be due to continued exposure to noise as well as vascular changes.

Otosclerosis
Otosclerosis is a fixation of the small bones in the middle ear, which conduct vibrations from the eardrum to the inner ear. Its cause is unknown, and it most commonly occurs in young women, resulting in gradual hearing loss. Operative mobilization of these tiny bones may improve sound conduction.

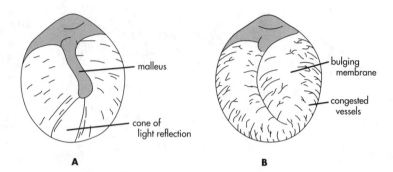

Figure 13–6. Eardrum: normal (A) and otitis media (B). In otitis media, normal landmarks on the eardrum (visualization of the malleus through the eardrum and the light reflex) disappear and bulging of the membrane and vascular congestion become evident.

Hyperplastic/Neoplastic Diseases

Squamous Cell Carcinoma

Carcinoma of the lip usually occurs on the lower lip because exposure to sunlight is the most important etiologic factor. Smoking is the most important factor in the genesis of laryngeal cancer. Some poorly differentiated pharyngeal cancers are associated with the Epstein-Barr virus. Most importantly, mouth cancers are greatly potentiated by the combined use of alcohol and tobacco and appear to be related to the dose of each. The early precancerous lesions in alcohol/tobacco abusers appear as reddened areas on thin, nonkeratinized areas of squamous epithelium (floor of mouth, ventrolateral tongue, and soft palate). Chewing tobacco has a high association with the development of oral cancer.

Squamous cell carcinomas present as expanding, ulcerating, and encrusted lesions (Figure 13–7). Most lip cancers (90 percent) are cured because the lesion can be detected early before lymph node metastasis has occurred and because resection or irradiation are relatively easy procedures. About two-thirds of laryngeal carcinomas are cured by resection, which is sometimes combined with irradiation. Carcinomas of the mouth and pharynx have the worst prognosis (about 50 percent) because lymph node metastasis is often present by the time of diagnosis.

Salivary Gland Tumors

Most salivary gland neoplasms arise in the parotid gland, and the majority are benign. The so-called *mixed tumor,* or pleomorphic adenoma, is the most common of several types.

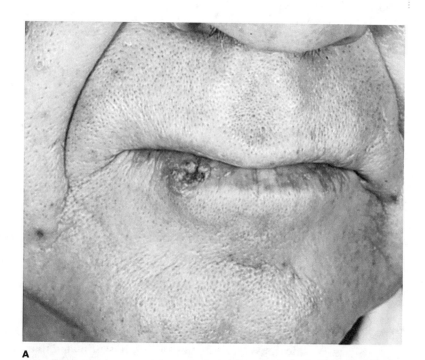

A

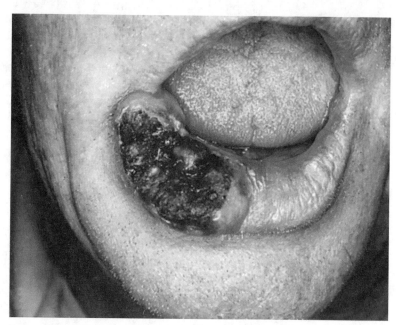

B

Figure 13–7. Squamous cell carcinoma of the lower lip; early lesion (A) and advanced lesion (B).

ORGAN FAILURE

Loss of ability to masticate (chew) is associated with loss of teeth, fractures of the mandible, extensive cancer operations, and severe congenital abnormalities. Swallowing may be defective with paralysis from poliomyelitis or stroke. Obstruction of the airway may be due to allergic nasal polyps or enlarged lymphoid tissue in the pharynx. Impaction of a large piece of meat in the lower pharynx is an occasional cause of sudden death.

Any person with a detectable hearing impairment may be described as relatively deaf, although the essence of deafness as we generally use the word is the inability to hear and understand the spoken voice. The types of deafness are usually divided into *nerve deafness*, in which there is interruption of the cochlear nerve, and *conduction deafness*, in which there is disease of the middle ear or occlusion of the external auditory canal. This separation is somewhat artificial, as many conditions, such as infection, can damage several components of the ear.

The true incidence of deafness as well as the relative causes of deafness are difficult to assess. It is estimated that there is a prevalence rate of up to 16 cases of deafness per 1000 school children in which the hearing loss is severe enough to at least require a hearing aid. About half of these cases are due to genetic conditions, whereas in the other half deafness is acquired. Most of the acquired cases in the past have been due to rubella in which there is inner ear damage. The prevalence of deafness increases linearly with age to the point where over 60 percent of persons above the age of 65 have a major impairment of hearing. The most common cause of hearing loss in the elderly is usually ascribed to presbycusis; however, this is begging the question, as presbycusis simply means hearing loss in the elderly. It is generally agreed that continued noise exposure, degeneration of ossicles, trauma, and infection are the most common contributing factors to deafness in adults; however, the relative incidence of each of these factors is unknown. Other known causes of deafness in persons of all ages include otosclerosis, cholesteatoma, Meniere's syndrome, neoplasms, psychogenic causes, and toxins. Some of the drugs that are known to produce sensorineural hearing loss are aspirin, neomycin, quinine, and streptomycin.

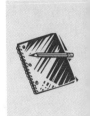

Review Questions

1. What are the most common diseases of the mouth, ear, and upper respiratory tract? How are they usually diagnosed?
2. Why is a throat culture such an important laboratory test?
3. What are the causes, lesions, and major manifestations of each of the specific diseases discussed in this chapter?
4. How does cleft lip differ from cleft palate?
5. What are the similarities and differences between dental caries and periodontal disease?
6. What are the major complications of upper respiratory infections?
7. How do squamous cell carcinomas of the lip, mouth, and larynx differ as to cause and prognosis?
8. What is the difference between nerve deafness and conduction deafness?
9. What do the following terms mean?
   Dental plaque
   Coryza
   Croup
   Mastoiditis
   Cholesteatoma
   Tinnitus
   Vertigo
   Presbycusis
   Mixed tumor

14.
Alimentary Tract

REVIEW OF STRUCTURE AND FUNCTION
Esophagus • Stomach • Small Intestine • Large Intestine, Including Vermiform Appendix • Anus • Propulsive Movement Through the Alimentary Tract • The Digestive Process • Effects of Removal of Parts of the Alimentary Tract

MOST FREQUENT AND SERIOUS PROBLEMS
Constipation • Diarrhea • Functional Bowel Syndrome • Viral Enteritis • Overindulgence in Alcohol • Hemorrhoids • Pilondal Sinuses and Abscess • Duodenal and Gastric Ulcer • Carcinoma of the Colon • Polyps of the Colon • Diverticulosis • Reflux Esophagitis • Inguinal Hernia • Acute Appendicitis • Pruritis Ani • Inflammatory Bowel Disease • Carcinoma of the Esophagus • Carcinoma of the Stomach • Esophageal Varices • Infarction of the Bowel • Peritonitis

SYMPTOMS, SIGNS, AND TESTS
Manifestations of Bleeding
Hematemesis • Melena • Hematochezia • Occult Focal Blood Test
Manifestations of Altered Motility
Distention • Vomiting • Hyperactive Bowel Sounds • Ileus • Adynamic Ileus • Diarrhea • Constipation • Dysphagia
Manifestations of Perforation
Pain • Rigid Abdomen • Adynamic Ileus • Fever • Leukocytosis
Tests and Procedures
Upper GI Series • Barium Enema • Sigmoidoscopy • Upper Gastrointestinal Endoscopy • Gastric Analysis • Absorption Tests • Fecal Ova and Parasites • Fecal Culture for Bacterial Pathogens

SPECIFIC DISEASES
Genetic/Developmental Diseases
Malformations
Congenital Pyloric Stenosis
Hirschsprung's Disease

Inflammatory/Degenerative Diseases
Infectious Diarrheas and Food Poisoning
Viral Enteritis • *Traveler's Diarrhea* • *Staphylococcal Food Poisoning*
• *Salmonella Food Infection* • *Shigellosis* • *Amebiasis* •
Campylobacter Enteritis
Reflux Esophagitis
Gastritis
Peptic Ulcer
Malabsorption Syndrome
Acute Appendicitis
Pseudomembranous Enterocolitis
Inflammatory Bowel Disease
Colonic Diverticulosis
Inguinal Hernia
Hyperplastic/Neoplastic Diseases
Carcinoma of Stomach
Colonic Polyps
Carcinoma of the Colon

ORGAN FAILURE

REVIEW QUESTIONS

REVIEW OF STRUCTURE AND FUNCTION

The *digestive* or *gastrointestinal system* includes the *oral region* (mouth, salivary glands, pharynx), the *alimentary tract* (esophagus, stomach, small intestine, large intestine, including the vermiform appendix, and anus), and the *pancreaticobiliary tract* (liver, gallbladder, bile ducts, pancreas). The function of the alimentary tract is to digest masticated food, to absorb digestion products, and to excrete the residue along with certain waste products excreted by the liver through the bile duct. The segments of the alimentary tract are reviewed in Figure 14–1.

The esophagus is a straight tube that serves to carry food from the pharynx to the stomach. The stomach is a distensible organ, particularly in its upper part, or body. The stomach body mucosal cells secrete hydrochloric acid and proteolytic enzymes, which aid in digestion. The mucosa of the lower part of the stomach, or antrum, is lined by mucous cells. The extreme distal end of the stomach is often called the *pylorus.* The small intestine is artificially divided into duodenum, jejunum, and ileum. Although some digestion occurs at the surface of the small intestinal mucosa, its major function is absorption. The large intestine, or colon, is also artificially divided into segments consisting of cecum, ascending colon, transverse colon, descending colon, sig-

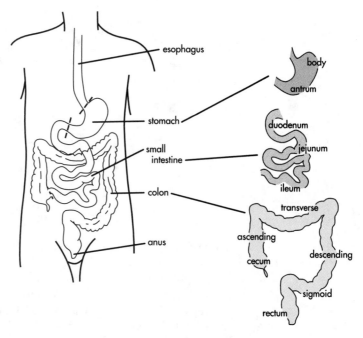

Figure 14–1. Major parts of the alimentary tract.

moid colon, and rectum. The vermiform appendix is a nonfunctional vestigial structure attached to the cecum. The colon is a storage reservoir for undigested food and also is a site of water absorption.

The alimentary tract has four layers—mucosa, submucosa, muscularis, and serosa (Figure 14–2A). The mucosal layer has three components—*epithelium* lining the surface, supporting connective tissue called the *lamina propria*, and a unique thin muscular layer called the *muscularis mucosae* (Figure 14–2B). The structure of inner mucosal layer is varied to provide the specialized function of each level of the tract: the esophagus is lined by stratified squamous epithelium, which promotes rapid gliding of masticated food from the mouth to the stomach; the stomach is lined by a thick glandular mucosa, which provides mucus, acid, and proteolytic enzymes to help break up food; the small intestinal mucosa has a villous structure, which provides a large surface of cells for active absorption; and the large intestinal mucosa is lined by abundant mucus-secreting cells, which facilitate storage and evacuation of the residue. Beneath the mucosa is the submucosa, a layer unique to the alimentary tract, which provides structural support to the tract because of the abundant collagenous tissue present. The muscle layer contracts rhythmically to move materials through the alimentary tract. The serosal layer is a thin, smooth membrane present on the outer surface of those parts of the alimentary

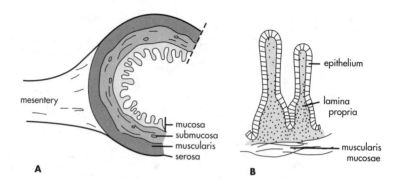

Figure 14–2. A. Layers of the wall of the alimentary tract. B. Components of the mucosal layer.

tract that lie within the abdominal cavity. It keeps the highly tortuous loops of bowel from becoming tangled. The serosa is continuous with the mesentery—the connective tissue attachment of the bowel that contains blood vessels, lymphatics, and nerves.

In order for the intestinal tract to carry out its job of digestion, absorption, and excretion, the contents of the lumen must be propelled along the tract at the appropriate rate, and reverse movement must be prevented. A wave of muscle contractions (peristalsis) carries a bolus of swallowed food down the esophagus, and a sphincter at the lower end of the esophagus prevents regurgitation. Contractions in the stomach emanate as waves from the body of the stomach and proceed toward the distal stomach (pylorus). They serve to mix the digesting food and push the partially digested contents into the duodenum. The greater the distention of the stomach, the stronger the contractions and the more rapid the emptying.

The muscle of the pylorus only partially closes the outlet to the stomach, so intestinal contents can regurgitate into the stomach, particularly when the small intestine is not emptying normally. Excessive distention of the stomach may result in vomiting, a process in which the esophageal sphincter opens to allow abdominal contractions to forcibly propel gastric and small intestinal contents upward through the esophagus. Under normal conditions, movement of lumenal contents of the small intestine is most rapid in the upper small intestine and decelerates distally. Contents gradually pass from the ileum to the cecum, and reverse movement is partially prevented by the ileocecal valve. The rate of movement in the colon depends on the amount of solid material that remains and the water content. Water is absorbed in the colon to make the contents solid, and the solid residue is moved to the left side of the colon and rectum. When the rectum becomes distended, an urge for voluntary relaxation of the anal sphincter to induce defecation occurs.

The digestive process begins in the mouth, where carbohydrate-splitting enzymes (amylases) from the salivary glands mix with food during mastication. In the stomach, proteolytic enzymes (pepsin) and hydrochloric acid are added to speed the digestive process. The greatest volume of digestive enzymes are added to the digesting mixture of food in the duodenum and originate from the pancreas. These include more amylases, more proteolytic enzymes (trypsins), and fat-splitting enzymes (lipases). In addition, bile salts, which are contained in bile secreted by the liver and stored in the gallbladder, are added to emulsify lipids into small water-soluble packets called *micelles*. The final phase of the digestive process occurs in the surface of small intestinal epithelial cells, where carbohydrate-splitting enzymes (disaccharidases) and protein-splitting enzymes (dipeptidases) are present. Complex endocrine and nervous mechanisms coordinate the timing of the secretion and storage of digestive enzymes, hydrochloric acid, and bile salts so that appropriate amounts are available when needed. For example, the sight of food may induce salivation and gastric secretions via nervous stimulation; distention of the gastric antrum causes release of gastrin, a hormone that stimulates acid production and gastric emptying; and emptying of food into the duodenum causes secretion of the hormones secretin and pancreozymin, which, in turn, cause the pancreas to secrete more fluid and enzymes and the gallbladder to empty bile into the duodenum.

Because many lesions of the alimentary tract are treated by surgical removal, it is important to know what parts can be removed and the physiologic consequences of removal. Short segments of large intestine, small intestine, and stomach and the entire vermiform appendix can be removed without significant functional impairment. Mild to moderate disability may be encountered with removal of all of the large intestine, large segments of small intestine, large segments or all of the stomach, and any part of the esophagus. Continuity of the alimentary tract with the pancreas and liver is essential for survival. Of the major operations that cause functional impairment, the two most common are removal of the distal two-thirds of the stomach for treatment of peptic ulcer and removal of the colon for inflammatory bowel disease.

MOST FREQUENT AND SERIOUS PROBLEMS

The most common problem confronting patients is functional alteration of movement through the alimentary tract. *Constipation* refers to infrequent and/or difficult evacuation of feces. *Diarrhea* refers to abnormally frequent and liquid stools. Constipation is frequently associated with a low-bulk diet and with aging. Diarrhea may be a manifestation of anxiety or due to organic disease. The most common functional alteration of the alimentary tract is called *functional (irritable) bowel syndrome,* or *spastic colon.* The symptoms are variable and include constipation, diarrhea, and crampy abdominal pain. The functional bowel syndrome mimics many organic diseases and is the most common malady of the alimentary tract.

There are many organic diseases of the alimentary tract that cause temporary or prolonged disability but are rarely fatal. The most common of these is viral enteritis (intestinal flu). Manifestations include nausea, vomiting, and diarrhea. The course is self-limited and the cause is most often a virus. Acute overindulgence in alcoholic beverages produces an illness similar to viral enteritis, although muscle aches and pains and fever are less frequent and the duration is often shorter. Diverticulosis of the colon and esophageal hiatal hernia are common conditions in older people but only occasionally cause symptoms. Inguinal hernia is an outpouching of the abdominal cavity into the groin that may trap loops of bowel. Preventative repair of inguinal hernias is the most common abdominal operation. Acute appendicitis is the most frequent indication for operations on the alimentary tract itself. Diseases of the anus are very common and an important source of discomfort to patients. Mild anal problems include itching in children due to pinworms, simple itching in adults (pruritis ani), and hemorrhoids. More severe anal lesions include thrombosed hemorrhoids, fissures, abscesses, and pilonidal sinuses.

Common conditions that require more extensive health care include duodenal and gastric ulcers, carcinoma of the colon, polyps of the colon, and inflammatory bowel disease (ulcerative colitis and Crohn's disease). Of these lesions, carcinoma of the colon is fatal about 40 percent of the time, the others being infrequently fatal. Lesions of the alimentary tract with a very low survival rate include carcinoma of the esophagus, carcinoma of the stomach, esophageal varices, infarction of the bowel due to occlusion of the mesenteric artery, and perforation with generalized peritonitis regardless of cause.

SYMPTOMS, SIGNS, AND TESTS

Many manifestations of alimentary tract disease can be related to hemorrhage, altered motility, and perforation. Hemorrhage may be mild or severe and may originate from the upper or lower part of the tract. Severe hemorrhage from the upper alimentary tract (esophagus, stomach, duodenum) leads to *hematemesis* (vomiting of blood). Vomited blood is bright red if fresh or has the appearance of coffee grounds if it has been altered by acid in the stomach. Severe upper tract bleeding will also produce melena (black tarry stools) due to alteration of the blood as it passes down the tract. Severe bleeding from the lower alimentary tract produces bright red blood in the stool (*hematochezia*). Mild bleeding from the upper or lower tract will not be noticed by the patient or produce gross color changes in the feces, but can be detected by chemical tests of the feces for hemoglobin (occult fecal blood test). In any patient with severe gastrointestinal bleeding, it is most important to look for evidence of low blood volume so that transfusions can be given before shock develops. Mild, prolonged bleeding will lead to loss of iron and eventually to iron-deficiency anemia. Mild bleeding tends to be an early manifestation of gastrointestinal cancers, so fecal blood tests and blood counts constitute important routine screening tests for persons in the cancer age range (over 40).

Manifestations of altered motility may be due to obstruction or altered activity of the bowel. Obstruction of the alimentary tract may be partial or complete. Complete obstruction will lead to distention of the bowel proximal to the obstruction and then to vomiting. The distended segment will be muscularly active in its attempt to overcome the obstruction, producing a sloshing of the liquid contents with resultant increase in "bowel sounds." The two most common causes of intestinal obstruction are trapped bowel in an inguinal hernia and twisting of bowel around a fibrous adhesion resulting from a previous abdominal operation. Obstruction usually requires surgical operation for diagnosis and treatment.

Altered motility without obstruction may be responsible for vomiting, ileus, diarrhea, constipation, or dysphagia. Vomiting is a common nonspecific symptom that may be associated with generalized illness, central nervous system disease, or intestinal disease. *Ileus* refers to dilation of the intestines. *Adynamic ileus* refers to ileus with absent bowel sounds because the intestinal musculature is hypoactive; the bowel is not physically obstructed. Adynamic ileus occurs most commonly during the first few days after abdominal operations and is one of the reasons for intravenous feeding following operation. When ileus is present, gastrointestinal contents may be vomited and aspirated producing pneumonia.

Diarrhea and constipation are most commonly functional; however, organic diseases of the colon must be considered if these symptoms are severe or prolonged.

Dysphagia is difficulty in swallowing. It may be caused by a variety of esophageal lesions.

Perforation of the intestinal tract into the peritoneal cavity is life threatening because of the massive seeding of intestinal bacteria and ease of spread of the peritonitis within the cavity. Inflammation of the peritoneal lining causes pain, muscle contraction leading to a rigid abdomen, and adynamic ileus. Systemic manifestations include fever and leukocytosis. Causes of perforation include peptic ulcer, trauma to the abdomen, infarcts, and untreated appendicitis.

Pain is also an important manifestation of gastrointestinal disease. The location, duration, and time sequence of pain may help localize the cause. Sudden severe abdominal pain suggests the possibility of perforation or sudden twisting of bowel. Duodenal ulcers produce a chronic, nonradiating, burning, epigastric pain perceived as deep to the abdominal wall. Heartburn, a burning substernal discomfort, is a typical symptom of esophagitis. The initial manifestation of appendicitis is pain in the umbilicus, which shifts to the right lower quadrant of the abdomen as it becomes more severe.

Because there is a wide variety of lesions that can produce the major manifestations described above, it is usually necessary to search for specific lesions using radiologic and endoscopic procedures. The radiologist can outline the normal and abnormal anatomic features of most segments of the gastrointestinal tract by placing a radiopaque material (barium) in the lumen. *Upper GI series* refers to radiologic examination of esophagus, stomach, and upper small intestine. *Barium enema* refers to radiologic examination of the colon. *Endoscopic procedures* refers to the use of a tube or scope to look inside a body passageway. Most endoscopes are equipped with biopsy forceps to obtain tissue so that the pathologist can make a specific histologic diagnosis. *Sigmoidoscopy,* the most common endoscopic procedure, is used to visualize the rectum and lower sigmoid colon. Using highly developed instruments, the specialized gastroenterologist may also directly visualize and biopsy lesions at higher levels of the colon and at all levels of the upper gastrointestinal tract. *Upper gastrointestinal endoscopy* is used to visualize and biopsy lesions of the esophagus, stomach, and the first portion of the duodenum. *Colonoscopy* is used to visualize and biopsy lesions of the entire colon and distal ileum.

The measurement of acid in the stomach is called *gastric analysis.* Its use is limited except to demonstrate the absence of acid (achlorhydria) or rare patients with very high acid output. Laboratory tests on gastrointestinal contents, blood, and urine may be used to evaluate absorption from the alimentary tract by calculating oral intake and output from feces and urine or rise and fall of blood levels of the nutrient under study. Several types of tests for carbohydrate and fat may be used to detect malabsorption. Examination of feces for ova and parasites is used to find ameba and helminths in the gastrointestinal tract. Fecal culture is used to identify specific bacterial pathogens.

SPECIFIC DISEASES

Genetic/Developmental Diseases

Developmental abnormalities include a number of embryonic malformations that are usually surgically correctable unless they are associated with other more serious malformations or are associated with problems of prematurity. In addition to malformations, pyloric stenosis, a condition of uncertain cause, and Hirschsprung's disease, a disease of defective innervation, will be discussed.

Malformations

Meckel's diverticulum is an outpouching of the ileum (Figure 14–3A) that results from a failure of the embryonic connection with the yolk sac to disappear. It occurs in 2 percent of the population and is usually discovered at autopsy. Occasionally, disease in a Meckel's diverticulum leads to hemorrhage, inflammation, or obstruction of the ileum.

Esophageal atresia is the absence of part of the esophagus so that the upper esophagus ends as a blind pouch (Figure 14–3B). Usually there is a connection of the trachea to the distal esophagus (tracheoesophageal fistula).

Congenital diaphragmatic hernia is a hole in the diaphragm separating the abdomen from the thorax (Figure 14–3C). Portions of the alimentary tract may herniate through the hole at birth or later to compress the lungs and impair breathing.

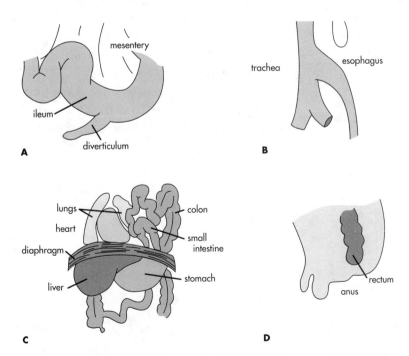

Figure 14–3. Four examples of embryonic anomalies of the alimentary tract. A. Meckel's diverticulum of the ileum. B. Tracheoesophageal fistula. C. Diaphragmatic hernia. D. Imperforate anus.

Imperforate anus is a failure of the anus to connect with the rectum (Figure 14–3D). There may be associated openings (fistulae) from the rectum to the bladder, urethra, or vagina.

These malformations as well as others that either compromise breathing or obstruct the intestinal tract must be repaired surgically to prevent a fatal outcome.

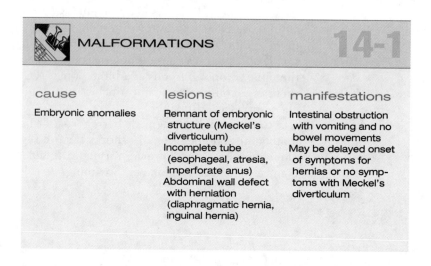

MALFORMATIONS   14-1

cause	lesions	manifestations
Embryonic anomalies	Remnant of embryonic structure (Meckel's diverticulum) Incomplete tube (esophageal, atresia, imperforate anus) Abdominal wall defect with herniation (diaphragmatic hernia, inguinal hernia)	Intestinal obstruction with vomiting and no bowel movements May be delayed onset of symptoms for hernias or no symptoms with Meckel's diverticulum

Congenital Pyloric Stenosis

Congenital pyloric stenosis is a narrowing of the outlet of the distal stomach due to hypertrophy of the muscle (Figure 14–4). The cause is unknown, and for some reason, symptoms of projectile vomiting after feeding do not begin until 2 to 4 weeks after birth. Other than

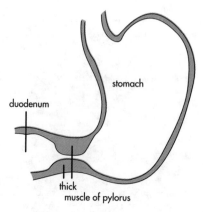

Figure 14–4. Pyloric stenosis.

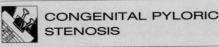

CONGENITAL PYLORIC STENOSIS		14-2
cause	**lesion**	**manifestations**
Unknown	Thickened muscle or distal stomach (pylorus)	Onset at age 2 to 4 weeks Usually in boys Dehydration and weight loss Relieved by splitting thickened muscle

Meckel's diverticulum, this is the most common developmental abnormality of the alimentary tract. It occurs almost exclusively in boys. A simple operation to split the thickened pyloric muscle effects a cure.

Hirschsprung's Disease

A lack of nerve (ganglion) cells in the rectum results in defective evacuation of feces from the rectum, with consequent massive distention of the colon with feces (megacolon) (Figure 14–5). Hirschsprung's disease is suspected in children with chronic constipation and distended abdomen, diagnosed by rectal biopsy to demonstrate absence of ganglion cells, and treated by surgical removal of the aganglionic segment.

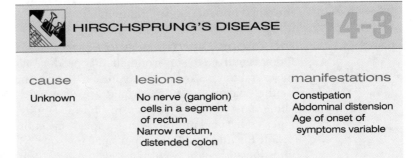

HIRSCHSPRUNG'S DISEASE		14-3
cause	**lesions**	**manifestations**
Unknown	No nerve (ganglion) cells in a segment of rectum Narrow rectum, distended colon	Constipation Abdominal distension Age of onset of symptoms variable

Inflammatory/Degenerative Diseases

The diseases discussed in this section illustrate the great variety of conditions that involve the alimentary tract. Infectious diarrheas and food poisoning are diseases acquired from the environment. Esophagitis,

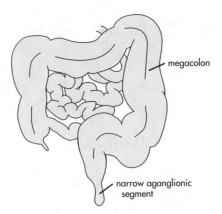

Figure 14-5. Hirschsprung's disease.

gastritis, and peptic ulcers are nagging, mostly chronic problems. The malabsorption syndrome, although relatively uncommon, illustrates the many ways that small intestinal function can be interfered with. Acute appendicitis is well known because it is frequent and strikes suddenly without warning. Pseudomembranous enterocolitis is an acute, life-threatening condition usually induced by antibiotic therapy. Ulcerative colitis and Crohn's disease, collectively known as inflammatory bowel disease, are chronic, usually lifelong conditions that require a lot of medical care. Colonic diverticulosis is an acquired structural defect with inflammatory complications. Inguinal hernia may be either congenital or acquired and is important as a cause of intestinal obstruction and infarction.

Infectious Diarrheas and Food Poisoning

Organisms from the environment may produce gastrointestinal disease in several ways. Most microorganisms that are ingested are destroyed by the acid in the stomach and are digested or pass through the alimentary tract without causing harm. Highly virulent organisms ingested in small numbers can escape destruction in the stomach and invade the mucosa of the upper small intestine (viruses) or distal small intestine and colon (*ameba, shigella, campylobacter*). The intestines may also serve as a portal of entry for systemic disease (e.g., typhoid fever). Intestinal diseases caused by highly virulent organisms are typically spread by the fecal–oral route. Small amounts of fecal material contaminate much of people's immediate environment and, in many areas of the world, the water supply is also contaminated. Microorganisms that are less virulent and/or are more susceptible to destruction in the stomach must be ingested in larger numbers in order to get sufficient numbers into the intestines to cause disease. Intestinal disease caused by microorganisms of low or intermediate virulence (e.g., most salmonellae) are typically associated with food poisoning—sufficient numbers of organisms must proliferate in food and be ingested in order to overcome the host's defenses. Another form of food poisoning involves bacteria growing in food and producing a toxin. The toxin, not the bacteria, causes disease of the stomach and upper small intestine (staphylococcal food poisoning) or the toxin is absorbed and damages the nervous system (botulism).

Viral enteritis (intestinal flu) is the most common type of gastrointestinal infection and is caused by normal daily contact with infected individuals. Rotavirus (mostly in infants) and Norwalk agent are the most common causes, but a variety of other viruses may cause gastroenteritis. Viral enteritis is both seasonal (epidemic) and sporadic. Children are more commonly involved than adults. The virus grows in surface epithelial cells of the small intestine, leading in 1 to 2 days to nausea, vomiting, diarrhea, and malaise (a vague feeling of discomfort) that lasts from one to several days. Diagnosis is presumptive, because there are no routine tests for viral enteritis. Prevention is not practical, and treatment is not needed unless there is excessive fluid loss from vomiting and diarrhea.

Traveler's diarrhea refers to any acute diarrheal illness in travelers to foreign countries. Natives can obviously be affected by the same disease, but they are more likely to be immune or have a low-grade chronic involvement. Causes are multiple. Recent studies have implicated enterotoxin-producing strains of *Escherichia coli* as the most common cause. These strains are not easily separated from harmless strains of *E. coli* normally present in the colon. Enterotoxin-producing *E. coli* proliferate in the small intestine and liberate their enterotoxin, which in turn causes outpouring of fluid into the intestinal lumen. The affected person may be mildly inconvenienced by diarrhea and abdominal cramps or completely incapacitated for one to several days. Traveler's diarrhea is most frequent in places where the water supply is contaminated by sewage. Prevention consists of avoidance of nonsterile fluids and uncooked foods such as salads. Specific diagnosis is difficult.

Staphylococcal food poisoning and salmonella food infection are both caused by contamination of food. When several people who have eaten together become ill with vomiting and diarrhea, food poisoning should be suspected. If the time from exposure to illness is short (1 to 4 hours), it is likely that toxins produced by certain strains of staphylococci have caused the illness. The bacteria can contaminate unrefrigerated food and liberate their enterotoxins. The enterotoxins, when ingested with the food, injure the mucosal lining of the stomach and small intestine, producing an illness that usually lasts less than 1 day. Salmonella food infection occurs when large numbers of salmonella are ingested and reach the distal alimentary tract, where these bacteria are capable of invading the mucosa and causing illness. Because large

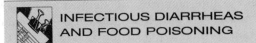

INFECTIOUS DIARRHEAS AND FOOD POISONING

14-4

	causes	lesions	manifestations
Viral enteritis	Viruses	Superficial damage to small-intestinal mucosa	Acute onset Diarrhea and vomiting Dehydration if severe Often epidemic 1- to 2-day duration
Traveler's diarrhea	Toxigenic *Escherichia coli* Many other possible agents	Often none	Acute onset Diarrhea Abdominal cramps Generalized malaise 1- to 2-day duration
Staphylococcal food poisoning	Toxin produced by staphylococci growing in food	Superficial damage to gastric and upper small-intestinal mucosa	Vomiting and diarrhea Acute onset 1 to 4 hours after eating food Usually several people involved 1-day duration
Salmonella food infection	Eating food contaminated by large numbers of salmonella	Mild inflammation of colonic mucosa	Acute onset 1 to 2 days after eating contaminated food Diarrhea and vomiting Malaise Duration of several days Resolves without treatment
Shigellosis	Bacterial infection by shigella	Severe inflammation of colonic mucosa with ulcers	Acute onset Bloody diarrhea Abdominal cramps Malaise Unsanitary environment Positive stool culture Lasts several days and occasionally fatal if untreated
Amebiasis	Protozoal infection by *Entameba histolytica*	Discrete colonic ulcers	Gradual onset Bloody diarrhea Unsanitary environment or recent travel to endemic areas Ameba seen on fecal smear Gradual recovery accelerated by treatment

numbers of organisms are required to induce the infection, growth of the organisms in food is usually required. The illness begins 1 to 2 days after ingesting contaminated food. The longer time from exposure to illness, as compared to staphylococcus food poisoning, is the result of the time needed for the bacteria to traverse the intestinal tract and initiate an infection in the mucosal lining. Outbreaks of food poisoning are investigated by public health authorities, who search for food handlers (carriers) who harbor the causative organism, thus contaminating food. Staphylococcal food poisoning can be prevented by keeping food refrigerated. Salmonella food infection can be prevented by keeping food refrigerated or by cooking contaminated food. Staphylococcal food poisoning is diagnosed by culturing the food; salmonella gastroenteritis is diagnosed by stool culture.

Shigellosis and amebiasis are infections of the colon caused by high virulent bacteria of the genus *Shigella* and the protozoan *Entameba histolytica*, respectively. The inflammation of the mucosal lining is often severe, leading to ulceration and *dysentery* (bloody diarrhea). Shigellosis has an acute onset and lasts for several days, whereas amebiasis has a gradual onset and may be chronic. These are classic diseases of overcrowding and poor sanitation such as occurs in mental institutions and war situations. The occurrence of dysentery calls for a search for shigella by culturing feces and for ameba by direct smear examination of feces. Of the infectious diarrheas discussed, shigellosis and amebiasis are the only ones that clearly require antimicrobial therapy to prevent complications and shorten the illness.

Campylobacter enteritis, due to bacteria of the genus *Campylobacter*, has been found to be among the more common causes of colitis with diarrhea or dysentery.

Reflux Esophagitis

Reflux esophagitis is inflammation of the mucosa and submucosa of the lower esophagus due to reflux of acid gastric contents into the lower esophagus. It is caused by incompetence of the sphincter at the lower end of the esophagus. In many, but not all, cases there is an associated esophageal hiatal hernia. Hiatal hernia is a sliding (herniation) of the stomach through the hole (hiatus) in the diaphragm normally occupied by the esophagus (Figure 14–6). Esophageal hiatal hernia is a common finding that increases in frequency with age. Most hiatal hernias are asymptomatic and not associated with an incompetent lower esophageal sphincter.

Reflux esophagitis may be a mild inflammation or may progress to ulceration. The ulcerative area of the esophagus may undergo metaplasia to a gastric-type or intestinal-type epithelium (*Barrett's esophagus*), and after many years adenocarcinomas may arise in the metaplastic epithelium. If persistent, ulceration leads to scarring, and contraction of the

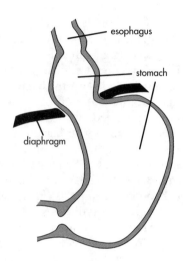

Figure 14–6. Esophageal hiatal hernia. Proximal stomach is herniated through the diaphragm into the chest.

scar tissue causes *stenosis* (stricture) of the esophagus in some patients. The most common symptom of reflux esophagitis is heartburn, a burning sensation in the chest beneath the sternum. Bleeding may also occur from the ulceration. Stricture causes dysphagia. In severe cases, an operation to repair the incompetent sphincter may be carried out.

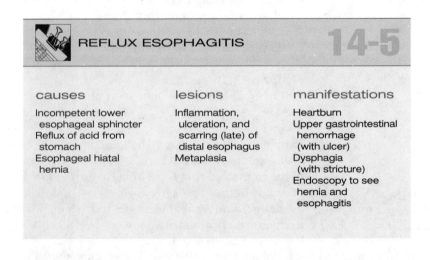

REFLUX ESOPHAGITIS 14-5

causes	lesions	manifestations
Incompetent lower esophageal sphincter Reflux of acid from stomach Esophageal hiatal hernia	Inflammation, ulceration, and scarring (late) of distal esophagus Metaplasia	Heartburn Upper gastrointestinal hemorrhage (with ulcer) Dysphagia (with stricture) Endoscopy to see hernia and esophagitis

Gastritis

Acute gastritis may be caused by injurious agents, such as aspirin, alcohol, and staphylococcal enterotoxin, that produce acute superficial injury to the mucosa that rapidly heals in a day or so and requires no specific treatment.

There are two major forms of chronic gastritis: fundal gastritis and helicobacter gastritis. Fundal gastritis involves the proximal stomach where the acid and pepsinogen-secreting cells are located. Over many years, these secretory cells are destroyed and replaced by metaplastic gastric antral or intestinal epithelium. In humans, extensive loss of acid-secreting cells leads to atrophic gastritis and achlorhydria (lack of hydrochloric acid) and to associated deficiency of intrinsic factor secretion, which is the cause of pernicious anemia. The cause of fundal gastritis is believed to be autoimmune. See Chapter 10 for more information on pernicious anemia.

Helicobacter gastritis is so prevalent that for most people it can almost be considered a normal condition associated with a commensal organism. *Helicobacter pylori* is a small curved bacterium that lives in the mucous layer of the gastric epithelial surface and incites an active low-grade acute and chronic inflammatory reaction most prominent in the distal (antral) part of the stomach. The condition becomes more frequent with age and affects about one-fifth of adults in the United States and probably more in many areas of the world. Gastritis is usually asymptomatic, and so-called symptoms of gastritis (epigastric discomfort, nausea, bloating) do not correlate well with the presence of gastritis histologically. Helicobacter gastritis may play some role in the development of gastric and duodenal ulcers and gastric carcinoma. Elimination of helicobacter may tip the balance in favor of ulcer healing; however, the organism should not be considered the most important factor in causing the ulcer. The cancer relationship is mild and likely related to the regenerative metaplastic changes resulting from prolonged chronic gastritis. Helicobacter gastritis is usually diagnosed by seeing the organisms in biopsy specimens, but the organism can be cultured and urease production in gastric juice is presumptive evidence that the organism is present. Helicobacter can be reduced or eliminated with various antibiotic regimens, but treatment of all persons with this condition is impractical and unnecessary.

Peptic Ulcer

Peptic ulcers are chronic ulcers due to injury produced by gastric secretions containing hydrochloric acid and proteolytic enzymes. They occur most commonly in the first part of the duodenum, where the stomach empties its acid contents onto the more susceptible intestinal mucosa. Less frequently, ulcers occur in the stomach (Figure 14–7). In men, duodenal ulcers are approximately seven times more common than gastric ulcers. In women, the ratio of duodenal to gastric ulcer is two to one. A peptic ulcer consists of a sharply punched out area of tissue necrosis that is covered by inflammatory exudate with underlying granulation tissue and fibrosis.

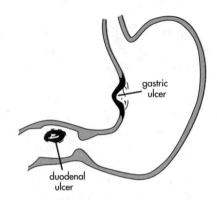

Figure 14–7. Peptic ulcer, typical location of duodenal and gastric ulcers.

Many peptic ulcers cause pain, but occasionally they are asymptomatic until one of the more serious complications such as massive bleeding, perforation, or obstruction occurs. Usually there is not a direct explanation of why the ulcer developed, but sometimes severe stress or heavy intake of drugs, such as aspirin, non-steroidal anti-inflammatory agents, or corticosteroids, are implicated as contributory factors. Although acid is necessary to produce peptic ulcers, this relationship cannot be quantitated in a particular individual. Although most duodenal ulcers heal with medical therapy, recurrences are common. Some patients require surgical therapy. Gastric ulcers are more likely to recur than duodenal ulcers and may require surgical treatment. Bed rest and abstinence from smoking are well-documented factors that promote healing. Antacids to neutralize gastric acid, H_2-histamine receptor antagonists to reduce histamine stimulation of gastric acid production and proton pump inhibitors

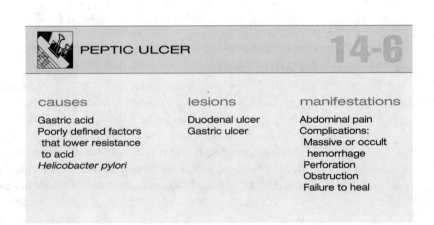

PEPTIC ULCER   14-6

causes	lesions	manifestations
Gastric acid	Duodenal ulcer	Abdominal pain
Poorly defined factors	Gastric ulcer	Complications:
that lower resistance		Massive or occult
to acid		hemorrhage
Helicobacter pylori		Perforation
		Obstruction
		Failure to heal

(omeprazole) all aid in ulcer healing. Elimination of helicobacter is helpful (see gastritis above).

Some patients have recurrent or chronic duodenal ulcers, which may lead to one of the four complications requiring an operation—severe hemorrhage, perforation, obstruction, or unrelieved pain.

Operations on the stomach are designed to reduce the effects of gastric acid by removing the gastric antrum, which secretes the acid-stimulating hormone gastrin, and by partial removal of the gastric body to remove a portion of the acid-secreting glands. In addition, vagotomy (cutting the vagus nerves) helps reduce the nervous stimulation to acid production.

Malabsorption Syndrome

Failure to digest and/or absorb food, leading to weight loss and steatorrhea (fat in the stool) is called the *malabsorption syndrome.* There are many diseases that cause the malabsorption syndrome. Specialized knowledge and procedures are required for their diagnosis. Severe malabsorption is rare but should be suspected when there is unexplained weight loss and the stools are large and bulky and very foul smelling (owing to bacterial action on unabsorbed fats). *Celiac* disease, one of the most common causes of severe malabsorption, is a sporadic, apparently genetic disease with onset at any age. In celiac disease, gluten, a protein found in grains (especially wheat), causes a mild prolonged injury to the small intestinal mucosa. This injury causes degeneration of surface epithelial cells, resulting in loss of villi and inflammatory cell infiltration of the lamina propria (Figure 14–8). A gluten-free diet effects a remission of the disease. As a gluten-free diet is expensive and because there are many other causes of malabsorp-

MALABSORPTION SYNDROME 14-7

causes	lesions	manifestations
Gluten sensitivity (celiac disease) Pancreatic insufficiency Altered continuity of gastrointestinal tract Many other causes	Mucosal degeneration with atrophy and inflammation (celiac disease) Inflammation of the pancreas with atrophy Surgical alteration or removal of parts of alimentary tract	Large, bulky, foul-smelling stools Weight loss Abnormalities of tests for fat and carbohydrate absorption May be abnormal intestinal biopsy (celiac disease)

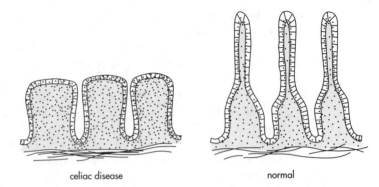

celiac disease   normal

Figure 14–8. Small intestinal mucosa with celiac disease compared with normal small intestine.

tion and weight loss, a diagnosis of celiac disease should be firmly established by a specialist before treatment is started. Chronic pancreatitis causes malabsorption when enough pancreatic tissue is destroyed to deplete the production of digestive enzymes.

Acute Appendicitis

The vermiform appendix is a vestigial outpouching of the proximal colon that has no known function but may become acutely inflamed at any time for no obvious reason. The bacteria causing the inflammation are those normally present in the colon. Sometimes a calcified mass of feces (fecalith) blocks the lumen of the appendix, thus predisposing to infection (Figure 14–9). It has been learned through experience that surgical removal of the acutely inflamed appendix is less risky than the complications that might develop from leaving it in. The complications include abscess formation, perforation leading to peritonitis, and spread of the infection to the liver. Appendicitis begins with pain, usually starting in the umbilical region and moving to the right lower quadrant of the abdomen. The inflammatory irritation of the peritoneum causes tenderness to palpation, and the

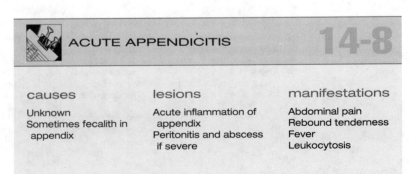

ACUTE APPENDICITIS   14-8

causes	lesions	manifestations

Unknown
Sometimes fecalith in
  appendix
	Acute inflammation of
	  appendix
	Peritonitis and abscess
	  if severe
		Abdominal pain
		Rebound tenderness
		Fever
		Leukocytosis

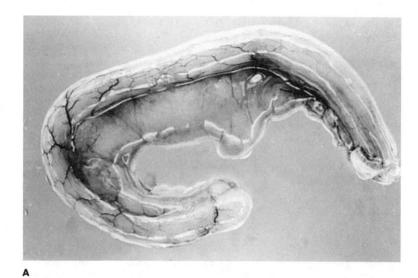

A

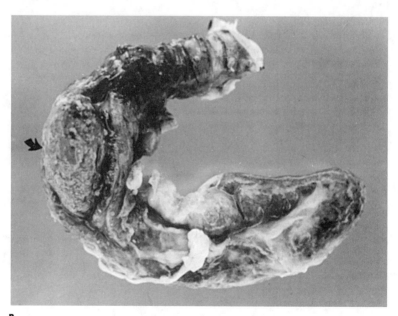

B

Figure 14–9. A. Normal appendix. B. Swollen, inflamed appendix with exudate on surface and fecalith (*arrow*) in lumen.

abdominal muscles become rigid. Appendicitis is the most common indication for laparotomy (surgically opening the abdominal cavity). However, diseases of adjacent organs, such as the right ovary and fallopian tube, distal ileum, and mesenteric lymph nodes, can closely mimic appendicitis. Appendicitis is prevented in those individuals who have their appendix removed during abdominal operations carried out for other reasons. This is called incidental appendectomy.

Pseudomembranous Enterocolitis

The false membrane of pseudomembranous enterocolitis is caused by superficial mucosal injury with necrotic cells, mucus, fibrin, and acute inflammatory cells forming a sticky exudate on the mucosal surface of colon and/or small intestine. Although there are several causes that will induce this type of injury, the most clinically important is the production of a necrotizing toxin by *Clostridium difficile*. The typical situation for this disease occurs in patients on prolonged antibiotic therapy. The therapy suppresses the normal intestinal flora and allows the toxigenic *Clostridium difficile*, which is normally present in small numbers, to proliferate and produce its toxin. Hospital transmission is a problem. The rapidly developing diarrheal disease may be fatal if not suspected and treated with change in antibiotics and fluid replacement.

Inflammatory Bowel Disease

Inflammatory bowel disease refers collectively to two chronic inflammatory diseases of the distal intestinal tract called *ulcerative colitis* and *Crohn's disease*. Both diseases are of unknown cause and produce weight loss and variable degrees of diarrhea, hemorrhage, and abdominal pain. Owing to the similarity of presentation, the specific diagnosis may not be immediately obvious, hence the need for the more general term inflammatory bowel disease. Pathologically, ulcerative colitis is a diffusely distributed mucosal disease of the colon (Figure 14–10A). Crohn's disease is a patchy disease involving all layers of the bowel wall; it occurs most commonly in the distal ileum but

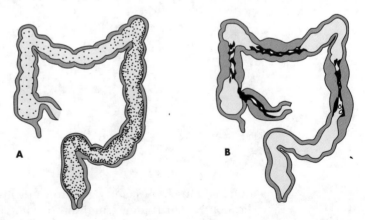

Figure 14–10. Inflammatory bowel disease. A. Ulcerative colitis with diffuse involvement of colonic mucosa. B. Crohn's disease with marked thickening of the wall of the ileum and patchy thickening of the wall of the colon.

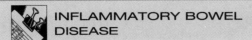

INFLAMMATORY BOWEL DISEASE

14-9

cause	lesions	manifestations
Unknown	Ulcerative colitis— diffuse chronic mucosal inflammation of colon Crohn's disease— localized inflammatory thickening anywhere in the alimentary tract	Chronic diarrhea Chronic hemorrhage leading to anemia Weight loss Exacerbations and remissions Interference with life style Cancer as late complication

also often involves the colon in a patchy manner (Figure 14–10B). About half of the cases have a granulomatous component to the chronic inflammatory reaction. Both diseases occur most commonly in young adults and disrupt their lives to a variable degree as the severity waxes and wanes. In ulcerative colitis, the risk of adenocarcinoma developing in the chronically inflamed and often dysplastic mucosa rises rapidly after 10 years. Total removal of the colon cures the disease and prevents cancer and the resulting permanent ileostomy is much preferable to the continuing risk of cancer. Complications of Crohn's disease resulting from the full wall inflammation and fibrosis include obstruction of the bowel and development of fistula tracts through the bowel wall and into adjacent tissues or organs. Perianal fistulas are particularly common. Resection of the diseased segment often relieves the complications, but recurrence may occur in previously normal segments. Drugs (azulfidine and corticosteroids) are used as anti-inflammatory agents with variable degrees of success. *Regional enteritis* and *granulomatous colitis* are synonyms for Crohn's disease of the small intestine and colon, respectively.

Colonic Diverticulosis

Multiple outpouchings (diverticula) of the colon develop frequently with advancing age at points of weakness in the muscular wall of the colon, especially the sigmoid colon. They are readily diagnosed by barium enema (Figure 14–11). *Diverticulosis* is usually an asymptomatic anatomic alteration but occasionally a diverticulum becomes inflamed producing diverticulitis. The inflammation may subside or persist leading to operative removal of the diseased segment. More rarely the artery overlying a diverticulum is eroded producing massive rectal bleeding.

COLONIC DIVERTICULOSIS 14-10

causes	lesions	manifestations
Not clearly defined Related to aging	Outpouchings of colonic mucosa through muscularis Most common in left colon, excluding the rectum	Usually none Infection produces diverticulitis with pain and altered bowel function Occasionally massive bleeding occurs

Inguinal Hernia

Inguinal hernia, commonly referred to as a *rupture*, is an outpouching of the outer peritoneal lining of the abdominal cavity into the groin (inguinal region). Loops of bowel can enter the pouch (Figure 14–12), and if they become caught or twisted, the intestine may be obstructed or the blood supply may be cut off causing infarction of the intestine. Because obstruction and/or infarction of the intestine is life threatening, it is better to surgically repair the hernia before, rather than after, the bowel gets caught. Inguinal hernias are much more common in men due to a congenital defect resulting from the peritoneum being

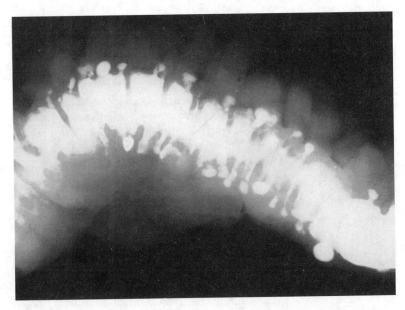

Figure 14–11. Colonic diverticulosis. X-ray of barium enema study shows barium-filled lumen and diverticula.

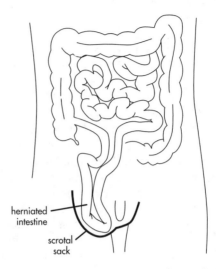

Figure 14–12. Inguinal hernia with entrapped loop of the bowel.

carried into the inguinal region as the testes descend from the abdomen into the scrotum. Some inguinal hernias in older people are due to a weakness in the wall of the abdomen without a congenital hernia sac. As a person ages and as a result of pressure, the hernia sac may enlarge and allow entrapment of bowel. In spite of the fact that symptoms usually develop in the aged, repair of congenital hernia sacs in males is best carried out in infancy or childhood.

INGUINAL HERNIA   14-11

causes	lesion	manifestations

Congenital defect
Weakness of abdominal
  wall
	Peritoneal pouch
	  extends into inguinal
	  region
		Pouch felt on physical
		  exam
		May be intestine or
		  other organ in pouch
		Intestinal obstruction
		  and infarction as
		  complications

Hyperplastic/Neoplastic Diseases

Alimentary tract cancers account for 20 percent of all cancers (skin cancers excluded). Colon cancer is by far the most common and also the most curable type. In addition, there are many benign tumors of the intestines, the most common occurring as polyps in the colon. There are many other types of neoplastic and non-neoplastic tumors of the alimentary tract. Most present with bleeding or obstruction and are diagnosed by the pathologist after removal of the tumor by the surgeon. Only carcinomas of the colon and stomach and polyps of the colon will be discussed here.

Carcinoma of the Stomach

Carcinoma of the stomach is less than half as common as carcinoma of the colon in the United States, although in some parts of the world it is the most common cancer. Dietary factors are suspected as the cause, but no specific agent has been proven. Helicobacter is also suspected. Carcinomas arise from the gastric mucosa, spread into the gastric wall, and metastasize to regional lymph nodes, liver, and other distant sites (Figure 14–13). Symptoms, such as loss of appetite, weight loss, pain, anemia, or abdominal mass, occur late, so that surgical cure is effected in only 15 percent of patients.

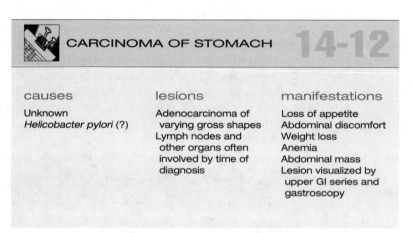

CARCINOMA OF STOMACH		14-12
causes	**lesions**	**manifestations**
Unknown	Adenocarcinoma of	Loss of appetite
Helicobacter pylori (?)	varying gross shapes	Abdominal discomfort
	Lymph nodes and	Weight loss
	other organs often	Anemia
	involved by time of	Abdominal mass
	diagnosis	Lesion visualized by
		upper GI series and
		gastroscopy

Colonic Polyps

A polyp is any protrusion from a mucosal surface and could represent an inflammatory lesion, a benign neoplasm, or a malignant neoplasm. Several types of polyps occur in the colon, the most common being hyperplastic polyps and two types of adenomas.

Hyperplastic polyps are small, slightly raised exaggerations of normal mucosal crypts. They are more common than adenomas and are totally innocuous. They are sometimes biopsied because they cannot always be distinguished from small adenomas.

The two types of adenomas (tubular and villous) are distinguished on the basis of their size, growth pattern, and malignant potential. *Tubular adenomas* (Figure 14–14A) are small (usually under

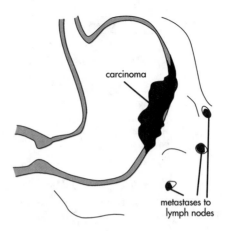

Figure 14–13. Carcinoma of the stomach.

2 centimeters), pedunculated (large head with narrow stalk), composed predominately of glands, and uncommonly contain cancer at the time of diagnosis.

Villous adenomas (Figure 14–14B) are large (usually over 2 centimeters), grow as a raised broad-based mass, composed predominately of villous type epithelium, and frequently (about 20 percent) contain cancer at the time of diagnosis. Adenomatous polyps are removed by excisional biopsy because they cannot be accurately separated from other types of polyps without histologic examination and because they are believed to be precancerous. If feasible, villous adenomas are removed by surgical resection, because they may already contain cancer and because they often recur if not completely removed.

COLONIC POLYPS

14-13

cause	lesions	manifestations
Unknown	Pedunculated (tubular) adenoma (most common type)	Often none—many discovered at sigmoidoscopy
	Large sessile villous tumor (villous adenoma), which may contain cancer	Bleeding Altered bowel movements (villous adenoma)
	Other types	

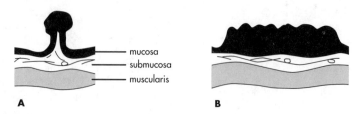

A **B**

Figure 14–14. Two types of colonic polyps. A. A pedunculated tubular adenoma. B. A sessile villous adenoma.

Carcinoma of the Colon

Adenocarcinoma of the colon is the most common internal cancer. It usually develops spontaneously without evident cause, but it also occurs as a complication of *familial adenomatous polyposis*, ulcerative colitis, and villous adenoma. Early diagnosis is important, because the disease is potentially curable by surgical resection. The cancer arises in the mucosa and gradually increases in size as it grows through the colonic wall to the serosa and expands into the lumen (Figure 14–15). At any time after it has invaded beyond the mucosa, it may spread through lymphatic channels to the lymph nodes in the pericolonic fat. Cancer cells may gain access to the bloodstream by further spreading up the lymphatic system to the thoracic duct or by directly invading veins. Blood-borne metastases are most frequently found in the liver; most patients with advanced colonic cancer have a large nodular liver filled with metastatic cancer. If surgical removal is carried out before the lymph nodes are involved, the cure rate is high. Once the liver is involved, there is no chance for cure.

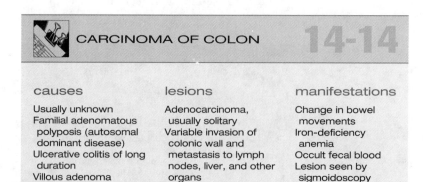

CARCINOMA OF COLON 14-14

causes	lesions	manifestations
Usually unknown	Adenocarcinoma, usually solitary	Change in bowel movements
Familial adenomatous polyposis (autosomal dominant disease)	Variable invasion of colonic wall and metastasis to lymph nodes, liver, and other organs	Iron-deficiency anemia
Ulcerative colitis of long duration		Occult fecal blood
Villous adenoma		Lesion seen by sigmoidoscopy
		Lesion felt by rectal exam
		Lesion visualized by barium enema
		Abdominal mass (uncommon)

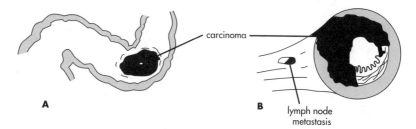

Figure 14–15. Carcinoma of the colon. A. Mucosal surface view. B. Cross-section with invasion through the muscle layer and metastasis to lymph nodes.

The main manifestations of colonic carcinomas are bleeding and altered bowel habits. Almost all colon cancers bleed due to ulceration of their surface. This may be detected by the patient noting gross blood in the stool, by the development of iron-deficiency anemia, or by screening the stool for occult blood. Because bleeding occurs from the surface, the cancer may still be in an early stage when bleeding is detected. Altered bowel habits resulting from colonic carcinoma may take the form of diarrhea, constipation, or narrow pencil-like stools. Development of colonic obstruction or pain implies more extensive tumor growth. Diagnosis is made in one of two ways—endoscopy (sigmoidoscopy or colonoscopy) or barium enema (Figure 14–16).

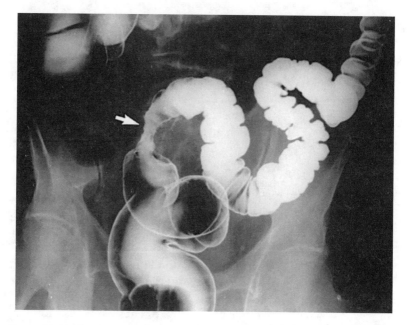

Figure 14–16. Barium enema illustrating a constricting colon cancer (*arrow*) with proximal dilated, air-filled colon due to obstruction of the lumen by the cancer.

ORGAN FAILURE

Acute failure of the absorption process can be tolerated for a number of days. Severe vomiting or diarrhea, however, may lead to fatal loss of fluids. Infants are most susceptible to fluid loss and much more frequently require intravenous fluid replacement for vomiting and diarrhea than do adults. The most striking acute organ failure occurs when the small intestine is massively damaged, such as with occlusion of the mesenteric artery by a thrombus, leading to infarction and death. The alimentary tract functions amazingly well in the face of chronic diseases unless obstruction develops. Ulcerative lesions of the intestinal tract are quite resistant to infection unless there is perforation into the peritoneal cavity.

Review Questions

1. What is the functional bowel syndrome and why may it be difficult to distinguish from organic disease?
2. What are the common alimentary tract diseases that cause mild or short-lived disability and few deaths?
3. Which alimentary tract diseases cause serious prolonged illnesses or are frequently fatal?
4. What are the manifestations of bleeding, altered motility, and perforation of the alimentary tract?
5. How are radiologic and endoscopic procedures used to diagnose alimentary tract diseases?
6. What are the causes, lesions, and manifestations of each of the specific diseases discussed in the chapter?
7. How are most developmental abnormalities of the alimentary tract treated and what is the likely outcome?
8. How do the infectious diarrheas and food poisonings differ in terms of causative agents, likely situation for their occurrence, and timing of onset and recovery?

9. What conditions may mimic appendicitis?

10. What is the relationship between reflux esophagitis and esophageal hiatal hernia?

11. Why is carcinoma of the colon a more important medical problem than carcinoma of the stomach?

12. What do the following terms mean?

    Digestive or gastrointestinal system

    Alimentary tract

    Diarrhea

    Constipation

    Hematemesis

    Hematochezia

    Melena

    Ileus

    Adynamic ileus

    Upper GI series

    Barium enema

    Sigmoidoscopy

    Upper gastrointestinal endoscopy

    Gastric analysis

    Hernia

    Tubular adenoma

    Villous adenoma

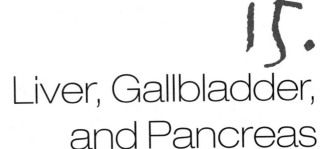

15.

Liver, Gallbladder, and Pancreas

REVIEW OF STRUCTURE AND FUNCTION
Liver
Blood Supply • Hepatocytes • Bile Canaliculi and Ducts • Kupffer Cells • Bile Salt Production • Bilirubin Excretion • Metabolism of Nitrogenous Substances • Serum Protein Production • Detoxification of Drugs and Poisons
Biliary Tree and Gallbladder
Pancreas
Acini and Ducts • Islets of Langerhans

MOST FREQUENT AND SERIOUS PROBLEMS
Gallstones • Viral Hepatitis • Cirrhosis • Metastatic Carcinoma of the Liver • Pancreatitis • Carcinoma of the Pancreas

SYMPTOMS, SIGNS, AND TESTS
Jaundice • Pain • Hepatomegaly • Serum Amylase • Serum Lipase • Serum Bilirubin • Serum Protein • Alkaline Phosphatase • Aspartate Aminotransferase • Prothrombin Time • Liver Biopsy • Ultrasound • Cholecystogram

SPECIFIC DISEASES
Genetic/Developmental Diseases
Neonatal Liver Disease
Cystic Fibrosis of the Pancreas
Inflammatory/Degenerative Diseases
Viral Hepatitis
Chemical Injuries to the Liver
Alcoholic Liver Disease
Cirrhosis
Cholecystitis and Gallstones
Pancreatitis

Hyperplastic/Neoplastic Diseases
  Metastatic Cancer of the Liver
  Carcinoma of the Pancreas
ORGAN FAILURE
REVIEW QUESTIONS

REVIEW OF STRUCTURE AND FUNCTION

The liver and the pancreas are glandular organs with excretory ducts emptying into the second portion of the duodenum, usually at a common site called the *papilla of Vater* (Figure 15–1). The excretory ducts of the liver are called *bile ducts*. The gallbladder is a storage reservoir connected to the bile ducts by the cystic duct.

The liver is the largest glandular organ in the body. Most of the blood from the abdominal organs is carried to the liver via the portal veins so that it can be filtered past the glandular cells of the liver (hepatocytes) before being returned to the heart via the hepatic vein. Because portal blood has little oxygen left after passing through the abdominal organs, the liver has a second source of blood, the hepatic artery, to provide oxygenated blood. The bulk of the liver is composed of hepatocytes, large epithelial cells capable of carrying out many metabolic functions. The hepatocytes are aligned in cords or plates with sinusoids between the plates to percolate the blood from the portal areas to the central vein (Figure 15–2). Between the cell membranes of adjacent hepatocytes are tiny canaliculi that carry bile produced by the hepatocytes to the portal area, where they empty into epithelial-lined bile ducts. Thus, blood flows into the liver through the hepatic artery and portal vein and enters the sinusoids from the widely dispersed portal areas. In the sinusoids, waste products and nutrients

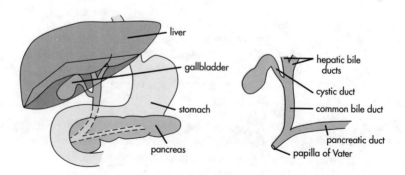

Figure 15–1. Major components of the liver, biliary tract, and pancreas.

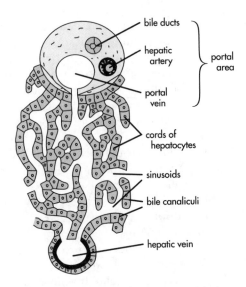

Figure 15–2. Basic histologic structure of the liver.

are removed and metabolized by the hepatocytes. The metabolites may be returned to the blood, stored in the hepatocytes, or excreted into bile canaliculi to form bile. The bile is carried through the canaliculi to the portal areas, where it enters the bile ducts and later is emptied into the intestine after storage in the gallbladder.

The liver also contains many mononuclear phagocytic cells, which are present in the form of fixed macrophages called *Kupffer cells.* Kupffer cells line the sinusoids and are normally inconspicuous. They phagocytize particulate material from the blood.

Of the many metabolic functions of the liver, five will be briefly reviewed: (1) production of bile salts, (2) excretion of bilirubin, (3) metabolism of nitrogenous substances, (4) production of serum proteins, and (5) detoxification of drugs and poisons.

The liver's main contribution to the gastrointestinal tract function is bile salts. Bile salts are bipolar molecules derived from cholesterol that aggregate into spherical masses (micelles). Lipids are soluble in the inside of the micelle, whereas the outer surface is water soluble. Bile salts render cholesterol soluble in bile to prevent the formation of cholesterol crystals, and in the intestine, they dissolve other lipid molecules so that they can be absorbed.

The most notable of the liver's excretion products is bilirubin, a hemoglobin breakdown product, which is produced from worn out red blood cells. Approximately $\frac{1}{120}$ of a person's red blood cells die every day. The liver cannot remove all of the bilirubin from the blood immediately, so in the normal state of equilibrium between bilirubin production and its removal by the liver there is about 1 mg/dL of bilirubin in the blood. After the liver cells remove bilirubin from the blood, they conjugate it with glucuronide molecules to make it water soluble and excrete it into the bile. Many other substances are handled in a manner similar to that for bilirubin, but bilirubin is more important because of the large amount excreted and because it is yellow. When bilirubin accumulates in the blood, the patient's skin and eyes appear yellow (*jaundiced*), indicating illness. This may result from too many red cells dying, from failure of liver cells to remove and excrete bilirubin, or from blockage of bile ducts.

Another important metabolic product of hepatocytes is urea nitrogen. This is handled differently from bilirubin. The breakdown of dead cells produces nitrogenous products such as ammonia. Also, the breakdown of protein by bacteria in the intestines produces ammonia, which can be absorbed into the blood by the portal vein. The liver converts these nitrogenous products to urea nitrogen and returns the urea nitrogen to the bloodstream, because it cannot excrete urea nitrogen effectively in the bile. It remains for the kidney to excrete urea nitrogen. From these considerations, it is easy to see that severe liver failure results in accumulation of ammonia in the blood and severe kidney failure results in accumulation of urea nitrogen in the blood.

Another notable chemical product of the liver is the production of serum proteins, particularly albumin and the specific globulins necessary for blood coagulation. Prothrombin is one of the specific globulins that is important for blood coagulation. The liver requires vitamin K to produce prothrombin; consequently, low prothrombin levels in the blood may be due to severe liver disease or vitamin K deficiency.

Many drugs and poisons are metabolized in the liver by way of conjugation with other compounds to increase their solubility or aid in their excretion. Thus, severe liver disease is likely to delay the excretion of drugs and enhance the effects of poisons.

The excretory ducts of the liver (bile ducts) form a long tree-like network with the trunk (common bile duct) emptying into the duodenum at the same point as the pancreatic duct. The gallbladder is an outpouching of the common bile duct that acts as a storage reservoir for bile. The gallbladder empties its contents into the duodenum at a time (after meals) when bile salts are needed for fat absorption. This reservoir function is not essential, as the gallbladder can be removed without loss of digestive function.

The pancreas is a long, narrow glandular organ lying horizontally in the midabdomen behind the peritoneum. Its tail stretches toward the spleen on the left, and its head nestles behind the proximal duodenum and distal stomach. The pancreatic duct runs the length of the pancreas and empties into the duodenum after joining the bile duct. The bulk of the pancreas is made up of glands (acini) that secrete digestive enzymes into the pancreatic duct. When activated by intestinal juices, these enzymes digest carbohydrate (amylase), fat (lipase), and protein (trypsins). Pancreatic enzymes are essential to life. When the pancreas is destroyed, it is not possible to give enough enzymes orally to restore normal function, so a state of chronic malnutrition ensues.

Scattered among the pancreatic glands are clusters of endocrine cells known as the *islets of Langerhans*, which produce insulin and other hormones. Removal of the entire pancreas or severe destruction will produce diabetes mellitus due to lack of insulin. Insulin therapy is then vital to life.

MOST FREQUENT AND SERIOUS PROBLEMS

The most common problem occurs in the gallbladder, namely, the formation of gallstones. Gallstones are usually asymptomatic but have the potential of producing serious complications such as obstruction of bile flow due to migration of stones into the common bile duct.

Viral hepatitis is probably the most common liver disease, particularly in younger people. It usually resolves completely but occasionally persists for many months or more rarely develops into a serious chronic inflammation leading to cirrhosis. *Cirrhosis* refers to fibrosis and nodular regeneration of the liver and is the characteristic lesion of serious chronic liver disease regardless of cause. Chronic alcoholism is the most common cause of cirrhosis, but only a fraction of chronic alcoholics develop cirrhosis. The most common neoplastic condition of the liver is metastatic carcinoma.

Inflammation of the pancreas is uncommon and usually mild; however, there are serious acute, often fatal forms and chronic forms that lead to destruction of the pancreas. The more severe acute and chronic forms are usually associated with alcoholism, whereas mild forms are often associated with gallstones. Carcinoma of the pancreas ranks sixth in frequency among carcinomas and is one of the most lethal of all cancers. Although insulin is produced in the pancreas, the relative lack of insulin (diabetes mellitus) is not usually related to any obvious pancreatic disease. Therefore, diabetes is treated as a metabolic/endocrine disorder rather than a pancreatic disorder.

SYMPTOMS, SIGNS, AND TESTS

Jaundice is an obvious and often serious symptom or sign of liver disease. It may be caused by increased hemoglobin breakdown, liver disease, or bile duct obstruction. Nonspecific digestive disturbances may be associated with acute hepatitis and gallstones. Pain is a feature of acute cholecystitis (inflammation of the gallbladder), gallstones in the common bile duct, pancreatitis, and late stages of carcinoma of the pancreas. Enlargement of the liver (hepatomegaly) is particularly prominent in alcoholic fatty liver and metastatic cancer to the liver.

Laboratory tests are often used to diagnose the type of liver disease. They are somewhat inappropriately referred to as *liver function tests* because they are not usually specific for liver function. Serum tests related to liver disease usually include a routine screening battery of bilirubin, total protein, albumin, aspartate aminotransferase (AST), and alkaline phosphatase. The causes of elevated bilirubin are the same as the causes of jaundice. The serum bilirubin is at least twice normal when jaundice becomes apparent. Low levels of serum protein, particularly albumin, occur with severe chronic liver disease such as cirrhosis. Aspartate aminotransferase is elevated with liver necrosis (as in hepatitis), and alkaline phosphatase is usually elevated with bile duct obstruction (often before the bilirubin is elevated). Prothrombin time is a blood coagulation test that reflects serum levels of prothrombin. Prothrombin deficiency may be caused by very severe liver disease or vitamin K deficiency.

Biopsy of the liver can be performed with a needle inserted through the skin or at the time of surgical opening of the abdomen (laparotomy or laparoscopy). Biopsy is the most reliable way of establishing the nature of the more serious liver diseases such as cirrhosis, chronic hepatitis, granulomas, and cancer.

Tests for gallbladder disease are designed to visualize gallstones. Twenty percent of gallstones are calcified and can be seen on an x-ray of the abdomen. Ultrasound is the preferred method of demonstrating gallstones because it is noninvasive, demonstrates most stones, and gives an immediate answer. Cholecystography involves swallowing a radiopaque dye and waiting for it to be absorbed, excreted by the liver, and concentrated by the gallbladder. Stones will then appear as holes on roentgenograms of the radiopaque gallbladder. If a stone blocks the cystic duct, no bile or radiopaque dye can enter the gallbladder; thus, the gallbladder is said to be nonfunctional.

Tests for pancreatic disease include measurement of serum amylase and lipase as indicators of acute or active pancreatic injury and tests for intestinal malabsorption as indicators of chronic damage with inadequate production of digestive enzymes.

SPECIFIC DISEASES

Genetic/Developmental Diseases

Neonatal Liver Disease

Jaundice at or shortly after birth may be due to increased breakdown of red blood cells, parenchymal liver disease, or atresia of bile ducts.

Normally there is an increased breakdown of red blood cells at birth producing an elevated serum bilirubin. This is accentuated by prematurity, because the liver is less able to remove and excrete bilirubin, and by erythroblastosis fetalis, because of the presence of maternal antibodies to the neonate's red blood cells. Neonatal infections and rare genetic metabolic defects may produce parenchymal injury at this time. Absence of bile ducts (biliary atresia) usually leads to progressive damage to the liver and death within a year. Occasionally extrahepatic atresia can be repaired surgically. Recent evidence suggests that biliary atresia is due to fetal inflammatory disorders rather than an embryonic anomaly.

Cystic Fibrosis of the Pancreas

This recessively inherited autosomal disorder will occur in about one-fourth of siblings when both parents are carrying the gene that causes cystic fibrosis. The pancreatic ducts are filled with thick mucoid material, leading to cystic dilatation of the ducts and fibrosis of the parenchyma. This leads to malabsorption and weight loss of variable severity. As described under lung, bouts of pneumonia also occur, and the pancreatic or pulmonary deficiencies lead to death in childhood. Treatment is directed at preventing pneumonia and replacing pancreatic enzymes.

Inflammatory/Degenerative Diseases

The liver is involved to a variable extent by many systemic diseases producing nonspecific changes such as fatty change (fatty metamorphosis), chronic inflammation of portal areas, and enlargement of Kupffer cells. In this section, we will concentrate on the major primary diseases of the liver, gallbladder, and pancreas.

Viral Hepatitis

Several viruses may affect the liver as part of systemic viral infections and a few have their major effect on the liver. The diseases caused by the latter group are yellow fever, a very serious disease that occurs in the tropics, and viral hepatitis, a term applied to at least five viral infections that have a similar clinical illness and liver lesions. Viral antigens and/or antibodies have been identified for viral hepatitis A, B, C, and delta.

Patients with viral hepatitis feel ill with loss of appetite (anorexia) and distaste for cigarettes (if they smoke). Jaundice may be the first clue to the presence of liver disease, although not all patients become yellow. Physical examination reveals an enlarged tender liver and the urine appears dark. In the acute stage of the illness, serum AST is always strikingly elevated (over 1000 units versus a normal of less than 40), indicating liver cell necrosis. There is no specific treatment other than rest and a good diet. Unlike many other viral illnesses, the disease runs a prolonged or subacute course, with 85 percent of patients having recovered by 6 weeks. Although viral hepatitis causes considerable disability, it is the long-term complications and potential for spread of the disease that make it a major health problem.

Hepatitis A, caused by an RNA virus, is the most benign form. The virus is spread sporadically or in epidemics by fecal contamination of water and food. The incubation period (2 to 6 weeks) is the shortest of the three forms and the onset of symptoms is the most abrupt. Diagnosis is made by finding elevated IgM anti-hepatitis A antibodies in the serum a few days to 3 months after onset of illness. Elevated IgG anti-hepatitis A antibodies without IgM antibodies indicates past illness and lifetime immunity to the disease. Hepatitis A is rarely fatal in the acute stage and does not lead to chronic hepatitis. The virus is shed in the feces for about 2 weeks before and 1 week after onset of illness; after that the patient is no longer a carrier of the disease.

In contrast, hepatitis B, caused by a DNA virus, is potentially a much more serious disease. The incubation period is long (1 to 6 months) and the onset of symptoms more gradual. Diagnosis is made by detecting serum antigens and antibodies, but is much more complex than for hepatitis A. The antigen in the surface coat of the virus is called hepatitis B surface antigen (HBsAg) and two antigens in the core of the virus are called core antigen and e antigen (HBcAg and HBeAg). The surface antigen is shed into the blood for several weeks before onset of illness and persists into the recovery period. Antibody to HBs rises sometime after recovery and is a good indication of recovery and lifelong immunity. Presence of the e antigen parallels disease activity and its persistence suggests chronic disease. Anti-HBc and anti-HBe indicate current or recent infection and do not confer immunity. These markers have proved useful in sorting out the various clinical forms of hepatitis B.

The most severe form of hepatitis B is massive or fulminant hepatic necrosis, an uncommon but often fatal form that kills most of the liver's cells. Chronic forms of hepatitis B, which may or may not be associated with an acute stage, are divided into two types. Chronic persistent hepatitis is a mild illness with prolonged (more than 6 months) elevations of aspartate aminotransferase levels. It is not associated with permanent liver damage and eventually recovery occurs. Chronic active hepatitis is clinically similar but liver biopsy reveals beginning fibrosis and progression to cirrhosis is expected in many cases. Finally, the carrier state occurs in asymptomatic patients and in those with chronic hepatitis. The carrier state is diagnosed by elevated serum HBsAg and anti-HBc. The presence of anti-HBe suggests that the carrier has active disease.

Hepatitis B is a major health problem because about one of every 1000 persons is a carrier and the potential effects of the disease are serious. Hepatitis B virus may be spread by feces, urine, and body secre-

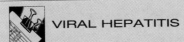

VIRAL HEPATITIS   **15-1**

cause	lesions	manifestations
Hepatitis viruses A, B, C, delta	Necrosis and swelling of hepatocytes Inflamed liver	Anorexia Malaise Jaundice Large tender liver High AST

tions, but more commonly it is spread by blood transfusion, contaminated breaks in the skin, or transplacentally. Drug addicts, homosexual men, institutionalized children, blood recipients, dentists, and selected other health care workers are particularly at risk. A vaccine prepared from surface antigen is available for persons at high risk for the disease.

Hepatitis C is caused by an RNA virus, has an incubation period that overlaps hepatitis A and B (2 weeks to 6 months), and is spread in a fashion similar to hepatitis B. After immunologic markers were found for hepatitis B, hepatitis C became the cause of most cases of post-transfusion hepatitis. Now that C can be recognized in blood, the incidence of post-transfusion hepatitis will greatly diminish. Hepatitis C is even more likely than B to become chronic and can lead to cirrhosis.

Delta agent, a rare cause of hepatitis, requires the presence of hepatitis B (usually a chronic infection) in order to cause hepatitis. The frequency of fulminant or chronic hepatitis is greater with delta agent than with hepatitis B alone. Other forms of hepatitis may be recognized such as a rare epidemic form identified epidemiologically as hepatitis E.

Chemical Injuries to the Liver

Many drugs and toxic chemicals have been associated with liver injury, but the degree of injury is usually mild, and the cause and effect relationship is difficult to prove. Some agents cause injury in selected individuals only (hypersensitivity), whereas other agents cause injury directly related to the dose of the injurious substance. Among the former type, the most important and serious is the reaction to a commonly used anesthetic agent, halothane. A very small percentage of patients anesthetized with halothane, particularly when used for a second operation, develop very severe massive necrosis of liver cells much like that occurring in acutely fatal cases of viral hepatitis. Isoniazide, a drug used for long-term treatment of tuberculosis, is also associated with occasional idiosyncratic cases of massive hepatic necrosis. Serious, although very uncommonly encountered, examples of direct toxic injury include ingestion or inhalation of carbon tetrachloride or chloroform and

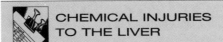

CHEMICAL INJURIES TO THE LIVER   15-2

causes	lesion	manifestations

Hypersensitivity to drugs
Chemical action of drugs
  or toxic chemicals
	Inflamed liver with
	  variable necrosis
		Jaundice
		Abnormal laboratory test
		  values
		History of exposure
		  to agent

mushroom poisoning. Because the liver metabolizes many drugs and toxic chemicals, it is not surprising that patients with severe acute liver disease (hepatitis) or severe chronic liver disease (cirrhosis) may be more susceptible to drugs and toxins regardless of the site at which they produce injury.

Alcoholic Liver Disease

Prolonged heavy ingestion of alcoholic beverages leads to acute and chronic liver disease in some individuals. Experimentally, mild histologic changes can be produced in persons ingesting "socially acceptable" amounts of alcohol. Three types of changes occur in the liver during the long time interval required for development of cirrhosis—fatty change, hepatitis, and fibrosis. *Fatty change* is reversible but is usually found to a variable extent at all stages of the disease. Fatty change appears to be the most universal effect of alcohol. Although more severe changes are also dose related, there appears to be some degree of individual susceptibility that is not adequately explained by our current knowledge. Acute cell damage occurs with bouts of heavy drink-

ALCOHOLIC LIVER DISEASE   15-3

causes	lesions	manifestations

Alcoholism
Other unknown factors
  that make some
  people susceptible
	Fatty metamorphosis
	Alcoholic hepatitis
	Fibrosis
	Finely nodular fatty
	  cirrhosis
		Long history of heavy
		  alcohol intake
		Enlarged liver
		Altered liver function
		Findings of cirrhosis

ing and results in inflammation of the liver called *alcoholic hepatitis*. After repeated episodes of injury, fibrosis develops and gradually causes the disruption of the hepatic architecture. Regenerative nodules of hepatocytes and fibrosis constitute the end stage of the disease, called *cirrhosis* (discussion follows). Clinically, alcoholic liver disease is often asymptomatic until advanced. Advanced disease presents as cirrhosis. Some patients present with a large fatty liver and jaundice. Others develop bouts of delirium tremens, especially upon withdrawal from alcohol. *Delirium tremens* is characterized by tremors, combative behavior, and hallucinations (often the patient sees strange objects).

Cirrhosis

Cirrhosis is the term used to describe the end stage of most serious chronic types of liver disease. It is characterized by fibrosis and nodular regeneration of hepatocytes. Normally, the liver can easily replace damaged hepatocytes. If the delicate connective tissue framework is destroyed or replaced by bands of fibrous tissue, the replacement process results in clusters of regenerated hepatocytes to form grossly visible nodules.

Of the many causes of cirrhosis, alcoholism and chronic hepatitis account for a large portion of the cases, but in many patients with cirrhosis, the exact cause cannot be determined. Other types of cirrhosis, which are uncommon, include biliary cirrhosis, resulting from prolonged bile duct obstruction; pigmentary cirrhosis of hemochromatosis, resulting from massive storage of iron; Wilson's disease, with cirrhosis resulting from an inherited defect in copper metabolism; and cirrhosis associated with α-1-antitrypsin deficiency.

The morphology of the cirrhosis may be helpful in determining its cause. Most instances of alcoholic cirrhosis produce a finely nodular liver (Figure 15–3A). Histologically, many hepatocytes are filled with fat. The finely nodular cirrhosis of alcoholism is sometimes called *Laennec's cirrhosis*. Idiopathic cirrhosis and cirrhosis associated with chronic hepatitis generally have larger regenerative nodules and broader and more irregular bands of fibrous tissue (Figure 15–3B). This is called *postnecrotic cirrhosis*.

The development of cirrhosis takes months to years. It is usually asymptomatic until serious irreversible changes in the architecture of the liver lead to any of several possible complications, including portal hypertension, esophageal varices, ascites, and hepatic encephalopathy. These complications usually result from altered blood flow through the liver. Blood may flow through the fibrous septae with reduced flow through hepatic sinusoids, and thus, blood has reduced contact with hepatocytes. The altered flow also leads to elevated blood pressure in the portal vein (portal hypertension). Failure of blood to flow past liver cells may lead to accumulation of nitrogenous breakdown products

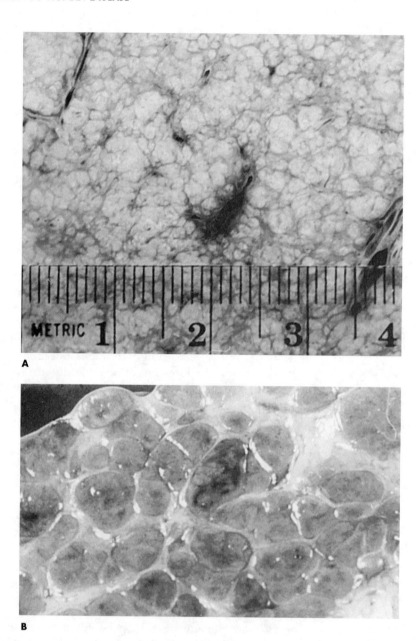

Figure 15–3. Comparison of finely nodular alcoholic cirrhosis (A) with the coarsely nodular irregular postnecrotic cirrhosis (B).

(such as ammonia) in the blood. This is associated with hepatic encephalopathy characterized by depression of the central nervous system, with stupor or coma. The shunting of blood away from the hepatocytes also explains why drugs are poorly metabolized in cirrhotic persons. Portal hypertension leads to development of the collateral venous connections to the vena caval system. Most notably, the veins of the lower esophagus become dilated (esophageal varices) by increased collateral blood flow, and they may rupture to produce massive hemorrhage into the alimentary tract. Another common feature of portal hypertension is passive congestion of the spleen leading to splenomegaly. Occasionally, the splenomegaly of portal hypertension is associated with increased destruction of blood cells by the spleen leading to anemia, leukopenia, and for thrombocytopenia (hypersplenism). Ascites also occurs. *Ascites* is the accumulation of massive amounts of watery fluid in the peritoneal cavity so that the abdomen becomes bloated. Its causation is complicated and involves low serum protein levels, increased back pressure in the portal vein and lymphatics of the liver, and retention of salt. Jaundice is a variable feature of cirrhosis and is caused by compression of bile ducts due to the fibrosis and to depressed function of the hepatocytes due to altered blood flow. Altered metabolism of sex hormones by the liver leads to estrogenic effects, including small dilated blood vessels in skin (spider angiomas) and breast enlargement in men (gynecomastia).

The average alcoholic cirrhotic patient comes to medical attention because of the development of one or more of the following: jaundice, ascites, bleeding esophageal varices, delirium tremens, or hepatic encephalopathy. If the cirrhosis is well advanced, the patient will die within a few years of encephalopathy, bleeding, or superimposed infection. If the diagnosis is made at an early stage of alcoholic liver disease, abstinence from alcohol can greatly prolong life for some individuals. Most nonalcoholic types of cirrhosis are progressive. Biopsy is the best way to evaluate the extent of the disease. Operations to relieve the portal hypertension and thus decrease the risk of esophageal varices are sometimes carried out.

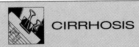

CIRRHOSIS   15-4

causes	lesions	manifestations
Alcoholism	Fibrous bands	Jaundice
Viral hepatitis	Regenerating nodules	Hepatic encephalopathy
Unknown causes	of hepatocytes	Bleeding esophageal
Bile duct obstruction		varices
Hemochromatosis		Ascites
Wilson's disease		Spider angiomas
α-1-antitrypsin		Gynecomastia
deficiency		Cirrhosis by biopsy

Cholecystitis and Gallstones

Bile is rich in cholesterol, which is barely held in solution by bile salts and phospholipids. In the gallbladder, bile is concentrated by absorption of its water content. If the cholesterol comes out of solution, it forms crystals, which, along with the bilirubin pigment and calcium in the bile, form stones (Figure 15–4). The stones vary greatly in number, size, shape, and color. The reasons why some people develop gallstones and others do not is not clear, although women are much more prone to develop gallstones than men, and the likelihood of developing gallstones increases with age. Native Americans have a very high rate of gallstone formation.

The stones in the gallbladder are associated with a very low-grade inflammation, which we label *chronic cholecystitis*. Gallstones are important because of their complications. The two most common complications of gallstones are acute cholecystitis, which is painful and makes the patient quite ill, and migration of gallstones down the cystic duct into the common bile duct, obstructing its distal narrow end to produce jaundice. The main reason for removing the gallbladder (cholecystectomy) is to prevent or treat these two serious complications.

Uncomplicated chronic cholecystitis with gallstones is usually asymptomatic but may be associated with symptoms such as pain fol-

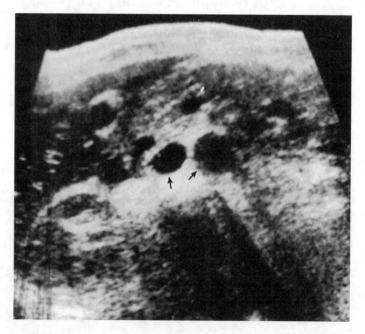

Figure 15–4. Ultrasound image of abdominal wall (*skin at top*) demonstrating gallstones (*arrows*) in gallbladder (*light area*).

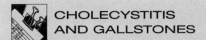

CHOLECYSTITIS AND GALLSTONES

15-5

cause	lesions	manifestations
Unknown, but strong association with increasing age and higher incidence in females	Gallstones Mild chronic inflammation	Usually none Pain after meals Obstruction of bile duct with jaundice Acute cholecystitis with pain, fever, and leukocytosis

lowing meals, especially when fatty or spicy food is ingested. Cholecystectomy may relieve symptoms of uncomplicated cholecystitis. Symptoms attributed to cholecystitis are sometimes due to other causes and are not relieved by cholecystectomy.

The diagnosis of gallstones is usually established by radiologic procedures. Roentgenograms of the abdomen usually fail to reveal gallstones, because only 20 percent of patients have enough calcium in their stones to make them radiopaque. The classic method of demonstrating gallstones, called a cholecystogram, involves ingestion of a radiopaque dye that is absorbed by the liver and excreted into the bile. If the gallbladder is normal, the dye is concentrated along with bile. Radiolucent gallstones produce less dense filling defects. If the cystic duct is blocked by a stone, dye cannot enter into the gallbladder and it is said to be nonfunctional. A newer technique for demonstrating gallstones, ultrasound, involves the creation of an image of sound waves as they are deflected from the stones (Figure 15–4). Ultrasound can be done rapidly and without ingestion of drugs or exposure to x-rays, but as with cholecystography, it produces some false-negative results.

Pancreatitis

Inflammation of the pancreas differs from inflammation in other organs, because the powerful digestive enzymes produced by acinar cells may escape from the cells or ducts to digest the pancreas itself and surrounding adipose tissue. This is called *enzymatic necrosis*. The mechanisms by which pancreatic enzymes escape into tissue are not well understood, although obstruction of the pancreatic duct and stimulation of secretion, such as occurs following a heavy meal, are thought to be important factors.

Most cases of severe pancreatitis are associated with alcoholism. Acute hemorrhagic pancreatitis results in extensive necrosis and hemorrhage into the pancreas, leading to pain and shock. This form usually follows a heavy, alcohol-laden meal and is often fatal in spite of attempts to decrease pancreatic secretion by evacuating food from the stomach and administering drugs that block secretion. Severe chronic pancreatitis occurs in chronic alcoholics and is a slowly progressive disease much like cirrhosis. After many years of heavy drinking, these patients develop malabsorption due to replacement of pancreatic acini by fibrous tissue and diabetes mellitus due to destruction of the islets of Langerhans. Severe abdominal pain may occur with chronic pancreatitis. End-stage pancreatitis in the alcoholic is less common than cirrhosis, and the two conditions may or may not be present together.

Other diseases associated with pancreatitis include gallstones and trauma. Patients with gallstones frequently have episodes of mild pancreatitis, which may either be asymptomatic or associated with abdominal pain. These episodes cease when the gallbladder is removed. It is likely that small gallstones migrate from the gallbladder down the bile duct and temporarily block the pancreatic duct before passing into the duodenum. Obstruction of the pancreatic duct may be the cause of pancreatitis. This form of pancreatitis is much milder than that seen with alcoholism. Trauma to the pancreas, whether caused by accident or surgical operation on the pancreas, can also lead to pancreatitis due to release of enzymes.

The manifestations of pancreatitis usually include pain in the midabdomen, that may bore through to the back. Acute or active pancreatitis is associated with increased levels of amylase and lipase in the blood and amylase in the urine. In severe chronic pancreatitis, the acini may be destroyed, so that enzyme levels are no longer elevated. In chronic pancreatitis, there may be evidence of malabsorption or diabetes. Also, stimulation of the pancreas with secretin, a hormone that causes fluid secretion by the pancreas, produces subnormal amounts of pancreatic secretions in the duodenum (secretin test).

PANCREATITIS 15-6

causes	lesions	manifestations
Alcoholism	Enzymatic necrosis of	Abdominal pain
Gallstones	pancreas and surrounding	Malabsorption (late)
Trauma	adipose tissue	Diabetes mellitus (late)
	Fibrosis (chronic)	

Hyperplastic/Neoplastic Diseases

In the liver, metastases are much more common than primary cancer. Hepatocarcinoma is the most common primary tumor of the liver, and it most often occurs as a complication of nonalcoholic types of cirrhosis. Gallbladder cancer is rare, usually fatal, and is usually associated with gallstones. Cancer of the pancreas accounts for 3 percent of cancers and is almost always fatal.

Metastatic Cancer of the Liver

Abdominal cancers, such as carcinoma of the colon, stomach, and pancreas, characteristically metastasize to the liver, but metastases of other neoplasms, such as leukemias and lymphomas, are also common. A few patients present with liver metastases without symptoms referrable to the primary cancer site. They have large, nodular livers and may have jaundice (Figure 15–5). Liver metastases are not curable.

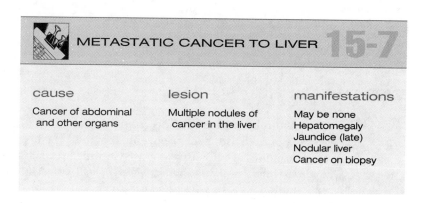

METASTATIC CANCER TO LIVER		15-7
cause	lesion	manifestations
Cancer of abdominal and other organs	Multiple nodules of cancer in the liver	May be none Hepatomegaly Jaundice (late) Nodular liver Cancer on biopsy

Carcinoma of the Pancreas

Most cases of carcinoma of the pancreas develop in the head of the pancreas, producing jaundice due to obstruction of the common bile duct and pain due to involvement of nerves in surrounding tissues.

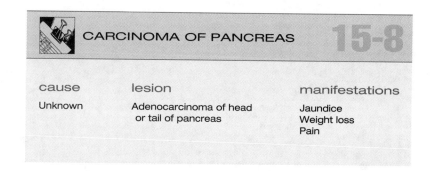

CARCINOMA OF PANCREAS		15-8
cause	lesion	manifestations
Unknown	Adenocarcinoma of head or tail of pancreas	Jaundice Weight loss Pain

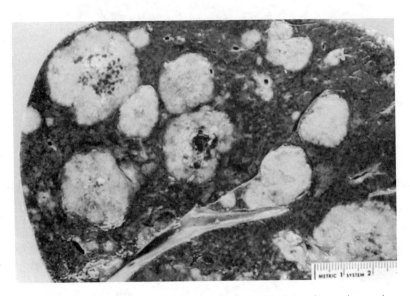

Figure 15–5. Liver metastases in a patient who presented with jaundice and an undiagnosed carcinoma of the colon.

ORGAN FAILURE

Acute liver failure results from massive death of hepatocytes and is associated with hepatic encephalopathy. Viral hepatitis and halothane reactions are the usual causes. Chronic liver failure is associated with cirrhosis. *Nonfunctioning gallbladder* is defined by a failure to take up radiopaque dyes designed to visualize the gallbladder. Stones wedged at the neck of the cystic duct are the usual cause. Acute pancreatic failure is not a recognized condition. Chronic pancreatic failure leads to the malabsorption syndrome if pancreatic acini are extensively destroyed and to diabetes mellitus if islets of Langerhans are extensively destroyed.

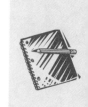

Review Questions

1. What are the most frequent diseases of the liver, gallbladder, and pancreas? Which are likely to be fatal?
2. What are three mechanisms by which jaundice may be produced?
3. What tests are used to detect liver disease? How do abnormalities of the tests correlate with changes in the liver?
4. How is a liver biopsy performed and what is its value?
5. How are gallstones demonstrated?
6. What are the causes, lesions, and manifestations of the diseases discussed in this chapter?
7. What is the most common outcome of viral hepatitis? What other outcomes occur?
8. What are the effects of alcohol on the liver and pancreas?
9. What are the causes and effects of portal hypertension, esophageal varices, ascites, and hepatic encephalopathy?
10. How do gallstones produce problems?
11. What do the following terms mean?
    Cholecystography
    Delirium tremens
    Jaundice
    Laennec's cirrhosis
    Nonfunctioning gallbladder
    Postnecrotic cirrhosis

16.

Kidney, Lower Urinary Tract, and Male Genital Organs

REVIEW OF STRUCTURE AND FUNCTION
Kidneys
Blood Supply • Glomeruli • Tubules • Juxtaglomerular Apparatus
Lower Urinary Tract
Ureters • Bladder • Urethra
Male Genital Organs
Testes • Prostate

MOST FREQUENT AND SERIOUS PROBLEMS
Cystitis • Prostate Enlargement • Renal Calculi • Glomerular Diseases • Carcinoma of Bladder and Prostate

SYMPTOMS, SIGNS, AND TESTS
Frequency • Dysuria • Nocturia • Hematuria • Proteinuria • Oliguria • Anuria • Urinalysis • Blood Urea Nitrogen • Creatinine • Renal Biopsy • Cystogram • Pyelograms • Catheterization • Cystoscopy

SPECIFIC DISEASES
Genetic/Developmental Diseases
Agenesis and Hypoplasia
Polycystic Kidneys
Dysplastic (Multicystic) Kidney
Cryptorchism
Inflammatory/Degenerative Diseases
Glomerular Diseases
Acute Poststreptococcal Glomerulonephritis
Chronic Glomerulonephritis
Pyelonephritis
Interstitial Nephritis

Cystitis
Prostatitis
Kidney Stones (Calculi)
Hyperplastic/Neoplastic Diseases
Benign Prostatic Hyperplasia (BPH)
Adenocarcinoma of the Prostate
Transitional Cell Carcinoma of the Bladder
Cancers of the Kidney
Cancers of the Testis

ORGAN FAILURE
Acute Renal Failure
Chronic Renal Failure

REVIEW QUESTIONS

REVIEW OF STRUCTURE AND FUNCTION

Disease of the male genital organs are discussed with diseases of the urinary tract because of the intimate anatomic relationship of the male genital organs and lower urinary tract (Figure 16–1).

The kidneys are bilateral retroperitoneal organs that receive blood from the renal arteries and are drained by the renal veins. Urine

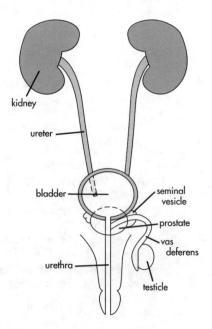

Figure 16–1. Components of urinary tract and male genital system.

formed by the kidney leaves through the ureter. The kidneys themselves consist of cortex, medulla, and pelvis (Figure 16–2). The cortex contains all of the glomeruli and most of the tubules. The medulla contains specialized parts of the tubules (loops of Henle) and the collecting tubules. The pelvis is a space lined by transitional epithelium that transmits urine from the collecting tubules to the ureters.

The kidneys' function is to regulate the concentration of salt, water, and hydrogen ions in the body and to excrete waste products such as urea and creatinine or foreign substances such as drugs and their metabolites. To accomplish this, the kidneys receive 20 percent of the circulating blood each minute. The main renal arteries branch several times into smaller arteries and arterioles, which eventually supply the renal glomeruli of the organ's cortex.

The basic functional unit of the kidney is called a *nephron* and consists of glomerulus, tubules, and associated vessels (Figure 16–3). Each glomerulus is a tuft of capillaries that are lined by endothelial cells. The entire tuft is covered with a layer of thin epithelial cells (Figure 16–4). Separating the two cell layers is an important basement membrane, which participates in the filtration function of the glomerulus. Blood leaving the glomerulus passes into a capillary network that surrounds epithelial-lined tubules. The waste materials that have been filtered through the glomeruli pass into these tubules. The tubules eventually merge to form collecting ducts, which carry urine to the renal pelvis. Throughout the length of the tubules there is constant exchange between the tubules and the capillary networks that surround them. Consequently, the urine that emerges from the kidney has a much different chemical composition than the initial filtrate emerging from the glomeruli. Many substances, such as glucose, chloride, and drugs,

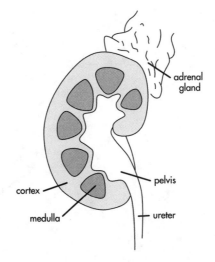

Figure 16–2. The kidney and adjacent structures.

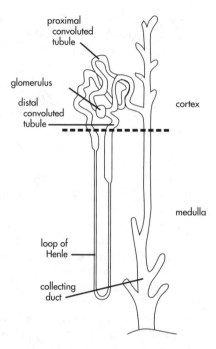

Figure 16–3. Components of a nephron.

continually pass back and forth between the tubules and the capillaries that surround them. Passage of substances from the capillaries to the tubules is termed *secretion*, while the opposite, passage from the tubules to capillaries, is termed *resorption*. The final concentrations of any substance in the urine is partly determined by the amount of secretion ver-

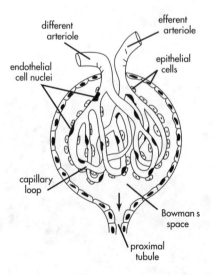

Figure 16–4. Components of a glomerulus.

sus resorption. One of the most important exchanges between renal tubular epithelium and surrounding capillaries takes place in the distal tubules and involves exchange of potassium for sodium. The kidney also contributes to the regulation of the body's acid-base balance by either secreting or absorbing hydrogen ion as required to control blood pH. The final composition of the urine is determined in the collecting tubules, where water is absorbed from urine back into the blood under the influence of antidiuretic hormone derived from the pituitary gland. The urine then passes through the pelvis of the kidneys and the ureters to the bladder. All the supporting tissue between the tubules and glomeruli is referred to as the interstitium of the kidney.

In the walls of arterioles supplying the glomerulus, there is a collection of cells called the *juxtaglomerular apparatus*. These cells secrete renin, an enzyme that acts on a protein secreted by the liver (renin substrate), converting it to angiotensin I. Angiotensin I is converted to angiotensin II by another enzyme (converting enzyme) produced by endothelial cells of the lung and kidney. Angiotensin II stimulates vasoconstriction (thereby elevating blood pressure) and enhances sodium and potassium absorption (by stimulating release of aldosterone from the adrenal cortex).

The lower urinary tract consists of the ureters, bladder, and urethra plus accessory glands of the tract. The tract is essentially similar in both male and female with regard to the ureters and the bladder. The ureters descend from the pelvis of the kidneys in the retroperitoneal tissue to the bladder. The function of the ureter is solely to transmit urine from the kidney to the bladder. No absorption of urine, or any of its contents, occurs along this muscular tubule. The bladder is a large muscular organ in which urine is collected from the ureters and passed down the urethra through the urethrovesicular outlet. The bladder outlet involves a complex intertwining of muscle fibers, which on contraction open the sphincter to allow discharge of bladder contents. The urethra of the female passes directly from the bladder through the urogenital diaphragm to the urethral meatus. In the male, however, the urethra consists of several additional segments that pass through the center of the prostate gland and extend on into the penis. In the prostate gland, the ejaculatory ducts penetrate through the substance of the prostate to connect the vas deferens to the urethra.

The testes consist basically of the seminiferous tubules where sperm are produced. Sperm are stored in the epididymis and vas deferens and are propelled along the vas deferens during ejaculation by muscular contraction. Sperm are also stored in the seminal vesicles, which lie along the vas deferens just posterior to the prostate.

The male prostate encircles the neck of the bladder in the retroperitoneal space. It is composed of three lobes and is a glandular organ, the ducts of which empty into the urethra as it passes through the prostate gland. Prostatic secretions comprise the major portion of seminal fluid and have a high antibacterial activity.

MOST FREQUENT AND SERIOUS PROBLEMS

Bacterial infections are the most frequent problems affecting the kidney and the lower urinary tract. Bladder infection (cystitis) is common in females, because bacteria from the perineum gain access to the bladder via the short female urethra. Prostatitis is fairly common in younger men. Prostatic enlargement is very common in older men and the consequent obstruction of the urethra predisposes to kidney as well as bladder infections. Renal calculi (stones) are not uncommon problems in adults. Diseases of the renal glomeruli are collectively of major importance, since they are the major cause of chronic renal failure. Transitional cell carcinoma of the bladder and adenocarcinoma of the prostate are relatively common in older individuals. Cancers of the kidneys and testes are uncommon.

SYMPTOMS, SIGNS, AND TESTS

Most patients with cystitis or urethritis experience *frequency of urination, dysuria* (painful urination), or *nocturia* (increased night time urination). In addition, the urine may be clouded by pus. Prostatitis may manifest simply as low back pain. Pyelonephritis may be asymptomatic or may present acutely with intense flank pain in addition to systemic signs of infection such as fever and leukocytosis. Diseases of the renal glomeruli may present with *hematuria* (blood in the urine), *proteinuria* (protein in the urine), or systemic signs such as edema and hypertension. Renal calculi characteristically present with intense, sharp *flank pains* that radiate toward the groin as the calculi migrate from the renal pelvis to the bladder. Acute necrosis of the renal tubules may result from either renal ischemia or the action of certain toxins and often is manifest by decreased output of urine (*oliguria*) or even complete absence of urine (*anuria*).

The nephrotic syndrome is a constellation of signs and laboratory abnormalities resulting from damage to the glomerular filtering apparatus. Proteinuria and hypoproteinemia are caused by excessive loss of protein through the defective glomerular basement membrane. Edema results from lowered plasma oncotic pressure due to protein loss. Hyperlipidemia is also present in the nephrotic syndrome for poorly understood reasons; it may be due to decreased lipid transport by proteins.

The most common causes of the nephrotic syndrome are lipoid nephrosis, amyloidosis, diabetes, focal glomerulosclerosis, and membranous glomerulonephritis, which will be discussed later in this chapter.

Physical examination of the urinary tract and genital organs consists of inspection of the penis or vulva for signs of exudation or ulceration from venereal infections, palpation of the abdomen for tumors of the kidney or a distended bladder, and, in the male, palpation of the inguinal ring for hernia or undescended testis, palpation of the testes for tumors, and rectal examination to feel for enlargement of the prostate.

Urinalysis is the most important routine laboratory test performed, because it can detect the presence of many common urinary tract disorders, especially infections. A urinalysis normally includes tests for the specific gravity, pH, and presence of protein, sugar, blood, and ketones, as well as microscopic examination to check for the possible presence of red blood cells, white blood cells, bacteria, crystals, and *casts* from damaged renal tubules (Figure 16–5).

Urine culture for bacteria may be performed when there are symptoms of urinary tract infection or increased amounts of white blood cells in the urine. Roughly, when there are over 100,000 bacteria per milliliter of urine, a diagnosis of urinary tract infection may be made. Lesser numbers suggest contamination of the specimen during collection. Bacterial antibiotic sensitivity studies help determine the most rational antibiotic therapy.

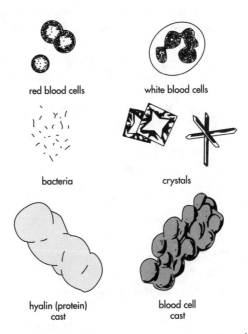

red blood cells   white blood cells

bacteria   crystals

hyalin (protein)   blood cell
cast   cast

Figure 16–5. Possible findings on microscopic examination of urine.

Renal function is most commonly evaluated by measuring levels of two substances in the blood that are excreted by filtration through the glomerulus, namely, *urea nitrogen* and *creatinine*. The normal blood levels of these substances are determined by an equilibrium between normal breakdown of nitrogenous compounds to produce urea nitrogen and normal muscle breakdown to produce creatinine, as well as the ability of the glomeruli to filter and the tubules to resorb these substances. Significant renal disease often raises the blood levels of these substances, because they are inadequately filtered in glomerular diseases or inadequately secreted and resorbed in tubular diseases.

Renal biopsies are often performed for the evaluation of glomerular disease by inserting a thin needle through the skin of the flank and extracting a core of renal tissue. Immunofluorescent techniques and electron microscopy, in addition to light microscopy, are usually performed on renal biopsies. A better understanding of glomerular diseases has been reached by this procedure.

Other examinations used in evaluating renal and urinary tract disease include *cystograms*, in which a radiopaque dye is introduced into the bladder by catheter and x-rays are taken to elucidate bladder morphology and function.

The intravenous urogram (IVU) is a commonly used test to look for gross structural changes in the kidneys and ureters. Radiopaque (iodinated) contrast material, injected intravenously, is filtered by the glomeruli into the tubules and concentrated in the renal pelvis and ureters. Distortion of the normal pattern of dye in the collecting system suggests a mass or cyst. Calculi in the renal pelvis appear as filling defects. Obstruction of the urinary tract dilates the pelvis and/or ureter.

Catheterization of the bladder refers to the process of placing a tube in the bladder, usually for the purpose of draining the bladder or collecting a urine sample. An indwelling catheter is one that is left in place for some time. *Cystoscopy* is the visualization of the bladder using a scope and is used to detect and biopsy bladder lesions. Seminal fluid examination is useful in detecting inflammatory cells and bacteria in cases of prostatitis and in evaluating sperm counts for determination of fertility.

CT and *ultrasound* techniques are used for diagnosis of renal masses such as cancer or cystic disease. *Doppler* ultrasound is used to evaluate blood flow.

SPECIFIC DISEASES

Genetic/Developmental Diseases

There are numerous developmental abnormalities of the genitourinary system, many of which occur in conjunction with anomalies of other organ systems. A few of the more common anomalies will be discussed.

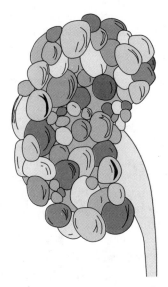

Figure 16–6. Adult polycystic kidney.

Agenesis and Hypoplasia

Complete agenesis of the kidney occurs very infrequently and is obviously incompatible with life if bilateral. Various degrees of hypoplasia may also be rarely encountered, and the final outcome of these cases depends upon the degree of hypoplasia plus the increased risk of superimposed insults such as pyelonephritis.

Polycystic Kidneys

Adult polycystic disease is a fairly common (1 in 500 persons) autosomal dominant disease in which thin-walled cysts of various size cause massive bilateral renal enlargement (Figure 16–6). The disease is usually

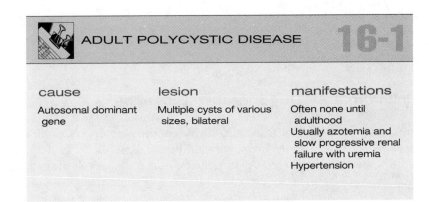

ADULT POLYCYSTIC DISEASE		16-1
cause	**lesion**	**manifestations**
Autosomal dominant gene	Multiple cysts of various sizes, bilateral	Often none until adulthood Usually azotemia and slow progressive renal failure with uremia Hypertension

not discovered until adulthood when hypertension or chronic renal failure occur. Although cysts occur in other organs, especially the liver, these are of little consequence, thus these patients are good candidates for renal dialysis and/or renal transplantation. *Infantile polycystic disease* is a rare, fatal autosomal recessive condition associated with bilateral renal cysts and hepatic fibrosis.

Dysplastic (Multicystic) Kidney
Malformation of embryonic development of nephrons with formation of cartilage and cysts may be unilateral or bilateral and is often associated with other anomalies and obstruction of the urinary tract. Prognosis for this common noninherited condition depends on the amount of normal renal parenchyma and seriousness of the associated anomalies.

Cryptorchism
Cryptorchism is a failure of the testes to descend into the scrotum. It is not uncommon. Bilateral cryptorchism will cause sterility if not surgically corrected in childhood. Descent normally does not occur until after birth and absence of descent 6 months after birth is not unusual. If surgical descent must be tried, it is usually undertaken around 5 years of age. If not surgically corrected, testicular cancer becomes a risk.

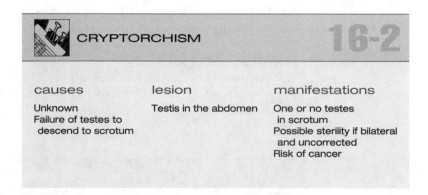

CRYPTORCHISM 16-2

causes	lesion	manifestations

Unknown
Failure of testes to
  descend to scrotum
	Testis in the abdomen	One or no testes
		  in scrotum
		Possible sterility if bilateral
		  and uncorrected
		Risk of cancer

Inflammatory/Degenerative Diseases

In this section, diseases of the glomeruli, infections of the kidney and lower urinary tract, interstitial nephritis, and kidney stones are considered. Acute degeneration and necrosis of renal tubules is discussed under Organ Failure.

Glomerular Diseases

Diseases of glomeruli may be divided into those that are primary diseases of the glomeruli and those that are secondary to systemic diseases such as diabetes mellitus or lupus erythematosus. *Nephritis* means inflammation of the kidney, and *glomerulonephritis* specifically designates inflammatory disease of the glomeruli. Many important primary diseases of glomeruli are inflammatory and are triggered by allergic (immune) injury of either of two types. In immune complex glomerulonephritis, antigen-antibody complexes form in the blood and are deposited on the basement membrane of the glomerulus as the glomerulus attempts to filter these complexes. In this context, the kidney is a passive recipient of these damaging antigen-antibody complexes. The second type is anti-basement membrane glomerulonephritis, in which antibodies are formed against the basement membrane itself, which acts as the antigen. The antibodies in this type of nephritis may be generated to react against a foreign protein (possibly a virus) that shares common antigenic properties with the glomerular basement membrane. This sharing of common antigenic properties is termed cross-reactivity. Both immune complex deposition and anti-basement membrane deposition damage the glomerular capillary structures, allowing excessive filtration of protein. In acute glomerulonephritis, red blood cells also leak through the glomerular structures, producing hematuria. A prototype immune complex disease is acute poststreptococcal glomerulonephritis.

Acute Poststreptococcal Glomerulonephritis

This disease is an immune complex glomerulonephritis that follows an antecedent infection with certain strains of group A streptococci anywhere in the body, usually a pharyngitis. One to 4 weeks following the initial streptococcal infection, antibodies are formed against the streptococcus antigens, and these antigen–antibody complexes are deposited on the glomerular basement membrane (Figures 16–7 and 16–8). The subsequent inflammation of the basement membrane leads to the cardinal clinical signs and symptoms of hematuria and proteinuria due to incompetence of the glomerular filtering apparatus. Generalized edema occurs because of loss of protein, and hypertension occurs because of stimulation of the juxtaglomerular apparatus. The diagnosis is made on the basis of hematuria, edema, and hypertension, plus a history of streptococcal infection. Other findings may include elevated urea nitrogen and creatinine in the blood, because these breakdown products cannot be excreted in normal amounts. The lesion is an inflamed glomerulus secondary to immune complex deposits. The recovery rate is approximately 95 percent in children and slightly lower in adults; the remainder in both groups develop progressive renal failure. Although numerous drugs, as well as other

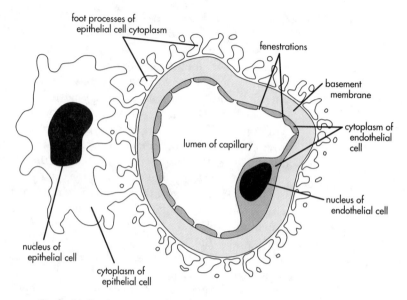

Figure 16–7. Components of a normal glomerulus by electron microscopy.

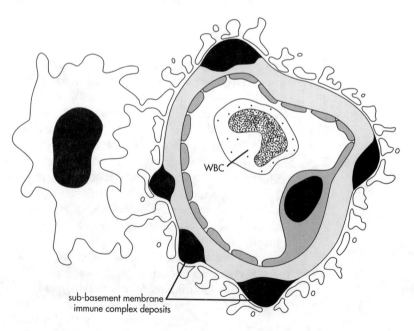

Figure 16–8. Glomerulus with immune complex deposits. WBC = white blood cell.

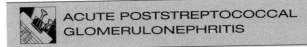

ACUTE POSTSTREPTOCOCCAL GLOMERULONEPHRITIS   16-3

cause	lesion	manifestations
Antigen—antibody complexes lodge in glomeruli	Inflamed glomeruli	Hematuria Proteinuria Hypertension Edema Possible progression to chronic renal failure

infectious agents, may also cause immune complex glomerulonephritis, the disease is no longer very common because of antibiotic treatment of group A streptococcal infections.

Chronic Glomerulonephritis

Chronic Glomerulonephritis refers to a variety of prolonged, often progressive, renal diseases. They may be initiated by immune complex deposition, by anti-basement membrane antibodies, or by nonimmunologic degeneration of unknown cause. Many of these diseases do not occur in an acute phase as does poststreptococcal glomerulonephritis; rather, the inflammation or degeneration and consequent scarring proceed slowly and insidiously. Often the diagnosis is made only after the patient complains of fatigue or edema and subsequent urinalysis reveals proteinuria. At this time, the kidney may be so severely damaged that the ordinary clues as to the cause of the disease are lost. Consequently, many patients are said to have chronic glomerulonephritis without regard to cause. However, using immunofluorescence and electron microscopy, the majority of cases of chronic glomerulonephritis can be classified as specific diseases.

Many patients, especially children, initially manifest chronic renal disease by the *nephrotic syndrome*. The nephrotic syndrome is not a disease per se but a complex of signs and symptoms (syndrome), which includes hypoproteinemia, proteinuria, hyperlipidemia, and edema. The syndrome may be associated with lipoid nephrosis, membranous glomerulonephritis, focal glomerulosclerosis, diabetes mellitus, amyloidosis, progressive poststreptococcal glomerulonephritis, and many other less common diseases. Of these, lipoid nephrosis and membranous glomerulonephritis are deserving of further description.

Lipoid nephrosis (also called minimal change glomerulopathy) is the most common cause of the nephrotic syndrome in children and adults. It accounts for 80 percent of the nephrotic syndrome in children and 30 percent in adults. The lesion of lipoid nephrosis is damaged epithelial foot processes adjacent to the glomerular capillary membrane (Figure 16–9) associated with leakage of protein into Bowman's space and thus into the urine. The damage can only be seen by electron microscopy. Further, there are no antibody deposits in the glomeruli of patients with lipoid nephrosis, and the cause as well as the pathogenesis of the disease are not known.

The second most common cause of the nephrotic syndrome in adults is *membranous glomerulonephritis.* Membranous glomerulonephritis is characterized by deposits of antigen-antibody embedded within the thickened glomerular basement membrane as observed in the electron microscope. These deposits disturb the normal permeability of the glomerular basement membrane, resulting in a large amount of protein, particularly albumin, passing from the vascular to the urinary space. In most cases, the nature of the antigen as well as the cause of the glomerulonephritis is unknown, and the disease is consequently termed *idiopathic membranous glomerulonephritis.* In a few instances, the antigen is known. Occasionally, the antigen is hepatitis virus. A bout of hepatitis may be associated with membranous glomerulonephritis with the nephrotic syndrome. In some instances, membranous glomerulonephritis may follow treatment

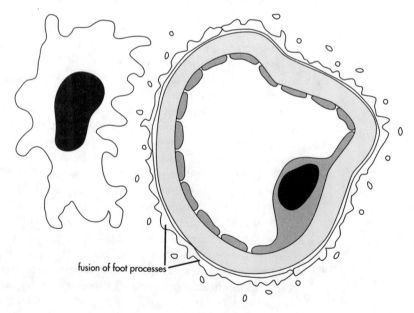

fusion of foot processes

Figure 16–9. Glomerulus in lipoid nephrosis with foot process fusion and no immune complex deposits.

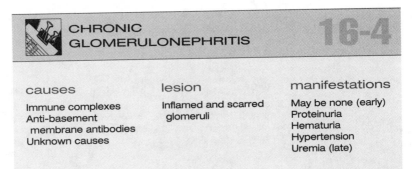

CHRONIC GLOMERULONEPHRITIS   16-4

causes	lesion	manifestations

Immune complexes
Anti-basement
  membrane antibodies
Unknown causes
	Inflamed and scarred
	  glomeruli
		May be none (early)
		Proteinuria
		Hematuria
		Hypertension
		Uremia (late)

with certain drugs such as gold salts, which are used to treat rheumatoid arthritis, or may be associated with certain other diseases such as syphilis.

Diabetes mellitus commonly causes chronic renal damage because of its effect on small blood vessels and often results in the nephrotic syndrome.

Some patients with the nephrotic syndrome will recover spontaneously, while others appear to respond to steroid therapy. Some will progress to chronic renal failure and may be kept alive for variable periods by *dialysis*—the so-called artificial kidney. Renal transplantation is possible in some patients with chronic renal disease.

Pyelonephritis

The most important inflammatory kidney disease is pyelonephritis, an acute or chronic bacterial infection predominantly involving the renal tubules and most commonly caused by *Escherichia coli* or other gram-negative bacteria such as proteus, pseudomonas, enterobacter, and klebsiella. The organisms may enter the kidney via the bloodstream or, most commonly, in retrograde fashion through the bladder and ureters. In the latter case, obstruction often plays an important role in the pathogenesis of the infection, because stagnation of urine consequent to urethral obstruction at any level favors the multiplication of bacteria and obviates their chances of being washed downstream. The patient with acute pyelonephritis will have more or less acute onset of flank pain as well as fever. Microscopically, the kidney will show variable amounts of acute inflammatory cells in the interstitial and tubular tissue, with relative sparing of the glomeruli. Later, the kidney will show scars in these areas. The patient's urine will have increased amounts of protein, casts, white blood cells, and bacteria. Often, the white cells will be so numerous as to constitute *pyuria* (pus in the urine). The casts are cylindrical protein deposits from damaged

PYELONEPHRITIS		**16-5**

causes	lesion	manifestations
Bacterial infection often resulting from obstruction Organisms from blood	Acutely and/or chronically inflamed renal tubules and pelvis	Flank pain Fever Leukocytosis Pus and casts in urine Possible renal failure

tubular epithelium (casts of the tubular lumens). The offending organism can usually be cultured from the urine. The treatment of pyelonephritis is antibiotic therapy and alleviation of the obstruction. In some patients, the disease may smolder for a long time in spite of antibiotic therapy. These are called *chronic pyelonephritis* and are often fostered by continued or intermittent obstructions of the urinary tract, although in some cases the reason for the perpetuation of the disease is not known.

Interstitial Nephritis

Chronic renal inflammations limited for the most part of the interstitium are encountered in patients who give a history of ingesting excessive amounts of analgesics, especially those containing phenacetin, or certain antibiotics.

Cystitis

Infection of the bladder is called *cystitis* and is usually caused by the same organisms that cause pyelonephritis. It is one of the more common infections encountered. The symptoms of cystitis are dysuria (painful urination), frequency (frequent urination), and urgency (repeated or continuous urge to urinate). The urine findings are the same as in pyelonephritis, except that casts are not found in cystitis. Infectious microorganisms invade the urinary tract by two major pathways—up the urethra or, rarely, via the circulatory system. The urethral route is the one most plaguing to women. In the male, the long penile urethra plus the presence of antibacterial secretions from the prostate discourage this route. Fecal soiling of the urethral meatus and sexual activity are common factors allowing organisms to enter the urinary tract in females. Instrumentation such as catheterization or cystoscopy is commonly complicated by infection in both sexes.

CYSTITIS 16-6

cause	lesion	manifestations
Bacterial infection often secondary to obstruction	Inflamed bladder mucosa	Dysuria Urgency Frequency White blood cells in urine Bacteria

Prostatitis

Prostatitis may be an acute or chronic infection and is often associated with considerable pain and discomfort. Leukocytes are encountered in the urine in prostatitis.

Kidney Stones (Calculi)

Crystallization of minerals in the urine to form hard, stone-like masses is common. Kidney stones are most often composed of calcium and various other substances excreted by the kidney such as oxalates. Stones containing calcium are visible on x-ray. Other stones, such as those composed of urates or cystine, are not visible by x-ray. Most commonly, small stones form in adults without clear-cut cause; however, low urine volume due to dehydration, chronic urinary tract infection, and prolonged bed rest with liberation of calcium from the bones can be precipitating factors. Less commonly, stones are caused by serious underlying diseases, including hyperparathyroidism and severe bone disease, which result in increased calcium in the urine. Gout and cystinosis are metabolic diseases that cause increased excretion of urates and cystine, respectively, leading to stone formation in some instances.

Passage of a small stone from the renal pelvis into the ureter produces sudden severe flank pain, which patients describe as worse than anything they have ever experienced. Immediate treatment consists of pain medications with the hope that the stone will pass down the urinary tract and be recovered in the urine. *Lithotripsy*, a non-invasive procedure utilizing *electroshock* waves to break up the stone, is often performed. If the stone fails to dislodge from the ureter, a urologist may have to remove the stone using catheters passed through the urethra, bladder, and ureter to dislodge the impacted stone. A stone impacted in the ureter may lead to hydronephrosis (Figures 16–10 and 16–11). Occasionally, large stones are encountered that fill the renal pelvis. These are referred to as *staghorn calculi* because of their appearance.

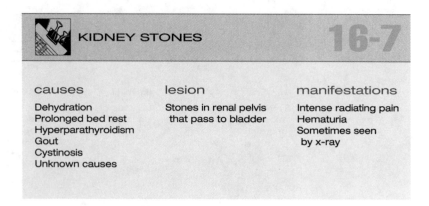

KIDNEY STONES

16-7

causes

Dehydration
Prolonged bed rest
Hyperparathyroidism
Gout
Cystinosis
Unknown causes

lesion

Stones in renal pelvis
that pass to bladder

manifestations

Intense radiating pain
Hematuria
Sometimes seen
by x-ray

Hyperplastic/Neoplastic Diseases

Hyperplasia of the prostate and carcinoma of the prostate and bladder are common and very significant diseases of the elderly. Cancers of the testis and kidney are much less common, are of several types, and occur in younger individuals.

Benign Prostatic Hyperplasia (BPH)

Enlargement of the prostate is caused by hyperplasia of the glandular parenchyma and its fibromuscular stroma in the periurethral area, probably due to relative hormonal imbalance in the elderly. As

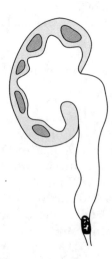

Figure 16–10. Renal stone lodged in ureter with dilated ureter and renal pelvis (hydronephrosis).

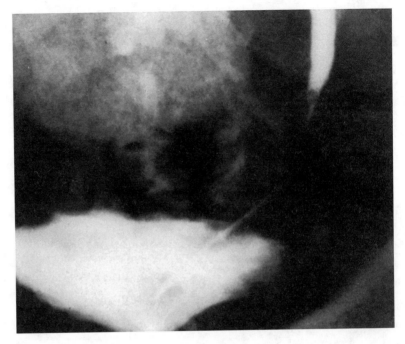

Figure 16–11. Intravenous urogram demonstrating a calculus lodged in the ureter (*arrow*) with dye-filled, dilated ureter above and dye-filled urinary bladder below.

the bulk of this central tissue enlarges, the peripheral tissue begins to atrophy. The hyperplastic process does not take place evenly throughout the affected regions but occurs as multiple nodules. The cause of prostatic hyperplasia is not known. The most popular theories involve imbalances in the blood androgen–estrogen ratios. The most common symptom of prostatic hyperplasia is difficulty in initiating and stopping urination. The major complication of prostatic

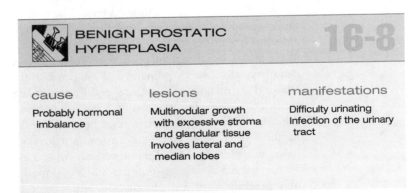

BENIGN PROSTATIC HYPERPLASIA

16-8

cause	lesions	manifestations
Probably hormonal imbalance	Multinodular growth with excessive stroma and glandular tissue Involves lateral and median lobes	Difficulty urinating Infection of the urinary tract

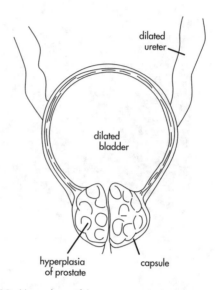

Figure 16–12. Hyperplasia of the prostate with obstruction of the urethra.

enlargement is obstruction of the urinary tract at the outlet of the bladder (Figure 16–12). Urinary tract infections frequently occur as a consequence of the obstruction. The most common surgical procedure for BPH is the *transurethral resection* (TUR) of excessive prostatic tissue. This operation entails the use of a special instrument inserted through the penis to cut away chips of prostatic tissue surrounding the urethra. Medical treatment is becoming more common and consists of anti-androgens or 5α-reductose inhibitors which block conversion of testosterone to dihydrotestosterone, thereby decreasing the influence of this androgen on the gland.

Adenocarcinoma of the Prostate

Cancer of the prostate is rare under the age of 50 but progressively more common thereafter, attaining a very high incidence in the elderly. Carcinoma of the prostate presents as a hard irregular nodule in the gland, usually in the posterior lobe (Figure 16–13). Its presence can often be found by palpation of the prostate from the rectum. An elevated serum level of prostate specific antigen (PSA) can aid in diagnosis. PSA is commonly used as a screening test for prostatic carcinoma but is somewhat controversial because of false positive and false negative tests. Low back pain and weight loss, x-ray appearance of pelvic bone lesions, and elevated serum acid and alkaline phosphatase all suggest metastatic dissemination. Occasionally, prostatic carcinomas produce urethral obstruction and may require transurethral resection to relieve the obstruction. Prostatic carcinoma preferentially

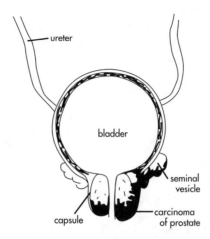

Figure 16–13. Carcinoma of the prostate with invasion of capsule and seminal vesicle.

metastasizes to bone. Carcinomas found while still contained within the prostate itself can sometimes be successfully treated by surgical excision. When metastatic spread has occurred, estrogen therapy with or without castration to remove the source of testosterone may be employed as palliative therapy. It is not uncommon for elderly men to live 10 years or more with prostatic cancer. On the other hand, in some patients the disease progresses rapidly, especially in younger ones with normal testosterone levels.

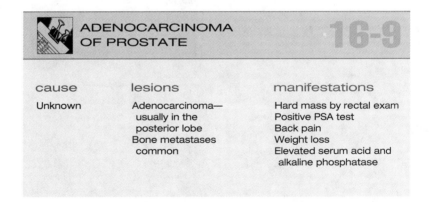

ADENOCARCINOMA OF PROSTATE

16-9

cause	lesions	manifestations
Unknown	Adenocarcinoma— usually in the posterior lobe Bone metastases common	Hard mass by rectal exam Positive PSA test Back pain Weight loss Elevated serum acid and alkaline phosphatase

Transitional Cell Carcinoma of the Bladder

Carcinoma of the urinary bladder is the fifth most common cancer, occurs much more commonly in males, and has an age peak in the seventies. In the United States, cigarette smoking may be the most important etiologic factor. There is a high incidence among employees of

TRANSITIONAL CELL CARCINOMA OF BLADDER   16-10

causes	lesions	manifestations
Usually unknown Possibly chemical carcinogenesis in some instances	Papillary growths of bladder mucosa Variable degrees of invasiveness	Hematuria Infection

industries that manufacture certain chemicals, notably aniline dyes. Transitional cell carcinomas usually present with painless hematuria. Diagnosis is made by cystoscopy and biopsy. Prognosis varies greatly depending on whether the tumor is superficial and well differentiated or extends into the muscularis propria and is poorly differentiated (Figure 16–14). Superficial lesions can be removed by transurethral resection, but they tend to recur or be multiple.

Cancers of the Kidney

Cancer of the kidney is relatively uncommon. In children, malignant tumors of primitive renal elements occur and are called *Wilm's tumor.*

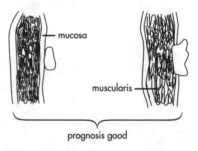

mucosa

muscularis

prognosis good

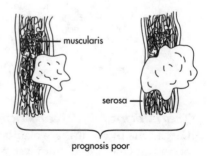

muscularis

serosa

prognosis poor

Figure 16–14. Transitional cell carcinoma of the bladder with varying degrees of invasion.

Adenocarcinomas of renal epithelial origin comprise most of the renal carcinomas in adults. Both types of tumors often present with hematuria and/or a flank mass. Treatment consists of surgical removal of the affected kidney plus chemotherapy or radiation therapy if extension beyond the kidney has occurred.

Cancers of the Testis

Several types of cancers of the germ cells of the testis occur. The most common is called *seminoma*. These cancers are uncommon but tend to occur most often in young adult men. They are usually detected as a mass. Seminomas have the most favorable outcome; however, other types are often cured by aggressive chemotherapy and radiation therapy even in the presence of metastases.

ORGAN FAILURE

Acute Renal Failure

The common life-threatening lesion of the renal tubules is *acute tubular necrosis*, an acute degeneration and necrosis of renal epithelial cells in the proximal and/or distal convoluted tubules. The common mechanisms of acute tubular necrosis are ischemic and toxic injury. Ischemic necrosis results from shock, with diversion of blood flow away from the kidney and insufficient oxygen to keep the tubular cells alive. Toxic necrosis is caused by a variety of poisons, the most common of which are methyl alcohol, ethylene glycol (antifreeze), mushroom poisons, chloroform, carbon tetrachloride, several antibiotic agents, and many heavy metals, especially mercury. Necrosis of the renal tubular epithelium rapidly leads to oliguria and even anuria. Consequent water and potassium retention in the patient results in a life-threatening situation. The clinical course of such a patient is monitored by following levels of the blood urea nitrogen and creatinine. The higher the values, the worse the patient's condition. If the patient can be kept alive by careful monitoring of blood electrolytes and possible dialysis (artificial kidney) for about 2 weeks, then the renal epithelium begins to regenerate. This regeneration is attended by significant diuresis (excessive urinary output), because the immature epithelium cannot efficiently reabsorb water.

Chronic Renal Failure

Most renal failure is chronic and insidious. Often the first detectable evidence of compromised renal function is the retention of the nitrogenous breakdown products of protein metabolism, reflected by elevated serum levels of creatinine and urea nitrogen. The retention of nitrogenous wastes in the blood is called *azotemia.* Progressive renal failure will result in body water disturbances, electrolyte (sodium, potassium, chloride, calcium) imbalances, and retention of acids; with profound effects on the body, including slowed mental activity, muscle weakness, and anemia. The sum total of all these effects of advanced renal failure is called *uremia.* Chronic renal failure is most often the result of chronic glomerulonephritis but may occasionally be due to severe pyelonephritis, long-standing obstruction of the urinary tract, or severe vascular disease of the kidney (arteriosclerosis).

In acute renal failure, the patient may be dialyzed if there is reasonable hope that kidney function may return to a near normal state. With chronic renal failure, the patient may be dialyzed at regular intervals on a permanent basis, or depending on the nature of the underlying disease, a kidney transplant may be considered.

Review Questions

1. What are the most common diseases of the kidney, lower urinary tract, and male genital system? What is the major effect of each?

2. What is the significance of each of the following signs or symptoms?
    Hematuria
    Dysuria
    Nocturia
    Frequency
    Anuria
    Flank pain
    Pyuria

3. What are the following tests and procedures used for?
    Urinalysis
    Blood urea nitrogen
    Creatinine

Intravenous urogram
Cystogram
Cystoscopy
Renal biopsy
Lithotripsy

4. What are the causes, lesions, and major manifestations of each of the specific diseases discussed in this chapter?

5. How do immune complex glomerulonephritis and anti-basement membrane glomerulonephritis differ in terms of cause and lesion?

6. How do acute and chronic glomerulonephritis differ?

7. What is the usual cause and pathogenesis of pyelonephritis?

8. What are the common causes and predisposing factors of kidney stones?

9. How do prostatic hyperplasia and prostatic carcinoma differ in terms of causes, lesions, manifestations, and possible complications?

10. How do acute and chronic renal failure differ in terms of causes, lesions, and manifestations?

11. What do the following terms mean?
Juxtaglomerular apparatus
Casts
Nephritis
Calculi
Transurethral resection
Wilm's tumor
Seminoma
Oliguria
Diuresis
Azotemia
Uremia

17.

Female Genital Organs

REVIEW OF STRUCTURE AND FUNCTION
Vulva • Vagina • Uterus • Fallopian Tubes • Ovaries

MOST FREQUENT AND SERIOUS PROBLEMS
Birth Control • Sexual Counseling • Prenatal Care and Childbirth • Menopausal Symptoms • Infections • Cancer

SYMPTOMS, SIGNS, AND TESTS
Bleeding • Pain • Discharge • Endocrine Effects • Pelvic Examination • Mass • Pap Smear • Biopsy • Laparoscopy

SPECIFIC DISEASES
  Genetic/Developmental Diseases
  Inflammatory/Degenerative Diseases
    Gonorrheal and Chlamydial Infections
    Syphilis
    Herpes Infection
    Condyloma Acuminatum
    Superficial Vaginal Infections
  Hyperplastic/Neoplastic Diseases
    Endometriosis
    Leiomyoma of the Uterus
    Carcinoma of the Endometrium
    Carcinoma of the Cervix
    Ovarian Tumors
  Diseases of Pregnancy
    Spontaneous Abortion
    Ectopic Pregnancy
    Septic Abortion
    Toxemia of Pregnancy
    Gestational Trophoblastic Neoplasms

ORGAN FAILURE
Infertility: Voluntary and Involuntary

REVIEW QUESTIONS

REVIEW OF STRUCTURE AND FUNCTION

Female genital organs include the vulva (labia majora, labia minora, clitoris), vagina, uterus (cervix, body), fallopian tubes, and ovaries (Figure 17–1). The vulva, vagina, and outer aspects of the cervix are lined by a protective stratified squamous epithelium. Bartholin's glands at the outlet of the vagina produce a mucoid secretion.

The uterine cervix is the distal, narrow portion of the uterus that projects into the vagina. The vaginal surface of the cervix is covered by stratified squamous epithelium. At the os (opening), there is a transition to the columnar mucus-secreting epithelium of the endocervix. The glandular mucosa lining the uterine cavity (endometrium) is the site for implantation of a fertilized ovum. The body (fundus) of the uterus is a muscular organ with a glandular epithelial lining. The muscular wall stretches and hypertrophies during pregnancy, and its contraction is important in accomplishing childbirth.

The ovaries and endometrium function synchronously to provide opportunity for pregnancy to occur. The menstrual cycle is timed from the onset of bleeding because this date is easily determined. However, the critical events are more accurately timed from the day of ovulation as determined by a rise in basal body temperature. In the 14 days following ovulation, the endometrium, under the influence of progesterone secreted by the ovary, undergoes secretory changes leading to sloughing if implantation does not occur. During and after the 3 to 5 days of menstruation, the endometrium is in proliferative phase for about 14 days, but the length of this phase is less predictable than the secretory phase. If implantation occurs, the stromal cells

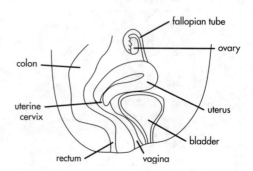

Figure 17–1. Female genital organs in relationship to colon and rectum.

of the secretory endometrium become large and plump producing decidualized endometrium or decidua. The complex endocrine control of the menstrual cycle and pregnancy involves hormones from the pituitary glands, adrenal glands, ovaries, and placenta. The details of these mechanisms and pathologic variations will be left to other sources.

MOST FREQUENT AND SERIOUS PROBLEMS

The most frequent health problems relating to the female genital system include birth control, sexual counseling, prenatal care and childbirth, menopausal symptoms, infections, and cancer screening.

Serious conditions associated with pregnancy include ectopic pregnancy, septic abortion, toxemia of pregnancy, hemorrhage, complications of delivery, and endometritis following delivery. Spontaneous abortion (miscarriage) and elective abortion are common.

Sexually transmitted (*venereal*) infections produce both acute and long-term problems in females. Gonorrhea is the most commonly reported communicable disease, but infections due to chlamydia, although less commonly reported, may be even more common. Gonorrhea and chlamydia infection produce urethritis and cervicitis. When they spread to the fallopian tubes they produce a more serious infection called *pelvic inflammatory disease*. Viral infections caused by human papilloma virus is an important factor in the genesis of carcinoma of the cervix. Herpes simplex commonly affects the cervix, vagina, and vulva.

Cytologic diagnosis of precancerous lesions has led to a decrease in carcinoma of the cervix so that it is now less common than endometrial carcinoma. Ovarian cancer is less common than uterine cancer, but much more likely to be fatal. Leiomyoma, a benign tumor, of the uterus is more common than cancer, but usually requires no treatment.

SYMPTOMS, SIGNS, AND TESTS

Major symptoms include bleeding, pain, vaginal discharge, and endocrine effects. Normal vaginal bleeding (menstruation), which occurs for 3 to 5 days at intervals of approximately 28 days from menarche to menopause (except during pregnancy) must be distinguished from abnormal uterine bleeding. Bleeding may be abnormal in amount, timing, or character. Hormonal changes are the most common cause of abnormal bleeding, but bleeding is also one of the principal symptoms of cancer. Several names have been coined to describe patterns of bleeding: menorrhagia (excessive menses), metrorrhagia (irregular bleeding from the uterus between menses), vaginal spotting (small amounts of blood not associated with menses), dysmenorrhea (painful menstruation), dysfunctional uterine bleeding (abnormal bleeding without causative lesion).

Cramping pain is common during menstruation (dysmenorrhea). Many women experience a sharp, one-sided abdominal pain at midcycle due to peritoneal irritation caused by rupture of an ovarian follicle at the time of ovulation. Causes of severe pain include ruptured ectopic pregnancy, acute pelvic inflammatory disease (salpingitis), and twisted or ruptured ovarian cysts. Pruritis (itching) is a form of pain that is commonly associated with atrophic changes in the vulvar skin in postmenopausal women and infections of the vulva and vagina in younger women.

Nonbloody vaginal discharge is associated with mild superficial infections, such as trichomonas and candida vaginitis. Symptoms related to endocrine changes are common prior to onset of menstruation (often called premenstrual syndrome) and at the time of menopause (hot flashes).

Signs of gynecologic disease are discovered by systematic examination of the female genitalia referred to as *pelvic examination.* This involves direct inspection of the vulva, examination of the vagina and cervix through a speculum (a device used to spread the vaginal wall), and bimanual palpation of the uterus, fallopian tubes, and ovaries. Bimanual examination is so named because one of the examiner's hands is placed on the abdomen and the fingers of the other hand are inserted into the vagina and the organs are palpated between the two hands. Bimanual rectal examination allows palpation of posterior uterine lesions.

The most common signs are pelvic mass and flat or raised lesions of the vulva and cervix. Pregnancy is the most common mass. Leiomyomas of the uterus are also common and the various ovarian tumors are usually discovered by palpation of a mass. Carcinomas of the vulva and cervix are visible by inspection. Condylomata acuminata are common venereal warts of the vulva, vagina, and cervix. The vulva may be involved by many skin diseases.

The most common test is the Papanicolaou smear (Pap smear) of the uterine cervix. (Figure 17–2). Pap smears at regular intervals allow detection of cervical cancer before it becomes invasive and can be credited with a sharp reduction in mortality from this disease. Blood counts are important for detection of iron-deficiency anemia, a common condition in women due to loss of iron in menstrual blood and transfer of iron to the fetus during pregnancy. Pregnancy tests involve the measurement of chorionic gonadotropin, a hormone, in urine or blood.

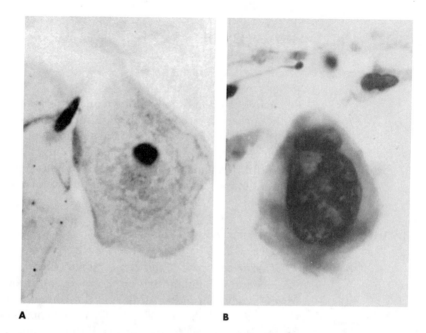

A   **B**

Figure 17–2. Photomicrograph of cells on a Pap smear from the uterine cervix. A. Normal surface squamous epithelial cell with small nucleus and abundant cytoplasm. B. Neoplastic squamous epithelial cell with large atypical nucleus and scant cytoplasm.

The female genital tract is rivaled only by skin in the frequency of use of biopsy as a diagnostic tool. Biopsy is used to define the nature of vulvar lesions, especially those with malignant potential. The cervix is biopsied whenever there is a visible lesion or a positive Pap smear. Staining of the cervix and examination at high magnification with a colposcope aids in selecting the most appropriate biopsy sites. Cone biopsy refers to the removal of a cone of tissue including the cervical os and endocervical lining for systematic histologic evaluation. Endometrial biopsy is essential for evaluation of endometrial lesions and to exclude endometrial carcinoma (cytology is much more reliable in detecting cervical lesions). One procedure for endometrial biopsy is called dilation and curettage (D & C) and involves dilating the cervical os and scraping out tissue with a curette. Small samples of endometrium can be obtained without dilating the cervix.

Diseases of the fallopian tubes and ovaries may be evaluated by ultrasound, a noninvasive procedure, and by *laparoscopy*, a procedure involving the insertion of an endoscope into the peritoneal cavity through an incision at the umbilicus. These procedures are particularly useful in diagnosis of ectopic pregnancy, endometriosis, and pelvic inflammatory disease.

SPECIFIC DISEASES

Genetic/Developmental Diseases

Compared to other organ systems, congenital anomalies of the female genital organs are relatively uncommon. Various degrees of uterine duplication occur. Resection of a uterine septum that divides the endometrial cavity into two compartments may improve chances for a successful pregnancy. Cysts formed from embryonic remnants occur adjacent to the fallopian tubes and in the lateral wall of the cervix and vagina.

Inflammatory/Degenerative Diseases

Gonorrheal and Chlamydial Infections

Gonococcal and chlamydial organisms account for millions of cases of venereally transmitted disease in the United States each year (see Chapter 26 for discussion of these diseases). Females with asymptomatic urethritis and cervicitis are carriers. If the organisms spread to the fallopian tubes, acute or chronic salpingitis may occur. Acute salpingitis with abdominal pain and fever must be differentiated from acute appendicitis since the treatment for the latter is surgical. Acute salpingitis is treated with antibiotics. Resolution of acute salpingitis often leads to scarring of the fallopian tube. Scarring of the tube leads to two important complications: infertility and ectopic pregnancy.

Syphilis

The painless primary ulcer of syphilis (chancre) will go unnoticed if located in the vagina or on the cervix. The key to control of syphilis is finding and treating such asymptomatic carriers. (For further discussion of this disease see Chapter 26).

Herpes Infection

Herpes simplex viruses cause blistering lesions of the squamous epithelium of the vulva and cervix. Most genital herpes is caused by herpes simplex virus type II, but some infections are caused by type I virus. At birth the virus may rarely be spread to the newborn producing a fatal disseminated infection.

Condyloma Acuminatum

Several serotypes of human papilloma viruses can cause multiple squamous papillomas of the vulva, anus, vagina, and cervix. These lesions are similar to the common skin wart (verruca vulgaris) except that they are commonly venereally transmitted and they tend to occur on moist mucous membranes in both males and females. Lesions on the cervix are usually flat. The papilloma virus and condylomatous changes in the cervix have been statistically associated with the development of carcinoma of the cervix.

Superficial Vaginal Infections

Trichomonas vaginalis (Figure 17–3A) is a protozoan that commonly produces a bubbly vaginal discharge and may cause small reddened areas in the vagina and cervix. Trichomoniasis does not cause any serious problems, is easily diagnosed by microscopic examination of a fresh drop of vaginal fluid, and can be treated with drugs. Candida (Figure 17–3B) are fungi that are normally present in small numbers but can proliferate to produce a superficial vaginitis, especially during pregnancy, in association with oral contraceptive therapy, in diabetic women, and as a complication of antibiotic therapy. Candidiasis can be diagnosed by smear or culture of vaginal discharge. Treatment consists of antimicrobial agents and control of the underlying condition.

Hyperplastic/Neoplastic Diseases

There is a wide variety of neoplasms, hyperplasias, and cystic diseases of the female genital system. Carcinomas of the vulva, cervix, endometrium, and ovary account for the vast majority of cancers. Leiomyoma of uterus is important because of its frequency. Endometriosis, a condition of uncertain cause, represents ectopic endometrium that responds to hormonal stimulation. Collectively, ovarian tumors are fairly common. They present as masses and are diagnosed by a pathologist after removal.

Endometriosis

Endometriosis is the occurrence of endometrial tissue outside the uterus, usually in the ovary, but also on the peritoneal surface of

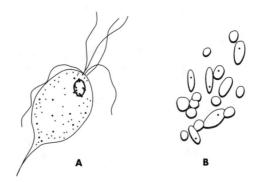

Figure 17–3. A. *Trichomonas vaginalis* organism. B. Yeast form of candida organisms.

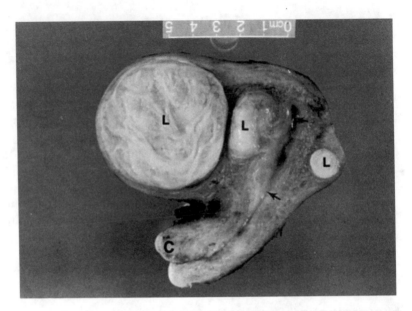

Figure 17–4. Uterus with three leiomyomas (L). Arrows indicate endometrial cavity. C is cervix.

adjacent organs. The origin of this tissue is unclear (metaplasia or ectopia). Bleeding may occur at the time of menstruation with the resultant hematoma producing severe dysmenorrhea. The hematoma may be walled off by fibrous tissue with the liquid contents forming a "chocolate" cyst. In addition to pain, endometriosis is often associated with infertility.

Leiomyoma of the Uterus

Solitary or multiple benign neoplasms of uterine smooth muscle are estrogen dependent, i.e., they develop during childbearing years and undergo atrophic changes after menopause. Atrophy with fibrous replacement accounts for the common synonym, *fibroid*. Leiomyoma may become quite large and distort the uterus (Figure 17–4). They

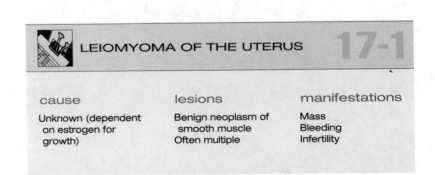

LEIOMYOMA OF THE UTERUS   17-1

cause	lesions	manifestations
Unknown (dependent on estrogen for growth)	Benign neoplasm of smooth muscle Often multiple	Mass Bleeding Infertility

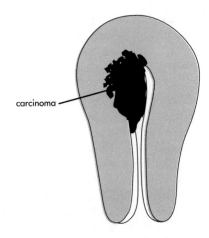

Figure 17–5. Carcinoma of the endometrium.

are usually asymptomatic but may cause pelvic pressures, bleeding, or infertility.

Carcinoma of the Endometrium

Adenocarcinoma of the endometrium is now the most common female genital cancer. Prolonged estrogen stimulation is associated with increased frequency of endometrial carcinoma such as occurs in patients with breast cancer being treated with hormones, estrogen-secreting ovarian tumors, and obesity. Current types of oral contraceptive therapy do not predispose to endometrial cancer. Other conditions associated with endometrial cancer include diabetes, hypertension, and infertility. Endometrial carcinomas, which are often well differentiated, begin in a normal or hyperplastic endometrium. They gradually grow into the wall of the uterus (Figure 17–5), but usually bleed and are diagnosed before they metastasize.

Radiation therapy and surgical removal of the uterus and ovaries can be combined to give an overall survival rate of about 80 percent

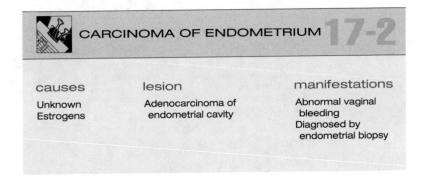

CARCINOMA OF ENDOMETRIUM 17-2

causes	lesion	manifestations
Unknown Estrogens	Adenocarcinoma of endometrial cavity	Abnormal vaginal bleeding Diagnosed by endometrial biopsy

because most of the cancers are confined to the body of the uterus at the time of diagnosis. The high cure rate may in part be due to the fact that most of the cancers develop after menopause so that bleeding is recognized by the patient as abnormal.

Carcinoma of the Cervix

Squamous cell carcinomas of the cervix almost always arise near the os at the junction of ectocervix and endocervix. Fortunately, carcinoma of the cervix usually develops in stages over a number of years so that Pap smears at regular intervals should provide a diagnosis in time for a cure. The evidence is overwhelming that human papillomavirus, a sexually transmitted virus, is involved in the pathogenesis of carcinoma of the cervix; women who have not had intercourse do not develop the cancer. The changes in the cervical epithelium that precede overt cancer with invasion represent a continuum, but for convenience are graded as follows: cervical intraepithelial neoplasia grade I (CIN-I or mild dysplasia), CIN-II (or moderate dysplasia), CIN-III (encompassing severe dysplasia and carcinoma-in-situ), and invasive squamous cell carcinoma. It is not clear exactly when the developing lesion becomes a cancer, but metastases cannot occur before microinvasion occurs and rarely occurs before a grossly visible cancer is present.

The grading of the developing lesion is done by cytology and biopsy and is subject to observer variability. CIN-I lesions are usually followed to see if they regress or become more severe. CIN-III lesions are removed by hysterectomy, cone biopsy, or laser cautery. CIN-II lesions are variably treated. Cone biopsy is used for treatment when the patient wishes to preserve childbearing potential. Invasive lesions are treated by surgical removal and/or radiation depending on the stage of the disease. Advanced carcinoma of the cervix (Figure 17–6)

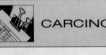

CARCINOMA OF THE CERVIX   17-3

causes	lesion	manifestations

Unknown
Sexually transmitted
  agent (human
  papillomavirus)
	Squamous cell
	  carcinoma
		Abnormal cells on
		  Pap smear by
		  routine examination
		Abnormal vaginal
		  bleeding
		Cervical mass

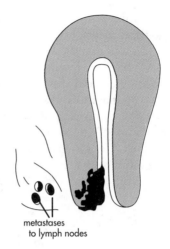

Figure 17–6. Carcinoma of uterine cervix.

usually kills by local invasion leading to obstruction of the ureters and renal failure.

Ovarian Tumors

The ovary has the potential to produce a greater variety of tumors than any other organ. These take the form of cysts and neoplasms of varying malignancy. Of the neoplasms, epithelial neoplasms derived from surface cells are most common. These epithelial neoplasms differentiate along several lines, with the three most common types including serous tumors, mucinous tumors, and endometrioid tumors. Serous tumors form from simple ciliated columnar epithelium, mucinous tumors have cells containing a drop of mucus, and endometrioid tumors are glandular tumors resembling endometrium. The serous and mucinous tumors are usually cystic and are classified into three groups: cystadenoma (a benign epithelial-lined cyst), lesions with low malignant potential (cysts with more cellular lining and capacity to implant in the peritoneum, but limited growth potential), and cystadenocarcinoma (obviously invasive). The survival rate for the carcinomas is very low; thus ovarian cancer kills more women than endometrial and cervical cancers combined. Tumors with low malignant potential are usually cured if localized to the ovary, but they are often large and may spill into the peritoneum where they have a tendency to recur. The endometrioid tumors are usually malignant.

Ovarian tumors derived from ovarian stroma or germ cells tend to be benign, although a few have malignant potential. The stromal tumors may secrete female or male hormones. The most common germ cell tumor is a benign teratoma, often called a *dermoid cyst.* Teratomas are composed of a variety of tissues including skin, various types of glands, cartilage, brain, and even teeth.

Non-neoplastic cysts are quite common and include follicular cysts (enlarged graafian follicles), corpus luteum cyst (enlarged corpus luteum), and chocolate cyst of endometriosis.

The diagnosis of ovarian tumors is based on pathologic examination after removal. Since most ovarian tumors are small and benign, professional judgment is required to decide which ones should be removed. Hemorrhage from a cystic tumor or twisting and infarction of the tumor may produce an acutely painful abdomen and require operative removal of the cyst or tumor.

Diseases of Pregnancy

The number of problems that can complicate pregnancy is so large that they are separately dealt with by the subspecialty of obstetrics. We will discuss a few important problems that arise at various times during and after pregnancy. Numerous other abnormal conditions, many of which occur at the time of labor and delivery, are beyond the scope of this text.

Spontaneous Abortion

At least one out of five pregnancies terminates spontaneously during the first third of pregnancy. These abortions usually result from a major defect in embryonic development due to abnormal chromosomes. The chromosome abnormality is usually confined to the individual sperm or ovum involved, so the next pregnancy is likely to be normal. The patient presents with cramps and bleeding, and the placental tissue either passes spontaneously or is found in the cervical os or vagina. Dilation and curettage may be needed to remove remaining placental tissue to prevent infection. The pathologist frequently finds only placental tissue without evidence of the embryo.

Ectopic Pregnancy

This results from implantation of the fertilized ovum before it reaches the endometrium. It most often occurs in a fallopian tube (Figures 17–7 and 17–8) but may occur in the abdominal cavity. As the placenta enlarges, blood vessels are likely to rupture and produce serious internal hemorrhage. The symptoms include pain from hemorrhage into the fallopian tube, vaginal bleeding, and light-headedness from blood loss. Laparoscopy leads to a specific diagnosis, and surgical removal of the ectopic pregnancy prevents fatal hemorrhage. Ectopic pregnancies are more likely to occur in fallopian tubes that have been partially obstructed by previous pelvic inflammatory disease.

ECTOPIC PREGNANCY   **17-4**

causes	lesions	manifestations
Implantation of fertilized ovum in fallopian tube or abdominal cavity	Fetus and placenta in fallopian tubes or abdominal cavity	Pain
		Vaginal hemorrhage
	Internal hemorrhage	Hemorrhage or mass seen by laparoscopy
Often follows pelvic inflammatory disease		

Septic Abortion

This refers to infection of the uterus superimposed on abortion and more commonly occurs when abortions are carried out by untrained persons using nonsterile technique. The infection may spread to the peritoneal cavity and cause death. Treatment consists of the removal of the infected tissue along with antibiotics.

Toxemia of Pregnancy

This common syndrome of unknown cause develops in the last third of pregnancy and is characterized by high blood pressure, edema, and proteinuria. Toxemia may progress to a severe, life-threatening stage with convulsions. Toxemia with convulsions is called *eclampsia*. Toxemia is most common in first pregnancies, in pregnancies with multiple fetuses, and in patients with previous high blood pressure or renal disease. It has been postulated that release of thromboplastin (tissue factor) from the placenta causes a low-grade disseminated intravascu-

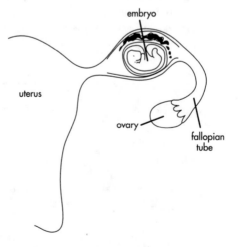

Figure 17–7. Ectopic pregnancy in fallopian tube.

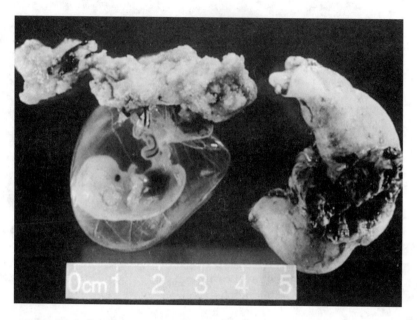

Figure 17–8. Ruptured ectopic pregnancy. Fallopian tube is on right, embryo on left.

lar coagulation with thrombotic lesions in the renal glomeruli leading to protein loss and activation of the renin-angiotensin mechanism to produce high blood pressure. Medical measures may lessen the effects to some extent, but termination of pregnancy is the only cure. In making the decision to terminate pregnancy, the danger of eclampsia to the mother must be weighed against dangers of prematurity to the fetus. Amniocentesis with measurement of surfactant levels may be helpful in determining the maturity of the fetus. Toxemia may or may not recur in a subsequent pregnancy. Detection of toxemia is a major reason for frequent medical visits in the last third of pregnancy.

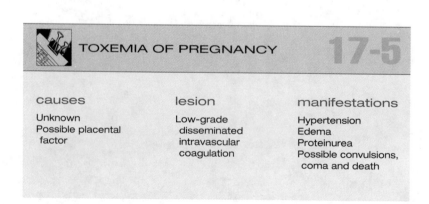

TOXEMIA OF PREGNANCY 17-5

causes	lesion	manifestations

Unknown
Possible placental
  factor
	Low-grade
	  disseminated
	  intravascular
	  coagulation
		Hypertension
		Edema
		Proteinurea
		Possible convulsions,
		  coma and death

Gestational Trophoblastic Neoplasms

Neoplastic placental tissue, which results from genetic material entirely derived from sperm, presents a spectrum of lesions whose behavior can be benign or malignant. Most are benign, grape-like masses of edematous placental villi that are noninvasive and are named *hydatidiform mole.* Some are locally invasive into the uterine wall (invasive mole). A malignant metastasizing variant, *choriocarcinoma,* occurs in about 2 percent of these neoplasms. Gestational trophoblastic neoplasms secrete chorionic gonadotropin that can be measured in blood or urine. This provides an effective diagnostic test and a test for determining when all of the neoplasm has been removed. Further, choriocarcinoma is one of the few cancers that can be cured by chemotherapy even when metastases are present.

ORGAN FAILURE

Fertility and infertility are both major health care problems. The majority of women desire temporary or permanent infertility at some time during the childbearing years. Temporary infertility can be produced by mechanical blockage of the cervix (diaphragm), spermicidal chemicals, mechanical prevention of implantation (intrauterine device), hormonal prevention of ovulation (oral contraceptives), and by hormonal prevention of implantation (the morning-after pill). Permanent infertility in the female can be accomplished by clamping or resecting a portion of the fallopian tubes or by hysterectomy. Occasionally tubes can be repaired to restore fertility. The condom is the major means available to produce temporary infertility in the male. Vasectomy provides permanent infertility. All of these techniques have desirable and undesirable features. Medical expertise and counseling are extensively used in order to reach optimum solutions.

Undesirable, involuntary infertility is also a common problem. Lesions that cause infertility in the female include polycystic ovaries, endometriosis, chronic salpingitis, leiomyomas, and congenital anomalies of the uterus. A low-grade endometritis of unknown cause may cause infertility and antibiotic therapy sometimes results in a successful pregnancy. Imbalance in the normal endocrine cycle may also lead to infertility. An infertility evaluation involves examination of male seminal fluid for number and quality of sperm, injection studies to determine the patency of the fallopian tubes, body temperature measurements to determine whether ovulation has occurred, and endometrial biopsy to evaluate the hormonal response of the endometrium, and search for evidence of endometritis. Sometimes the cause of infertility cannot be found.

Review Questions

1. What are the most frequent health problems of the female genital system?
2. What are the typical causes of abnormal vaginal bleeding, pelvic pain, vaginal discharge, and pelvic mass?
3. How are each of the following tests or procedures helpful in evaluation of a patient with health problems referable to the female genital system?
   Pelvic examination
   Pap smear
   Cone biopsy
   Dilation and curettage
   Laparoscopy
4. What are the causes, lesions, and manifestations of each of the specific diseases discussed in this chapter?
5. What are the possible complications of the various infections of the female genital tract?
6. Why is cervical carcinoma preventable?
7. Why is ectopic pregnancy life threatening?
8. What are the methods of voluntary infertility and causes of involuntary infertility?
9. What do the following terms mean?
   Menarche
   Menopause
   Menorrhagia
   Dysmenorrhea
   Human chorionic gonadotropin
   Fibroid
   Dermoid cyst
   Follicular cyst
   Eclampsia
   Hydatidiform mole
   Choriocarcinoma

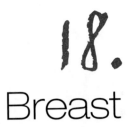

Breast

18.

REVIEW OF STRUCTURE AND FUNCTION
Glands and Ducts • Connective Tissue • Changes with Puberty,
Menstrual Cycle, Pregnancy, Menopause

MOST FREQUENT AND SERIOUS PROBLEMS
Carcinoma • Fibrocystic Changes • Fibroadenoma

SYMPTOMS, SIGNS, AND TESTS
Mass • Galactorrhea • Mammography • Biopsy •
Estrogen/Progesterone Receptors

SPECIFIC DISEASES
  Genetic/Developmental Diseases
    Supernumerary Nipples
    Accessory Breast Tissue
  Inflammatory/Degenerative Diseases
    Acute Mastitis
  Hyperplastic/Neoplastic Diseases
    Fibroadenoma
    Fibrocystic Changes (Fibrocystic Disease)
    Intraductal Papilloma
    Carcinoma of the Breast
    Lesions of the Male Breast

REVIEW QUESTIONS

REVIEW OF STRUCTURE AND FUNCTION

The mature female breast is composed of eight to ten separate sets of glandular units, each of which empties into the nipple by means of an excretory duct (Figure 18–1). The branching ducts of each unit connect with many glandular lobules. Within each glandular lobule, there are epithelial buds surrounded by loose connective tissue. Between glandular lobules, there is a variable amount of dense connective tissue and adipose tissue.

At birth, male and female breasts consist only of ducts. The ducts may be hypertrophied at birth, producing slight breast enlargement due to the influence of maternal hormones. Otherwise, the breasts remain quiescent until puberty, when both male and female breasts undergo ductal hyperplasia. The reaction is of minimal extent and regresses in the male. Proliferation of ducts, glandular buds within lobules, and, to a great extent, connective tissues account for the enlargement of the female breast at puberty. The cyclic hormonal stimulation of the menstrual cycle results in mild hyperplasia and regression of glandular buds and edema of the connective tissue. In some women, this results in a feeling of fullness at the end of the menstrual cycle. High levels of the hormones estrogen, progesterone, and prolactin produced during pregnancy cause a striking change in the structure of the breast. The glandular buds become glands with luminal secretion. The glandular proliferation compresses connective tissue so that the entire breast appears to be composed of glands, as compared to the nonlactating breast, which appears to be predominantly connective tissue. Following the period of lactation, the physiologic glandular hyperplasia gradually regresses, although glands are somewhat more abundant than before the first pregnancy. After menopause, there is gradual atrophy of glands, so that in very old women the breasts consist mainly of ducts, dense connective tissue, and some adipose tissue.

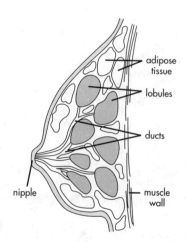

Figure 18–1. Structures of normal mature breast.

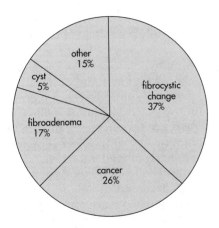

Figure 18–2. Relative frequency of breast lesions as diagnosed at the time of operation. (*Data from Postgraduate Medicine 60:653, 1984*).

MOST FREQUENT AND SERIOUS PROBLEMS

Carcinoma of the breast is by far the most important breast disease. About 1 of every 9 women will develop breast cancer and about 44,000 die from it each year. Other lesions of the breast are important because they may be causally related to breast cancer (epithelial hyperplasia) or need to be differentiated from it (fibroadenoma fat necrosis, fibrocystic disease). The relative frequency of breast problems that are biopsied is shown in Figure 18–2. The age range and final diagnosis at the time of evaluation of breast problems (including patients with and without biopsies) is shown in Figure 18–3.

Infection of the breast (acute mastitis) is usually a complication of lactation. The extreme variation in normal size of the breasts is a problem for some women who undergo reduction mammoplasties (to remove tissue) or insertion of prostheses (to increase the apparent size).

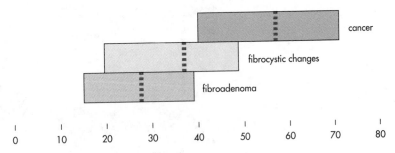

Figure 18–3. Age frequencies of major breast lesions, with mean represented by dashed line. (*Data from Postgraduate Medicine 60:653, 1984*).

SYMPTOMS, SIGNS, AND TESTS

Symptoms and signs of breast disease are similar as patient and physician make the same observations. The most important finding is a painless lump, which is usually discovered by the patient, particularly if she practices routine self-examination. The probability of the lump being cancer increases with age (Figure 18–3), but most lumps that are biopsied are not cancer (Figure 18–2). Further, many lumps that are clinically judged to be benign are not biopsied. Other signs of breast cancer will be discussed later.

Secretion of milk unassociated with pregnancy is called *galactorrhea*. It may be associated with oral contraceptive therapy; otherwise, investigation for the presence of a prolactin-secreting pituitary tumor or other cause should be undertaken.

X-ray examination of the breast (*mammography*) is used to evaluate breast lumps and to screen patients for early breast cancer. Mammography may demonstrate masses (Figure 18–4) and is particularly

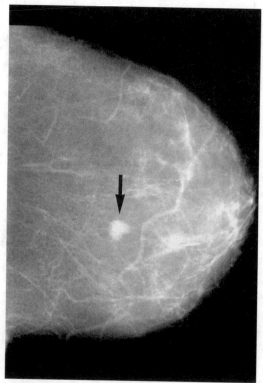

Figure 18–4. Mammogram demonstrating a small radiodense cancer in breast (*arrow*).

useful because cancer tends to have foci of dystrophic calcification that are easily seen radiologically.

Biopsy is the definitive test of breast disease. The tissue may be obtained by fine needle aspiration biopsy, core needle biopsy, or open biopsy. The decision to biopsy lies in the hands of the surgeon who must judge the likelihood of a mass being carcinoma. It is impractical to biopsy all breast masses and unwise to biopsy too few.

Measurement of estrogen and progesterone receptor sites on breast cancer cells is often performed on biopsy tissue to predict the likely response of the cancer to hormone manipulation therapy.

SPECIFIC DISEASES

Genetic/Developmental Diseases

Supernumerary Nipples
Extra nipples may be located anywhere along the milk line, which extends from clavical to midgroin.

Accessory Breast Tissue
Breast tissue may extend into the axilla. Enlargement of the tissue occasionally may be confused with metastatic carcinoma in axillary lymph nodes.

Inflammatory/Degenerative Diseases

Inflammatory conditions of the breast are not common. In addition to acute mastitis, there is an unusual form of chronic inflammation of unknown cause called duct ectasia (*comedomastitis*), which affects one or more of the major ducts and occurs in women near the time of menopause. Trauma to the breast can produce localized *fat necrosis*, which becomes scarred and may produce a hard lump simulating carcinoma. Trauma and infection, however, do not cause cancer.

Acute Mastitis
Ordinary bacteria from the skin, such as *Staphylococcus aureus*, may gain access to the breast through the nipple and cause an acute inflammatory reaction. This is most likely to occur during lactation. The involved area becomes painful, red, hot, and swollen. Abscesses often form, with drainage of pus. If not severe or excessively painful, breast feeding can continue since the organisms likely originated from the baby's mouth anyway and decompression of the breast aids the healing process.

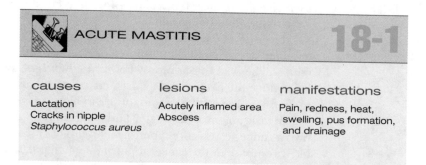

ACUTE MASTITIS   18-1

causes	lesions	manifestations
Lactation Cracks in nipple *Staphylococcus aureus*	Acutely inflamed area Abscess	Pain, redness, heat, swelling, pus formation, and drainage

Hyperplastic/Neoplastic Diseases

Fibroadenoma

This benign tumor is peculiar in that it is composed of both glandular and fibrous elements, which form a well-circumscribed nodule (Figure 18–5). It occurs as a painless, movable lump, most commonly in women 15 to 35 years of age. Excisional biopsy results in diagnosis and cure.

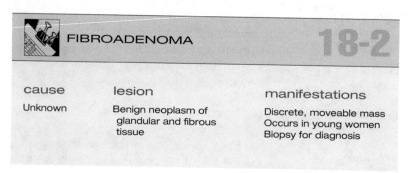

FIBROADENOMA   18-2

cause	lesion	manifestations
Unknown	Benign neoplasm of glandular and fibrous tissue	Discrete, moveable mass Occurs in young women Biopsy for diagnosis

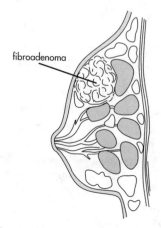

fibroadenoma

Figure 18–5. Fibroadenoma of breast.

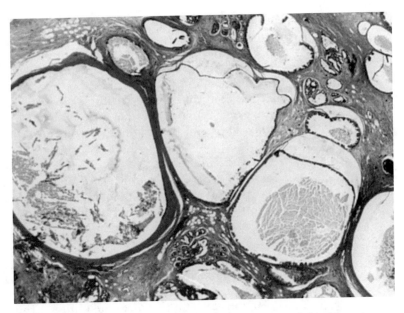

Figure 18–6. Fibrocystic change with many large cysts surrounded by fibrous tissue.

Fibrocystic Changes (Fibrocystic Disease)

Fibrocystic change is a general term used to encompass a variety of alterations that occur in the breast. The most conspicuous changes are fibrosis and cystic dilation of ducts (Figure 18–6). The most important changes, however, relate to hyperplasia of breast ducts because ductal hyperplasia may be a precursor of carcinoma. It is assumed that the stimuli for ductal hyperplasia also promote the development of cancer. The greater the extent of ductal hyperplasia and the more atypical the cells are, the more one is concerned about the future likelihood of cancer. Overall the association between fibrocystic changes and cancer is low. In examining biopsies of fibrocystic changes, pathologists try to identify those patients who are at higher risk for cancer.

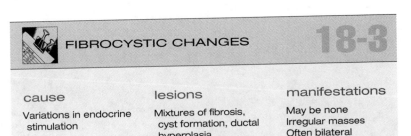

FIBROCYSTIC CHANGES   18-3

cause	lesions	manifestations
Variations in endocrine stimulation	Mixtures of fibrosis, cyst formation, ductal hyperplasia May be premalignant epithelial hyperplasia	May be none Irregular masses Often bilateral Biopsy for definitive diagnosis

This is of aid to the surgeon in deciding to biopsy the breast again when another lump is found.

The cause of fibrocystic changes appears to be fluctuating estrogen stimulation of the breast. Combined oral contraceptive therapy with estrogens and progesterones appears to decrease the extent of this condition. Mild degrees of fibrocystic changes are so frequent and nonspecific histologically that it is difficult to interpret statistical findings of possible associations with cancer.

Intraductal Papilloma

A localized hyperplasia within a large duct is called intraductal papilloma. A serous or bloody nipple discharge or a small mass call attention to these lesions. Removal is indicated because they cannot be distinguished clinically from carcinoma.

Carcinoma of the Breast

Breast carcinoma is the most common cancer in women in the United States, but not in all areas of the world. It increases in frequency after age 30, thus affecting many women in the prime of life. The 5-year survival rate is 75 percent. Carcinoma of the breast can arise from the ductal epithelium or from the glandular epithelium of the lobules. Carcinoma may develop in any area of the breast. Genetic factors, hormonal imbalances, and environmental factors may all play a role in the development of breast cancer.

Grossly, a breast cancer may be of any size. It usually can be felt on physical examination when it reaches 1 to 2 centimeters in diameter. When advanced, it may cause dimpling of the skin, changes in skin texture, retraction of the nipple, bloody discharge from the nipple, or even a protruding mass with ulceration (Figure 18–7).

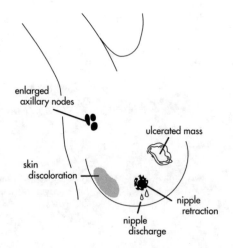

Figure 18–7. Signs produced by carcinoma of the breast.

Microscopically, carcinomas of the breasts are composed of cells in a more or less glandular arrangement (adenocarcinoma) and surrounded by variable amounts of connective tissue. The neoplastic cells invade and replace normal breast tissue and often induce more fibrosis around the invading neoplastic cells. The histology varies from well-differentiated glands to undifferentiated masses of cancer cells. The natural history of untreated breast cancer includes metastasis to axillary lymph nodes and widespread metastasis to many organs. Occasionally, tumors are more selective in their site of metastasis, such as those that spread to bone, producing bone pain and sometimes fractures.

Carcinoma of the breast may be confined to ducts or lobules (in situ), or it may be invasive (infiltrating) (Figure 18–8). Ductal carcinoma in situ and lobular carcinoma in situ increase a woman's risk of developing invasive carcinoma by 10 or 11 times. Invasive carcinomas are subclassified into several types, with infiltrating ductal and lobular being the most common. The vast majority of breast carcinomas are the infiltrating ductal type. Infiltrating lobular carcinomas are much less common than infiltrating ductal, are more often bilateral, and tend to have a slightly better prognosis.

Treatment of breast cancer is variable and subject to constant study to find the optimum methods. Nevertheless, the primary goal is to remove or destroy all of the cancer cells. Wide excision of the mass or mastectomy may be combined with radiation therapy. Resection of axillary lymph nodes provides information on the stage of the disease and may improve the cure rate when only a few of the nodes nearest to the breast are involved. Some patients with widespread disease are treated with bone marrow transplantation following total body radiation.

The progress of metastatic breast cancer can be delayed, but the long-term outlook is not favorable once the cancer has spread beyond

CARCINOMA OF THE BREAST   18-4

causes	lesions	manifestations
Unknown	Adenocarcinoma	Mass
Fibrocystic changes	Metastases to	Changes in overlying skin
mildly predisposing	regional lymph nodes	Nipple discharge
Genetic predisposition	and other organs	Enlarged axillary lymph
Hormonal imbalances		nodes
Environmental factors		Mammography
		Biopsy

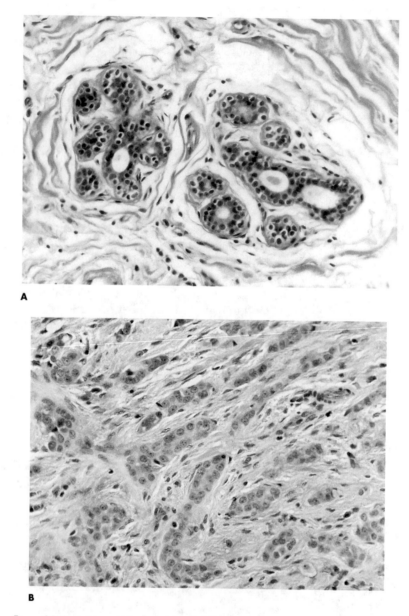

Figure 18–8. A. Normal breast ductules. B. Infiltrating carcinoma. Note that the carcinoma cells do not form channels but rather spread wildly through the connective tissue of the breast.

the regional lymph nodes. Bone metastases, which are relatively common, often can be ameliorated by radiation therapy. Hormones affect the growth rate of many breast cancers. At the time the cancer is first removed, cancer cells can be evaluated for the presence of receptor sites for estrogen and progesterone. The majority of cancers with these receptors regress when the level of estrogen in the body is reduced by anti-estrogen therapy, tamoxifen, or removal of ovaries.

The clinical course of breast cancer is quite variable. The majority are cured by removal of the primary lesions. Some cancers grow rapidly and are fatal within months, others are very slow growing and may recur years after removal of the primary lesion. Thus 5- and 10-year survival rates do not adequately reflect the overall mortality and morbidity of this disease. The variable survival rates and long duration make it difficult to evaluate the efficiency of various therapies.

Lesions of the Male Breast

Enlargement of the male breast due to proliferation of ducts and connective tissues is called *gynecomastia*. If bilateral, gynecomastia is usually due to estrogen simulation such as occurs with estrogen-secreting neoplasms, estrogenic drugs such as digitalis and marijuana, cirrhosis of the liver with decreased metabolism of the normally small amounts of estrogen produced by males, Klinefelter's syndrome, and aging with decreased countereffects of androgens. Unilateral gynecomastia typically occurs in younger men, is idiopathic, and is of no particular consequence. Pseudogynecomastia is an increase in adipose tissue in the region of the male breast, a common finding in the obese and elderly.

Carcinoma of the male breast accounts for 1 percent of all breast cancers. It is a disease of the elderly with a somewhat worse prognosis than cancer of the female breast.

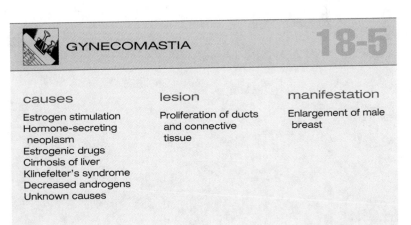

GYNECOMASTIA   18-5

causes	lesion	manifestation

Estrogen stimulation
Hormone-secreting
  neoplasm
Estrogenic drugs
Cirrhosis of liver
Klinefelter's syndrome
Decreased androgens
Unknown causes
	Proliferation of ducts
	  and connective
	  tissue
		Enlargement of male
		  breast

Review Questions

1. What is the most significant manifestation of breast disease and why?
2. How are breast masses detected and evaluated?
3. What are the causes, lesions, and major manifestations of the diseases discussed in the chapter?
4. Why is fibrocystic change clinically important?
5. What steps are involved in the development, diagnosis, treatment, and outcome of carcinoma of the breast?
6. What do the following terms mean?
    Mammography
    Galactorrhea
    Fat necrosis
    Gynecomastia

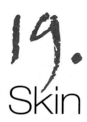
Skin

REVIEW OF STRUCTURE AND FUNCTION
Functions • Epidermis • Dermis

MOST FREQUENT AND SERIOUS PROBLEMS
Cuts • Abscesses • Acne • Nevi • Warts • Eczematous Dermatitis • Seborrheic Dermatitis • Seborrheic Keratosis • Actinic Keratosis • Psoriasis • Skin Cancer • Burns • Drug Reactions • Lesions of Systemic Diseases

SYMPTOMS, SIGNS, AND TESTS
Pruritus • Pain • Rash • Macule • Nodule • Papule • Pustule • Vesicle • Wheal (Hive) • Scale • Crust • Biopsy • Culture • Smear

SPECIFIC DISEASES
Genetic/Developmental Diseases
Hemangiomas
Hair Disorders
Disorders of Pigmentation
Inflammatory/Degenerative Diseases
Viral Exanthems
Verruca (Warts)
Acne
Abscess
Impetigo
Syphilis
Superficial Fungal Infections
Dermatitis in General
Contact Dermatitis
Poison Ivy
Atopic Dermatitis
Seborrheic Dermatitis
Urticaria (Hives)
Psoriasis

Hyperplastic/Neoplastic Diseases
Senile (Solar) Degeneration and Actinic Keratosis
Seborrheic Keratosis
Melanocytic Nevus
Malignant Melanoma
Other Pigmented Lesions
Basal Cell and Squamous Cell Carcinomas

ORGAN FAILURE

REVIEW QUESTIONS

REVIEW OF STRUCTURE AND FUNCTION

The skin functions as a barrier between the body and its external environment, protecting the body from injury by external forces and preventing excessive loss of body fluids. The skin also constitutes a major sense organ; cutaneous sensation of touch, temperature, pressure, and pain is essential for man to maintain orientation with his environment. In addition, the skin plays a vital role in regulation of body temperature, both by controlling the amount of blood brought near the surface for heat exchange and through the process of sweating, which lowers skin temperature through vaporization.

Histologically, as depicted in Figure 19–1, the skin consists of an outer covering of stratified squamous epithelium (epidermis); an underlying layer of fibrous connective tissue (dermis), which contains the hair follicles, sebaceous and sweat glands, blood vessels, and sen-

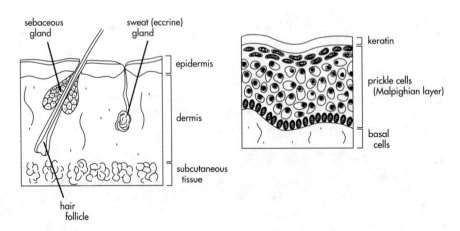

Figure 19–1. Histologic components of the skin.

sory nerves; and a deep layer of adipose tissue (subcutis or subcutaneous tissue).

The epidermis has three major morphologic divisions. The deepest, the basal layer, is a single layer of columnar germinative cells that gives rise to all other epidermal cells by mitotic division. The broad middle Malpighian zone consists of several layers of prickle cells undergoing progressive maturation to become keratinized surface cells. As cells migrate upward through the Malpighian layer they become flattened, acquire keratin fibrils, keratohyaline granules, and form rows parallel to the skin surface. The outermost layer consists of anuclear keratinized cells. The thickness of the keratin layer varies greatly in different body sites; for example, the keratin layer is very thick over the palm and fingers and thin over the skin of the forearm. Scattered throughout the basal layer are larger, pale cells which may contain brown granules. These cells, called *melanocytes*, produce brown melanin pigment, which helps protect the skin from sunlight damage and contributes to skin color. The concentration of melanocytes varies widely, with melanocytes being twice as numerous on the face as on the trunk.

The dermis consists of fibrous tissue intermixed with elastin fibers. The high collagen concentration provides great skin resistance to mechanical force and the elastin allows the skin to return to its normal form after mechanical deformation. When elastin fibers are destroyed with aging or disease, the skin becomes loose and wrinkled. A gel-like ground substance holds the dermal fibers together and permits the skin to change shape slowly, as with changes in body weight. *Eccrine glands* are present in the deep dermis all over the body and are responsible for the production of sweat in response to heat stress. *Apocrine glands* occur in a restricted distribution (axillae, pubis, perineum, nipple region, ear canal) and produce a sticky proteinaceous fluid in response to hormonal stimuli; apocrine glands are not functional until puberty. With the exception of palms, soles, and portions of the genitalia, the entire body surface is covered by hair; the hairs are produced by division of cells lining the hair follicle. Each bulb (follicle) undergoes recurring cycles of hair growth, regression, and rest. Attached to each hair follicle is a *sebaceous gland*, which secretes lipid-rich sebum; the function of sebum in man is not known.

MOST FREQUENT AND SERIOUS PROBLEMS

Among the most common dermatologic problems that may prompt a person to seek medical attention are cuts, abscesses, acne, nevi (moles), warts (verruca vulgaris), eczematous dermatitis, seborrheic dermatitis (dandruff), and rashes of various types. Small, greasy, warty lesions (seborrheic keratoses) commonly occur on the face, trunk, and extremities of persons past middle age and are usually multiple. Older persons who have been exposed to sunlight for many years frequently have small precancerous lesions (actinic or solar keratoses) or early skin cancers on exposed surfaces. Psoriasis is a chronic, scaling skin disease, which sometimes is quite distressing to the patient.

Life-threatening skin conditions include extensive burns, severe drug reactions with sloughing of portions of the epidermis (exfoliative dermatitis), and malignant melanomas. Loss or destruction of large areas of epidermis is always potentially lethal because of the resulting loss of body fluids and because of the high risk of secondary infection, usually by pseudomonas or *S. aureus*.

Skin lesions may be important indicators of systemic disease. Cutaneous lesions, most commonly a red rash over both cheeks and the bridge of the nose, occur in most patients with systemic lupus erythematosus and often constitute the first sign of disease. Deposits of urate crystals frequently occur in patients with gout; these chalky deposits most commonly occur in the subcutis of the helix of the ear and over the elbows and digits of hands and feet. Well-circumscribed areas of brown atrophic skin and foci of dermal connective tissue degeneration with ulcers are common on the lower extremities of diabetics. Small, soft, yellow papules (xanthomas) are common on the face and extremities of persons with consistently elevated plasma lipid levels (hyperlipidemia and uncontrolled diabetes) and may be the first sign of disease. Some degree of hyperpigmentation of skin occurs in 90 percent of pregnant women, with the most striking manifestation being mask-like pigmentation of the face. Freckles and nevi commonly appear darker during pregnancy.

SYMPTOMS, SIGNS, AND TESTS

Most skin diseases are not life threatening, but many are distressing to patients because of unsightly appearance, itching (*pruritus*), or pain. Unlike diseases of other body systems, skin diseases are readily visible both to the patient and the doctor. The mere discovery of a skin lesion may bring the patient to a doctor, or he/she may seek medical attention because of pain or itching. Distress over the appearance of skin lesions and fear of cancer are perhaps the most common concerns of patients with skin disease.

Often, the gross appearance of the lesions and the history of their development is sufficient to make a diagnosis. The gross appearance is described in terms of size, location on the body, multiplicity, color, shape, and texture. Lesions that are flat are termed *macular* and those that are raised are called *papular*. Rashes are temporary eruptions on the skin that have a multitude of causes. General causes of rashes include systemic infections (measles, rubella, chicken pox, scarlet fever, secondary syphilis), hypersensitivity reactions to food or drugs, and local reactions to surface contact with topical drugs and allergenic or irritating substances. The following terms are commonly used to describe the gross appearance of skin lesions. Their appearance is depicted in Figure 19–2.

- *Macule*—Change in skin color; not raised or depressed
- *Nodule*—Knot or lump; elevated solid lesion (>5mm)
- *Papule*—Very small lump (<5 mm)
- *Pustule or abscess*—Elevated skin lesion containing pus
- *Vesicle or blister*—Bubble-like swelling containing air or fluid
- *Wheal or hive*—Ridge-like reddened elevation caused by edema and congestion
- *Plaque*—Elevated, flat-topped lesion (>5 mm)
- *Scale*—Flaky superficial material (keratin) that easily separates from the skin
- *Crust*—Hardened, adherent serum on skin surface over a lesion

Biopsies are used in evaluation of many chronic eruptions and nodular lesions. Excisional biopsy may be used in the evaluation of neoplastic lesions and often constitutes the sole treatment. Laboratory tests are only indicated under selected circumstances, such as culturing a purulent lesion for bacteria, preparing a smear when fungal infection is suspected, or ordering blood tests when systemic disease is suggested.

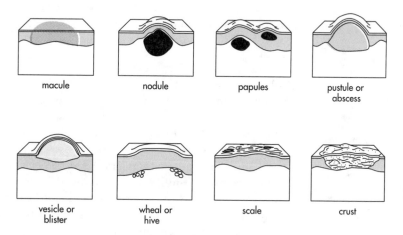

Figure 19–2. The appearance of various types of skin lesions.

SPECIFIC DISEASES

Genetic/Developmental Diseases

Hemangiomas have been mentioned previously in Chapter 9. Neuro-fibromatosis is discussed in Chapter 22. Major inherited disorders of hair distribution and pigmentation are included in this category, because they can be considered specific diseases. Acquired problems of hair distribution and pigmentation are possible manifestations of a wide variety of diseases and will not be specifically discussed.

Hemangiomas

These congenital proliferations of small blood vessels in the dermis present as elevated red or purple lesions. They increase slowly in size, usually commensurate with body growth. Even small hemangiomas, if located on the face, may be important for cosmetic reasons. Large hemangiomas (*port wine stains*) that cover the forehead and cheek on one side are genetically determined. Port wine stains that involve one side of the forehead may be associated with vascular lesions in the brain, seizure disorders, and mental retardation.

Hair Disorders

The distribution, color, and texture of scalp and body hair are genet-ically determined and influenced by hormones. Excessive body hair (*hirsutism*) may be particularly distressing to female patients. The early onset of baldness (*alopecia*) in men is often inherited as a dominant trait. It is not manifest in women, because its expression is influenced by male sex hormones.

Disorders of Pigmentation

Albinism is an uncommon autosomal recessive hereditary condition in which melanocytes are unable to produce normal amounts of melanin pigment. Patients lack normal pigmentation in skin, hair, and irides. The absence of normal cutaneous melanin renders the patient mark-edly sensitive to sunlight and predisposes to increased incidence of basal and squamous cell cancers. *Xeroderma pigmentosum* is a rare auto-somal recessive condition characterized by intolerance of skin and eyes to sunlight, with development of skin cancers in childhood or early adult life. These patients lack enzymes necessary to repair dam-age to DNA caused by sunlight.

DISORDERS OF PIGMENTATION **19-1**

cause	lesions	manifestations
Autosomal recessive inheritance	Lack of skin pigment (albinism) Skin degeneration with low-grade inflammation and pigmentation (xeroderma pigmentosum)	White skin, hair, irises (albinism) Pigmented patchy skin lesions with multiple skin cancers (xeroderma pigmentosum)

Inflammatory/Degenerative Diseases

The first part of this section will deal with the various types of skin infections and the situations in which they occur. This will be followed by a discussion of the various forms of dermatitis. Although *dermatitis* literally means inflammation of the skin, the term is usually used in a narrower sense to describe patchy noninfectious inflammations that may be chronic and often are allergic in nature. Finally, acute edema (urticaria) and chronic scaling skin diseases will be discussed.

Viral Exanthems

Rashes of various viral diseases are most often seen in children, and their clinical appearance and distribution are the basis for diagnosis of measles, rubella, and chicken pox. See Chapter 26 on infectious diseases for further discussion.

Verruca (Warts)

Human papilloma viruses of several strains cause benign neoplastic proliferations of stratified squamous epithelium called squamous papillomas. Three different patterns of disease, presumably caused by different strains of papilloma virus, are verruca vulgaris, condyloma acuminatum, and juvenile laryngeal polyps.

Verruca vulgaris (common wart) occurs on exposed body parts, particularly the fingers and back of the hand, and is a raised, horny, dry lesion (Figure 19–3A). Warts on the palms and soles (palmar and plantar warts) are flat or elevated dry lesions that may be very painful. Warts on the face and neck may form tiny finger-like projections (filiform warts). Verruca vulgaris are common in children but may occur at any age. Although warts eventually regress spontaneously, they may

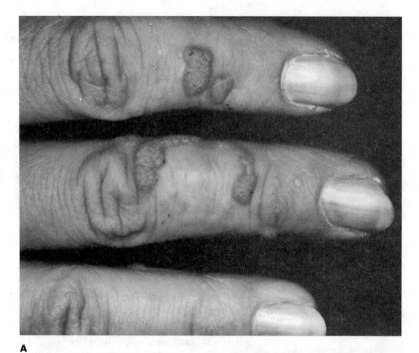

A

B

Figure 19–3. A. Verruca vulgaris on fingers. B. Condyloma acuminatum on vulva.

VERRUCA (WARTS) 19-2

cause	lesion	manifestations
Virus	Discrete raised proliferation of squamous epithelium	Nodules on exposed parts of body (verruca vulgaris) Nodules in anogenital region (condyloma acuminatum)

cause considerable pain and discomfort, especially when frequently traumatized. Various techniques are used to destroy the lesions, but eradication may be difficult due to repeated autoinoculation.

Condyloma acuminata occurs on anogenital mucous membranes and is spread by venereal contact, particularly in young adults (Figure 19–3B). Juvenile laryngeal papillomas occur in selected patients and are strikingly prone to recur but eventually disappear in adulthood.

Acne

Multiple recurrent crops of nodules and pustules on the face and upper back during puberty and early adulthood are called acne (Figure 19–4). The basic lesion in acne is plugging of hair follicles and associated sebaceous gland ducts with lipid and keratin material, producing slightly raised white heads or blackheads (comedones). The inflammatory reaction of acne is thought to be due to irritating fatty acids liberated from the sebaceous material by *Propionibacterium acnes*, a bacteria that is

ACNE 19-3

causes	lesions	manifestations
Pilosebaceous plugs *Proprionibacterium acnes* Chemical irritation Secondary infection Endocrine factors Hereditary factors	Multiple plugged sebaceous glands with surrounding inflammation Pustules when secondarily infected	Multiple facial lesions, with whiteheads, blackheads, pustules Occurs in adolescents and young adults Facial scarring (late)

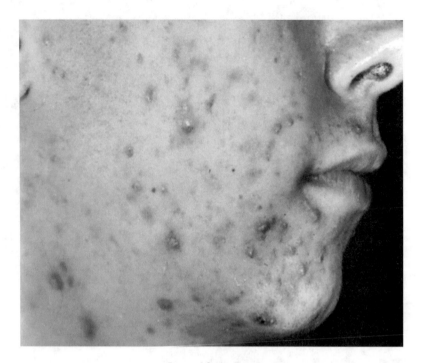

Figure 19–4. Acne.

able to grow when it is trapped in the plugged hair follicle. Other more virulent organisms may infect the lesions producing tiny abscesses. The severity of acne varies greatly among individuals, suggesting hereditary and hormonal influences on sebaceous glands. Acne may be aggravated by emotional stress and administration of adrenocorticosteroids. Severe cases lead to facial scarring, which may be disfiguring. Treatment is directed toward reduction of greasiness of facial skin to avoid plugging of sebaceous glands and, in severe cases, toward reduction of bacteria in the lesions.

Abscess

Skin abscesses when small and solitary are called *furuncles* or *boils*. *Staphylococcus aureus* is the most common offending organism in skin abscesses. Skin abscesses occur at sites of skin trauma, in obstructed skin appendages, and around embedded foreign material. Abscesses commonly occur in the folds around the nails (*paronychia*) (Figure 19–5), around the nose, around splinters, in the hairy skin over the tip of the spine between the buttocks (*pilonidal abscess*), around the anus, and on the back of the neck. Abscesses commonly develop in obstructed hair

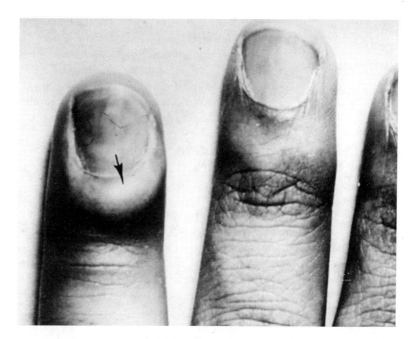

Figure 19–5. Paronychia, with swelling due to collection of purulent exudate around the nail (arrow).

follicles and enlarge to form painful, elevated, red areas, which subsequently develop a pale, soft center that represents liquefaction necrosis of tissue with accumulation of purulent exudate. If uncomplicated, the furuncle is gradually walled off, ruptures to release the exudate, and then collapses to heal with a small scar. Healing may be accelerated by puncturing the abscess to release the exudate, but this should

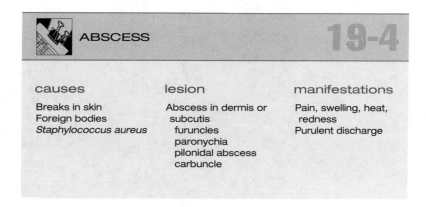

ABSCESS   19-4

causes	lesion	manifestations

Breaks in skin
Foreign bodies
Staphylococcus aureus
	Abscess in dermis or
	  subcutis
	  furuncles
	  paronychia
	  pilonidal abscess
	  carbuncle
		Pain, swelling, heat,
		  redness
		Purulent discharge

not be undertaken until liquefaction necrosis is well established and granulation tissue has formed to line the abscess cavity. Recurrent abscesses, such as pilonidal abscesses, may require an operation to remove the infection. Splinters and other foreign materials should be removed, preferably before an abscess develops.

A *carbuncle* is a group of confluent furuncles with associated connecting sinus tracts and multiple openings on the skin. This uncommon lesion usually occurs on the back of the neck. Diabetics are especially prone to develop carbuncles because of their reduced resistance to infection.

Impetigo

This is a superficial bacterial skin infection that occurs predominantly in children and is characterized by oozing, crusty blisters, and pustules, usually on the face (Figure 19–6). The pustules often rupture to exude purulent material. Group A streptococci are the offending organisms. *Staphylococcus aureus* may also be present.

Impetigo is contagious and may spread rapidly among very young children in crowded conditions.

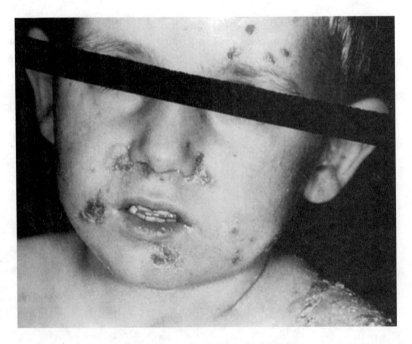

Figure 19–6. Impetigo on face and shoulder.

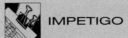

IMPETIGO 19-5

causes	lesion	manifestations
Unknown factors	Multiple superficial	Occurs in children
Group A streptococci	facial inflammatory	Facial lesions in
	foci developing into	varying stages from
	pustules	mild inflammation to
		blisters to pustules

Syphilis

The primary lesion of syphilis, known as a *chancre*, occurs at the site of entry of the causative organism, *Treponema pallidum*, and takes about 3 weeks to develop. Common sites of chancres include the mucous membranes of the penis, vagina, cervix, anus, and mouth. The chancre is usually a single, painless, superficial papule with superficial central ulceration that heals spontaneously in 4 to 12 weeks. The chancre contains many spirochetes and is highly contagious even though serologic tests for syphilis may be negative at this stage. The secondary stage of syphilis may be associated with a variety of cutaneous manifestations, most commonly a faint rash on the trunk or extremities, often with involvement of the palms and soles. For further discussion of syphilis see Chapter 26.

Superficial Fungal Infections

In the superficial fungal infections, the fungi are located in the keratin layers of the skin, nail, or hair and can often be demonstrated in a smear prepared from skin scrapings. The dermis is not affected. The two main types of superficial fungal infection of the skin are *ringworm* (*tinea*) and *candidiasis*. Ringworm is not caused by a worm but by various fungal species. Regardless of the site affected, the lesions are typically itchy, brown or red scaly patches; blisters, cracks or localized thickenings may also occur. Some forms of ringworm are transmitted from person to person or animal to person; in other forms, the mode of acquisition is not known. The most common form of ringworm is athlete's foot (*tinea pedis*), which affects the soles and interdigital spaces of the feet. Hereditary and immunologic factors, sweating, and type of foot covering all appear to play a part in the etiology of this infection. *Tinea cruris* (jock itch) produces symmetric involvement of the perineum, buttocks, and inner thighs. Ringworm of the scalp (*tinea capitis*) and beard (*tinea barbae*) produce breaking of hairs and focal hair loss. Ringworm infections of the nails produce opaque, discolored

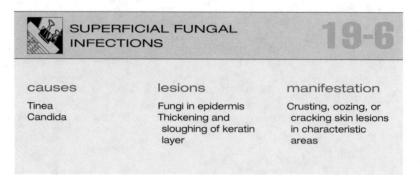

causes	lesions	manifestation

Tinea
Candida
	Fungi in epidermis
	Thickening and
	  sloughing of keratin
	  layer
		Crusting, oozing, or
		  cracking skin lesions
		  in characteristic
		  areas

SUPERFICIAL FUNGAL INFECTIONS 19-6

painless patches within the nail; in late stages of infection, the nail is deformed and eventually destroyed. Most ringworm infections are eradicated by treatment with topical agents.

Superficial infections with *Candida albicans* (candidiasis) may be focal or diffuse and produce red, itchy, scaly patches, often with blisters or pustules at the margin. Factors that predispose to superficial candida infection include diabetes mellitus, leukemia, and lymphoma; treatment with antibacterial or immunosuppressive drugs; and chronic immersion in water. Involvement of intertriginous and interdigital skin is likely in diabetics. Candidiasis of the perioral skin (perleche) produces red cracks and fissures at the corners of the mouth. People who chronically have their hands in water (bartenders, dishwashers) may develop candidiasis of the fingernails manifest by painless, red swelling of the skin around the nail and brown discoloration and ridging of the nail. Superficial candidiasis may be difficult to eradicate.

Dermatitis in General

Dermatitis is a generic, clinical term used to describe a wide variety of skin conditions all characterized by inflammation of the skin. *Eczema* is a term often used to describe dermatitis, particularly that of nonspecific type that evolves slowly from an acute to a chronic dermatitis. Dermatitis occurs in response to a wide variety of stimuli, including drugs, chemical allergens, ultraviolet radiation, local trauma, and various metabolic and immunologic disorders. Dermatitis accounts for about one-third of patients who consult a dermatologist. Acute dermatitis is red and oozing, with many small blisters and crusts (Figure 19–7A); in later stages, the skin becomes reddened and thickened, with accentuation of normal skin lines (Figure 19–7B). Severe pruritus may accompany any stage of disease. Thickening of the lesion is largely a reaction to prolonged scratching.

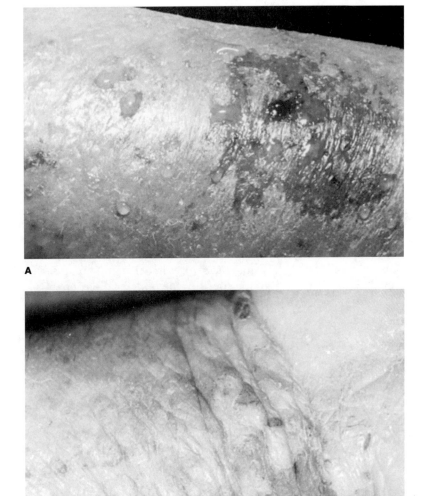

Figure 19–7. A. Acute stage of dermatitis. B. Chronic stage of dermatitis.

TABLE 19–1. CLASSIFICATION AND CHARACTERISTICS OF DERMATITIS

Type	Morphologic Pattern	Location	Frequency	Severity
Contact	Eczema	Site of allergen contact	Most common	Distressing recurrent
Atopic	Eczema	Begins on face, extremities late	Common	Disfiguring, impaired function
Seborrheic	Greasy, scaling	Scalp, face, trunk	Common	Widely variable
Light-induced	Eczema or rash	Exposed skin	Common	Usually mild
Exfoliative	Sloughing of superficial epidermis	Total body	Uncommon	May be fatal

Histologic features in dermatitis are usually nonspecific, and diagnosis of the specific type of dermatitis depends primarily on the clinical evolution and distribution of the lesions.

Ideally a classification of dermatitis would be based on cause. In many patients, however, cause cannot be determined, and some clinical types are of unknown cause. The types described in Table 19–1 represent a mixed classification based on cause and morphology. Contact, atopic, and seborrheic dermatitis will be discussed below. Light-induced dermatitis is diagnosed by history of exposure to sunlight and location on exposed surfaces. Exfoliative dermatitis is the most severe and least common type. Drugs are the cause in many cases of dermatitis.

Contact Dermatitis

This is a type of eczematous dermatitis that occurs as a delayed hypersensitivity reaction to chemical allergens such as clothes, cosmetics, jewelry, and various metals. Since skin changes occur at the site of allergen contact, the location and configuration of the skin eruption often provides an important clue to the causative agent. A suspected substance can be placed on a patch on the patient's back to test for reactivity (*patch test*). A local reaction to the offending substance will occur under the patch after 24 to 28 hours. Avoidance of the causative allergen cures the eruption; avoidance of the allergen often entails a change in work or personal activities. Contact dermatitis may be subclassified by the causative agents. Poison ivy is a common example.

CONTACT DERMATITIS   19-7

cause	lesion	manifestation
Environmental allergens, such as clothes, cosmetics, metals, plants, chemicals	Low-grade, usually chronic, inflammation of skin	Red, slightly raised, pruritic area corresponding with area of contact

Poison Ivy

Poison ivy is an example of allergic contact dermatitis. Vesicles, often linear, and redness of the skin develop at the site of contact with the oil of poison ivy leaves (Figure 19–8). This reaction occurs in previously sensitized persons about 24 hours after contact. Oozing from the vesicles may spread the eruption to other body parts. When poison ivy is severe, it may be advisable to treat the patient with systemic corticosteroids to reduce the inflammatory reaction. Poison oak plants and sumac bushes may produce a similar allergy.

 POISON IVY   19-8

cause	lesion	manifestations
Chemical produced by poison ivy plant	Inflamed areas, with degeneration and blister formation in epidermis	Red streaks with blisters Pruritus Location of exposed areas Begins about 24 hours after exposure

Atopic Dermatitis

Atopic allergy occurs by a different mechanism from contact dermatitis (see Chapter 27 for discussion of mechanism). Descriptively, atopic dermatitis is a type of eczematous dermatitis that occurs in individuals having other manifestations of atopic allergy (asthma, hayfever, urticaria). Atopic dermatitis usually begins in infancy with

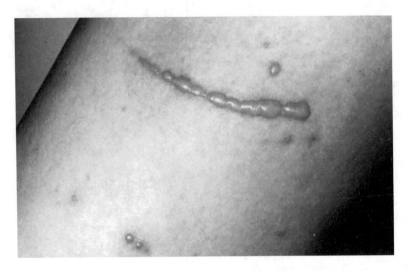

Figure 19–8. Poison ivy blisters.

eczema of the face and scalp, then recurs in children and adults with more generalized involvement of the trunk and extremities. This condition is characterized by severe itching. Vesicular lesions predominate in infants, while children and adults develop dry, thickened skin lesions. A specific offending substance is not identified, but exacerbations of this disease have been related to substances in the environment, temperature variation, and emotional stress, as well as by hereditary predisposition. Patch testing is not useful in atopic dermatitis.

ATOPIC DERMATITIS   19-9

cause	lesions	manifestations
Hereditary predisposition to atopic allergies	Eczematous dermatitis early Disfiguring skin thickening	Multiple patchy skin lesions varying from moist to dry, with or without vesicles Pruritus Other atopic allergies

Seborrheic Dermatitis

This common form of dermatitis occurs in sites of greatest concentration of sebaceous glands—scalp, face, ears, neck, axillae, breasts, umbilicus, and anogenital regions. Seborrheic dermatitis usually begins in childhood as fine scaling of the scalp (*cradle cap*) and may continue throughout life with variable extension to other areas. The scaly lesions often resemble psoriasis but are usually yellow and greasy. In men, severe seborrheic dermatitis may be associated with a chronic pustular eruption in the beard area. The specific cause is unknown.

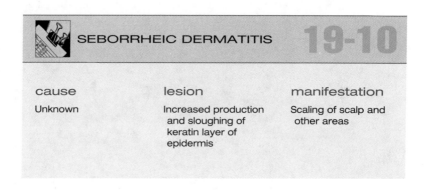

SEBORRHEIC DERMATITIS   **19-10**

cause	lesion	manifestation
Unknown	Increased production and sloughing of keratin layer of epidermis	Scaling of scalp and other areas

Urticaria (Hives)

Urticaria is an acute patchy eruption with raised edematous areas (*wheal*) surrounded by red margins (*flare*). The lesions itch. The lesions seldom persist for more than 48 hours but may recur in successive episodes. Urticaria results from local release of histamine in the skin and is usually due to an atopic type of allergic reaction commonly caused by an allergen in food such as chocolate or shellfish or by a drug such as penicillin.

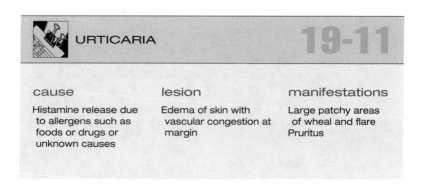

URTICARIA   **19-11**

cause	lesion	manifestations
Histamine release due to allergens such as foods or drugs or unknown causes	Edema of skin with vascular congestion at margin	Large patchy areas of wheal and flare Pruritus

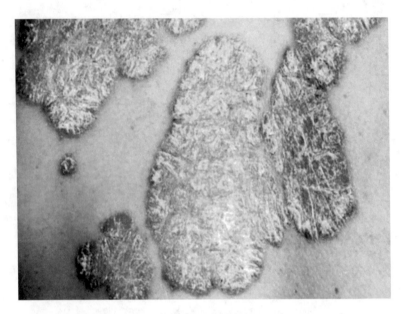

Figure 19–9. Well-demarcated, raised, red, scaly lesions characteristic of psoriasis.

Psoriasis

Psoriasis is a chronic inflammatory disease of skin of unknown cause that varies greatly in severity and is characterized by thickened areas of skin with silver-colored scales (Figure 19–9). Lesions are most common on the extensor surfaces of the knees and elbows. Proliferation of the epidermis is a prominent feature of this disease. In severe cases, various ointments and ultraviolet light are used to control the proliferative activity. Psoriasis may be quite distressing to the patient but is usually not life threatening.

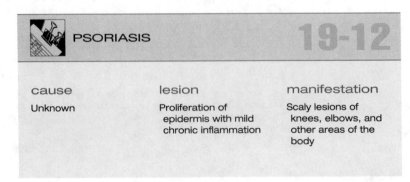

PSORIASIS   19-12

cause	lesion	manifestation
Unknown	Proliferation of epidermis with mild chronic inflammation	Scaly lesions of knees, elbows, and other areas of the body

Hyperplastic/Neoplastic Diseases

The skin is the most common site of neoplastic and preneoplastic change. Long exposure to sunlight in association with aging is important in the vast majority of these lesions. Although some of the lesions discussed are degenerative in nature, they are discussed here because they represent a spectrum of changes. The neoplastic lesions involve two separate cell lines—the squamous cells and the melanocytes of the epidermis. Melanocytes are epithelial-like cells that are derived embryologically from neural elements. The relative frequency of the three major types of cancer of the skin is shown in Figure 19–10.

Senile (Solar) Degeneration and Actinic Keratosis

With age, a number of changes occur in exposed skin, predominantly as a result of years of exposure to sunlight. The degree of skin change is directly related to the duration and intensity of solar exposure. The most characteristic change is degeneration of dermal collagen and elastic fibers, which results in excessive wrinkling of the skin. Other skin changes attributed to solar degeneration include skin atrophy, areas of decreased pigmentation (*vitiligo*), areas of increased pigmentation (*lentigo*), collections of small blood vessels (*telangiectasia*), and keratoses. Thus, the face of an elderly farmer or seaman is likely to have areas of pigmentation and depigmentation as well as a ruddy complexion due to telangiectasia and keratoses (Figure 19–11).

Actinic keratoses (also called senile or solar keratoses) occurs as multiple, scaly lesions on sun-exposed skin of persons in or past mid-

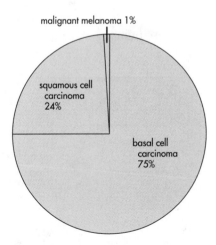

Figure 19–10. Relative frequency of skin cancers derived from squamous cells (basal and squamous cell carcinomas) and from melanocytes (malignant melanoma).

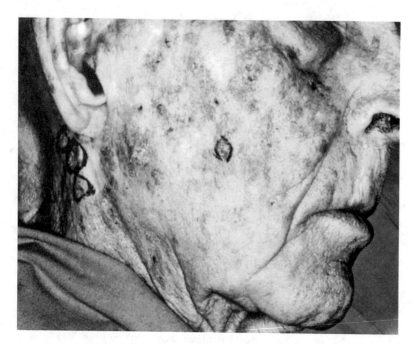

Figure 19–11. Multiple actinic keratoses and solar degeneration of the face. Circles are sites to be biopsied to distinguish actinic keratosis from early cancer.

dle life; they are more common in fair-skinned persons. The actinic keratosis is an area of atypical epidermal proliferation usually accompanied by thickening of the keratin layer (*hyperkeratosis*). Squamous cell carcinoma frequently arises in an actinic keratosis. About one-fourth of patients with actinic keratosis eventually develop squamous cell carcinoma.

 SENILE DEGENERATION   19-13

causes	lesions	manifestations
Long exposure to sunlight Aging	Degeneration of collagen and elastic fibers Telangiectases Increased or decreased pigmentation Actinic keratoses	Wrinkling of skin of face and hands Pigmented or depigmented spots on exposed areas Ruddy complexion Small hyperkeratotic foci

Seborrheic Keratosis

Seborrheic keratoses are benign neoplastic proliferations of basal cells of the epidermis that occur on the trunk, face, and arms of persons in middle life and beyond. The seborrheic keratosis is a warty, brown, greasy lesion that appears to be tacked on to the skin and can often be easily scraped off (Figure 19–12). The stimulus that triggers this proliferative response is not known. Seborrheic keratoses are not premalignant.

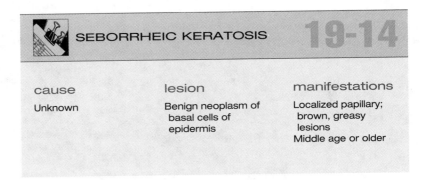

SEBORRHEIC KERATOSIS		19-14
cause	lesion	manifestations
Unknown	Benign neoplasm of basal cells of epidermis	Localized papillary; brown, greasy lesions Middle age or older

Melanocytic Nevus

The common nevus (*melanocytic nevus, nevocellular nevus,* mole) results from a benign proliferation of melanocytes of the epidermis. At first the melanocytes or nevus cells proliferate at the junction of the epidermis

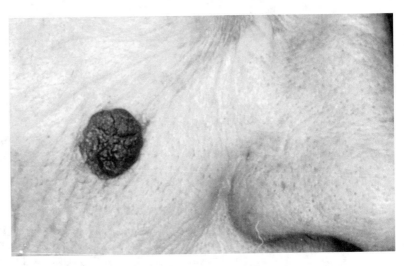

Figure 19–12. A large seborrheic keratosis of the face.

and dermis (*junctional nevus*); later the cells migrate into the dermis and form clumps of nevus cells (*intradermal nevus*). When both components are present they are called *compound nevi*. Melanocytic nevi develop in most light-skinned individuals any time from childhood to early adulthood and evolve from junctional to intradermal nevi over a number of years. They may eventually disappear. They may be brown to black or even colorless, depending on the amount of melanin pigment produced. They vary from flat to pedunculated depending on the number of nevus cells present (Figure 19–13).

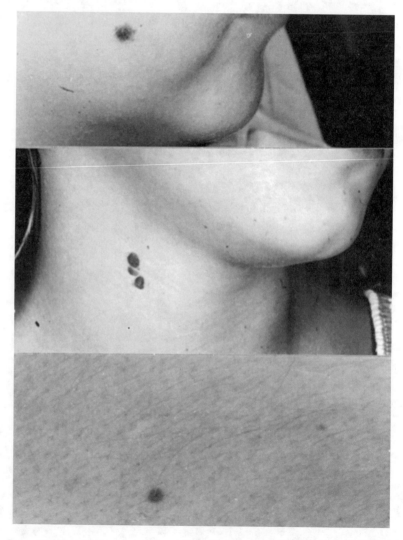

Figure 19–13. *Melanocytic nevi varying from flat to raised and sharply demarcated to less discrete.*

MELANOCYTIC NEVUS 19-15

causes	lesion	manifestation
Congenital malformation ?Hereditary	Clusters of melanocytes at dermal/epidermal junction and/or in dermis	Small brown spots; may be flat, raised, or pedunculated

The vast majority of melanocytic nevi are harmless and are only occasionally removed for cosmetic reasons. It is estimated that about 30 percent of malignant melanomas arise from melanocytic nevi, but the chance of any one nevus becoming malignant is extremely small. The risk is considerably greater in large congenital nevi (*giant hairy nevi*). Dysplastic nevi are nevi with architectural and cytologic atypia; some are thought to be precursors of malignant melanoma. A mole that increases in size, has irregular borders, ulcerates, bleeds, or undergoes color changes should be evaluated by a physician for possible malignant melanoma.

Malignant Melanoma

Skin cancers composed of melanocytes are much more dangerous than those derived from squamous cells (*basal cell* and *squamous cell carcinomas*). Currently it is estimated that about 20 percent of patients with malignant melanoma die from metastases. This number would be much greater if many lesions were not removed at an early stage. Once metastases have occurred, malignant melanoma has a tendency to spread widely and rapidly to many organs in the body, but occasionally malignant cells will lie dormant for several years before producing obvious metastases.

Four forms of malignant melanoma are recognized based on clinical and histologic appearance and behavior of the lesions. *Superficial spreading melanoma* is characterized by spreading growth of malignant cells within the epidermis producing a flat to slightly raised lesion, often with central regression of the lesion and a variegated color pattern (Figure 19–14A). If not removed, downward growth into the dermis and metastases will occur after months to years of superficial growth. *Lentigo maligna melanoma* also spreads radially in the epidermis and eventually invades the dermis; however, it develops on the exposed skin of the face of older persons and becomes very large because it grows for years before invading. Before it invades the dermis it is called lentigo maligna or Hutchinson's freckle. *Acral-lentiginous melanoma* is

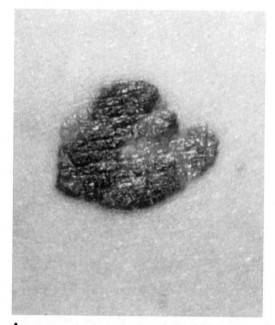

A

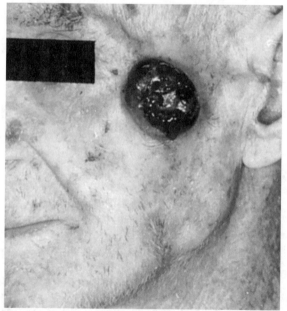

B

Figure 19–14. A. Superficial spreading melanoma of trunk. B. Nodular malignant melanoma of the face.

MALIGNANT MELANOMA 19-16

causes	lesion	manifestations
Unknown Influenced by long exposure to sunlight	Proliferation of malignant melanocytes	Enlarging pigmented skin lesion, either superficial or nodular Lymph node metastasis Widespread metastasis

composed of more spindle-shaped melanocytes that tend to grow into the dermis without producing a nodule. They tend to occur on the hands and feet and mucous membranes such as the vulva. Acral-lentiginous melanoma is less likely to be discovered early and more dangerous than the preceding types. *Nodular melanoma* grows downward and expands outward to form a nodule (Figure 19–14B). The likelihood of metastasis in nodular melanoma, as well as with other types, correlates with the vertical thickness of the tumor. Classification and staging of malignant melanomas are done by a pathologist after a wide excisional biopsy of the lesion is performed.

Other Pigmented Lesions

Freckles are localized areas of hyperpigmentation that occur in response to sunlight. Freckles begin in childhood and usually increase in number with repeated exposure to sunlight. On the other hand, *lentigo senilis* (age spots) are localized areas of increased melanocytes in the epidermis or exposed areas of skin in persons past middle age. Actinic keratoses, seborrheic keratoses, and basal cell carcinomas may also be dark colored when they contain increased amounts of melanin.

Basal Cell and Squamous Cell Carcinomas

Skin cancer is the most common type of cancer in man and in most instances is related to exposure to sunlight. Skin cancers are often multiple and occur most frequently on the face and hands of older adults. There are two distinctive cellular types of skin cancer—basal cell carcinoma and squamous cell carcinoma. Basal cell carcinoma is more common (75 percent of skin cancers) and is made up of cells that resemble those of the basal cell layer of epidermis (Figure 19–15A). The basal cell carcinoma usually presents as a slowly enlarging, raised lesion that does not ulcerate until advanced (Figure 19–16A); if untreated, it will slowly enlarge and destroy normal tissue,

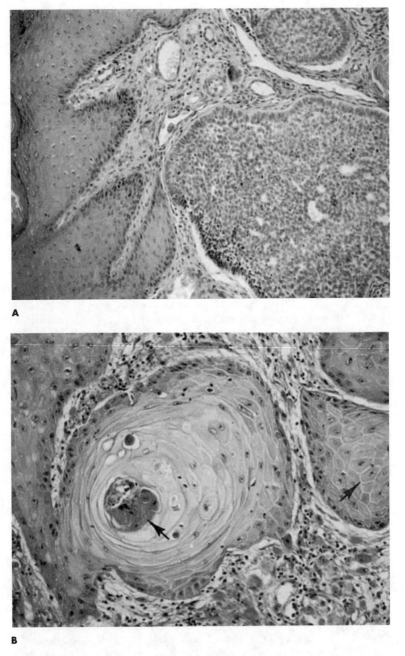

Figure 19–15. Histology of basal cell (A) and squamous cell (B) carcinomas. Compare with normal epidermis in A (*left*). The squamous cell carcinoma exhibits keratin formation (*left arrow*) and prickle cells with intercellular spaces (*right arrow*).

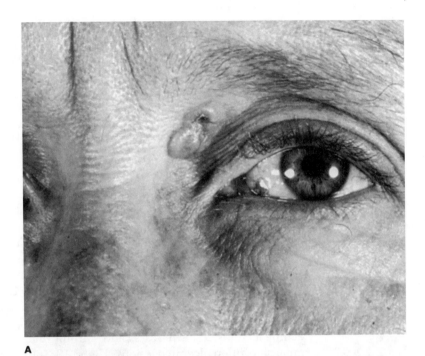

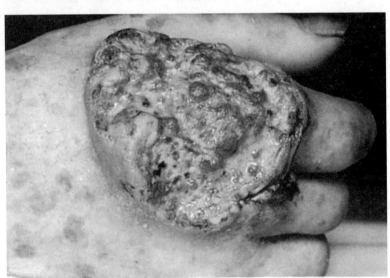

Figure 19–16. A. A basal cell carcinoma of the eyelid. B. A large, ulcerated squamous cell carcinoma of the hand.

BASAL CELL AND SQUAMOUS CELL CARCINOMAS 19-17

cause	lesion	manifestation
Long exposure to sunlight or x-rays	Malignant proliferation of basal cells or differentiating squamous cells to form small nodular lesions	Enlarging nodule on exposed areas of skin

but it does not metastasize. Basal cell carcinoma usually does not arise in any pre-existing skin lesion.

Squamous cell carcinoma is composed of clumps of cells in layers that resemble the layers of the epidermis (Figure 19–15B) and has a slightly greater growth potential than basal cell carcinoma. Squamous cell carcinomas commonly arise in pre-existing skin lesions, such as actinic keratoses, burn scars, and chronic ulcers, and present as enlarging, often ulcerated lesions (Figure 19–16B). If untreated, some skin carcinomas may metastasize, usually only to regional lymph nodes. Large, untreated skin cancers may cause death from secondary infection or, rarely, from hemorrhage.

Cancers can also arise from the skin appendages, blood vessels, and connective tissue, but these neoplasms are all rare.

ORGAN FAILURE

Lethal failure of skin function occurs with extensive, severe burns and rare cases of diffuse blistering diseases such as epidermolysis and pemphigus vulgaris. In these conditions, there may be inability to control fluid loss and to prevent infection.

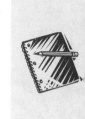

Review Questions

1. What kinds of skin diseases are most common?
2. Which skin conditions are likely to be fatal?
3. Which systemic diseases commonly have skin manifestations?
4. What do the following descriptive terms used to describe skin lesions mean?
   Macule
   Nodule
   Papule
   Pustule
   Vesicle
   Wheal
   Eczema
   Scale
   Crust
5. What are the causes, lesions, and manifestations of the specific diseases described in this chapter?
6. How do verruca vulgaris and condyloma acuminatum differ?
7. What are the various types of skin abscesses?
8. What infectious agents cause skin lesions and what is the nature of the lesions they cause?
9. What are the similarities among the various types of dermatitis?
10. What are the skin lesions associated with exposure to sunlight?
11. How do neoplasms of squamous cells and melanocytes differ in frequency and prognosis?
12. How can extensive skin lesions lead to a fatal outcome?

20.

Eye

REVIEW OF STRUCTURE AND FUNCTION
Layers of the Globe
Sclera • Uvea • Retina
Anterior Segment of the Globe
Conjunctiva • Cornea • Anterior Chamber • Iris • Ciliary Body • Posterior Chamber • Lens
Posterior Segment of the Globe
Vitreous Cavity • Retina • Optic Nerve

MOST FREQUENT AND SERIOUS PROBLEMS
Myopia • Hyperopia • Presbyopia • Strabismus • Cataract • Glaucoma

SYMPTOMS, SIGNS, AND TESTS
Decreased Visual Acuity • Visual Field Defects • Pain • Blurred Vision • Nystagmus • Funduscopic Examination • Clinical Eye Tests • Tonometry • Slit-Lamp Examination

SPECIFIC DISEASES
Genetic/Developmental Diseases
Inflammatory/Degenerative Diseases
Trauma and Chemical Injury
Conjunctivitis and Dry Eyes
Strabismus (Heterotropia)
Cataract
Glaucoma
Hypertensive Retinopathy
Diabetic Retinopathy
Myopia (Nearsightedness)
Hyperopia (Farsightedness)
Presbyopia
Astigmatism

Hyperplastic/Neoplastic Diseases
Retinoblastoma
Malignant Melanoma

ORGAN FAILURE

REVIEW QUESTIONS

REVIEW OF STRUCTURE AND FUNCTION

The *globe* of the eye (eyeball) sits inside the bony orbit and is protected anteriorly by the eyelid. The extraocular muscles attach to its outer surface. The optic nerve together with blood vessels enter the globe posteriorly. The globe is composed of three layers (Figure 20–1)—the outer *scleral layer*, a tough fibrous coating; the *choroid* or *uveal layer*, a pigmented layer of connective tissue through which nerves and blood vessels course; and the inner, *retinal layer*.

Anteriorly, the scleral layer is continuous with the cornea, the transparent structure through which light first passes into the globe. The *cornea* is the initial refracting surface of the eye. The exterior of the sclera is covered by the *conjunctiva*, a sheet of cells that reflect onto the inner surface of the eyelids at approximately 1 centimeter posterior to its origin at the corneoscleral junction. The *lens*, the suspending ligaments of the lens, the *iris*, and the muscular *ciliary body* are

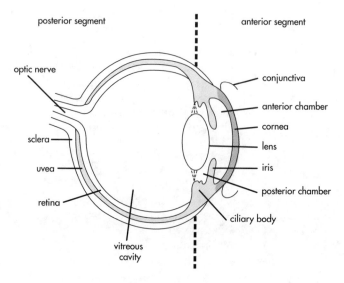

Figure 20–1. Anatomy of the eye.

all located in the anterior portion of the eye. Contraction of the ciliary body controls the focal length of the lens. The iris controls the amount of light reaching the lens by varying the size of its aperture (*pupil*). Decrease in pupil size (*miosis*) is achieved by contraction of the circular smooth muscles in the iris, which are stimulated by autonomic nerve fibers from the third cranial nerve, the oculomotor.

Posteriorly, the retina is the site of the light- and color-sensing rod and cone neurons. Impulses generated in these cells by light are transmitted by a chain of neurons back through the optic nerve to the visual cortex of the cerebrum. The macula is the spot on the retina of greatest visual acuity. The fovea is the central portion of the macula. The ciliary body and the lens and its ligaments mark the boundary between the anterior and posterior segments of the globe. Within the anterior segment is the anterior chamber, which is filled with a watery fluid, *aqueous humor*. Aqueous humor is secreted by the ciliary body and diffuses forward, around the lens, from the posterior to the anterior chamber and serves to nourish and cleanse the avascular lens and retina. It drains out of the anterior chamber slowly through a series of tissue spaces at the periphery of the chamber. The posterior segment is filled with a clear gelatinous substance, the *vitreous humor*.

MOST FREQUENT AND SERIOUS PROBLEMS

The most common overall problem affecting the eyes is a decrease in visual acuity (indistinct focusing of the visual image on the retina) from refractive error. Age-related macular degeneration is the most common cause of legal blindness in persons over 65. Approximately one-third of the population wears eyeglasses for correction of the main types of refractive error, which include myopia, hyperopia, presbyopia, and astigmatism. Trauma to various parts of the eye, especially to the cornea, are very common problems and can lead to significant pain and disability. Acute conjunctivitis, colloquially called *pink-eye*, may occur by itself or be associated with another bacterial or viral infection such as an upper respiratory infection. Infections in the adjacent sinuses can spread to the orbit resulting in serious complications. Strabismus is deviation of one or both eyes that cannot be overcome by the patient. Strabismus is relatively common and is due to several causes. Cataract is an opacity of the lens leading to decreased visual acuity. Cataracts may be the result of birth defect, infection, or trauma, but most commonly they arise de novo in elderly persons. Glaucoma is a disease caused by an increase in intraocular pressure, with resultant damage to the optic nerve and its fibers inside the eye. Afflictions of the small retinal vessels occur commonly in individuals with hypertension and diabetes. Tumors of the eye itself are relatively rare.

SYMPTOMS, SIGNS, AND TESTS

The most common manifestation of eye disease is decreased visual acuity. Decreased visual acuity may be a symptom when experienced by a person or a sign when manifested as a result of a visual acuity test. Decreased visual acuity may result from macular degeneration, cataracts, and vascular diseases, as well as from myopia or hyperopia. Visual field defects (focal areas of blindness) also may be signs or symptoms and result from diseases affecting the optic pathways of the central nervous system or from diseases of the retina. Pain is often a manifestation of trauma, infection, or acutely increased intraocular pressure from closed-angle glaucoma. Blurring of vision accompanies various systemic diseases, especially those of toxic and metabolic origin. *Papilledema* (swelling of the head of the optic nerve as seen through the ophthalmoscope) may reflect an increase in intracranial pressure, usually due to an expanding intracranial mass. *Photophobia* (uncomfortable sensitivity to light) is commonly seen with inflammation inside and outside the eyeball. *Nystagmus* (flickering eye movements) may be caused by a variety of central nervous system lesions.

Clinical tests for eye disease include the utilization of eye charts for testing *visual acuity*. The person being examined reads letters or numbers from a chart at a distance of 20 feet. Normal visual acuity (20/20) means that the person can accurately read with either eye the smallest figures that are readable to a normal control population. A visual acuity of 20/40 means that the affected eye can accurately read at 20 feet what a normal eye can read at 40 feet. These charts are widely used as screening devices for school children and for persons applying for drivers' licenses.

Tests for mapping visual field defects are employed to detect area(s) of the retina or optic pathways affected by a particular disease process (Figure 20–2). In administering *visual field tests*, the person being examined is asked to focus on a small stationary spot while a test spot is moved to different points of a circular map. In those areas where the person cannot see the test spot, he or she has a visual field defect.

The *ophthalmoscope* is a hand-held, light-projecting instrument used to examine the retina by utilizing lenses of various refractive powers to focus the image for the examiner. Visualization of the retina with the ophthalmoscope is referred to as a *funduscopic examination*. A *tonometer* is a small instrument that is placed directly on the eyeball to measure the intraocular pressure, which may be elevated in glaucoma. A *slit-lamp* is a binocular magnifying instrument that projects a beam of light into the eye and is used for detailed examination of the cornea, anterior chamber, iris, and lens, and is useful in the evaluation of glaucoma, trauma, inflammation, and other conditions. Various types of lenses are utilized in the evaluation of myopia and hyperopia to deter-

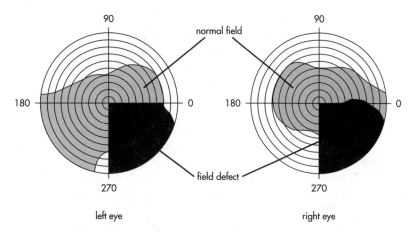

Figure 20–2. Visual field chart with visual field defects marked in black.

mine the *refractive error* (degree by which the cornea, lens, and humor fail to focus light rays on the retina).

SPECIFIC DISEASES

Genetic/Developmental Diseases

Isolated congenital eye defects are rare, but genetic factors appear to predispose individuals to certain eye disorders such as myopia, glaucoma, strabismus, cataracts, and retinoblastoma (a malignant neoplasm). *Cyclopia*, a very rare condition in which a single, malformed eye is centrally situated, may occur in conjunction with severe brain malformation.

Inflammatory/Degenerative Diseases

Except for injuries and infections, the diseases discussed here represent a heterogenous group of developmental and acquired conditions. Although not discussed further, it should be noted that infections of the maxillary, ethmoid, and frontal sinuses can extend into the orbit and cause damage to the eye.

Trauma and Chemical Injury

The eye is susceptible to many different types of injuries, which include penetrating injuries, blunt injuries, and chemical injuries. The most common penetrating injury occurs when metal strikes metal. The manifestations of penetrating injuries are usually readily apparent and receive the immediate attention of an ophthalmic surgeon. The manifestations of blunt injuries are usually less apparent, but may be no less severe. When the eye is hit directly by a blunt object (e.g., a paddle ball), compression/decompression occurs, which can produce damage to several intraocular structures. Such damage can, in time, result in retinal detachment, intraocular hemorrhage, dislocation of the lens, and/or glaucoma. Of the different types of chemicals that can damage the eye, concentrated alkali solutions such as nitrogen fertilizers produce the most damage to the cornea and adjacent tissues. Complications of severe chemical burns include corneal ulcer and corneal perforation.

Conjunctivitis and Dry Eyes

Inflammation of the conjunctiva with vascular congestion producing a red or pink eye (Figure 20–3) may be secondary to viral, chlamydial, bacterial, and fungal infections or allergy. Symptoms include irritation, blurred vision, and photophobia. Conjunctivitis most often occurs in association with an upper respiratory infection but may occur by itself. Measles often present with conjunctivitis. Conjunctivitis associated with hay fever may be very troublesome because of photophobia and itching. Viral and allergic types of conjunctivitis are prone to secondary bacterial infections; hence, the treatment of conjunctivitis often consists of administration of eye drops that contain antibiotics and topical antihistamines. Conjunctivitis caused by *trachoma* (a chlamydial disease) is one of the most common causes of blindness in many parts of the world because it results in corneal scarring. Inflammation of other parts of the eye are less common, but keratitis (corneal inflammation), uveitis, and retinitis can be very devastating to sight.

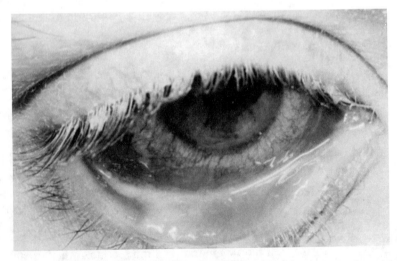

Figure 20–3. Conjunctivitis with congested conjunctival vessels and exudate on lower lid.

CONJUNCTIVITIS 20-1

causes	lesion	manifestations
Bacteria	Inflamed conjunctiva	Red eye
Viruses		Irritation
Chlamydia		Blurred vision
Fungi		Photophobia
Allergy		
Drugs		

Dry eyes are a common similar problem occasionally associated with systemic immune disorders such as rheumatoid arthritis, but more often secondary to systemic drugs such as antihypertensive, antidepressant, and antihistamine medications. Dry eye symptoms are itching, burning, photophobia, "sandy" sensation, blurred vision, and vascular congestion. Treatment consists of eye drops plus alleviation of the primary condition.

Strabismus (Heterotropia)

Strabismus is an improper alignment of the visual axis (the line of vision), with one or both eyes at fault. The result is that each eye points in a different direction and the eyes cannot fixate on the same visual object simultaneously (Figure 20–4). Strabismus is a common condition, most often manifest in childhood and often referred to as crossed eyes in layman's terms. Normally children attain alignment by 3 to 4 months of age. A variety of factors may cause strabismus—paralysis of an extraocular muscle, refractive errors, opacities of the cornea or lens, diseases of the retina, and diseases of the optic nerve or brain. Some types of strabismus may be corrected with lenses; others are corrected

STRABISMUS 20-2

causes	lesion	manifestation
Extraocular muscle defects	Varies with cause	Deviation of eyes
Refractive errors		
Corneal opacities		
Retinal disease		
Nerve or brain disease		

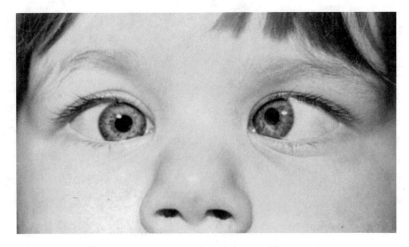

Figure 20–4. Strabismus.

surgically by altering the insertions of extraocular muscles to realign the eyes. If not discovered and treated early, strabismus can cause irreversible loss of vision in one eye called *amblyopia* (lazy eye).

Cataract

Cataract is an opacification of the lens (Figure 20–5) that most commonly occurs in older individuals (*senile cataract*). Less commonly, cataracts may be secondary to trauma or may be accelerated by diabetes mellitus in poor control. Congenital cataracts are rare, and some types have a familial tendency. Most cataracts develop slowly, resulting in progressive diminution of vision. In most cases, treatment of cataracts consists of surgical extraction of the opacified portion of the lens followed by placement of a prosthetic intraocular lens inserted inside the preserved outside capsule of the natural lens.

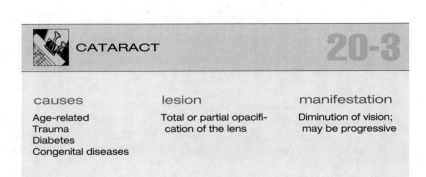

CATARACT 20-3

causes	lesion	manifestation
Age-related Trauma Diabetes Congenital diseases	Total or partial opacification of the lens	Diminution of vision; may be progressive

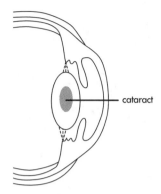

Figure 20–5. Cataract.

Glaucoma

Glaucoma is a condition characterized by a rise in intraocular pressure sufficient to damage optic nerve fibers. The increase in intraocular pressure is almost always due to obstruction of the normal exit of anterior chamber fluid (aqueous humor) in the angle where the iris meets the corneal-scleral junction. Glaucoma is divided into open-angle, closed-angle, and rare congenital forms. In *open-angle glaucoma,* there are gross or microscopic abnormalities of the angle tissues. Open-angle glaucoma is the much more common type and is chronic and insidious in onset. The patient is unaware of slowly progressive damage to the optic nerve with consequent peripheral visual loss until the condition is far advanced.

In *closed-angle glaucoma,* there is obstruction of the angle by the iris (Figure 20–6). The adhesion of the iris to the angle structures may be reversible or, if inflammation and scarring has occurred, permanent.

GLAUCOMA   **20-4**

cause	lesions	manifestations
Obstruction of exit flow of aqueous humor	Abnormal structure of angle (open angle) Obstruction of angle by iris inflammation and scarring (closed angle)	Increased intraocular pressure (open and closed angle) Pain Nausea and vomiting (closed angle) Progressive loss of vision (closed angle)

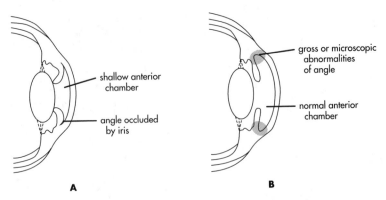

Figure 20–6. A. Closed-angle glaucoma. B. Open-angle glaucoma.

The symptoms of closed-angle glaucoma are usually acute, with pain, nausea, vomiting, and a sudden decrease in vision.

Glaucoma is diagnosed by demonstration of increased intraocular pressure as measured with a tonometer and by documented defects in peripheral visual fields. It is treated by various adrenergic and anticholinergic drugs, newer β-blockers, prostaglandins, and by carbonic anhydrase inhibitors, which partially inhibit the formation and secretion of aqueous humor and, to some degree, increase outflow.

Hypertensive Retinopathy

Hypertension causes progressive arteriolosclerosis of the retinal vessels, eventually resulting in loss of vision because of compromised oxygen delivery to the retinal neurons. Hypertensive retinopathy is diagnosed by funduscopic examination, because the sclerosis of the retinal arteries is seen as characteristic alterations in the light reflection from these vessels (Figure 20–7) along with "flame" hemorrhages and "cotton wool" spots when severe. Control of the hypertension will usually result in some visual improvement.

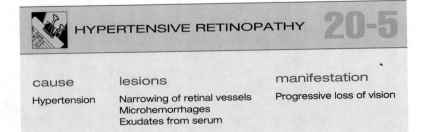

HYPERTENSIVE RETINOPATHY		20-5
cause	**lesions**	**manifestation**
Hypertension	Narrowing of retinal vessels Microhemorrhages Exudates from serum	Progressive loss of vision

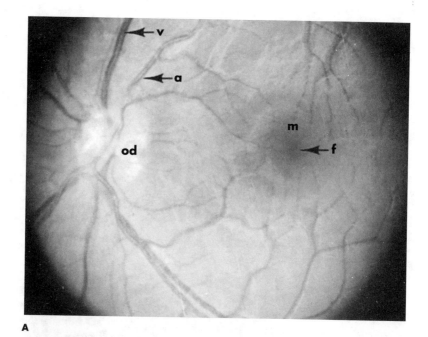

A

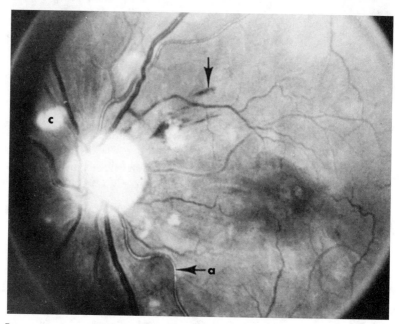

B

Figure 20–7. A. Normal retina, showing optic disk (od), macula (m) with fovea in center (f), artery (a), and vein (v). B. Hypertensive retinopathy, with flame-shaped hemorrhages (arrow), narrow, tortuous artery (a), and cotton wool patches (c) caused by focal ischemia.

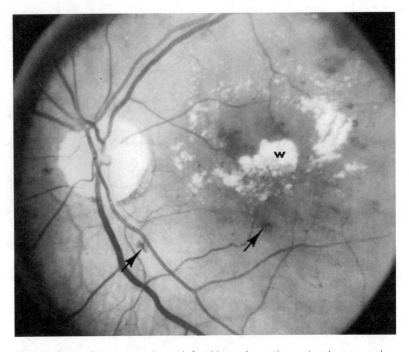

Figure 20–8. Diabetic retinopathy, with focal hemorrhages *(arrows)* and waxy exudates (W) forming a ring around the macula.

Diabetic Retinopathy

Long-standing diabetes mellitus leads to retinal vessel disease manifested by progressive arteriosclerosis similar to that which occurs with hypertension. In addition, diabetes is associated with the development of vascular abnormalities. Early vascular lesions consist of *capillary aneurysms* and *microhemorrhages*, the latter eventually resulting in visual loss (Figure 20–8). The most advanced vascular lesions consist of proliferation of newly formed abnormal vessels, which can cause retinal

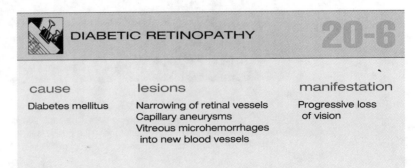

DIABETIC RETINOPATHY		20-6
cause	**lesions**	**manifestation**
Diabetes mellitus	Narrowing of retinal vessels Capillary aneurysms Vitreous microhemorrhages into new blood vessels	Progressive loss of vision

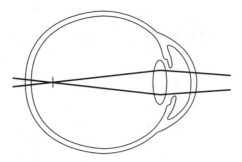

Figure 20–9. Myopic eye.

detachment and vitreous hemorrhage. Treatment of new retinal vessels may be effectively accomplished using a lasar beam to coagulate many areas of the retina by thermal energy.

Myopia (Nearsightedness)

Myopia is a condition of refractive error in which light entering the eye is focused at a point anterior to the retina (Figure 20–9). This may be due either to abnormal curvature and refractive power of the cornea and lens, or it may be due to relative elongation of the eyeball. Myopia often develops in childhood for poorly understood reasons and progresses until early adulthood, when the condition stabilizes because of normal loss of elasticity of the eye structures. Myopia tends to be familial and is usually treated successfully with corrective lenses. Severe myopia may be associated with multiple defects in intraocular structures, including the angle and retina.

MYOPIA		20-7
causes	**lesion**	**manifestation**
Unknown Tends to be familial	Abnormal configuration of cornea, lens, or globe allowing convergence of light in front of the retina	Decreased visual acuity for distant objects

Hyperopia (Farsightedness)

This condition is different from myopia in that light entering the eye tends to focus at a point posterior to the retina, with resultant poor vision for near objects and better vision for far objects (Figure 20–10).

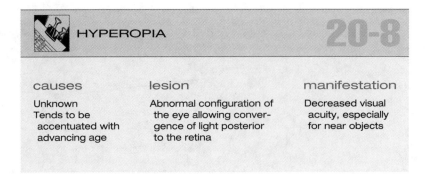

causes	lesion	manifestation
Unknown Tends to be accentuated with advancing age	Abnormal configuration of the eye allowing conver- gence of light posterior to the retina	Decreased visual acuity, especially for near objects

Hyperopia is the result of a relatively short eyeball or reduced refractive power of the cornea or lens. Children can often overcome an underlying mild hyperopic refractive error because of lens elasticity but often lose this ability as they grow older. The lens loses its elasticity and ability to adjust its focusing power *(accommodation)* with advancing age and is less able to focus light rays closer to the retina rather than behind it. Thus, a mild hyperopia can become manifest in later years and only then require corrective lenses.

Presbyopia

Presbyopia is a refractive error produced by loss of elasticity of the lens starting in the 40s for most persons. It represents an inability to accommodate. Accommodation means the ability of the lens to change its shape in order to focus light rays from nearby objects onto the retina. Although the optical defect of presbyopia is similar to that of hyperopia inasmuch as light rays are focused behind the retina, the pathogenesis of the two conditions is different. Hyperopia is due to the relatively short length of the eyeball, whereas presbyopia results from

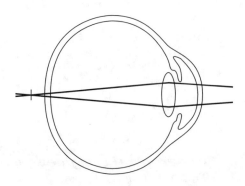

Figure 20–10. Hyperopic eye.

the degenerative effects of aging on the lens. Presbyopia is corrected by reading glasses or bifocals.

Astigmatism

Astigmatism is uneven focusing of light entering the eye due to unequal curvature of the cornea or acquired irregularities in the corneal surface or lens. Astigmatism may occur by itself or may accompany myopia or hyperopia. Unless unusually severe, astigmatism is correctable with appropriate lenses.

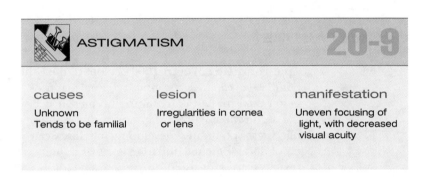

ASTIGMATISM		20-9
causes	**lesion**	**manifestation**
Unknown Tends to be familial	Irregularities in cornea or lens	Uneven focusing of light, with decreased visual acuity

Hyperplastic/Neoplastic Diseases

Retinoblastomas and melanomas comprise over 90 percent of all primary intraocular eye tumors. With rare exceptions, retinoblastoma occurs in children, while melanoma occurs in adults.

Retinoblastoma

This is a rare malignant tumor of primitive neurons, which are the precursors of the retinal ganglion cells. Retinoblastomas occur in chil-

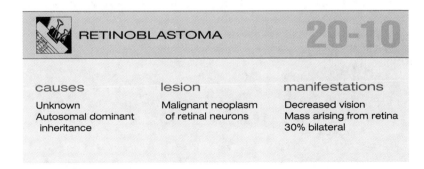

RETINOBLASTOMA		20-10
causes	**lesion**	**manifestations**
Unknown Autosomal dominant inheritance	Malignant neoplasm of retinal neurons	Decreased vision Mass arising from retina 30% bilateral

dren; they tend to be familial and have an autosomal dominant inheritance pattern with incomplete penetrance. Retinoblastomas are bilateral about 30 percent of the time. Treatment is removal of the eye *(enucleation)*, often combined with chemotherapy or radiation.

Malignant Melanoma

This is a malignant tumor arising from the choroid pigment-containing cells and is primarily a tumor of adults. Most ocular melanomas arise from the choroid layer, although they can arise from the iris or ciliary body. They carry a better prognosis than melanomas of the skin.

ORGAN FAILURE

Approximately 4 of every 1000 persons in the United States are legally blind. *Legal blindness* is defined as visual acuity of 20/200 or less in the better eye with best correction. Blindness may be caused by lesions of the cornea, lens, vitreous humor, retina, and optic nerve. Congenital blindness or blindness developing in infancy can be due to a wide variety of developmental, inflammatory, or traumatic conditions. Oxygen toxicity causes fibrosis of the retina, a condition called retinopathy of prematurity. Attention to the amount of oxygen given to newborns with respiratory distress syndrome has greatly reduced the incidence of this condition. The most common of the many causes of blindness in adults are glaucoma, diabetic retinopathy, macular degeneration, senile cataract, optic nerve atrophy, and retinitis pigmentosa. Degeneration of the macula with resultant loss of central vision may be due to several causes, the most common of which is an idiopathic condition called *senile macular degeneration* characterized by damage to retinal pigment epithelium with underlying vascular proliferation. Optic atrophy may be caused by occlusion of the small vessels supplying the optic nerve, by optic neuritis such as occurs in multiple sclerosis, and by masses that press on the optic nerve. Retinitis pigmentosa, usually a recessively inherited condition, results in progressive destruction of rods and cones beginning in childhood and leading to blindness.

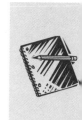

Review Questions

1. What symptom is common to most people wearing eye-glasses regardless of their underlying eye disorder?
2. How are each of the following instruments or procedures helpful in evaluation of eye problems?
   - Visual acuity tests
   - Visual field tests
   - Funduscopic examination
   - Tonometer
   - Slit-lamp
3. What are the causes, lesions, and major manifestations of each of the specific diseases or disorders discussed in this chapter?
4. How do abnormalities in the cornea, lens, or retina lead to strabismus?
5. What is the pathogenesis of visual loss in glaucoma?
6. How does diabetic retinopathy differ from hypertensive retinopathy?
7. What is the pathogenesis of decreased visual acuity in myopia, hyperopia, presbyopia, and astigmatism?
8. What are the leading causes of blindness?
9. What do the following terms mean?
   - Visual acuity
   - Papilledema
   - Photophobia
   - Nystagmus
   - 20/20 vision
   - Visual axis
   - Amblyopia
   - Capillary aneurysms
   - Microhemorrhages
   - Accommodation
   - Enucleation
   - Legal blindness

21.
Bones and Joints

REVIEW OF STRUCTURE AND FUNCTION
Major Bones and Joints • Functions of Bones and Joints • Long Bones • Large Joints • Spinal Column • Flat Bones • Bone Development and Regeneration

MOST FREQUENT AND SERIOUS PROBLEMS
Strains and Sprains • Low Back Problems • Degenerative Arthritis • Rheumatoid Arthritis • Gouty Arthritis • Fracture • Osteoporosis • Metastatic Cancer • Osteosarcoma

SYMPTOMS, SIGNS, AND TESTS
Pain • Joint Stiffness • Deformity • Decreased Mobility • X-rays • Serum Calcium, Phosphorus, and Alkaline Phosphatase

SPECIFIC DISEASES
Genetic/Developmental Diseases
Clubfoot (Talipes Equinovarus)
Intoeing
Congenital Dislocation of the Hip
Torticollis (Wry Neck)
Achondroplasia
Osteogenesis Imperfecta
Marfan's Syndrome
Inflammatory/Degenerative Diseases
Injuries to Joints and Muscles
Low Back Pain
Scoliosis and Kyphosis
Fractures
Acute Arthritis
Osteomyelitis
Osteoporosis
Osteomalacia and Rickets
Degenerative Arthritis
Rheumatoid Arthritis

Gout
Ganglion
Hyperplastic/Neoplastic Diseases
Paget's Disease of Bone
Osteosarcoma

ORGAN FAILURE

REVIEW QUESTIONS

REVIEW OF STRUCTURE AND FUNCTION

The human body contains 206 bones, many of which have joints at their ends to connect them to adjacent bones. The major bones and joints are labeled on Figure 21–1.

Bone provides a framework for the attachment of muscles, supports weight bearing, and protects internal organs from injury. It also plays a major role in calcium and phosphorus metabolism. Bone marrow, which may be considered part of bone, is discussed in Chapter 10. Joints allow movement of body parts and control the extent of movement.

The components of a typical long bone are shown in Figure 21–2. Between the epiphysis and metaphysis lies the epiphyseal plate, a layer of cartilage that undergoes growth and ossification (bone development) until the bone has reached its mature length.

Joints consist of the articular and adjacent surfaces of bone bridged externally by a fibrous capsule. The joint is lined by flattened mesothelial-like synovial lining cells and contains a small amount of serous fluid.

The knee joint (Figure 21–3) is more complex, but particularly important because it is a frequent site of injury and disease. Unlike other joints, the knee joint contains fibrocartilagenous pads called *menisci* and contains a bone, the patella, within an overlying tendon. The spinal column (Figure 21–4) has pads between vertebral bodies that consist of nucleus pulposis surrounded by fibrocartilage. The spinal canal, which houses the delicate spinal cord and emerging spinal nerves, lies posterior to the vertebral bodies and anterior to the more complex bony parts of the vertebrae. Like the knee, the spine is particularly vulnerable to the effects of weight bearing.

The flat bones such as ribs, sternum, pelvis, and cranium serve to protect the thorax, abdomen, and brain. They also (along with the vertebrae) are major sites of hematopoiesis.

Bone, in spite of its solid consistency, is an active tissue that responds to physical stress, metabolic conditions, injury, and disease.

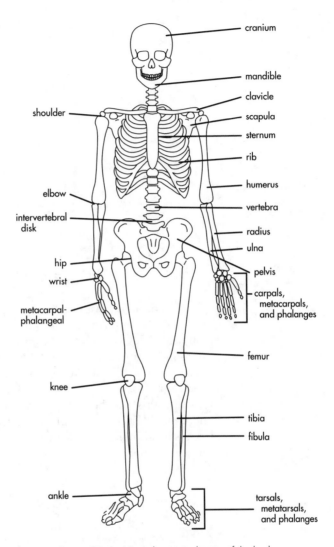

cranium
mandible
clavicle
scapula
sternum
rib
humerus
vertebra
radius
ulna
pelvis
carpals,
metacarpals,
and phalanges
femur
tibia
fibula
tarsals,
metatarsals,
and phalanges

shoulder
elbow
intervertebral
disk
hip
wrist
metacarpal-
phalangeal
knee
ankle

Figure 21–1. Major bones and joints of the body.

Bone is formed by osteoblasts, cells that lay down a collagenous matrix called osteoid and promote deposition of hydroxyapatite crystals within the collagenous matrix to form bone. During development, osteoblasts may differentiate from primitive mesenchymal cells and form bone directly (intramembranous bone formation) or invade and replace a growing cartilagenous plate with bone (enchondral bone formation). Intramembranous bone formation typically occurs in flat bones and endochondral bone formation typically occurs in long tubular bones with a dense cortex.

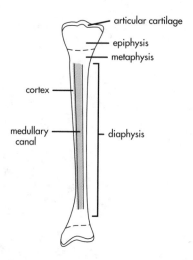

Figure 21–2. Structure of a long bone—the tibia.

In childhood, most of the increase in body height is due to enchondral bone formation in long bones. Disease or injury to epiphyseal plates will produce asymmetric body growth and deformity. Bone continues to remodel throughout adult life. When injured, such as by fracture, osteoblasts proliferate to form new bone. Chondrocytes may also produce cartilage at the site of injury and this may be invaded by osteoblasts and replaced by bone. Osteoblasts must be able to differentiate from more primitive cells in adult life, as metaplastic bone is seen in sites of injury remote from bone.

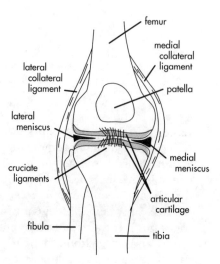

Figure 21–3. Structure of a large, complex joint—the knee.

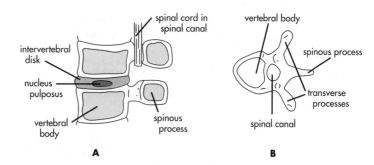

Figure 21–4. Structure of the spinal column. A. Sagittal plane. B. Transverse plane.

Osteoclasts, the cells responsible for bone destruction, are multinucleated cells seen at the edge of bony seams.

MOST FREQUENT AND SERIOUS PROBLEMS

By far the most frequent affliction of bone is fracture. Fractures may be caused by trauma alone or may be pathologic, meaning that the bone was already weakened by other disease such as metastatic cancer or osteoporosis. Sites commonly involved with fractures vary with age and sex. For example, traumatic fractures are most common in 20- to 40-year-old males and are common in the extremities. In children, the most common fractures are of the clavicle and the humerus. Elderly persons, especially women, are prone to fracture their hips or vertebrae due to osteoporosis.

If arthritis is considered to be primarily a disease of joints, then joint disease is much more prevalent than bone disease. This generalization also holds for traumatic injuries, as strains and sprains, which affect joint function, are more common than fractures of bone.

Strains and sprains are among the top ten causes of patients' seeking health care for acute disease, while low back problems and degenerative arthritis are among the top ten causes of patients seeking health care for chronic disease. The prevalence of these forms of arthritis is very high; 5 percent of the population suffers from degenerative arthritis, 1–2 percent from rheumatoid arthritis, and 0.5 percent from gouty arthritis.

Generalized loss of bone *(osteopenia)* may be due to a wide variety of causes such as osteoporosis, osteomalacia, rickets, hyperparathyroidism, and metastatic cancer. Osteoporosis in postmenopausal women is the most common of these conditions and the vertebral column is the most significant site of involvement by painful fractures.

Metastatic cancer is the most common malignancy of bone and often requires considerable health care because of associated pain and pathologic fracture. Of the several types of bone cancers, multiple myeloma is the most common in adults and osteosarcoma is the most common in young people, particularly adolescents.

SYMPTOMS, SIGNS, AND TESTS

The most common symptoms of bone and joint diseases are pain, decreased mobility, and deformity. Almost all fractures of bone are associated with pain due to disruption of sensory nerves. Usually, the fracture is obvious because of the attendant deformity, although in some fractures the bone is not displaced. The muscles surrounding a fracture site will undergo intense sustained contraction (spasm) in an attempt to protect the fractured area and this spasm will often cause additional pain.

Joint stiffness, decreased mobility, and varying degrees of pain are associated with chronic arthritis (rheumatoid and degenerative); whereas, the cardinal signs of inflammation (redness, heat, swelling, and pain) are associated with acute infectious arthritis.

Physical examination of patients with bone and joint disease involves careful attention to evaluation of joint mobility, gait, and neurologic examination (see Chapter 23 for description), as well as looking for deformity or masses.

X-ray films are the primary laboratory results used for evaluation of most bone and joint diseases. The metabolic activity of bone is evaluated by a battery of serum tests, including calcium, phosphorus, and alkaline phosphatase. Calcium and phosphorus are principal constituents of bone, and alkaline phosphatase is an enzyme present in the serum that is produced by the osteoblast and is elevated in many bone diseases involving proliferation of osteoblasts. The erythrocyte sedimentation rate may be used as an indicator of chronic inflammation and is useful in following patients with rheumatoid arthritis. Tests for rheumatoid factor (latex fixation titer) and serum uric acid levels may be useful aids in the diagnosis of rheumatoid arthritis and gout, respectively. Cultures are important in the diagnosis of acute arthritis and osteomyelitis. Biopsy is used to diagnose bone tumors.

SPECIFIC DISEASES

Genetic/Developmental Diseases

Developmental abnormalities fall into two broad groups. Selected structural defects include embryonic anomalies and localized deformities that arise during fetal development and childbirth. The most common types, many of which need early diagnosis and treatment to prevent permanent deformity, are discussed below. These include clubfoot, intoeing, congenital dislocation of the hip, and torticollis.

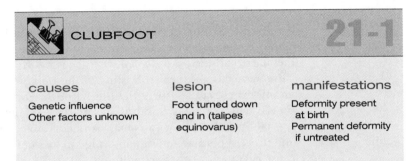

CLUBFOOT		**21-1**
causes	lesion	manifestations
Genetic influence Other factors unknown	Foot turned down and in (talipes equinovarus)	Deformity present at birth Permanent deformity if untreated

The wide variety of other types include conditions such as missing limbs and extra digits. The second major group of developmental abnormalities are generalized genetic disorders. These are much less common than the localized types, and their treatment is symptomatic rather than curative. Three types are discussed briefly—achondroplasia, osteogenesis imperfecta, Marfan's syndrome.

Clubfoot (Talipes Equinovarus)

Clubfoot occurs in approximately 1 of every 1000 births. Clubfoot consists of a downward (equino) and inward (varus) turning of the foot (Figure 21–5). It may occur bilaterally and is more frequent in males. Although the precise cause of clubfoot is not known, there is evidence that a genetic factor is involved. The deformity is evident at birth and can usually be corrected by placing the foot in casts for 2 to 6 months to gradually correct the deformity.

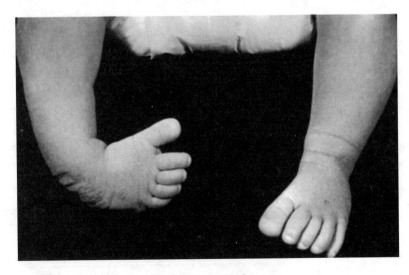

Figure 21–5. Clubfoot.

Intoeing

An inward turning of the toes is a very common finding in infants. Three common causes are femoral anteversion, tibial torsion, and metatarsus adductus. *Femoral anteversion* is a turning in of the femur. *Tibial torsion* is an internal twisting of the tibia. *Metatarsus adductus* is an inward curvature (varus deformity) of the forefoot. These conditions usually correct themselves. In some cases of metatarsus adductus, special braced shoes or casts may be needed to correct the deformity and prevent permanent intoeing (pigeon toes deformity). No specific cause is known for these conditions.

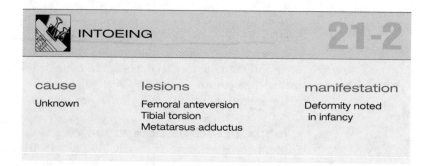

INTOEING		21-2
cause	**lesions**	**manifestation**
Unknown	Femoral anteversion	Deformity noted
	Tibial torsion	in infancy
	Metatarsus adductus	

Congenital Dislocation of the Hip

Congenital dislocation of the hip may be detected during infancy or childhood. It consists of a malformation of the acetabulum (hip socket) that allows displacement of the head of the femur in relation to the acetabulum (Figure 21–6). The occurrence is influenced by heredity and much more frequently involves girls than boys. The most common clinical signs are shortening of the involved extremity,

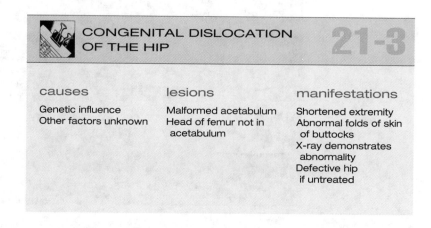

CONGENITAL DISLOCATION OF THE HIP		21-3
causes	**lesions**	**manifestations**
Genetic influence	Malformed acetabulum	Shortened extremity
Other factors unknown	Head of femur not in acetabulum	Abnormal folds of skin of buttocks
		X-ray demonstrates abnormality
		Defective hip if untreated

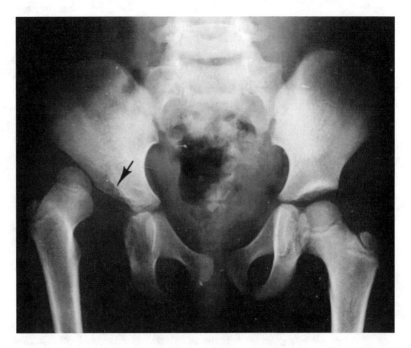

Figure 21–6. X-ray of congenital dislocation of the hip. Note irregularity of acetabulum on the involved side (*arrow*).

with abnormal folds of skin in the buttocks. Treatment with appropriate splinting, if done in time, prevents permanent deformity and crippling.

Torticollis (Wry Neck)

Torticollis means turned neck and presents within the first 3 months of infancy as a neck pulled to one side. Although the cause is usually not clinically evident, it is believed to be due to injury to the sternocleido-

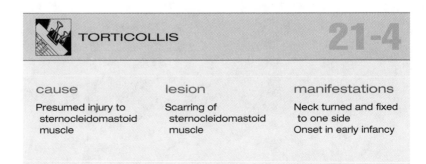

TORTICOLLIS		21-4
cause	**lesion**	**manifestations**
Presumed injury to sternocleidomastoid muscle	Scarring of sternocleidomastoid muscle	Neck turned and fixed to one side Onset in early infancy

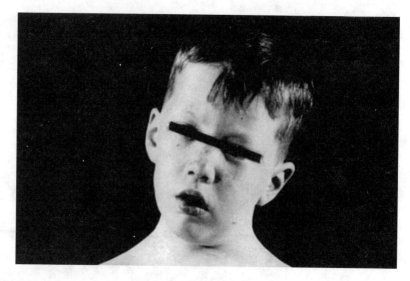

Figure 21–7. Torticollis.

mastoid muscle during the fetal period by abnormal intrauterine positioning or injury at birth. Scarring and contraction of the muscle leads to the pulling of the neck to one side (Figure 21–7). Treatment consists of manipulative stretching or surgical cutting of the muscle to prevent permanent facial deformity.

Achondroplasia

Achondroplasia is a rare autosomal dominant disorder most often arising by mutation. The anatomic defect consists of poorly organized epiphyseal cartilage, which results in reduced growth of long bones and short stature (Figure 21–8). A similar disorder is present in basset hounds. Persons affected may die before birth or during infancy, or they may have a normal life expectancy.

ACHONDROPLASIA		21-5
cause	lesion	manifestations
Autosomal dominant gene	Failure of growth of long bones due to defective epiphyseal cartilage	May be early death Dwarfism

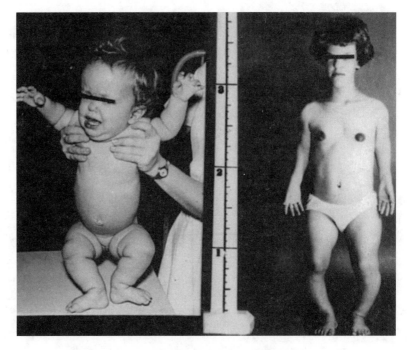

Figure 21–8. Achondroplastic dwarf as an infant and at age 13.

Osteogenesis Imperfecta

This genetic condition associated with abnormal collagen formation usually follows an autosomal dominant inheritance pattern. Severe forms cause death in utero or soon after birth. The more common delayed form is characterized by thin bones that fracture with minimal trauma. The abnormal collagen production results in thin blue sclera, fractures of the bony ossicles of the ear leading to deafness, and deformed, hypoplastic teeth.

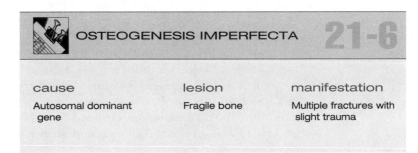

OSTEOGENESIS IMPERFECTA   21-6

cause	lesion	manifestation
Autosomal dominant gene	Fragile bone	Multiple fractures with slight trauma

Marfan's Syndrome

This is another autosomal dominant disorder, which involves elastic tissue of bone, blood vessels, and other sites. Unlike the conditions discussed above, it may go undetected, because the changes are subtle and only certain complications prove to be harmful. Involved individuals are tall and slender with long narrow fingers and toes and asymmetrical skulls. About half have dislocation of the lens of the eye. Weakening of the media of the aorta due to the defective connective tissue leads to the most serious complication, rupture of the aorta with fatal hemorrhage. This is likely to occur suddenly during exercise.

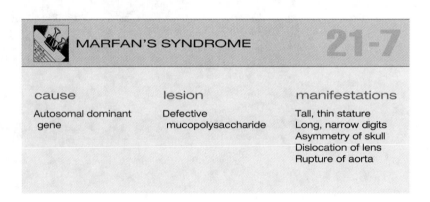

MARFAN'S SYNDROME   **21-7**

cause	lesion	manifestations
Autosomal dominant gene	Defective mucopolysaccharide	Tall, thin stature Long, narrow digits Asymmetry of skull Dislocation of lens Rupture of aorta

Inflammatory/Degenerative Diseases

Under this category, we will discuss the effects of trauma (strains, sprains, fractures), infection (acute arthritis, osteomyelitis), and chronic disorders of varied etiology. Low back pain and curvatures of the spine (scoliosis and kyphosis) are clinical syndromes with multiple causes. There are many other inflammatory and degenerative conditions of bones and joints, often made specific by their location and symptomatology, that are beyond the scope of this text.

Injuries to Joints and Muscles

An acute injury to a joint with tearing of the joint capsule and ligaments around the joint is called a *sprain*. Hemorrhage around or into the joint may also be present. Twisting of the ankle is a common cause of a sprain and usually involves rupture of a ligament on the lateral side of the foot. *Whiplash injury*, caused by sudden extension of the neck, is a sprain in which ligaments and other tissues supporting the cervical spine are torn.

SPRAINS AND STRAINS   21-8

causes	lesions	manifestations
Trauma	Tearing of joint capsule (sprain)	Swollen, tender, nonfunctional joint
Twisting		Muscle pain and tenderness
Excessive exercise	Tearing of muscle of tendon (strain)	

Tearing of a muscle and/or its tendon due to excessive use and stretching is called a *strain*. Muscle strains (pulled muscles) produce disruption of the muscle with hemorrhage and mild inflammation. Athletes use conditioning and warm-up exercises to prevent strains.

Bones may be traumatically dislocated from their joint sockets. A partial dislocation is called a *subluxation*.

The knee joint is a common site of acute injury, especially in athletes. Tears may occur in the menisci, cruciate ligaments, and medial and lateral ligaments. Arthroscopic surgery is an endoscopic technique used to examine the inside of the knee joint and remove torn fragments of tissue. This technique has much less morbidity than open knee operations.

Low Back Pain

Owing to an upright posture, humans are uniquely susceptible to low back pain. The problem of weight bearing thrust upon the lumbar spine is accentuated by obesity, weak abdominal muscles, poor posture, and sudden physical stresses. These factors, however, are more likely to cause problems when there is underlying disease of the spine. The evaluation of persistent low back pain, an extremely common problem, involves evaluation of the patient for underlying disease of the spine, which may or may not be found. Pain may be due to compression of nerves, muscle spasm (a protective mechanism), or sprained ligaments.

Generalized diseases that can cause or accentuate low back pain include degenerative arthritis, rheumatoid arthritis, ankylosing spondylitis, osteoporosis, and metastatic cancer. Diseases that are specific to the spine include herniated intervertebral disc and congenital fusion defects of vertebrae, especially the fifth lumbar vertebra. Neurologic examination to evaluate for nerve compression and roentgenograms of the lower spine will reveal most of these conditions, but one of the most common causes of back pain, herniated intervertebral disc, may require further study.

LOW BACK PAIN — 21-9

causes	lesion	manifestations
Strains	Depends on cause	Low back pain
Congenital defects of		Radiating pain to legs
spinal column		if nerves compressed
Herniated intervertebral		
disc		
Arthritis		
Cancer		

Herniated intervertebral disc, usually in the lumbar region, is a common and important cause of low back pain, because the herniated disc puts pressure on spinal nerves. The pain may radiate down the back of the leg, a condition called *sciatica* because the sciatic nerve is often involved. The soft central material (nucleus pulposus) is pushed out through the surrounding fibrocartilage (annulus fibrosus) and displaces the capsule to impinge on a spinal nerve (Figure 21–9). Radiologic examination after injection of radiopaque dye into the spinal canal (myelogram) is used to demonstrate compression of the spinal cord and nerve roots (Figures 21–10 and 21–11). Operative removal of the disc may be required to relieve pain and prevent paralysis.

Scoliosis and Kyphosis

Scoliosis is abnormal lateral curvature of the spine, and kyphosis is an abnormal forward bending of the upper spine producing a hunched back (Figure 21–12). By the age of 14, approximately 2 percent of

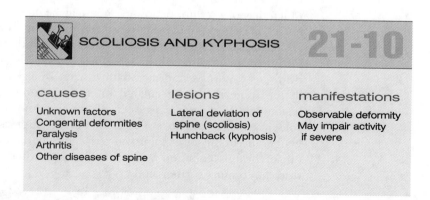

SCOLIOSIS AND KYPHOSIS — 21-10

causes	lesions	manifestations
Unknown factors	Lateral deviation of	Observable deformity
Congenital deformities	spine (scoliosis)	May impair activity
Paralysis	Hunchback (kyphosis)	if severe
Arthritis		
Other diseases of spine		

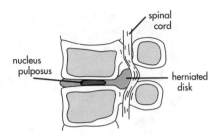

Figure 21–9. Herniated intervertebral disc.

people have some degree of scoliosis. Most of the time the cause is unknown. Known causes include congenital deformity, paralysis of one side of the body, and diseases involving the vertebrae. Kyphosis is most often due to arthritis of the spine but may be due to other spinal column diseases.

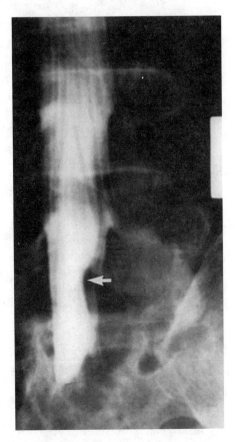

Figure 21–10. Myelogram demonstrating compression of the radiopaque dye in the spinal canal by a herniated intervertebral disc (*arrow*).

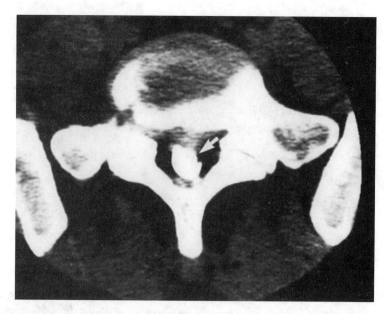

Figure 21–11. Magnetic resonance scan demonstrating compression of the radiopaque dye in the spinal canal (arrow) and failure of dye to fill around the nerve root on the right.

Fractures

A fracture is any disruption of the continuity of bone. Most fractures are caused by trauma. Spontaneous fractures or fractures resulting from slight trauma suggest the possibility that the fracture was caused by underlying disease of bone (pathologic fracture).

Many terms are used to describe the nature of the fracture (Figure 21–13). *Incomplete fractures* produce cracks without separation of the bone; with *complete fractures*, the bone is separated into two or more parts (Figure 21–14). *Comminuted fractures* are ones in which more than two fragments are produced. A *compression fracture* is one in which the bones are pushed together rather than apart. These commonly occur in vertebrae. *Open fractures* produce disruption of the skin; *closed fractures* do not. A stable fracture tends to maintain its position following fracture, an unstable one does not.

The sites of fractures vary in frequency with age and sex, because these factors are related to the likelihood of various types of injury and the possibility of underlying disease. For example, arm fractures are common in children due to pulling or falling; spine and hip fractures are common in elderly women because these weight-bearing bones are affected by osteoporosis. Bone has great power to heal, so that continuity can be accomplished in a few weeks and remodeling and return to normal strength can occur in a few months. Fracture healing is much more rapid in the young than in the elderly.

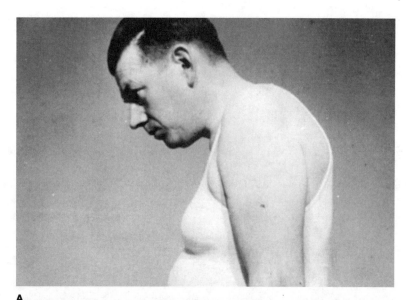

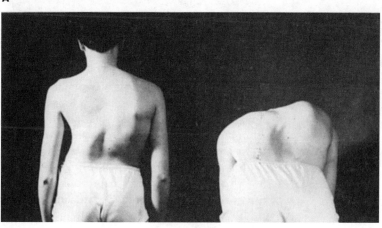

Figure 21–12. A. Kyphosis. B. Scoliosis, with winging of the scapula when bent forward.

The process of fracture healing involves the proliferation of osteoblasts from the fracture margins to form new cartilage and bone. The immature bone and cartilage is gradually remodeled into mature bone. Bone is usually produced in excess, but eventually, through the process of remodeling, the bone returns to normal structure.

There are several important factors that can prevent this normal healing sequence. The broken fragments must be close to each other or the ends will fail to unite (nonunion). The fracture must be a stable fracture or, if unstable, it must be artificially stabilized using splints,

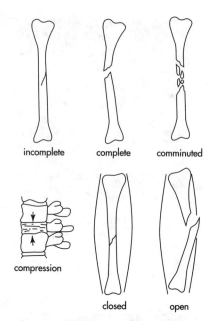

incomplete   complete   comminuted

compression

closed   open

Figure 21–13. Types of fractures.

casts, traction (steady pulling by means of weights), or operatively inserted metal pins, screws, or plates. With fractures of the neck of the femur, the head of the femur is sometimes removed and replaced with a metal ball. Nonstabilized fractures also lead to nonunion. One of the worst complications of fracture is infection. Open fractures, particularly those in which the trauma drives dirt into the wound, and fractures that are artificially opened in the operative room to accomplish immobilization are subject to the possibility of infection. Cleaning of the wound, removal of dead tissue, and antibiotics are used to prevent infection. The consequences of an infected fracture are chronic osteomyelitis, nonunion, and eventual deformity. Another factor affecting healing is the extent and location of the fracture. Commin-

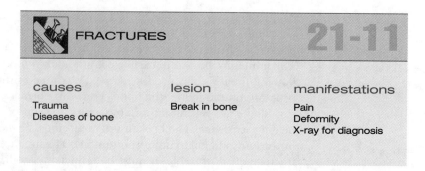

FRACTURES   **21-11**

causes	lesion	manifestations
Trauma	Break in bone	Pain
Diseases of bone		Deformity
		X-ray for diagnosis

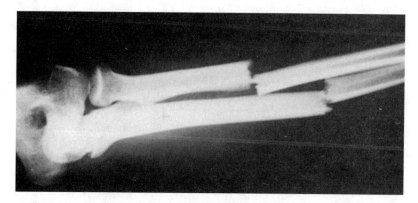

Figure 21–14. Complete fractures of radius and ulna.

uted fractures heal well unless they are displaced, involve joints, or cannot be stabilized. Fractures in the middle of long and flat bones generally heal well, while fractures involving joints are likely to produce problems with joint mobility. Fractures that disrupt the blood supply to the bone will not heal well. Finally, pathologic fractures may not heal, depending on the nature of the disease causing them.

Acute Arthritis

Severe acute arthritis is usually caused by pyogenic bacteria. Acute arthritis is occasionally associated with gonorrhea, as the gonococcus organism gains access to the blood and preferentially locates in the joint space, causing a swollen, painful, red joint. Staphylococci may be spread to the joint through the blood but more often may cause arthritis when the joint is opened due to trauma, adjacent disease, or operation. Acute arthritis produces rapid destruction of the joint lining and is likely to lead to permanent destruction and bony ankylosis of the joint.

ACUTE ARTHRITIS   21-12

cause	lesion	manifestations

Bacterial infection
  gonococcus
  staphylococcus
	Acutely inflamed joint
	  space
		Pain, heat, swelling,
		  redness,
		  leukocytosis, fever
		Nonfunction of joint
		  (acute)
		Destruction of joint
		  (chronic)

Osteomyelitis

Although *osteomyelitis* means inflammation of bone, the term is usually used in a more restricted sense to mean infection of bone. The route of infection is the basis of classification of the two major types of osteomyelitis. Hematogenous osteomyelitis involves spread of the causative organism through the blood to localize in one bone to set up a focus of infection. The site of entry of the organism is usually a skin infection (which may go unnoticed), the organism is usually *Staphylococcus aureus*, and the site of the osteomyelitis is usually the metaphysis of a long bone near but not involving the epiphysis. Children are most commonly affected. If untreated, the infection spreads, producing necrosis of the bone. The purulent infection may produce draining sinuses, and the necrotic bone must be removed, because antibiotics will not be effective against bacteria lurking in dead bone. The clinical findings are pain and other local and systemic signs of inflammation. By the time x-ray changes occur, the bone is necrotic. The outcome in advanced cases includes recurrence of the infection and bone deformity with crippling.

The other form of osteomyelitis, which is much more common, is called secondary osteomyelitis, because the infection spreads to bone secondarily from an adjacent site of infection or open wound. The most common causes are infected operative sites (most commonly involving repair of fractures), soft tissue infections adjacent to bone, and gangrene of the toes with ulceration and infection. Treatment consists of removal of dead tissue and bone, open drainage of the infected area, and antibiotics. Permanent damage is likely.

Osteoporosis

Osteoporosis is a generalized quantitative decrease in bone with the remaining bone having a normal amount of mineral and matrix (Figure 21–15). The osteopenia (quantitative loss of bone) is usually demonstrated by x-ray. The normality of mineral and matrix is suggested by finding normal serum levels of calcium, phosphorus, and

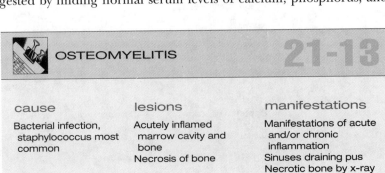

OSTEOMYELITIS   21-13

cause	lesions	manifestations
Bacterial infection, staphylococcus most common	Acutely inflamed marrow cavity and bone Necrosis of bone	Manifestations of acute and/or chronic inflammation Sinuses draining pus Necrotic bone by x-ray Recurrence common

alkaline phosphatase. Conditions that cause metabolic breakdown of bone, such as osteomalacia, hyperparathyroidism (see Chapter 26), and Paget's disease, typically have elevated alkaline phosphatase levels and altered calcium and phosphorus levels.

Thinning of bone occurs normally with aging, so the diagnosis of osteoporosis is relative. Most symptomatic osteoporosis occurs in post-

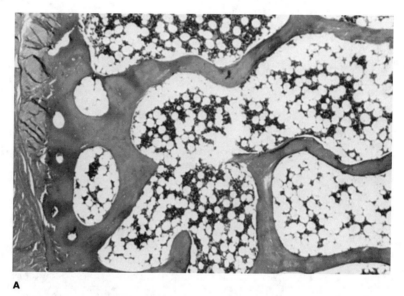

A

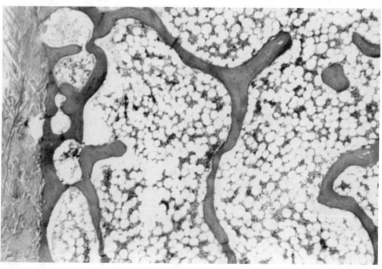

B

Figure 21–15. Histologic section of vertebra. A. Normal from 20-year-old. B. Osteoporosis from 80-year-old with narrow, widely separated bone spicules and thin cortex.

	OSTEOPOROSIS	21-14
causes	**lesion**	**manifestations**
Aging	Thin bone which is	Back pain
Reduction in female	otherwise normal	Fractures
hormone	appearing	Radiolucent bone
Corticosteroids		by x-ray
Immobilization of bone		Normal calcium,
		phosphorus, alkaline
		phosphatase

menopausal women, but it may occur in elderly men, in patients on long-term corticosteroid therapy, and with prolonged bed rest. Persons with large bones are less affected than persons with small bones and thin trabecular bones (such as vertebrae) are more affected than dense cortical bones.

No single specific cause for osteoporosis has been identified; multiple factors are likely involved in its pathogenesis. Once developed, reversion back to normal bone thickness does not appear to be possible. Therefore, prevention of the development of the disease is most important and this must be done years (decades) before the disease is likely to become manifest. Therapies that have been directed at this goal include high calcium intake, vitamin D supplements, estrogens in menopausal women, testosterone in men with low levels, exercise, and various other drugs. However, in most instances, preventive treatment is not employed and complications are treated as they develop.

The most common complications of osteoporosis are compression fractures of vertebra and hip fractures. Vertebral disease is associated with pain and height reduction. Hip fracture, which occurs with minimal trauma in osteoporotic persons, is a severe acute illness that is often fatal or leads to permanent disability, particularly in frail elderly women.

Osteomalacia and Rickets

These are relatively rare conditions characterized by softening of bone. They differ from osteoporosis in that there is inadequate deposition of calcium and phosphorus, leaving an excess of the protein matrix of the bone. Osteomalacia is the adult form characterized by bone softening. Rickets is the childhood form with both softening and decreased growth of bones. The majority of cases are secondary to poor intake or poor utilization of vitamin D, with consequent improper deposition of calcium and phosphorus in bone. In children, untreated rickets leads

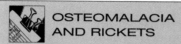

OSTEOMALACIA AND RICKETS		21-15
cause	**lesion**	**manifestations**
Vitamin D deficiency due to inadequate diet or malabsorption	Bone matrix without calcium present	Soft flexible bones Fractures Deformity and retarded bone growth (rickets)

to markedly deformed bones. Osteomalacia in adults may cause fractures. Serum levels of calcium, phosphorus, and alkaline phosphatase are abnormal.

Degenerative Arthritis

This very common disease is also called *degenerative joint disease* and *osteoarthritis*. It occurs most often in the middle aged to elderly and is estimated to be present in 20 million persons in the United States. The main manifestations are joint stiffness and often pain. The lesion consists of wearing of the articular joint cartilage, with subsequent deformity of the cartilage and of the bone, resulting in stiffness and decreased motion. New growth of bone at the margins of the joint lead to so-called lipping (osteophytes), which further limits movement of the joint (Figure 21–16B). Degenerative joint disease is more common in women and typically involves the weight-bearing joints and the distal finger joints (Figure 21–17A). This pattern of involvement, plus a typical x-ray picture, help distinguish degenerative from rheumatoid arthritis. Degenerative arthritis is likely to develop with time in injured joints or joints subject to undue stress, such as might occur with congenital dislocation of the hip or a knee subject to football injuries.

DEGENERATIVE ARTHRITIS		21-16
causes	**lesions**	**manifestations**
Aging Joint injury or deformity	Destroyed articular cartilage New bone formation with lipping	Pain Decreased mobility of joint Enlarged joint Bone and cartilage changes by x-ray

Rheumatoid Arthritis

This is a chronic inflammatory disease that predominantly affects joints, but may produce lesions in other organs. The joint lesions, which produce pain, stiffness, and deformity, are due to inflammation of the synovial lining. As the inflammation extends on to the joint surface, it destroys cartilage and produces a layer of granulation tissue called a *pannus*. Eventually the entire joint surface may be destroyed and replaced by fibrous tissue. Fusion of joints is called *ankylosis*.

Rheumatoid arthritis is three times more common in women than men and varies in severity from mild joint stiffness to severe cases, showing distortion and ankylosis of many joints, with almost total loss of function. Usually the metacarpal-phalangeal joints are initially affected, followed by wrists, knees, and elbows. Involvement of the metacarpal-phalangeal joints leads to characteristic ulnar deviation of the fingers (Figure 21–16B). Many patients with severe rheumatoid arthritis will also have chronic inflammation and vasculitis involving other organs such as the heart, muscle, lungs, skin, and possibly the eye.

Morphologically, the joint lesion consists of a low-grade chronic inflammation of the synovial lining and joint surface, with destruction

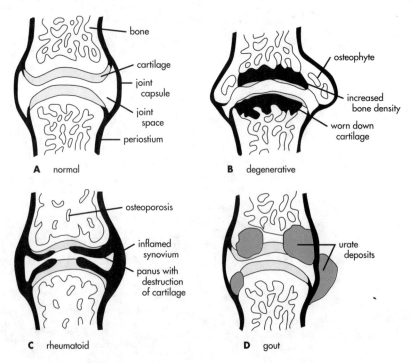

Figure 21–16. Schematic representation of normal joint (A) and lesions of degenerative arthritis (B), rheumatoid arthritis (C), and gout (D).

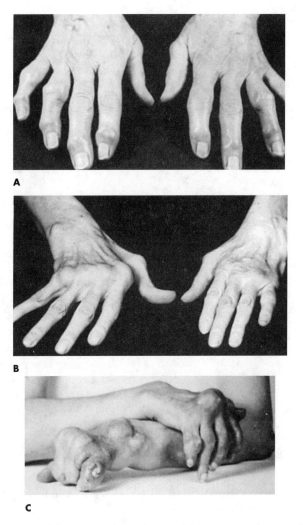

Figure 21–17. Hand changes in advanced cases of degenerative arthritis (A), rheumatoid arthritis (B), and gout (C). In degenerative arthritis, the distal interphalangeal joints show swelling due to formation of osteophytes. Rheumatoid arthritis is characterized by ulnar deformity and involvement of metacarpal-phalangeal joints. In gout, tophi produce irregular nodules about the joints. (*Reproduced from Clinical Slide Collection on the Rheumatic Diseases, produced by The Arthritis Foundation, New York, copyright 1972.*)

of the joint cartilage, fibrosis around the joint, and osteoporosis of the surrounding bone due to disuse (Figure 21–17C).

The cause of rheumatoid arthritis is not known, but it is associated with an abnormal immunoglobulin M, which is directed against the body's normal immunoglobulin G (in effect, an antibody against an antibody). This abnormal antibody is called the rheumatoid factor and

<table>
<tr><td colspan="3">RHEUMATOID ARTHRITIS 21-17</td></tr>
<tr><td>**cause**</td><td>**lesions**</td><td>**manifestations**</td></tr>
<tr><td>Probably an autoallergic reaction</td><td>Chronically inflamed joint lining with granulation tissue and scarring of joint surface
Atrophy of surrounding bone</td><td>Pain
Joint deformity
Decreased mobility of joints
Elevated erythrocyte sedimentation rate
Positive tests for rheumatoid factor
Changes seen by x-ray</td></tr>
</table>

may be tested for in the laboratory as an aid to diagnosis. It is thought that this abnormal immunoglobulin complex is deposited on the synovial membrane, eliciting an inflammatory response that results in proliferation and thickening of the synovium. Severe rheumatoid arthritis is often treated with corticosteroids, because these drugs inhibit both the formation of immunoglobulin complexes and inflammation.

In recent years, surgeons have had much success in replacing severely ankylosed joints with artificial (prosthetic) joints. Knee and hip joints can be replaced as well as finger joints. Variants of rheumatoid arthritis include *juvenile arthritis*, in which the involvement occurs very early in life and may be extremely severe.

Ankylosing spondylitis is an inflammatory arthritis predominantly involving the spine and sacroiliac joints. Long considered a variant of rheumatoid arthritis because the lesions are histologically similar, it is now considered by many to be a separate disease because it occurs in young men, has a strong association with the inherited HLA-B27 antigen, and has a familial tendency. The deformity of the spine with stooped posture often leads to severe disability.

Gout

This is an inherited disease in which there is abnormal metabolism of uric acid. The excess uric acid may be deposited in many tissues, particularly joints, and eventuates in painful arthritis. In the chronic stage, these urate deposits accumulate to form tophi (Figures 21–16D and 21–17C). Gout occurs almost exclusively (over 90%) in men over 30 and clinically manifests by bouts of painful arthritis, particularly in the fingers, wrists, ankles, knees, and toes, especially the great toe. Treatment of gout consists of long-term administration of agents that pro-

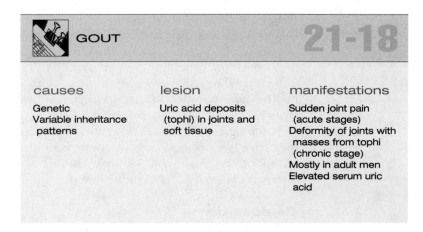

GOUT		21-18
causes	lesion	manifestations

Genetic
Variable inheritance
  patterns
	Uric acid deposits
	  (tophi) in joints and
	  soft tissue
		Sudden joint pain
		  (acute stages)
		Deformity of joints with
		  masses from tophi
		  (chronic stage)
		Mostly in adult men
		Elevated serum uric
		  acid

mote the excretion of uric acid or inhibit its production. See Chapter 7 for further discussion, including treatment.

Ganglion

A ganglion is a smooth cystic swelling that arises from joint capsules, most commonly on the wrist. They are often associated with continued trauma and may be painful, although they usually arise insidiously as a simple swelling. Surgical removal may be undertaken if the ganglion is bothersome to the patient.

GANGLION		21-19
cause	lesion	manifestation

Unknown	Outpouching of synovial
	  lining into soft tissue
		Fluctuant lump on back
		  of wrist

Hyperplastic/Neoplastic Diseases

There are many types of neoplasms and non-neoplastic tumors of bone, cartilage, joints, and tendon sheaths. Most are rare and will not be discussed. The most common malignant tumors are metastatic cancers from sites such as breast, lung, prostate, and kidney, as well as multiple myeloma and lymphomas. Paget's disease of bone is a peculiar hyperplastic disease.

Paget's Disease of Bone

Paget's disease or osteitis deformans is a localized or multifocal enlargement of bone of unknown cause that affects about 2 percent of the population, typically in persons over 40 years of age. It is thought to be related to paramyxovirus infection. Initially the affected bone may be more porous, but there is a gradual haphazard bony proliferation leading to some deformity of the bone and occasionally to pathologic fracture. High serum alkaline phosphatase reflects the active bone remodeling, but there is no defect in calcium and phosphorous metabolism. Most patients are asymptomatic. Rarely, osteosarcoma may develop in the lesion.

Osteosarcoma

This is a malignant bone-forming tumor arising in bone, thus it is to be considered a neoplasm arising from osteoblasts. Osteosarcoma arises most commonly in the long bones, especially near the knees (Figure 21–18), but it may be seen in other bones. Osteosarcoma occurs in children and in young adults and presents with pain or swelling. Most patients present with a bony mass and no evidence of metastasis, but occult metastases are probably present because amputation alone is followed by overt metastases and death in 80 percent of

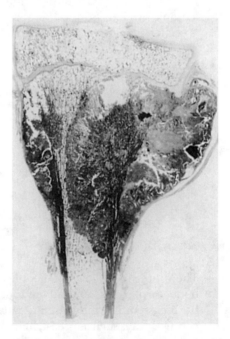

Figure 21–18. Large histologic section of a typical osteosarcoma of the distal femur involving metaphysis and spreading through the periosteum.

patients. This has led to aggressive radiation and chemotherapy at the time of removal of the mass and a cure rate of over 60 percent. Some cases occur in adult years after radiation of bone or in association with Paget's disease of bone.

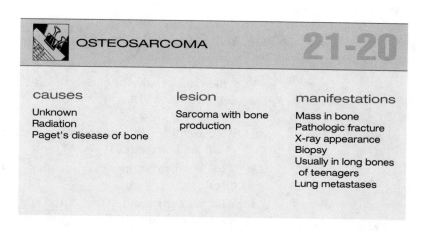

OSTEOSARCOMA 21-20

causes	lesion	manifestations
Unknown Radiation Paget's disease of bone	Sarcoma with bone production	Mass in bone Pathologic fracture X-ray appearance Biopsy Usually in long bones of teenagers Lung metastases

ORGAN FAILURE

The main function of the skeletal system is to maintain support and mobility for everyday activity. Injury or disuse of major joints and fractures of weight-supporting bones are likely to lead to considerable incapacity of movement. Extensive severe arthritis or widespread bone metastases may confine patients to a wheelchair or bed.

Review Questions

1. What is the relative frequency of joint disease as compared to bone disease? How are they likely to differ in their consequences?

2. What are the most common musculoskeletal problems and which are most serious?

3. What are the common manifestations of bone and joint disease?

4. What are the symptoms, signs, and laboratory abnormalities of each of the specific diseases discussed in this chapter?

5. How do localized developmental abnormalities differ from generalized genetic abnormalities of the skeletal system in terms of frequency and likely outcome?

6. What is a herniated intervertebral disc and what are its effects?

7. How do fractures heal? What factors impair healing?

8. How do hematogenous and secondary osteomyelitis differ in terms of cause, persons affected, and outcome?

9. How do osteoporosis and osteomalacia differ in terms of cause, histology, and laboratory findings?

10. How do degenerative and rheumatoid arthritis differ in frequency, cause, morphology, and location?

11. How do metastatic cancer of bone and osteosarcoma differ in frequency, age, and outcome?

12. What do the following terms mean?
    Pathologic fracture
    Rheumatoid factor
    Talipes equinovarus
    Femoral anteversion
    Tibial torsion
    Metatarsus adductus
    Whiplash injury
    Ankylosis
    Sciatica
    Incomplete fracture

Comminuted fracture
Compression fracture
Open fracture
Unstable fracture
Nonunion of a fracture
Senile osteoporosis
Juvenile arthritis
Ankylosing spondylitis
Paget's disease

22.

Skeletal Muscle and Peripheral Nerve

REVIEW OF STRUCTURE AND FUNCTION
Muscle Fibers • Innervation • Actin and Myosin • Type I and II Fibers •
Peripheral Nerves

MOST FREQUENT AND SERIOUS PROBLEMS
Muscle Wasting Secondary to Generalized Disease • Muscular
Dystrophies • Nervous System Diseases

SYMPTOMS, SIGNS, AND TESTS
Weakness and Atrophy • Pain • Serum Enzymes • Electromyography •
Muscle Biopsy • Nerve Biopsy

SPECIFIC DISEASES
  Genetic/Developmental Diseases
    Duchenne Dystrophy
    Myotonic Dystrophy
    Hereditary Motor and Sensory Neuropathies
    Other Dystrophies
  Inflammatory/Degenerative Diseases
    Autoimmune Diseases
    Neurogenic Disorders
    Amyotrophic Lateral Sclerosis
    Myasthenia Gravis
    Metabolic Myopathies
    Acute Inflammatory Demyelinating Polyradiculoneuropathy
      (Guillaín–Barré Syndrome)
    Diabetic Neuropathy
  Hyperplastic/Neoplastic Diseases

ORGAN FAILURE

REVIEW QUESTIONS

REVIEW OF STRUCTURE AND FUNCTION

Skeletal muscle is the largest organ in the body and utilizes about 10 percent of the body's oxygen in the resting state but as much as 80 percent or more with intense exercise. All skeletal muscles are separated into bundles called *fascicles*, which are enclosed in connective tissue. Fascicles are in turn composed of individual muscle fibers (cells), each of which courses the entire length of the muscle (Figure 22–1). Muscle fibers are innervated by branches of axons from anterior horn neurons in the spinal cord. In muscles that need fine discriminatory movements, such as the eye, one neuron may innervate as few as four to six muscle fibers; whereas in large muscles used for strength and weight bearing (gluteus or quadriceps), one neuron may innervate up to 2000 muscle fibers. Muscle maintains its tone by a complex system of nerves that wrap around special fibers (spindles) and send information regarding the degree of muscle contraction back to the spinal cord neurons. Chemically, muscle is composed primarily of two proteins called *actin* and *myosin*, which are filaments arranged alternately in parallel rows. These filaments slide back and forth beside each other, thereby performing the contraction and relaxation process. The overlapping of the filaments delineates the I and the A bands, which can be seen by light microscopy as striations (Figure 22–1).

Muscle fibers are divided into types I and II on the basis of their histochemical reactions (Figure 22–2). These types also correspond

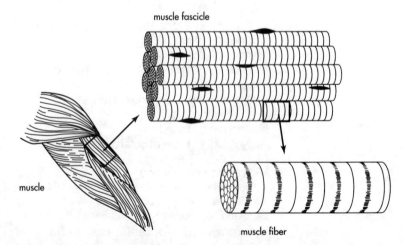

muscle fascicle

muscle

muscle fiber

Figure 22–1. Schematic representation of skeletal muscle, with a fascicle and an individual fiber. Each muscle fiber courses the entire length of the muscle. The alternating light and dark bands are called striations and can be seen by light microscopy.

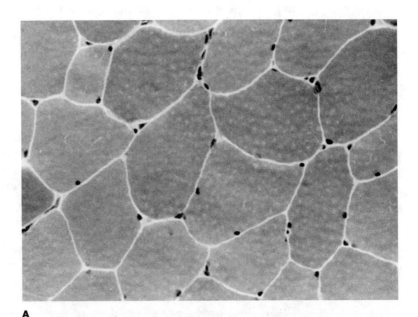

A

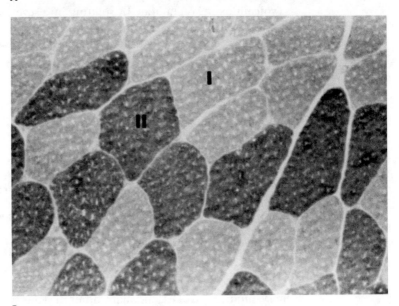

B

Figure 22–2. Cross-section of muscle fibers. A. Routine hematoxylin and eosin stained section. B. Stained with an enzyme stain (ATPase) to demonstrate type I and II fibers.

somewhat to physiologic properties. For example, type I fibers are more utilized for slow, sustained contractions, whereas type II fibers contract more quickly. Type II fibers respond to exercise by hypertrophy and to disuse by atrophy. In humans, the two fiber types are evenly distributed throughout all muscles, but in many animals an individual muscle may be composed entirely of one fiber type. For example, in domestic birds such as chickens, the dark muscles (leg, thigh) consist entirely of type I fibers, while the light muscles (wings, breast) are all type II fibers.

A peripheral nerve runs from the spinal cord to an organ where it receives either sensory input for return to the spinal cord or brain, or delivers a signal to skeletal muscle to contract. Some nerves belong to the autonomic nervous system. Sensory autonomic nerves transmit sensations from internal organs and motor autonomic nerves send signals to smooth muscle such as the vascular system, the intestinal tract, or the uterus. Autonomic nerve axons are characteristically unmyelinated whereas regular motor and sensory nerves contain a myelin sheath composed of several layers of lipid membranes wrapped around the axon with periodic constrictions called nodes of Ranvier. Axons and myelin sheaths are sustained by Schwann cells (Figure 22–3). Both myelin sheaths and axons can regenerate if damaged. Typically axons regenerate by splitting into several smaller axons and grow at a slow, finite rate back to their end organ. When myelin sheaths regenerate they usually do not contain as many lipid wrappings as formerly existed.

MOST FREQUENT AND SERIOUS PROBLEMS

Probably the most common affliction of muscle is simply weakness with or without muscle atrophy. This may occur as a part of a generalized disease such as cancer or any disease that results in prolonged immobilization. Muscular dystrophies are important muscle diseases because they are often inherited and, consequently, genetic counseling becomes an important aspect of disease prevention. The most frequently occurring and most severe dystrophy is Duchenne muscular dystrophy. Whenever there is disease of the nervous system, there will also be associated muscle weakness. Therefore, victims of traumatic nerve injuries, strokes, and many other nervous system diseases will all display muscle weakness. Trauma may result in muscle weakness from either muscle destruction or nerve damage.

Disruptions in peripheral nerve function constitute neuropathies and can result in various types of sensory loss or weakness if motor fibers are primarily involved. Inflammatory neuropathies are not common, but can be severe. The most important type of infectious

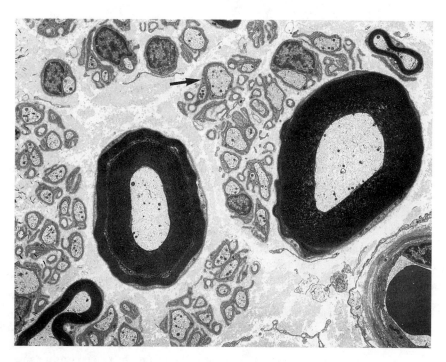

Figure 22–3. Cross-section of part of a nerve by electron microscopy. The large dark circles are the layers of the myelin sheath that encircle the axon. The arrow points to one of numerous unmyelinated axons. The three dark spots in the upper left corner are Schwann cell nuclei, two of the Schwann cells have axons in the cytoplasm. In the lower right corner is a small blood vessel containing a red blood cell in its lumen.

neuropathy worldwide is leprosy (Chapter 26). Diabetics commonly acquire peripheral neuropathies that can be severe and difficult to treat. Hereditary, motor, and sensory neuropathies can occur by themselves or be associated with other diseases. A variety of biologic toxins, industrial chemicals, heavy metals such as lead and arsenic, and drugs can result in toxic neuropathies. Some of the most common offending drugs are ethanol and acrylamides. Peripheral nerve tumors are rare but occasionally tumors called Schwannomas or neurofibromas arise from the Schwann cells in peripheral nerves. These are commonly associated with the disease called neurofibromatosis.

SYMPTOMS, SIGNS, AND TESTS

Weakness is the common denominator of muscle disease, whether it be primary disease of muscle (*myopathic*) or secondary to disease of the nervous system (*neurogenic*). The pattern of weakness often affords the physician an important clue as to the type of muscle disease present.

For example, muscular dystrophies most often involve proximal muscle groups, whereas diseases of nerves are more likely to result in atrophy and weakness of the more distal parts of the extremities. If weakness persists for any length of time, the muscle will become atrophic, irrespective of the cause of the disorder, simply because of disuse. Conversely, atrophy of muscle obviously will result in weakness. Pain is occasionally associated with muscle disease and when present often signifies muscle inflammation.

Although the presence of muscle disease is often obvious because of weakness and atrophy, many times the patient's symptoms may be nondescript or vague. In such cases, there are certain laboratory tests that aid in the diagnosis of muscle disease and at the same time help quantify the degree of muscle damage. *Creatine kinase* is an enzyme normally involved in the metabolism of muscle that is present in the serum in increased quantities following many disorders that damage muscle. It is usually more elevated in myopathic than in neurogenic disorders, and the degree of elevation of this enzyme will roughly parallel the extent of muscle damage. Electromyography will also help to separate intrinsic muscle disorders from neurogenic muscle disorders and to quantify the extent of muscle damage. *Electromyography* is accomplished by inserting a needle into a muscle and recording the electrical activity. The most reliable means of separating myopathic from neurogenic causes of muscle disease is muscle biopsy, a procedure that is easily performed on most muscles. The major differences between neurogenic and myopathic muscle disorders are summarized in Table 22–1.

TABLE 22–1. COMPARISON OF NORMAL, MYOPATHIC, AND NEUROGENIC MUSCLE DISORDERS

	Normal	Myopathic	Neurogenic
Symptoms or signs	None	Proximal weakness, possible pain	Distal weakness, often in a nerve distribution; possible sensory loss
Electromyography	No spontaneous activity in muscle	Asynchronous spontaneous activity	Synchronous activity of small amplitude
Serum enzyme (creatine kinase)	Normal	Often markedly elevated	Mildly elevated or normal
Biopsy	Normal fiber configuration	Variable size of fibers; degenerative fibers; possible fibrosis	Atrophic fibers in small groups

The peripheral nerve status of a patient is assessed first by a good neurologic examination in which the various sensory modalities such as touch, pain, temperature, and two-point discrimination are tested. Motor neuron integrity is assessed by examining the patient for weakness in the various muscle groups supplied by particular nerves. Electrophysiologic nerve conduction tests can determine the speed and amplitude of an impulse conducted along an axon that can help in determining whether damage to a nerve is primarily directed at the axon or the myelin sheath. More definitive evaluation can be obtained by a nerve biopsy. Commonly the sural nerve in the lower leg is examined because sacrifice of this nerve does not harm the patient. However, the sural nerve is predominantly sensory, and if motor function is to be evaluated a muscle biopsy is usually necessary. The most important direct examination of peripheral nerve is by electron microscopy because this can determine whether the damage is to the axon or myelin sheath, whether there is inflammation present, whether the unmyelinated nerves are involved, and what the status of the nerve vasculature is.

SPECIFIC DISEASES

Genetic/Developmental Diseases

There are numerous types of primary muscle degeneration collectively called *dystrophies*. Since many of the more common types of dystrophy are genetically determined, we will consider the entire group under developmental rather than under degenerative disorders, keeping in mind that the exact cause of some types of dystrophy is undetermined.

Dystrophy literally means poor nutrition and was originally applied to muscle disorders thought to be of simple cause and not due secondarily to disease of nerves. Today there are many diseases termed *dystrophic* that have various causes. Many are hereditary with onset at an early age. Others are definitely hereditary but do not become manifest until adult life. Still others do not appear to be hereditary at all. Dystrophies are classified according to the pattern of muscle involvement—group(s) of muscles affected—or according to the type of microscopic lesion. Different dystrophies initially show slightly different lesions, but eventually all will lead to muscle atrophy with replacement of muscle by adipose and fibrous tissue. Most of the dystrophies involve proximal muscles of the extremities and the pelvis and shoulder girdles in preference to distal muscles of the extremities. There is no known cure for any of the dystrophies, and all follow a variable but fairly predictable course. Therapy must be supportive. By light microscopy, most dystrophies show variable fiber size, fiber splitting,

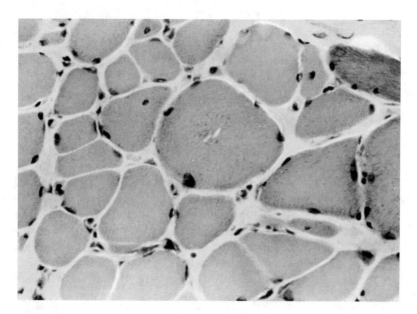

Figure 22–4. Photomicrograph of dystrophic muscle. Note the excessive amount of connective tissue, marked variation in fiber size, and large, rounded fibers. Central nuclei are present in some fibers.

increased amounts of connective tissue, and large rounded fibers (Figure 22–4). Other microscopic findings are more specific for particular types of dystrophy.

Duchenne Dystrophy

The most common and serious of the dystrophies is Duchenne dystrophy, which is inherited as a sex-linked recessive disorder with an incidence of 1 in 3,500 male births, and affects males within the first few years of life, with an expected lifespan of only 12 to 20 years. The Duchenne gene encodes for a muscle protein called dystrophin that normally links the cytoskeleton of the muscle cell to the extracellular matrix. Mutations in the gene result in dystrophin deficiency with consequent loss of stability and breakdown of the muscle fiber. As in most myopathic conditions, the weakness is predominantly of the proximal muscle groups. Boys with Duchenne dystrophy characteristically develop "pseudohypertrophy" of the calves, in which the calves appear large and muscular but are actually replaced by adipose tissue (Figure 22–5). The heart muscle may also be involved in this disease. A less severe variety of the disease is referred to as Becker's dystrophy. The diagnosis of Duchenne dystrophy is based upon typical age of occurrence, family history, and findings of intrinsic muscle disease (myopathic) by electromyography, genetic analysis, enzyme tests, and muscle biopsy. The biopsy shows disruption, loss of both type I and type

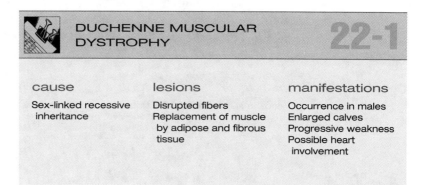

DUCHENNE MUSCULAR
DYSTROPHY

22-1

cause	lesions	manifestations
Sex-linked recessive inheritance	Disrupted fibers Replacement of muscle by adipose and fibrous tissue	Occurrence in males Enlarged calves Progressive weakness Possible heart involvement

II muscle fibers with replacement by connective tissue and absence of dystrophin by immunostaining.

Myotonic Dystrophy

This is an autosomal dominant disease associated with muscle weakness and a characteristic inability to release contraction (*myotonia*). Patients with myotonic dystrophy will shake hands with someone and

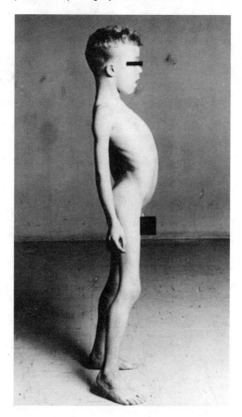

Figure 22–5. Child with Duchenne muscular dystrophy. Note the enlarged calves.

MYOTONIC DYSTROPHY   22-2

cause	lesions	manifestations
Autosomal dominant inheritance	Disrupted fibers Replacement of muscle by adipose and fibrous tissue	Myotonia Cataracts Heart disease Gonadal atrophy Progressive weakness

then are unable to let go. Patients with myotonic dystrophy also may have cataracts, frontal balding, heart disease, and gonadal atrophy.

Typical facial appearance is shown in Figure 22–6. Type I fibers are preferentially involved by atrophy, splitting, and encasement in fibrous tissue. In many fibers, nuclei migrate to the center of the fiber. The electromyographic findings are very characteristic in this disease. Patients may lead a long life but are often quite disabled.

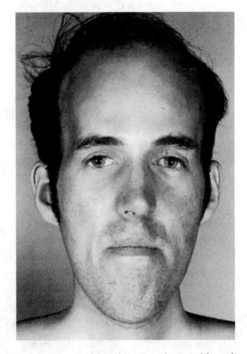

Figure 22–6. Patient with myotonic dystrophy. Note elongated face, frontal baldness, and lack of facial muscle tone.

Hereditary Motor and Sensory Neuropathies

This is a group of hereditary motor and sensory neuropathies that include neuropathies associated with familial amyloid and with porphyria, both uncommon diseases. Most cases of hereditary motor and sensory neuropathy however are those that used to be called Charcot–Marie–Tooth disease (peroneal muscular atrophy). This uncommon disease usually presents in childhood with progressive muscle atrophy of the calf and subsequent orthopedic problems related to the foot. This disease is not life threatening, but can result in considerable morbidity due to the crippling effect. The disease is usually inherited as an autosomal recessive trait with the affected gene located on chromosome 17.

Other Dystrophies

Other, less common dystrophies named by site of involvement include limb–girdle dystrophy (limbs, pelvic and pectoral girdles), facioscapulohumeral (face, scapula, and humerus), and oculopharyngeal. More recently discovered dystrophies, which are often called *congenital myopathies*, are named according to histologic appearance of the muscle. These include nemaline myopathy, in which small thread-like rods are found in the muscle; central core disease, in which each fiber has a central, pale-staining area on cross-section; and central nuclear myopathy, in which the muscle fiber nuclei are in the center of the fiber instead of at the normal, peripheral position. These disorders are all manifest by variable degrees and types of weakness.

Inflammatory/Degenerative Diseases

Neuroscience practitioners commonly divide diseases of muscle into myopathic types, in which there is primary affliction of muscle, and neurogenic types, in which the muscle affliction is secondary to disease of the nerves that innervate the muscle. The muscular dystrophies are one group of the myopathies category. Other types of myopathic disorders include all those conditions in which muscle weakness follows another disease process, such as immunologic disease, vascular disease, neoplasia, or metabolic disease.

Autoimmune Diseases

Polymyositis is an autoimmune inflammatory disease that affects muscle in preference to other organs and is characterized by a lymphocytic infiltrate. A similar lymphocytic infiltration of muscle fibers is seen in other autoimmune diseases such as lupus erythematosus and rheumatoid arthritis. These diseases, collectively referred to as autoimmune inflammatory myopathies, produce muscle weakness, often accompanied by pain and tenderness, and elevation of serum creatine kinase. Autoimmune inflammatory myopathies can often be successfully treated with corticosteroids because these drugs are antilymphocytic in addition to being anti-inflammatory. Paradoxically, muscle weakness and atrophy can also result from corticosteroid therapy in susceptible persons.

Neurogenic Disorders

As alluded to previously, any affliction of peripheral nerve or spinal cord motor neuron will result in muscle weakness and wasting. Acceptable treatment demands the separation of nervous system disease from that of primary muscle disease. Histologically, muscles that are atrophic secondary to lesions of the nervous system show a characteristic pattern of atrophy in which atrophic fibers have sharply angulated contours and occur in groups (Figure 22–7). The group occurrence is due to the fact that adjacent fibers are all innervated by the same axon.

In addition to laboratory tests, helpful clues to the presence of neurogenic disease include the pattern of muscle involvement and the presence of sensory symptoms such as decreased pain. For example, muscle weakness in the distribution of a motor nerve or loss of sensation in the same area as the weakness would indicate a neurogenic disorder. In addition, disease of nerves tend to affect the more distal muscles in the extremities first. Treatment of neurogenic muscular

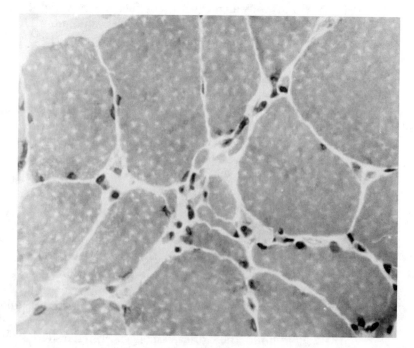

Figure 22–7. Photomicrograph of neurogenic atrophy. Note the small, angulated fibers in a group.

NEUROGENIC DISORDERS 22-3

cause	lesion	manifestation
Peripheral nerve disruption or spinal cord anterior horn cell degeneration	Angular atrophy of fiber in groups	Weakness in distribution of peripheral nerve or spinal cord involvement weakness often distal

diseases consists of dedicated physical therapy to prevent irreversible atrophy and fibrosis of muscle and contracture of joints.

The most common neurogenic disorder of muscle is that which is secondary to peripheral nerve injury. Other important primary neurogenic diseases that severely affect muscle are *Werdnig-Hoffman's disease* in infants and *amyotrophic lateral sclerosis* in adults.

Amyotrophic Lateral Sclerosis

Amyotrophic lateral sclerosis (ALS or Lou Gehrig Disease) is a sporadic disease with a prevalence rate of approximately 5 per 100,000 people, which means that there may be 10,000 cases in the United States. The disease may occur at any age, but rarely occurs before the age of 20 or after the age of 70. There is a 2:1 male:female ratio and approximately 10% of cases are familial. The clinical symptoms of ALS are muscle weakness, usually in the distal extremities, which are more or less symmetrical. The weakness progresses to involve the whole body, including areas supplied by the cranial nerve nuclei. Occasionally the disease may begin with bulbar (brainstem) involvement, usually starting with atrophy of the tongue. A noteworthy feature of the disease is the fasciculations, which are small vermiform movements seen under the skin or on the tongue of patients with the disease. These small movements are attributed to the irritation of dying neurons. The course of ALS is usually relentless and without remission. The average duration of the disease is 3 years, but may be prolonged. Without cortical motor neuron and corticospinal tract involvement, the disease process is referred to as spinomuscular atrophy. The lesion of ALS is the degeneration and eventual loss of motor neurons in the spinal cord, medulla, and cortex, accompanied by degeneration of the corticospinal tracts. Werdnig–Hoffman disease is an analogous disease of dying motor neurons but occuring in infants and small children.

Myasthenia Gravis

Myasthenia gravis is characterized by a progressive decrease in muscle strength associated with activity and a return of strength after rest. It is

MYASTHENIA GRAVIS   22-4

cause	lesions	manifestations
Autoimmune reaction	Biochemical defect without initial histologic change Atrophy of muscle—late	Decreased muscle strength with activity Diplopia often first symptom Associated thymoma in many cases

a disease of the junction of nerve endings with muscle, so it does not fall clearly into either of the myopathic or neurogenic categories discussed above. In myasthenia gravis, antibodies against the acetylcholine receptor are present in the serum of most affected persons, resulting in degeneration of the receptor. Consequently, the nerve impulse, which is normally transmitted by acetylcholine, is ineffectively transferred to the muscle resulting in progressively weaker muscle contractions.

The initiating cause of the antibody production is not known; therefore, the disease can be considered an autoimmune disease. In many cases the disease is associated with a neoplasm of the thymus. The onset of myasthenia gravis is usually insidious. Almost any muscle may be affected; however, half of the patients with this disease have *diplopia* (double vision) as a first symptom because of frequent involvement of extraocular muscles. Myasthenia gravis runs a course of years but is ultimately fatal in most cases due to slowly developing atrophy of muscles, especially those required for respiration.

The course of the disease may be improved by use of anticholinesterase drugs. Normally cholinesterase degrades acetylcholine; anticholinesterase drugs slow this process, thus making more acetylcholine available to initiate muscle contraction. If a thymoma is found by chest x-ray, its removal may be associated with clinical improvement.

Metabolic Myopathies

Many metabolic conditions can result in muscular weakness. Some of these are inherited, such as the glycogen storage diseases, lipid metabolism disorders, and familial periodic paralysis. Other metabolic disorders are situational, such as myopathy due to excessive alcoholic intake or uremia. The inherited metabolic myopathies may surface in childhood or adulthood depending on the relative amounts of key enzymes in the patient's system. In familial periodic paralysis, the patient may become profoundly weak within a matter of minutes due to poorly understood fluctuations in serum potassium. These episodes can occur irregularly throughout a patient's life. Metabolic myopathies are diagnosed by history and selected tests. The muscle biopsy may be helpful in some, such as glycogen storage disease.

Acute Inflammatory Demyelinating Polyradiculoneuropathy (Guillain–Barré Syndrome)

Guillain–Barré Syndrome (GBS) occurs in one to two persons per 100,000 population yearly in the United States. The disease is usually characterized by a rapid paralysis starting in the peripheral limbs and advancing to affect more proximal muscle functions including respiration. Over half of the cases of GBS appear to be triggered by an acute influenza-like illness from which the patient has just recovered. This indicates that the disease is probably an immune phenomenon triggered by T cells and antibodies directed against a virus that cross react with nerve tissue. This hypothesis is supported by experiments in which lymphocytes transferred from the GBS lesions of human patients to animals can produce the disease.

Diabetic Neuropathy

Diabetic neuropathy can occur in any patient with diabetes. It typically involves distal nerves and can be symmetrical or asymmetrical. Patients typically display decreased sensation in their hands and feet without significant motor abnormalities. Because these patients have diminished pain sensation in their extremities, combined with compromised microvasculature associated with this disease, they are predisposed to ulcers that heal poorly. The autonomic nerves are also affected in a high proportion of diabetic patients with neuropathies.

Hyperplastic/Neoplastic Diseases

Rhabdomyosarcoma is a rare primary malignant neoplasm of skeletal muscle. Metastases of carcinomas to skeletal muscle are uncommon; sarcomas will occasionally spread through skeletal muscle.

Neurofibromas and Schwannomas are more common tumors arising anywhere along the course of peripheral nerves. They are usually benign, but may rarely be malignant. A familial disease—neurofibromatosis—manifest by a plethora of these tumors, especially under the skin, was brought to public attention by the "elephant man."

ORGAN FAILURE

A single muscle or group of muscles may fail (*paralysis*) because of focal dystrophic, traumatic, neurogenic, or inflammatory involvement. Simultaneous failure of most of a person's muscle mass may be acute or chronic. Acute paralysis of all muscles follows administration of curare-like drugs, which block the myoneural junction. These drugs are often used during operative procedures when complete muscle relaxation is required. Acute paralysis of muscle may also follow rapidly progressive peripheral nerve diseases in which there is generalized inflammation of nerves or nerve roots. Chronic muscle failure is the end result of any neurogenic or myopathic disorder and consists of replacement of muscle by fibrous and adipose tissue. Whether acute or chronic, muscle failure eventually affects the diaphragm and intercostal muscles, and the patient will succumb to respiratory paralysis.

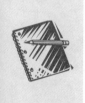

Review Questions

1. What are the two major divisions of muscle disease in terms of pathogenesis?
2. How are each of the following tests or procedures helpful in evaluation of a person with muscle disease?
    Serum aldolase and creatine kinase
    Electromyography
    Muscle biopsy
3. What are the causes, lesions, and major manifestations of each of the specific muscle and nerve diseases listed in this chapter?
4. How might the signs and symptoms of neurogenic muscle disorders differ from those of myopathic disorders?
5. Why is it important to separate dystrophic, inflammatory, and neurogenic causes of muscle weakness?
6. What do the following terms mean?
    Dystrophy
    Pseudohypertrophy of calves
    Myotonia
    Polymyositis
    Werdnig–Hoffman disease
    Amyotrophic lateral sclerosis
    Rhabdomyosarcoma
    Paralysis
    Neurofibromatosis

23.
Central Nervous System

REVIEW OF STRUCTURE AND FUNCTION
Cortex and White Matter • Meninges • Cerebrospinal Fluid • Vessels • Histology

MOST FREQUENT AND SERIOUS PROBLEMS
Cerebrovascular Accidents • Trauma • Infections • Neoplasms

SYMPTOMS, SIGNS, AND TESTS
Cognitive and Motor Dysfunction • Focal and Generalized Dysfunction • Increased Intracranial Pressure • Cerebrospinal Fluid Analysis • Angiograms • Electroencephalogram • Pneumoencephalogram • Computerized Tomography • Magnetic Resonance Imaging

SPECIFIC DISEASES
Genetic/Developmental Diseases
Malformations
Destructive Brain Lesions
Inflammatory/Diseases
Meningitis
Encephalitis
Rabies
Myelitis
Vascular Disease and Trauma
Cerebrovascular Accident (Stroke)
Trauma
Concussion
Contusion
Epidural Hematoma
Subdural Hematoma
Penetrating Injuries
Degenerative Diseases
Multiple Sclerosis
Creutzfeldt–Jakob Disease
Senile Dementia

Parkinson's Disease
Hydrocephalus
Epilepsy
Hyperplastic/Neoplastic Diseases
Brain Neoplasms

ORGAN FAILURE

REVIEW QUESTIONS

REVIEW OF STRUCTURE AND FUNCTION

The central nervous system consists of the brain and spinal cord (Figure 23–1). The brain consists of the cerebrum, cerebellum, and brain stem (midbrain, pons, and medulla). The cerebrum consists of an outer layer of gray matter (cortex), deep gray matter, and white matter (Figure 23–2). The cortex is replete with neurons that are employed for intellectual (cognitive) functions as well as for sensory and motor functions above the vegetative level. The deep gray matter consists of groups of neurons such as the thalamus and basal ganglia that perform the same type of functions as the cortex, albeit at a much more primitive level.

The white matter is composed primarily of the axons and their myelin sheaths. Brain axons are long processes of neurons that connect with neurons in other parts of the brain and spinal cord. Axons of spinal cord neurons innervate skeletal muscles. Thus a voluntary thought generated from neurons of the cerebral cortex can control movement of skeletal muscles. Of course, some axons convey sensory impulses in the opposite direction, from the spinal cord to various parts of the brain. The cerebellum, which is situated in the posterior inferior aspect of the skull, is mainly responsible for coordination of motor functions. The brain stem is a relay between brain and spinal cord and is also a control center for heart rate, respiration rate, sleep and wakefulness, integration of eye movements, and other functions.

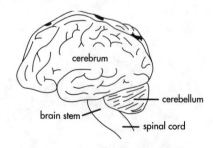

Figure 23–1. Parts of the central nervous system.

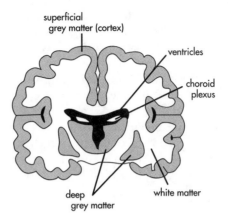

Figure 23–2. Coronal section of the brain.

The brain is covered by meninges, which include an outer, tough membrane called the *dura*, which is next to the skull, and an inner lace-like membrane, the *pia-arachnoid*, which lies directly over the cortex. Meninges also form a continuous covering over the spinal cord.

Cerebrospinal fluid is utilized for metabolic exchange, as an excretory vehicle, and as a means to absorb pressure changes in the central nervous system. The cerebrospinal fluid is formed in the ventricles of the brain by secretion from the choroid plexus and by filtration through the ependyma. It flows from the three ventricles in the anterior part of the brain, through a narrow aqueduct, to the area of the brain stem (medulla). At this point, it passes out of the ventricular system and percolates between the layers of the pia-arachnoid membrane, bathing the brain and spinal cord before being absorbed back into veins.

Most of the blood flows to the brain through the two internal carotid arteries anteriorly and the paired vertebral arteries posteriorly. The carotid arteries supply blood to the bulk of the cerebrum, whereas the vertebral arteries supply blood only to the brain stem, cerebellum, and posterior part of the cerebrum (occiput). Although the vertebral arteries carry much less blood than the carotids, they supply the vital areas in the brain stem, including cranial nerve nuclei and control centers for respiration and consciousness. These vessels all interconnect at the base of the brain, forming the *circle of Willis*. Consequently, occlusion of one major artery to the brain may not necessarily result in deprivation of blood to its area of distribution, because blood can be "borrowed" from other arteries via the circle of Willis. The major arteries branch into smaller arteries as they course through the pia–arachnoid membrane and eventually penetrate the cortex and deeper structures. The anatomy and physiology of the capillaries in the brain differ from those in the rest of the body. The brain capillaries are constructed and function in such a manner as to prevent passage of many substances into the brain that can easily reach other body tissues. This selective exclusion of substances is termed the *blood-brain barrier*. For example, certain antibiotics will not pass the barrier and consequently are not useful in the treatment of brain infections. The actual site of the blood-brain barrier is the endothelium but the astrocytes lying just outside of the capillaries give signals to the endothelium, which help to govern the passage of molecules between the blood and the brain. The capillaries entering the choroid plexus are different from those in the brain parenchyma; thus, some drugs that cannot enter the brain parenchyma may enter the cerebrospinal fluid. However, this blood–cerebrospinal fluid barrier does not allow indiscriminate passage of all drugs.

Microscopically, the important cellular constituents of the brain stem and spinal cord are the *neurons, astrocytes*, and *oligodendroglia*. Neurons are the large cells found in gray matter that conduct nervous impulses. Their efferent processes (axons) may extend for long distances in gray and white matter. Their short afferent processes (dendrites) connect to other neurons through synapses. Astrocytes with their spider-like processes provide structural support to the central nervous system. Astrocytes also regulate the blood–brain barrier and tissue electrolytes. When the brain is injured, astrocytes proliferate, much like fibroblasts, to form a glial scar composed of glial processes but lacking collagen. Oligodendroglia manufacture and maintain the myelin sheath that surrounds and protects axons and dendrites.

MOST FREQUENT AND SERIOUS PROBLEMS

The major diseases of the brain are cerebrovascular accidents (strokes), traumatic injuries, infections (meningitis, encephalitis, and abscess), Alzheimer disease, and neoplasms. Strokes are the third leading cause of death in the United States. Developmental disorders and other degenerative diseases, such as multiple sclerosis, Parkinson's disease, and senile dementia, are also significant. Headaches and epilepsy are very important in terms of prevalence and morbidity but may be manifestations of a variety of diseases.

SYMPTOMS, SIGNS, AND TESTS

The most common presenting symptoms of central nervous system disease are headache, diminution or loss of a motor function, sensory loss, seizures, and disturbances in intellectual or memory capabilities.

The neurologic examination of a patient presenting with one or more of these symptoms will include examination of the motor and sensory systems and testing of cognitive function. The motor system examination involves observation of the patient's gait, posture, and symmetry of muscle mass, as well as testing for muscle strength, coordination, and quality of reflexes. Abnormalities of any of these parameters could be due to lesions of the cerebrum, cerebellum, spinal cord, peripheral nerves, or muscle. Examination of the sensory system entails eliciting a careful history of abnormal sensations (*dysesthesias* and *paresthesias*) and testing for diminished or absent sensory perception on various areas of the body by means of pinprick or application of heat, cold, or vibration. Lesions causing abnormalities of sensation may be located in the peripheral nerves, spinal cord, or cerebral cortex. Testing of reflexes is an important part of a neurologic examination. A decreased reflex may indicate a lesion in the appropriate peripheral nerve, with resultant inability to either transmit the sensory impulse back to the spinal cord or to transmit the motor impulse out to the muscle. A hyperactive reflex, such as an exaggerated knee jerk, represents an intact nerve between the knee and the spinal cord, albeit without the modifying control of the reflex normally mediated by the central nervous system. Testing of cognitive (memory, intellect) functions of the cerebral cortex entails asking the patient to repeat special phrases and perform arithmetic tasks. Other aspects of the neurologic examination may include tests for the integrity of the cranial nerves, observations of abnormal movements, and specific tests for the ability to perform coordinated movements.

The neurologic examiner will attempt to categorize the findings as focal (referable to a specific area of nervous system involvement) or generalized (involving integrated functions of the whole brain). Examples of focal signs or symptoms are *hemiparesis* (weakness of one side of the body), localized areas of sensory deprivation, abnormalities of one or two cranial nerves, or localized headaches. Examples of generalized signs and symptoms are intellectual impairment, generalized headaches, stupor, or loss of consciousness (*coma*). One of the major causes of generalized signs and symptoms is increased intracranial pressure. Because the brain is enclosed in a rigid skull, an increase in volume anywhere within the cranial cavity will rapidly cause a generalized increase in pressure throughout the entire brain. This effect will follow the development of any mass lesion in the cranial cavity, such as a neoplasm, hematoma, abscess, or localized edema surrounding a lesion. The increased intracranial pressure may also be the result of generalized edema secondary to diffuse infection. The only major opening in the skull is the foramen magnum (the opening for the spinal cord), and the substance of the brain tends to be pushed toward this foramen as a consequence of any increased intracranial pressure (Figure 23–3).

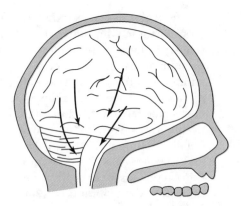

Figure 23–3. Forces resulting from increased intracranial pressure pushing the brain into the foramen magnum.

As the cerebrum is forced into the space where the cerebellum lies, the oculomotor nerve becomes pinched, resulting in pupillary dilation of the same side as the lesion. This affords the physician a valuable clue as to the side of the brain lesion. The downward and backward excursion of brain substance toward the foramen magnum will result in hemorrhage into the brain stem, with coma and rapid death due to involvement of respiratory and activating centers if the pressure is unrelieved. The treatment of increased intracranial pressure is removal of any space-occupying lesion. In addition, steroid drugs and osmotic agents, such as mannitol, may help relieve brain edema by drawing interstitial and intracellular fluid back into the vascular system.

The most important laboratory examination utilized in the evaluation of central nervous system disease is the analysis of cerebrospinal fluid. Cerebrospinal fluid is usually obtained by inserting a needle into the lumbar pia–arachnoid space in a sitting or reclining patient. As the fluid is being withdrawn, the pressure is measured with a manometer to detect elevations in intracranial pressure. The fluid is then examined under the microscope for the presence of leukocytes, red blood cells, neoplastic cells, and microorganisms. Chemical determinations are made for protein and sugar. Serologic tests are utilized for the detection of syphilis and certain viral agents. If an infectious agent is suspected, the fluid is cultured.

Several radiologic procedures are used in evaluation of the patient with a neurologic lesion. Skull x-rays are used to detect fractures of the skull. A skull fracture connotes an injurious force of sufficient magnitude to also damage the underlying brain. A patient presenting with a localized lesion in the brain often undergoes angiography. Radiopaque dye is injected into the appropriate artery (most often carotid) and a simultaneous x-ray is taken to look for abnormal distribution or distortion of vessels in the region of a lesion such as a neoplasm, abscess, or hematoma. Angiograms are also utilized to demonstrate vessel occlusion in the patient with a cerebrovascular accident and to find the site of rupture of an intracranial aneurysm.

The *electroencephalogram* (EEG) is a device for evaluating electrical activity simultaneously in various areas of the brain. Normal neurons discharge electrically in certain known patterns. Abnormalities in patterns denote neuronal disturbance, which may be predictive of injury in specific areas. Patients with seizures may have violent focal disturbances in neuronal electrical activity, thereby localizing the site where the seizure originates. A damaged area in the brain may generate abnormal electrical activity by EEG even when the disturbance is not of sufficient magnitude to cause a clinical seizure. The patient with generalized signs and symptoms may show diffuse EEG abnormalities. The EEG is also used to determine if brain death has occurred in some patients who are in a deep coma.

Computerized tomography (CT scan) is used extensively to study the brain, ventricles, and subarachnoid spaces. Plain CT scans will allow evaluation of ventricular size, the presence of blood, or an infarct. Intravenous contrast material may be injected to detect a brain tumor that has sufficient vascular supply to become enhanced. *Magnetic resonance* (MR) produces even better images than a CT scan, but is not as available.

SPECIFIC DISEASES

Genetic/Developmental Diseases

Developmental abnormalities are more important in the brain than in any other single organ, with the possible exception of the heart. Persons with brain developmental abnormalities may live for many years with very little functional deficit or may be quite retarded and require constant nursing care. Developmental abnormalities of the central nervous system are usually divided into malformations and destructive brain lesions.

Malformations
Malformations are the result of deleterious forces acting upon the embryonic or fetal brain roughly within the first half of gestation. Malformations may be mediated genetically or may be the result of infection or hypoxic or traumatic insult to the brain. Further brain development following an insult early in gestation will result in abnormal brain structure (malformation). Individuals with brain malfor-

mations are often severely retarded mentally, unable to care for themselves, and, consequently, confined to hospitals. Other persons with brain malformations function at various levels in society. Down syndrome is an example of a malformation caused by a chromosomal abnormality. Persons with Down syndrome vary widely in intellectual capabilities. The structural abnormalities of the brain in Down syndrome are not striking and consist of abnormal variation in brain shape and location of neurons.

One of the most common malformations is spina bifida, in which the posterior arches and spines of some vertebrae are absent. This defect is often discovered incidentally on x-rays, but if severe, a meningomyelocele will result. Meningomyelocele is a defect in the spinal column through which spinal cord and meninges protrude into the skin of the back. The cause of meningomyelocele is not known. It may result in severe paralysis of the legs but is compatible with life. Anencephaly is a severe malformation in which the entire forebrain is missing. Infants with anencephaly are stillborn or die soon after birth. Hydrocephalus may also result from a malformation that occludes the flow of cerebrospinal fluid. Hydrocephalus is discussed later in this chapter.

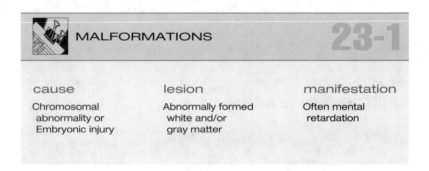

MALFORMATIONS		23-1
cause	**lesion**	**manifestation**
Chromosomal abnormality or Embryonic injury	Abnormally formed white and/or gray matter	Often mental retardation

Destructive Brain Lesions

These occur in the last half of gestational life or during the first 2 years after birth. Since the brain is reasonably well formed during the second half of gestation, injuries at this time result in destructive lesions with actual loss of brain substance in various areas. Most destructive lesions occur at the time of labor and delivery or in the neonatal period in premature infants and are due to anoxia from prolonged and difficult labor or to respiratory distress following delivery. Infections, especially meningitis, may also cause destructive brain lesions. Destructive brain lesions vary greatly in severity. Most patients have motor problems (weakness or incoordination), although one-third or more also are mentally retarded. Clinically, patients with destructive brain lesions are usually referred to as having *cerebral palsy*, which is defined as a nonprogressive condition manifested by motor retarda-

DESTRUCTIVE BRAIN LESIONS 23-2

cause	lesion	manifestation
Fetal injury in last half of pregnancy or at birth	Destruction of white and/or gray matter	Motor handicaps with some mental retardation (cerebral palsy)

tion and sometimes accompanied by mental retardation. Malformations may also be a cause of cerebral palsy, but more often the mental retardation they cause will overshadow the motor retardation. External influences such as maternal diet, drugs, radiation, and toxins can adversely affect brain development. The severity of the defect will depend upon the stage of development at the time of insult.

Inflammatory Diseases

Numerous infectious diseases involve the brain preferentially. Some of the more common processes and diseases will be discussed in this chapter, whereas, others, such as central nervous system syphilis, poliomyelitis, and HIV infection, are covered in the chapter on infectious diseases. The more common manifestations of degenerative diseases of the brain and spinal cord are also discussed in this section.

Meningitis

Meningitis means inflammation of the pia–arachnoid and is most often caused by bacteria. Meningitis most commonly occurs by itself but may be associated with other infections, such as pharyngitis or pneumonia. The onset is usually abrupt, and the major signs and symptoms are fever, headache, neck rigidity, and pain due to muscle spasm from nerve irritation. *Escherichia coli* is a common cause of meningitis in newborn infants, while *Haemophilus influenzae* commonly causes meningitis in small children.

Streptococcus pneumoniae and *Neisseria meningitidis* are more often the cause of meningitis in older children and adults. Neisseria meningitis is especially important, because it can occur in epidemics. Bacteria usually gain access to the brain and spinal cord via the blood. The diagnosis of acute meningitis is made on the basis of cerebrospinal fluid findings of neutrophilic leukocytes, decreased sugar, and the presence of organisms. Treatment consists of immediate antibiotic therapy. If treatment is not immediate or is inadequate, the presence of the bacteria and the leukocytes will result in alterations in the blood–brain barrier, leading to edema with consequent increased

MENINGITIS   23-3

cause	lesion	manifestations
Bacterial or fungal entry into the CNS, usually via the blood	Acute or chronic inflammation of the pia–arachnoid	Headache Neck rigidity and pain Fever Coma Neutrophils in spinal fluid Possible hydrocephalus

intracranial pressure and death of the patient. The lesion of acute meningitis is mainly that of purulent exudate in the subarachnoid space. Less commonly, bacteria will locate in the brain parenchyma rather than the meninges, forming an abscess that behaves as an expanding mass lesion and, if untreated, is almost always fatal.

Chronic meningitis may be caused by tuberculosis or several types of fungal organisms, the most common being *Cryptococcus neoformans.* The inflammatory cells in chronic meningitis are predominantly monocytes and lymphocytes rather than neutrophils, and the disease often smolders at the base of the brain for weeks to months, gradually affecting more and more cranial nerves at their point of exit from the brain. If a patient does not die from acute or chronic meningitis, there is always a danger of developing hydrocephalus from the obliteration of the subarachnoid space by fibrous tissue, with resultant failure to absorb cerebrospinal fluid.

Encephalitis

Encephalitis refers to a more or less diffuse inflammation of the brain. It is usually caused by viral infections. Bacterial, fungal, and protozoal infections usually affect the meninges or cause localized abscesses rather than encephalitis. Many viral encephalitides in the United States are mosquito-borne and occur in epidemics in the warm months of the year. Common types include St. Louis, equine, and Venezuelan encephalitis. Patients with any of these viral encephalitides usually present with generalized signs and symptoms of irritability, drowsiness, and headache. Specific diagnosis depends on culture and identification of the viral agent from the cerebrospinal fluid by serologic testing. In contrast to bacterial infections, viral encephalitis is usually accompanied by a cerebrospinal fluid lymphocytosis. There is no specific treatment for these diseases, and patients will either die, recover fully, or recover with variable neurologic deficit.

ENCEPHALITIS		**23-4**
causes	**lesion**	**manifestations**
Viral entry into the CNS Often epidemic	Inflammation of the brain and spinal cord parenchyma	Irritability Headache Drowsiness, coma Lymphocytes in spinal fluid

Herpes simplex virus type I also can cause an encephalitis. The same virus that causes oral blisters in susceptible persons may, on rare occasions, invade the brain and result in severe destruction of large areas of the brain, most often the temporal lobes.

HIV can cause a primary encephalitis and when HIV progresses to AIDS, encephalitis secondary to toxoplasma or cytomegalovirus is common.

Rabies

Although death from rabies occurs only rarely in the United States, it is such a feared disease that virtually every animal bite raises a concern for rabies. The reservoir of the virus is in wild animals, especially fox and skunk. These animals may transmit the disease to domestic pets, which in turn transmit the virus to humans via bites. The virus travels up the peripheral nerve to the brain and, once the brain is infected, death is virtually inevitable. The incubation period is proportional to the distance from the bite to the brain. After a bite by a domestic animal, the animal should be watched closely for 12 days. If the animal is still alive and well after 12 days, it is unlikely that it has rabies. However, if the animal shows signs of having rabies during the 12-day period, immunization of the victim should be initiated. If there is any suspicion by way of abnormal behavior or symptoms of rabies in the animal or the patient's bite is on the head or neck (close to the brain), immunization should start immediately, since it takes approximately 2 weeks after initiation of immunization to develop effective levels of antibody. Veterinarians are usually prophylactically immunized. If a person is bitten by a wild animal, especially one that displays abnormal behavior, every attempt should be made to locate the animal and submit it to an appropriate laboratory for rabies analysis. Rabies analysis consists of inoculating mice with brain tissue from the suspected animal plus a search for the viral inclusion bodies of rabies in the neurons of the suspected animal. These inclusion bodies are called *Negri bodies* and are found in the cytoplasm of neurons by light microscopy and by immunofluorescence, in which fluorescent-labeled antibodies are directed against the inclusions on tissue section and visualized with a microscope having an ultraviolet light source.

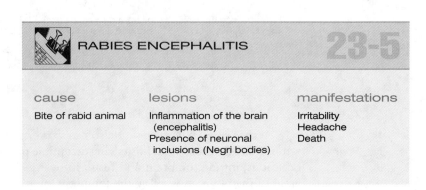

RABIES ENCEPHALITIS

23-5

cause	lesions	manifestations
Bite of rabid animal	Inflammation of the brain (encephalitis)	Irritability
	Presence of neuronal inclusions (Negri bodies)	Headache
		Death

Myelitis

Myelitis is an infection of the spinal cord. Poliomyelitis is a specific infection of the gray matter of the spinal cord. The poliomyelitis virus preferentially destroys the gray matter of the cord, killing the anterior horn motor neurons with resultant paralysis. Poliomyelitis is no longer the dreaded disease that it was prior to 1960 because of successful immunization programs.

Vascular Disease and Trauma

Cerebrovascular Accident (Stroke)

A stroke is a sudden neurologic deficit caused by either vascular occlusion from thrombosis or embolism or from hemorrhage into the brain. The majority of cerebrovascular accidents are caused by emboli, which arise by separating from a thrombus in a large vessel such as the carotid artery (Figure 23–4) or perhaps the heart. The embolus then travels distally, where it lodges in a brain vessel and results in an infarct. Most thrombi initially form because the endothelium of the vessel in which they arise has been damaged by atherosclerosis. Consequently, the common denominator of most cerebrovascular accidents is atherosclerotic vascular disease. This is why cerebrovascular accidents become increasingly prevalent in the elderly.

Whether from emboli or thrombi, vascular occlusions result in infarcts in the brain tissue supplied by the affected vessel. The damaged brain tissue loses function within minutes and becomes soft and necrotic within a few days. Later, tissue is lost from the area, leaving a cystic cavity (Figures 23–5 and 23–6).

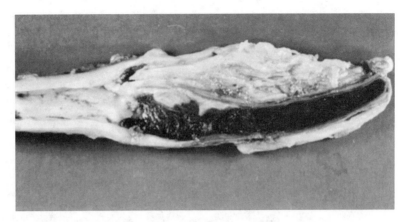

Figure 23–4. Laminated thrombus has filled the lumen of this carotid artery in a patient who died of a massive brain infarct.

The middle cerebral artery is the largest cerebral artery, and it is most often occluded by emboli, because it is a direct continuation of the carotid artery. Occlusion of the middle cerebral artery is important, because this artery supplies the part of the cortex controlling motor function. Involvement of the motor cortex will produce weak-

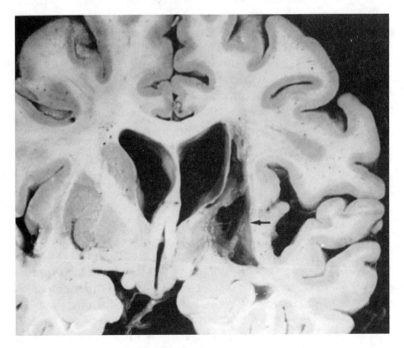

Figure 23–5. Coronal section of a cerebrum with an old infarct in the distribution of the middle cerebral artery with cystic changes.

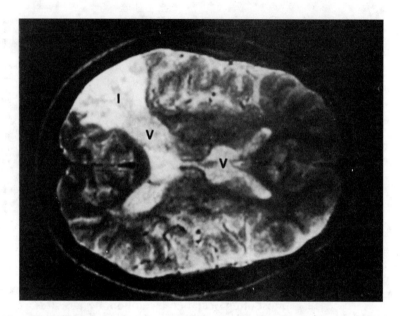

Figure 23–6. Magnetic resonance scan of large peripheral cystic infarct (I). Centrally, the fluid-filled ventricles can be seen (V).

ness (*paresis*) or paralysis on the opposite side of the body. If the dominant side of the brain (the side that primarily controls speech and motor function, usually the left side) is involved, the patient will also have *aphasia* (impaired language function).

Cerebrovascular accidents involving the vertebral arteries or their branches may also cause paralysis because of injury to motor fibers in the brain stem coursing between the brain and spinal cord. Large cerebrovascular accidents in the brain stem will usually kill the patient because of interruption of the nervous centers that control respiration.

Cerebrovascular accidents are also caused by rupture of vessels and bleeding into the brain (brain hemorrhage). The ruptured vessel has usually been weakened by arteriosclerosis, in a patient with hypertension. The signs and symptoms of a brain hemorrhage depend upon its location and size, but almost half of the patients with large brain hemorrhages will die within hours, because the accumulation of blood displaces adjacent tissue and rapidly elevates the intracranial pressure (Figure 23–7).

A third important cause of stroke is ruptured saccular *aneurysm*. Saccular (berry) aneurysms occur predominantly in the vicinity of the circle of Willis, where vessels branch (Figure 23–8 and 23–9). They are saccular outpouchings of vessels due to deficiencies in the blood vessel wall. The reasons for development of these aneurysms are poorly understood. Saccular aneurysms are present in 2 to 5 percent

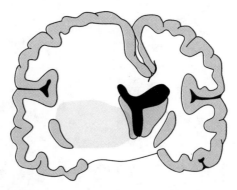

Figure 23–7. Area of hypertensive hemorrhage with displacement of adjacent brain tissues.

of the population, but most do not rupture. When they do rupture, blood is spilled into the subarachnoid space and can be detected in the cerebrospinal fluid. Consequently, examination of the cerebrospinal fluid following a stroke may distinguish ruptured aneurysm from the other important causes of strokes.

Overall, up to one-third of the patients with a cerebrovascular accident will die, one-third will be left with a serious neurologic deficit, and one-third will recover (Figure 23–10). The individual's prognosis depends upon the amount of brain involved and the quality of supportive care received. Many persons sustain small infarcts that never result in neurologic deficit, because they occur in noncritical, so-called "silent" areas of the brain. Little can be done to reverse the damage done by a cerebrovascular accident, but much can be done with good physical therapy to rehabilitate the patient who has sustained a cerebrovascular accident.

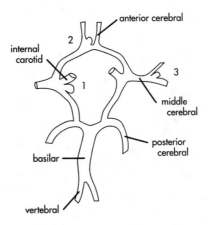

Figure 23–8. Circle of Willis and three most frequent locations of aneurysms.

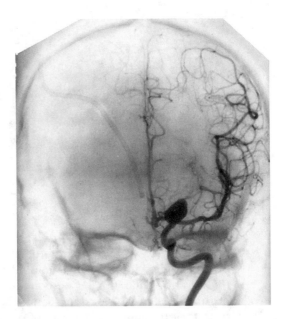

Figure 23–9. Carotid angiogram demonstrating radiopaque dye in a saccular aneurysm of the middle cerebral artery.

When the brain is damaged by ischemia following a cerebrovascular accident, the neurons die within minutes to hours and are never replaced. The oligodendroglia are likewise very vulnerable to injury and readily die following ischemia. The astrocytes proliferate rapidly and repair the injury structurally by forming a scar (glial scar). The astrocytes and their processes are the central nervous system analog of fibroblasts and connective tissue. Monocytes enter from the blood after injury and aid in clearing away the debris.

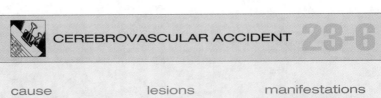

CEREBROVASCULAR ACCIDENT   23-6

cause	lesions	manifestations
Occlusion or rupture of a brain blood vessel	Brain infarct or Brain hemorrhage	Sudden paralysis of opposite side of body Possible aphasia Possible loss of consciousness Vascular occlusion by angiography

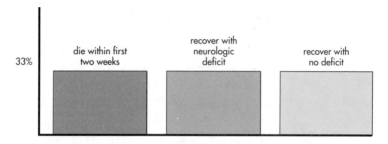

Figure 23–10. Prognosis for stroke patients.

Trauma

The brain is especially vulnerable to injuries in modern times with high-speed transportation. The more common types of brain injuries include concussion, contusion, epidural hemorrhage, subdural hemorrhage, and penetrating injury. Patients who have sustained head trauma may have a concussion and recover completely, only to lapse into coma several hours later. The usual reason for late deterioration is that a subdural or epidural bleed developed immediately following the injury but did not affect the patient until a critical amount of blood accumulated. For this reason, any patient who has had sufficient head trauma to sustain a concussion should be watched closely for 12 to 24 hours.

Concussion

Concussion is a momentary loss of consciousness and loss of reflexes following head trauma, with amnesia for the traumatic event and complete recovery. No structural damage can be detected in the brain.

CONCUSSION		23-7
cause	**lesion**	**manifestations**
Cranial trauma	None	Momentary loss of consciousness
		Momentary loss of reflexes
		Amnesia of the event

Contusion

Contusions are bruises of the surface of the brain sustained at the time of traumatic impact. Contusions occurring on the same side of the brain as the trauma are termed *coup lesions*, whereas those on the opposite side are *contrecoup lesions*. If the head is in motion at the time of

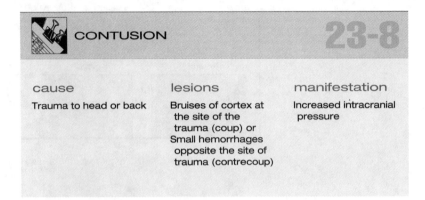

impact, the contrecoup lesion will often be larger than the coup lesion, because the force of the blow is magnified as it is transmitted to the opposite side. Contusions result in hemorrhages from small blood vessels in the brain. These hemorrhages cause further vessel occlusion and consequent edema, rendering the patient vulnerable to the sequelae of increased intracranial pressure.

Epidural Hematoma

Epidural hemorrhage occurs between the dura and the skull (Figure 23–11). It is associated with severe trauma in which the skull is usually fractured. Because an artery is ruptured (middle meningeal), the blood accumulates rapidly, and the patient will die within hours unless the hematoma is removed by an operation. Often the patient with an epidural hematoma sustains a concussion followed by a lucid interval prior to the onset of the signs of increased intracranial pressure.

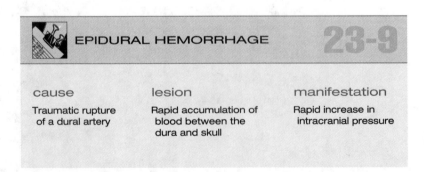

Subdural Hematoma

Subdural hematoma is a collection of blood beneath the dura (Figure 23–11). It is a common sequelae of head injury and is due to rupture of veins on the dorsum of the brain. Because this bleeding is

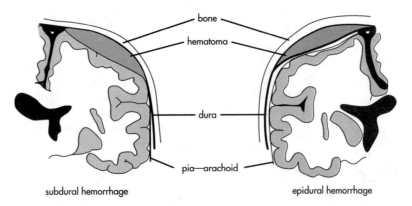

Figure 23–11. Comparative locations of epidural and subdural hematomas.

venous, the blood does not accumulate as rapidly as in an epidural hemorrhage and consequently is not quite as life threatening, although usually the blood must be removed by a surgical procedure to prevent compression of the underlying brain. Subdural hematomas are relatively more common in infants and elderly persons and often are discovered in patients who have no history of trauma. Infants have thin-walled veins and in the elderly, the brain shrinks away from the skull, allowing torsion and tearing of veins when there is brain movement with relatively mild trauma.

SUBDURAL HEMORRHAGE 23-10

cause	lesion	manifestation
Traumatic or atraumatic rupture of a vein between the dura and pia–arachnoid	Slow accumulation of blood beneath the dura	Slow increase in intracranial pressure

Penetrating Injuries

Most penetrating injuries are from bullets. The damage to the brain from a bullet is proportional to the square of the velocity of the bullet; consequently, high-speed bullets do much more damage to the brain than low-speed bullets. Other dangers from penetrating injuries are the impaction of fractured bone splinters into the brain plus the strong likelihood of introducing infection into the open wound.

Penetrating and crushing injuries of the spinal cord are very common and if severe may result in complete paralysis of the body below the lesion. A very common form of spinal cord injury is herniation of the cushioning material (disc) between vertebrae. Herniation of discs is discussed in Chapter 21. Spinal cord injuries are often surgical emergencies.

Degenerative Diseases

Multiple Sclerosis

Multiple sclerosis (MS) is a common disease that affects many young and middle-aged adults throughout the world, primarily in northern hemispheric countries. There are at least 100,000 persons in the United States with multiple sclerosis at any one time, and there is a slightly higher incidence among women than men. The basic lesion is focal loss of the myelin sheath (demyelination), which appears to render axons incapable of properly transmitting a nervous impulse. Because this loss of myelin can occur anywhere in the brain or spinal cord, the symptoms may vary considerably from one patient to another. Visual impairment is usually present to some degree, because multiple sclerosis preferentially affects the optic nerves as well as the tissue surrounding the brain ventricles and the spinal cord. The cause of multiple sclerosis is not known, although it is strongly suspected to be a virus or an immunologic reaction to a virus in persons who have a genetic predisposition. The disease span is usually 5 to 25 years, with the course of the disease alternately remitting and relapsing. The patient eventually becomes quite debilitated from muscle weakness. The diagnosis is made on the basis of clinical history and physical find-

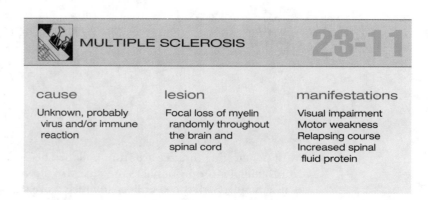

MULTIPLE SCLEROSIS   23-11

cause	lesion	manifestations
Unknown, probably virus and/or immune reaction	Focal loss of myelin randomly throughout the brain and spinal cord	Visual impairment Motor weakness Relapsing course Increased spinal fluid protein

ings that support a multifocal neurologic deficit plus the findings of increased IgG protein in the cerebrospinal fluid. The lesions can be seen using magnetic resonance imaging (Figure 23–12).

Creutzfeldt–Jakob Disease

Creutzfeldt–Jakob disease (CJD) is the human prototype of a group of diseases in animals and man that result in brain degeneration and have been referred to as "slow virus" diseases. "Mad cow" disease, allegedly acquired by eating infected beef in the United Kingdom, is a form of CJD. Persons who are afflicted with CJD become rapidly demented and usually die within 4–6 months after diagnosis with severe brain degeneration. A characteristic electroencephalogram often renders the diagnosis, but sometimes brain biopsy is necessary.

CJD is rare in its occurrence but, similar to rabies, strikes fear in the public disproportionate to its incidence. It is not caused by a virus at all but appears to be the result of transformation of a normal brain protein into an abnormal configuration allowing it to replicate. The abnormal protein (called a *prion*) then builds up in the brain and is associated with severe degeneration of the gray matter characterized by the formation of multiple vacuoles referred to as "spongiform" degeneration. CJD can be transmitted to animals by direct inoculation of brain tissue from a person with the disease. In fact, the disease can be transmitted after the affected brain tissue has been immersed in

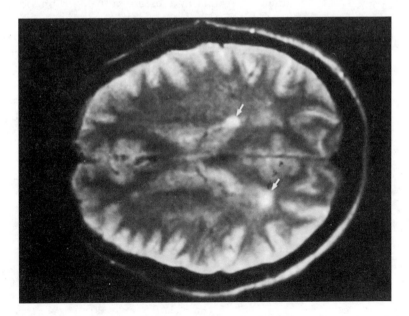

Figure 23–12. Magnetic resonance image of brain demonstrating two plaques (*arrows*) of multiple sclerosis in the white matter.

formaldehyde solution for years, accounting for part of the fear of the disease. On the other hand, transmission by simple contact is rare or non-existent as persons exposed to patients with CJD, including spouses, do not acquire the disease. A few known transmissions in humans have been via organ or tissue transplants. The importance of CJD is that it represents a remarkable type of protein proliferation, apparently undirected by either DNA or RNA, and the protein with its ability to replicate can be transmitted. There are familial varieties of CJD, each being associated with mutations in the prion gene. There is no known cure or effective treatment.

Senile Dementia

Dementia means a decrease in cognitive function, usually accompanied by loss of memory for recent events. *Senile dementia* is a descriptive term for a condition of elderly persons who have poor memory for recent events, pick at their clothes, get lost easily, and are often irritable.

The degree of dementia in a patient is proportional to the loss of substance in the frontal lobes, the region of the brain that is associated with higher cognitive function. The loss of substance may be due to trauma or stroke (infarct) but it is more often secondary to generalized atrophy and degeneration of the neurons in the gray matter (Figure 23–13). This latter condition is called *Alzheimer disease* and accounts for over 60 percent of cases of chronic dementia. Alzheimer disease is ordinarily a disease of the aged but occasionally affects persons in their forties. Characteristic silver-staining neuritic plaques and neurofibrillary tangles are found in the cerebral cortex and allow the neuropathologist to diagnose Alzheimer disease. A large number of these are found in the hippocampal formation in the temporal lobes, explaining the loss of recent memory associated with the disease. It is not known what causes neurons to degenerate resulting in Alzheimer disease. The social impact of this disease is significant. It is estimated that currently there are over four million persons with Alzheimer dis-

SENILE DEMENTIA

23-12

causes	lesions	manifestations
Alzheimer disease	Brain atrophy	Poor recent memory
Other organic brain diseases	Diffuse loss of neurons in the cerebral cortex	Irritability
		Lapses in social restraints

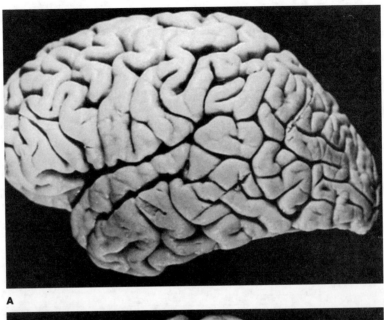

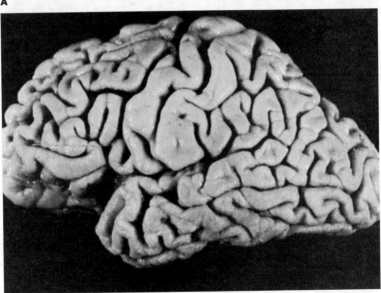

Figure 23–13. Atrophic brain of Alzheimer's disease (B) compared with normal (A).

ease in the United States and with an increasing population of elderly persons, there may be as many as eight million cases by the year 2020. A significant increase in the quantity and quality of resources necessary to care for these patients will be needed. These resources include more and better training of health care professionals in the home and nursing home care of these patients. Dementia may also accompany numerous metabolic conditions such as uremia or electrolyte and fluid imbalance. Many of these types of dementia are reversible.

Parkinson's Disease

Parkinson's disease is caused by degeneration of certain portions of the extrapyramidal (involuntary) motor system, especially the substantia nigra nucleus in the midbrain. A characteristic inclusion called the Lewy body in present in degenerating substantia nigra neurons. Parkinson's disease usually affects older people and results in tremors at rest, mask-like facial expression, and rigidity of skeletal muscles. A shuffling gait is characteristic. Many older people appear to have minor degrees of Parkinson's disease, and about 10 percent of persons with Parkinson's disease will also be demented. Treatment of Parkinson's disease with L-dopa results in some symptomatic relief in about half of the patients.

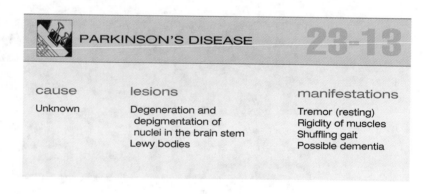

PARKINSON'S DISEASE 23-13

cause	lesions	manifestations
Unknown	Degeneration and depigmentation of nuclei in the brain stem Lewy bodies	Tremor (resting) Rigidity of muscles Shuffling gait Possible dementia

Hydrocephalus

Hydrocephalus literally means water brain, and it may occur congenitally or may arise at any time after birth from a variety of causes. In hydrocephalic individuals, the ventricles enlarge (Figure 23–14) secondarily to a block in the flow of cerebrospinal fluid at some level. The most common type of congenital hydrocephalus is stenosis (closure) of the aqueduct between the third and fourth ventricles. As the ventricles expand with accumulated cerebrospinal fluid, the head may enlarge enormously. In older children and adults, the causes of hydrocephalus are more often tumors that block the flow of cerebrospinal fluid and meningeal scarring secondary to meningitis or hemorrhage, with consequent failure of cerebrospinal fluid to be reabsorbed into the venous system. In older children and adults, the head does not

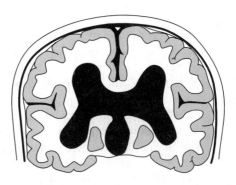

Figure 23–14. Expanded ventricles with hydrocephalus (compare with Figure 23–3).

usually enlarge, because the skull is well formed; rather, the increased pressure from the accumulated fluid in the ventricles causes pressure atrophy of the surrounding white and gray tissue, resulting in mental deterioration. If the increased pressure is not relieved, the brain may herniate toward the foramen magnum. Pressure may be relieved by placement of a tube that acts as a shunt between the ventricles and the veins, heart, or peritoneal cavity.

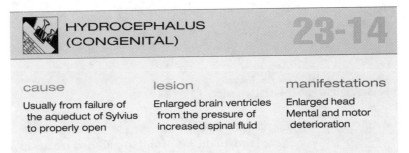

HYDROCEPHALUS (CONGENITAL)

23-14

cause	lesion	manifestations
Usually from failure of the aqueduct of Sylvius to properly open	Enlarged brain ventricles from the pressure of increased spinal fluid	Enlarged head Mental and motor deterioration

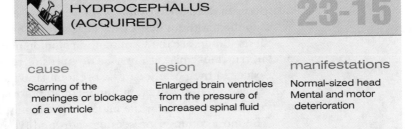

HYDROCEPHALUS (ACQUIRED)

23-15

cause	lesion	manifestations
Scarring of the meninges or blockage of a ventricle	Enlarged brain ventricles from the pressure of increased spinal fluid	Normal-sized head Mental and motor deterioration

Epilepsy

This is a condition of recurrent seizures. Seizures are focal and/or generalized disturbances of neuronal electrical activity, which may be manifested by abnormal movements or sensations and loss of reflexes, memory, or consciousness. Epilepsy may follow recovery from trauma or central nervous system infections or may be induced by malformations or neoplasms of the brain. In most cases, persons with epilepsy have a lifelong history of seizures without known cause. Seizures may also be due to more acute conditions such as electrolyte imbalance, high fever, uremia, and eclampsia. Seizure activity in persons with epilepsy is usually controlled with barbiturates or phenytoin-type drugs.

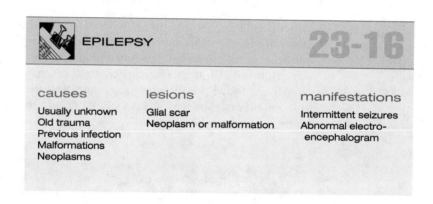

EPILEPSY   **23-16**

causes	lesions	manifestations
Usually unknown	Glial scar	Intermittent seizures
Old trauma	Neoplasm or malformation	Abnormal electro-
Previous infection		encephalogram
Malformations		
Neoplasms		

Hyperplastic/Neoplastic Diseases

Brain Neoplasms

Neoplasms of the brain and spinal cord are not as neatly separated into benign and malignant varieties as are tumors elsewhere. The reason is that small, slowly growing tumors of the brain that would be benign in other locations may readily disrupt vital functions in strategic locations such as the brain stem, killing the patient. Other benign brain tumors may occur in deep areas of the brain where the surgeon cannot gain access to them without destroying adjacent vital brain structures.

Brain tumors are the second most common neoplasms occurring in children (leukemias are first). Two-thirds of brain tumors in children occur in the posterior fossa, predominantly in the cerebellum. Conversely, two-thirds of brain tumors in adults occur in the anterior parts of the brain, in the white matter of the hemispheres.

The most common presenting signs and symptoms in patients with brain tumors are those of increased pressure because of the mass lesion, often with accompanying edema. Generalized symptoms such as headaches, vomiting, blurred vision, and seizures may all result from increased intracranial pressure, while focal signs may accompany brain tumors, depending upon where the tumor arises.

The treatment of brain tumors almost always entails an operation, because some of the tumor tissue needs to be examined in order to establish a histologic diagnosis. In general, if a tumor is of a slow-growing type, the surgeon will attempt to remove as much as possible. Whereas, if a tumor appears to be malignant, the surgeon will sample enough tissue to establish a definitive diagnosis and then further treat the patient with radiation and/or chemotherapy.

The most common brain tumors are those arising from astrocytes. Slower-growing types are called *astrocytomas*. The fast-growing malignant type is called *glioblastoma multiforme*. Glioblastomas are the most common brain tumor in adults and usually result in death within a year or two following diagnosis. As the tumors grow, they produce an expanding, poorly defined mass (Figure 23–15). Almost no patients survive.

The second most common brain tumor is the *meningioma*, a benign neoplasm that arises from the dura and is slow growing and well circumscribed without infiltration of surrounding brain (Figure 23–16).

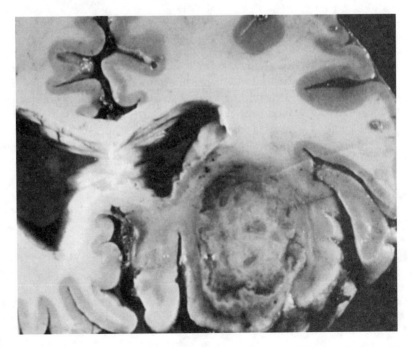

Figure 23–15. Glioblastoma multiforme, with mass infiltrating and displacing of surrounding structures.

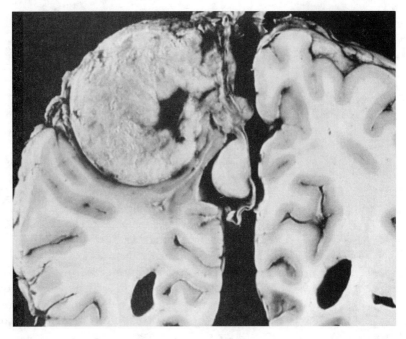

Figure 23–16. Meningioma arising from the dura, with displacement but no infiltration of the brain. (*Courtesy of Margaret Jones.*)

Since most meningiomas arise from the dorsum (top) of the head, the surgeon can usually excise the entire tumor, and the patient's prognosis is good. If a meningioma arises at the base of the brain, however, the surrounding vital structures such as hypothalamus, brain stem, and blood vessels make surgical excision much more difficult, and the prognosis is correspondingly worse.

Pituitary tumors (adenomas) are also common and likewise are difficult to remove because of location. Some pituitary adenomas secrete

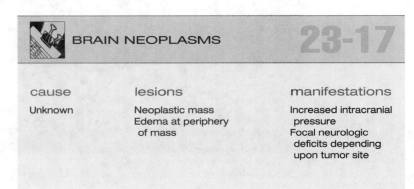

BRAIN NEOPLASMS 23-17

cause	lesions	manifestations
Unknown	Neoplastic mass Edema at periphery of mass	Increased intracranial pressure Focal neurologic deficits depending upon tumor site

growth hormone, resulting in gigantism or acromegaly, syndromes that are discussed further in Chapter 25. Brain tumors arising from oligodendroglia, ependymal cells and neuronal cell lines occur but are less common. One of the most important brain tumors in children is the *medulloblastoma,* which arises in the cerebellum from primitive cells that are neuronal precursors. These tumors are malignant but do respond well to radiation therapy, and 30 to 40 per cent of patients are now cured.

Metastatic tumors to the brain are common. They usually are removed only if there is just one focus of metastasis and the patient is in sufficiently good health to withstand the surgical procedure. Tumors of the spinal cord are much less common than brain tumors.

ORGAN FAILURE

As the brain is a composite of numerous groups (nuclei) of neurons with partially related functions, any group of neurons may fail, resulting in a focal neurologic deficit. Generalized brain failure results from diffuse brain disease and places the patient in a vegetative state, incapable of performing basic mental or motor functions (*coma*). The patient in coma is alive because of the continuing function of the brain stem, which is often the last part of the brain affected by diffuse disease. Coma may be reversible if structural damage to the brain has not taken place. In many areas of the United States, a patient is considered legally dead if two successive electroencephalograms taken 24 hours apart both show complete absence of electrical activity in the brain, irrespective of the status of the heart. Interpretation of the death of the patient by demonstrating death of the brain is somewhat controversial and poses ethical as well as legal dilemmas. Other criteria for determining brain death should include body temperature and reflex responses determined by neurologic examination. Since barbiturates may cause decreased or absent electrical activity in the brain that is reversible, blood levels of these substances should also be measured before pronouncing brain death.

Review Questions

1. What is the difference between a focal and a generalized neurologic deficit?

2. What are the causes of increased intracranial pressure? Why is increased intracranial pressure dangerous?

3. How is each of the following tests utilized in diagnosing central nervous system disease?
   Cerebrospinal fluid analysis
   Angiography
   Electroencephalogram
   Computerized tomography
   Magnetic resonance imaging

4. What are the causes, lesions, and manifestations of each specific disease listed in this chapter?

5. How does the pathogenesis and clinical expression of developmental brain malformations differ from developmental brain destructive lesions?

6. How does meningitis differ from encephalitis in terms of pathogenesis, location of lesion, and clinical expression?

7. When should rabies be suspected? How should it be diagnosed and treated?

8. What is the relationship between cerebrovascular accidents and atherosclerosis?

9. Which cells in the brain are most vulnerable to anoxia from cerebrovascular accidents?

10. Why should a patient who recovers from a brain concussion be closely watched?

11. What are the differences between epidural and subdural hematomas in terms of pathogenesis and development of symptoms?

12. How can senile dementia be distinguished from the dementia associated with Parkinson's disease?

13. Why is Creutzfeldt–Jakob disease so feared?

14. How does congenital hydrocephalus differ from acquired hydrocephalus in terms of pathogenesis and clinical expression?

15. Why should almost all patients with brain tumors be operated on?

16. What do the following terms mean?

   Down Syndrome
   Anencephaly
   Meningomyelocele
   Spina bifida
   Cerebral palsy
   Aphasia
   Astrocytoma
   Glioblastoma multiforme
   Meningioma
   Medulloblastoma

24.
Mental Illness

NATURE OF MENTAL ILLNESS
Definition • Functional Mental Illness • Organic Brain Syndromes • Mental Health Care Specialists

MOST FREQUENT AND SERIOUS PROBLEMS
Alcohol Disorders • Schizophrenia • Anxiety Disorders • Personality Disorders • Depression • Organic Brain Syndromes • Suicide • Psychiatric Emergencies

SYMPTOMS, SIGNS, AND TESTS
Physical Examination • Screening Tests • Psychologic Assessment • History • Mental Status Examination

SPECIFIC DISEASES
Organic Mental Disorders
Schizophrenia
Affective Disorders (Mood Disorders)
Anxiety Disorders
Personality Disorders
Disorders Arising in Childhood and Adolescence
Disorders with Symptoms Suggestive of Organic Disease
Autism
Psychophysiologic Disorders

REVIEW QUESTIONS

NATURE OF MENTAL ILLNESS

Mental or psychiatric illnesses are those that affect behavior, emotion, and cognition. There is no precise definition of what constitutes mental health; rather, it is a matter of experienced judgment whether a person has normal intellectual capacity and is functioning normally as a member of society. The degree to which a person is emotionally impaired (i.e., whether or not the patient receives a psychiatric diagnosis) depends primarily on (1) the degree to which the symptoms interfere with his or her ability to function appropriately and to obtain gratification in life experiences and (2) the degree to which the symptoms disturb others. For example, many persons who might be diagnosed as having schizophrenia function well as semi-isolates, holding a regular job and maintaining a restricted social life.

Psychiatric disorders have traditionally been separated from diseases of the nervous system because most mental illnesses have not been shown to be associated with demonstrable lesions. However, evidence acquired over the last decade has documented altered neurobiologic function in patients with major mental illnesses, in addition, many mental symptoms are known to occur as a result of neurologic, metabolic, or endocrinologic disorders. Mental illnesses that are caused by detectable brain lesions are called *organic mental disorders* or *organic brain syndromes.*

Health care specialists who deal primarily with mental and emotional illnesses include psychiatrists, psychologists, and social workers. Psychiatrists are physicians who are trained to diagnose and treat psychiatric illness. Psychologists usually hold advanced degrees in psychology and are concerned with the study of normal and abnormal behavior. Psychologists often play a role in diagnosis of subtle psychiatric illnesses, by using specific psychologic tests. Psychologists may also be involved in psychologic or behavioral aspects of treatment of patients. Social workers are especially concerned with the social and physical environments of patients with psychiatric illness, just as they are with patients having organic disease. Psychiatric illnesses are often first detected by primary care practitioners.

MOST FREQUENT AND SERIOUS PROBLEMS

Psychiatric illnesses collectively are a common and very serious problem. Each year at least 500,000 persons in the United States enter a mental hospital for the first time. At any given moment, approximately 1 out of every 1,000 persons is hospitalized under psychiatric care. Underscoring these high incidence and prevalence rates is the fact that in one recent year 6 billion doses of tranquilizers (1.2 million pounds) were produced.

Affective disorders are estimated to affect 7 percent of the population and are the most common severe psychiatric disorders. Affective disorders are a group of illnesses characterized by a disturbance of mood accompanied by a manic or depressive syndrome that is not due to any other physical or mental disorder.

Panic disorder, anxiety disorder, post-traumatic stress disorder, obsessive–compulsive disorder, and social phobia are all fairly common and, when severe, can be quite disabling.

Schizophrenia, another common severe psychiatric disorder, affects about 1 percent of the population. It usually begins between 15 and 24 years of age. At older ages the types of psychiatric diseases vary considerably among males and females. Alcoholic disorders are probably the most common psychiatric problem in males of all ages over 24, followed by the affective disorders, schizophrenia, and personality disorders. In females of comparable ages, schizophrenia and anxiety syndromes are much more frequent than alcoholic and personality disorders. In middle-aged and older people, depression is a frequent and serious psychiatric disorder. In the elderly, permanent organic brain diseases, often collectively referred to as *chronic brain syndromes,* become more prevalent. Although chronic brain syndromes are associated with brain atrophy, the symptoms are usually behavioral in nature. Dementia is discussed in Chapter 23.

Suicide may be associated with acute or chronic environmental stress, with alcoholism, with emotional disorders (especially those in which depression plays a major role), or with chronic illnesses (especially chronic lung diseases or illnesses in which chronic pain is a major factor). Suicide among patients with psychiatric illness is three to fifteen times more frequent than among the general population. The incidence of suicide varies considerably in different populations, being influenced by age, sex, population density, occupation, climate, and alcoholism. In the United States, suicide is the eleventh leading cause of death overall, but the third leading cause of death in the 18 to 30 age group. There are eight attempts for every suicide committed.

Psychiatric emergencies in addition to suicide attempts include acute toxic psychoses (delirium), alcohol and other drug withdrawal, manic excitement, and acute anxiety or panic attacks. Acute toxic psychoses may be secondary to intoxication with or withdrawal from drugs or alcohol, infection, metabolic disorders, or trauma.

SYMPTOMS, SIGNS, AND TESTS

Mental illnesses are manifested by a wide range of symptoms, subjective feelings, and behaviors, the majority of which are not specifically pathologic when viewed in isolation. Because the symptoms are nonspecific and because many are known to be associated with physical illnesses as well as with organic brain syndromes, a complete physical examination and screening laboratory tests are an essential part of a psychiatric evaluation. X-rays of the chest and skull, brain magnetic resonance imaging (MRI), electroencephalogram (EEG), and psychologic assessment, such as neuropsychologic testing and personality inventory, are usually a part of a thorough psychiatric evaluation. Hormonal studies may be important to rule out pituitary, thyroid, or adrenal disease with psychiatric manifestations.

As in physical illnesses, a detailed history is essential and is usually obtained from family members as well as the patient. The mental status examination, a specific component of the psychiatric evaluation, is of great value in differentiating between organic and nonorganic mental diseases. The mental status examination includes evaluation of (1) orientation to time, place, and person; (2) memory, both recent and remote; (3) intellectual functions, including general fund of information and arithmetic ability; (4) judgment; (5) mood and affect, (6) speech pattern; and (7) delusions and hallucinations.

Table 24–1 classifies and defines many of the manifestations of mental illness. It should be remembered that many symptoms and signs are experienced by normal people. When they are disproportionately intense or prolonged in relation to their stimulus or when they significantly interfere with the individual's ability to function in and gain gratification from his or her environment, they may indicate an abnormal mental state. Symptoms such as anxiety and depression are experienced by almost everyone at certain times. Not infrequently, an individual's symptoms are more troublesome to others than they are to the person with the symptoms.

SPECIFIC DISEASES

The classification of mental illness is based on several major parameters, including intelligence (for mental retardation), presence or absence of brain lesions, ability to correctly interpret reality, and duration of the condition.

Subnormal intelligence occurring before age 18 is referred to as *mental retardation*; loss of intellectual capacity after age 18 is termed *dementia*. Mental changes associated with demonstrable brain lesions are termed *organic brain disorders*; all others are classified as "functional disorders." The ability to correctly interpret reality is the fundamental consideration in separating psychoses from nonpsychotic illnesses. Reversible mental disorders of rapid onset are referred to as acute, while prolonged conditions are termed chronic.

The American Psychiatric Association has established criteria for the classification of mental illnesses in its *Diagnostic and Statistical Manual of Mental Disorders*. A modified classification used in this chapter is presented in Table 24–2. Some general comments are in order before proceeding with a discussion of specific categories.

TABLE 24–1. TYPES OF MANIFESTATIONS OF PSYCHIATRIC ILLNESS

I. Disturbances of consciousness
    Confusion—lack of orientation of time, place, or person
    Delirium—bewildered, restless, confused

II. Disturbances of affect
    Euphoria—feeling of well-being inappropriate to apparent events
    Depression—feeling of sadness inappropriate to apparent events
    Grief—sadness appropriate to a real loss
    Anxiety—feeling of apprehension with no known precipitant

III. Disturbance of motor behavior
    Compulsion—uncontrollable impulse to perform an act
    Hyperactivity—restless, aggressive
    Hypoactivity—slowed psychologic and physical function

IV. Disturbance of thinking
    Autistic thinking—thinking that gratifies unfulfilled desires without regard to reality
    Incoherence—run together thoughts without logical coherence
    Flight of ideas—rapid shifting of ideas
    Aphasia—loss of ability to comprehend language (sensory aphasia) or verbalize (motor aphasia)
    Delusion—false belief that cannot be corrected by reasoning
    Hypochondria—exaggerated concern over health not based on real disease
    Obsession—recurrent thought, feeling, or impulse
    Phobia—exaggerated fear of a specific situation

V. Disturbance of perception
    Agnosia—inability to recognize and interpret sensory impressions
    Hallucinations—false sensory perceptions not associated with real stimuli
    Illusions—false sensory perceptions of real stimuli

VI. Disturbances of memory
    Amnesia—partial to total inability to recall past experiences
    Paramnesia—falsification of memory by distortion of recall

VII. Disturbances of intelligence
    Mental retardation—developmental lack of intelligence that interferes with social and vocational performance (IQ less than 70)
    Dementia—loss of intellectual capacity occurring after developmental period and secondarily to organic disease

---

Emotional disorders may be associated with organic disease in several ways. First and most common is the emotional response of an individual to a physical illness or injury. While one would consider this a normal, if not expected, reaction, the severity of symptoms, usually depression and/or anxiety, may vary considerably, depending on such factors as the person's basic personality, prior level of activity, and seriousness of the illness. Often the symptoms are of sufficient intensity and persistence to justify a diagnosis of transient situational disturbance. Second, mental illness may occur secondarily

TABLE 24–2. CLASSIFICATION OF MENTAL ILLNESS

Organic mental disorders
    Drug-induced disorders
    Dementias
    Mental manifestations of other diseases
Schizophrenia
Affective disorders
    Bipolar (manic–depressive disorder)
    Unipolar (psychotic depression)
    Intermittent affective disorders
Anxiety disorders (neuroses)
    Phobias
    Panic reaction
    Obsessive compulsive neurosis

Personality disorders
Disorders arising in childhood and
    adolescence
    Mental retardation
    Generalized emotional disorders
    Specific disorders
Disorders with symptoms suggestive of
    organic disease
    Factitious disorder
    Malingering
    Somatoform (psychosomatic) disorder
    Autism
Psychophysiologic disorders

to organic disease of the central nervous system (organic brain syndrome). Third, certain physical illnesses are called *psychophysiologic disorders* because of their frequent association with emotional disturbances. In most instances, the nature of the association between emotional disturbance and physical illness is poorly understood, i.e., the causal relationship is not clear. The combination of emotional disturbance and organic disease can often be best represented by separate diagnoses for the mental and organic components of the illness.

In addition to considering the possible relationship of the patient's mental illness to organic disease, it is also important to judge whether the patient is psychotic or not. Psychosis entails altered perceptions (hallucinations), illogical beliefs (delusions), and illogical thinking (loose associations). Most functional psychoses fall into the categories of schizophrenia and affective disorders; less commonly they fall into the category of disorders of childhood and adolescence. Pure paranoid psychoses are rare, paranoid symptoms more often being a feature of schizophrenia. In addition to the functional psychoses, many organic mental disorders, such as acute drug-induced reactions and chronic dementias, are psychotic reactions.

Another important point to be made about the classification of mental illnesses is that most symptoms are not specific for any particular category. This is particularly true of depression and anxiety, which commonly occur with many different types of mental illness. For example, depression, one of the most common and important symptoms, may be associated with organic brain disease, schizophrenia, affective disorders, alcoholism, and transient situational disturbances. If depression occurs after the onset of one of those disorders, it may be termed a secondary depression. The criteria for and characteristics of the major categories will be discussed below.

Finally, there is no general agreement regarding diagnostic criteria for many psychiatric illnesses, thereby resulting in different classification schemes and different reported relative incidences for many of these illnesses. The criteria for classifying psychiatric illness is continuously evolving.

Organic Mental Disorders

The essential feature of this category is mental disturbance due to disease of the brain or widespread alteration of brain function due to drugs, toxins, or metabolic products. Acute forms of organic mental disorders often present with psychotic features, while chronic forms more often become psychotic in the late stages of the disease.

Acute organic brain syndromes are usually manifested by delirium and intoxication. Drugs such as alcohol, barbiturates, and narcotics are common causes as well as electrolyte imbalances and inflammatory processes. With some drugs, particularly alcohol, symptoms may be precipitated by withdrawal of the agent. For further discussion of alcoholism see Chapter 30.

Chronic brain syndromes are usually manifested by dementia, loss of recent memory, personality changes, and sometimes by depression, delusions, and hallucinations. Alzheimer's disease, a diffuse atrophy of the brain with loss of neurons of unknown cause, accounts for most cases of chronic irreversible dementia. The course is slowly progressive, with an average survival of about 5 years. See Chapter 23 for further discussion of Alzheimer's disease.

Repeated cerebral infarcts may produce dementia in some individuals but are a much less common cause of dementia than Alzheimer's disease. Multiple cerebral infarcts with dementia are more likely to be associated with a stepwise progression and findings that indicate focal neurologic damage.

Many other brain diseases and metabolic intoxications, such as acidosis, uremia, and hepatic failure, can present with mental disturbances. Organic disease with mental disturbance is usually separable from "functional disease" on the basis of abnormalities found by neurologic examination, laboratory tests, special procedures, and mental status examination. Occasionally, brain lesions, such as a brain tumor, will present as a psychosis and may be misdiagnosed as a "functional disease." Some symptoms and signs of organic psychosis may overlap other psychotic states, but the more common signs and symptoms of organic psychoses are delirium (mental confusion, disorientation, abnormal emotions, and altered consciousness) and dementia (loss of the intellectual processes, such as memory, reasoning, judgment, and problem solving, and the loss of the higher aspects of personality). It is extremely important to recognize organic psychosis because effective treatment is available for many of its causes.

Schizophrenia

Schizophrenia is a common psychosis. It affects approximately 1 percent of the population. Schizophrenia is primarily a thought disorder in which misinterpretation of reality can lead to delusions and hallucinations. Alterations in mood and behavior are also prominent in schizophrenia, and schizophrenic patients are often ambivalent, display inappropriate emotional responses, and become either aggressive or withdrawn. There are several different subtypes of schizophrenia, which are classified on the basis of the predominant symptoms (Table 24–3).

The cause of schizophrenia is unknown. The familial tendency suggests a poorly defined, possible multiple-gene, genetic influence in schizophrenia. General personality characteristics and environmental influences are possible contributing factors in the development of schizophrenia. Numerous biochemical and neurophysiologic abnormalities have been demonstrated in patients with schizophrenia, none of which have been demonstrated to be causative.

Schizophrenia usually has its onset in late adolescence and early adulthood, with fewer new cases occurring in middle age. The severity of the disease varies considerably. Some patients are able to maintain employment while being treated on an outpatient basis, while other require hospitalization. In general, schizophrenia is a chronic disabling illness that results in social and occupational decline. The

TABLE 24–3. SUBTYPES OF SCHIZOPHRENIA

Subtype	Characteristics
Disorganized (hebephrenic)	Marked incoherence Flat, incongruous, or silly affect
Catatonic	Stupor or mutism Rigid positioning Inappropriate excited motor activity Inappropriate or bizarre posturing
Paranoid	Persecutory delusions Grandiose delusions Delusions of jealousy Persecutory or grandiose hallucinations
Undifferentiated	Psychotic symptoms prominent (delusions, hallucinations, formal thought disorder, bizarre behavior) Does not fit other subtypes

predominant modes of medical therapy are medication with phenothiazine derivatives or other antipsychotic (neuroleptic) drugs and psychotherapy. Recent advances have resulted in new "atypical" antipsychotic medications that are proving to be more effective with fewer side effects. The aim of psychotherapy in the schizophrenic patient is more to aid coping behaviors and improve social adjustment rather than to uncover deep-seated feelings and motivations. Various forms of shock therapy are only rarely utilized today.

Affective Disorders (Mood Disorders)

This group of illnesses is called affective disorders because they are characterized by alteration of mood. *Mania* is a euphoric or irritable, hyperactive state, and *depression* is a sad or melancholy state with either decreased activity or agitation. It is estimated that 15 million persons in the United States have some form of mood disorder.

Clinically, the term depression is used to describe a cluster of symptoms that may include any of the following: poor appetite or weight loss, sleep disturbance, loss of energy, agitation or retarded motor activity, loss of interest in usual activities or decreased sexual drive, feelings of self-reproach or guilt, complaints of or actual diminished ability to think or concentrate, and thoughts of death or suicide.

Clinically, the manic syndrome includes elevated mood, hyperactivity, involvement in activities without recognizing potential for painful consequences, rapid speech with flight of ideas, inflated self-esteem, decreased need for sleep, and distractibility.

Affective disorders are usually episodic, with one or more episodes clearly distinguished from previous levels of function, or they may be intermittent, with periods of depressed mood having less clear onset and shorter duration. The episodic forms can be of psychotic proportions and fall into two major groups, termed *bipolar* and *unipolar*. The intermittent affective disorders are usually nonpsychotic and are similar in nature to personality disorders (see below).

The bipolar form of *manic–depressive psychosis* is inherited, has onset of symptoms in early adulthood, and is characterized by periods of mania and periods of depression alternating with periods of normal function. The inheritance pattern may be partly controlled by an X-linked dominant gene, although father-son transmission has been recorded also. In contrast to schizophrenia, manic-depressive illness occurs in persons of higher socioeconomic classes, and some individuals are highly productive, especially during periods of mania. Manics, however, tend to carry their ambitions beyond reality and end up in difficult situations, such as financial ruin.

The unipolar form of episodic affective disorder is five to ten times more common than the bipolar form and is characterized by depression without episodes of mania. Inheritance also plays a large role in unipolar depression. The cause is not known but aberrations in the levels of the neurotransmitters, norepinephrine or serotonin, have been identified in several patient studies. The onset can occur at any time in life with a preponderance in middle age. Approximately 50 percent of patients have more than one episode of psychotic depression. It is more common in females.

Anxiety Disorders

The anxiety disorders are characterized by symptoms such as exaggerated or inappropriate feelings of tension and nervousness, phobia, insomnia, obsession, or compulsiveness in which one symptom usually dominates and in which there is no evidence of psychosis or of reaction to a transient situation. Approximately 20 million persons in the United States suffer from anxiety disorders. Anxiety disorders frequently occur with affective disorders.

Sigmund Freud originally used the term neurosis to indicate a specific disease process but also to indicate unpleasant symptoms in a person with nonpsychotic mental illness. Currently, usage of the terms neurotic disorders or neurotic symptoms indicates a variety of psychiatric symptoms covering several specific disease categories including anxiety disorders.

Neurotic symptoms also occur to some degree in everyone and may be found in patients with other mental illnesses such as psychoses or personality disorders. Thus, neurotic symptoms are not specific. Nevertheless, at times one or more neurotic symptoms become sufficiently dominant as to interfere with an individual's ability to lead a gratifying or productive life. Under such circumstances, a diagnosis of anxiety disorder is often made. Neurotic symptoms may at times be very severe and immobilizing, requiring hospitalization. In anxiety disorders, the patient is aware that the symptoms are irrational but is unable to control them. Thus, this group of mental illnesses does not reflect a thought disorder as do the psychotic illnesses. In addition, persons with anxiety disorders maintain the ability to distinguish external reality from internal processes; thus, reality impairment is isolated to the symptom itself and does not, as in psychotic illnesses, pervade the individual's total awareness.

People with phobias persistently avoid specific objects, activities, or situations because of irrational fears. Patients with agoraphobia avoid being alone, whereas patients with social phobia avoid specific social situations due to overconcern about humiliation and embarrassment. Common simple phobias involve animals (particularly reptiles, insects, and rodents), tight places (claustrophobia), and high places (acrophobia).

Panic reactions involve sudden, short-lived, severe anxiety reactions without the patient being certain when the attack will occur. Symptoms relate to sudden autonomic nervous system discharge, producing dyspnea, palpitations, chest pain, choking, dizziness, paresthesias, hot and cold flashes, sweating, trembling, and fear.

Obsessive compulsive neuroses involve senseless and repetitive thoughts (obsessions), such as violence, contamination, and doubt, or compulsions to perform an act, such as handwashing, counting, checking, or touching, accompanied by a desire to resist such activity. However, attempts to resist the compulsion are accompanied by tension and anxiety.

It is estimated that 2 to 4 percent of all persons experience an anxiety disorder at some time during their life. Treatment usually consists of supportive therapy, environmental manipulation, and the use of minor tranquilizing drugs such as the benzodiazepines, antidepressant agents, or monoamine oxidase inhibitors.

Stress disorders are usually considered separately from anxiety disorders and are the consequence of stressful life situations—which are different for different people. Many types of aberrant behavior characterize stress disorders. A special type of stress disorder is *posttraumatic stress disorder* which may follow a physical beating, severe burns, rape, or other severe physical stress. In this disorder the person re-experiences the original event, sometimes after experiences that serve as a reminder of the original traumatic event. The person may experience difficulties in concentration, startle reactions, sleep problems and nightmares, illusions, and over-generalized associations. Treatment is supportive.

Personality Disorders

Personality disorders are lifelong patterns of behavior that are usually inconsistent with social norms and are often unacceptable to others. They account for a high proportion of nonpsychotic psychiatric problems. They often include or overlap with such problems as sexual deviation, alcoholism, and drug dependence.

The various types of personality disorders are defined in approximate order of frequency in Table 24–4. Personality disorders may be caused by organic brain disease or may be acquired functional disorders. Some persons with personality disorders experience brief periods of psychotic-like symptoms.

Disorders Arising in Childhood and Adolescence

Mental illness in children and adolescents differs sufficiently from that of adults to merit separate classification. The many conditions of

TABLE 24–4. TYPES OF PERSONALITY DISORDERS

Type	Characteristics
Histrionic	Excitability, emotional instability, overactivity, self-dramatization
Passive aggressive	Uses passive behavior to express hostility, obstructionism, pouting, procrastination, stubbornness, intentional inefficiency
Dependent	Need overtly expressed, compliant, eager to perform for others, clinging, immature
Avoidant	Withdrawn, overly sensitive, shy, low self-esteem
Antisocial	Lack of loyalty to individuals, groups or society; selfish, irresponsible, impulsive, lack of guilt, violation of rules
Compulsive	Overly conscientious, overly meticulous, perfectionistic
Inadequate	Ineffectual responses to social, psychologic, and physical demands; inept; social instability
Paranoid	Hypersensitive, rigid, unwarranted suspicion, jealous, excessive self-importance
Narcissistic	Grandiose sense of self-importance, exhibitionism, preoccupation with fantasies of unlimited success, power, brilliance, or beauty

these age groups will be briefly described below as mental retardation, generalized emotional disorders characteristic of childhood, and specific disorders, such as stereotyped movements and speech disorders.

Mental retardation is subnormal intellectual function (IQ below 70) with onset before age 18 but usually present from birth. Approximately 3 percent of the population of the United States is mentally retarded, and the majority of retarded people live in urban and rural slums. The cause is unknown 80 percent of the time. Known causes include prenatal infectious diseases, such as rubella, toxoplasmosis, cytomegalic inclusion disease, and syphilis; neonatal meningitis or encephalitis; Down syndrome; metabolic disease such as hypothyroidism and phenylketonuria; brain damage from perinatal diseases such as erythroblastosis fetalis, birth injury, and anoxia at birth; and external agents such as trauma, carbon monoxide poisoning, and lead poisoning. Approximately three-fourths of the mentally retarded are mildly so (IQ 55 to 70) and are educable to about the sixth grade level by the time they reach adult age.

Generalized emotional disorders of childhood are likely to affect social and intellectual development. Psychotic disorders are uncommon in childhood, although schizophrenia and manic-depressive psychoses may begin in late childhood and adolescence. Autism starts in childhood (see below). Attention deficit disorders are common and become particularly evident in school situations, where they are manifested by an inability to concentrate, hyperactivity, and impulsiveness. Conduct disorders resemble the antisocial personality disorder but are separated, because conduct disorders do not necessarily continue as an antisocial personality disorder. Conduct disorders are common in late childhood and adolescence and may be manifested by persistent lack of concern for others, delinquency, and illegal acts. Anxiety disorders in childhood commonly take the form of separation anxiety, relating to fear of being away from home or of shyness. Specific developmental disorders that are common include defective articulation, poor motor coordination, enuresis (bed wetting), motor tic (rapid spasmodic, involuntary movement), and stuttering.

Disorders with Symptoms Suggestive of Organic Disease

Factitious disorders involve the voluntary production of symptoms that are not real, genuine, or natural for a well-defined goal. These patients create symptoms and inflict physical changes upon themselves in order to receive medical attention and hospitalization. The term *malingering* is used if the symptoms are produced to avoid an obvious external circumstance, such as conscription into the military.

Somatoform disorders are distinguished from factitious disorders and malingering in that the symptoms suggestive of organic illness are not under voluntary control. The complaints, frequently referred to as *psychosomatic*, take the form of headache, fatigue, palpitations, fainting, nausea, loss of sensation, paralysis, blindness, vomiting, abdominal pain, bowel troubles, allergies, and menstrual and sexual difficulties. In its fully developed form, a patient with somatization disorder will have a lifelong pattern beginning in the teenage period of seeking medical evaluation, being hospitalized, and even having unnecessary surgery. The disorder is more common in women and is often associated with use of many potentially addicting prescription drugs obtained from multiple physicians and pharmacies. Pain, often the dominant symptom, accounts for the most common types of drugs obtained by these patients.

It is important to recognize that psychosomatic complaints may be dominant symptoms in other mental illness, especially depression and schizophrenia; however, the other features of these diseases will also be present. Another problem is that the expression of complaints associated with organic illness varies greatly among individuals; thus, the diagnosis of organic lesions may be delayed in persons with frequent psychosomatic complaints or in those that do not readily express pain.

A conversion disorder is a form of a somatization disorder in which there is involuntary loss of function suggestive of physical illness such as paralysis, loss of voice, blindness, anesthesia, or incoordination.

Autism

Autism is a probable organic developmental disorder that starts before 36 months of age and is marked by sustained impairment of verbal and non-verbal communication skills with restricted patterns of behavior. Children and adults with autism smile only rarely, display apparent indifference to human warmth, and do not interact socially well at all, appearing passive and aloof. Typically, when presented with a variety of stimuli, persons with autism respond to only one. Treatment includes specific programming to learn and enhance verbal skills.

Psychophysiologic Disorders

These are organic illnesses in which emotional factors are felt to play a significant role. These illnesses involve the autonomic nervous system and are usually isolated to a single organ system. Demonstrable organic lesions are present.

Since many emotions are expressed by way of the autonomic nervous system (blushing, sweating, increased heart rate, diarrhea, and nausea), it is not surprising that long-lasting, severe emotions may be expressed as chronic derangements of the autonomic nervous system that eventuate in structural (organic) lesions. The best known examples of psychophysiologic diseases are peptic ulcers, bronchial asthma, migraine, and hypertension. These diseases are all very complicated, and the emotional component in one individual may be much greater than in the next. Other examples of diseases that have variable psychophysiologic overlay are neurodermatitis, psoriasis, obesity, anorexia nervosa, visual disturbances, and sexual disorders such as dyspareunia, frigidity, premature ejaculation, and impotence.

GENERAL REFERENCE

Tasman A, Kay J, Lieberman JA (eds): *Psychiatry*. Philadelphia: W.B. Saunders, 1997.

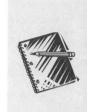

Review Questions

1. Are all mental or psychiatric disorders functional disorders? Why or why not?

2. How do the roles of psychiatrists, psychologists, and social workers differ?

3. Which six mental illnesses account for the most first admissions to mental hospitals?

4. Which mental illnesses account for 80 percent of long-term hospitalizations in mental illness?

5. At what ages do the major mental illnesses most frequently begin?

6. What factors predispose to suicide?

7. What are the major psychiatric emergencies?

8. How do the psychiatric history and mental status examination differ from the usual medical history and physical examination?

9. What are seven major categories of manifestations of psychiatric illness? What terms are used to define the specific manifestations in each category?

10. What criteria are used to classify the major categories of mental illness?

11. What are the causes, lesions (if any), and major manifestations of the specific diseases discussed in this chapter?

12. How do schizophrenia and manic-depressive illness differ?

13. How do anxiety disorders and personality disorders differ?

14. How do patients with symptoms suggestive of but not due to organic lesions create medical problems?

15. What is the meaning of the following terms?
    Organic brain syndrome
    Chronic brain syndrome
    Mental retardation
    Dementia
    Psychosis
    Depression
    Mania

Autism
Factitious disorder
Malingering
Somatoform disorder
Psychosomatic
Psychophysiologic

25.

Endocrine System

REVIEW OF STRUCTURE AND FUNCTION
Organs • Hormones and Their Effects • Feedback Control Mechanism

MOST FREQUENT AND SERIOUS PROBLEMS
Diabetes Mellitus • Goiter • Hyperparathyroidism • Cushing's Syndrome

SYMPTOMS, SIGNS, AND TESTS
Hyposecretion • Hypersecretion • Goiter • Measurement of Hormones • Measurement of Hormone Effects

SPECIFIC DISEASES
Diseases of the Pituitary Gland
Panhypopituitarism
Gigantism and Acromegaly
Diabetes Insipidus
Pituitary Tumors
Diseases of the Thyroid Gland
Hypothyroidism
Hyperthyroidism
Nontoxic Goiter
Thyroid Neoplasms
Diseases of the Parathyroid Glands
Hypoparathyroidism
Hyperparathyroidism
Diseases of the Adrenal Glands
Addison's Disease
Cushing's Syndrome
Conn's Syndrome
Pheochromocytoma
Neuroblastoma

Diseases of the Pancreatic Islets of Langerhans
  Diabetes Mellitus
  Pancreatic Endocrine Tumors
Endocrine Syndromes
  Multiple Endocrine Tumors
  Ectopic Hormone-Producing Cancers
ORGAN FAILURE

REVIEW QUESTIONS

REVIEW OF STRUCTURE AND FUNCTION

The endocrine system is so named because it includes all of those organs, or tissues within organs, that secrete their cellular products (hormones) directly into the bloodstream rather than into viscera, cavities, or outside the body, as is the case with the exocrine glands. Implicit in this definition is the fact that hormones exert their influence on tissues of the body remote from their site of origin. Major endocrine organs or tissues include hypothalamus, posterior and anterior pituitary gland, thyroid gland, parathyroid glands, adrenal cortex and medulla, islets of Langerhans, ovaries, testes, and placenta (Figure 25–1). The hormones produced at each of these sites and their effects are listed in Table 25–1.

The anterior pituitary produces trophic hormones, which serve as intermediates by stimulating hormone production in other organs—adenocorticotropic hormone (ACTH), thyroid-stimulating hormone (TSH), follicle-stimulating hormone (FSH), luteinizing hormone (LH), and others that act directly on target tissues (melanocyte-stimulating hormone, growth hormone [GH], prolactin). The pituitary tropic hormones control hormone production by other endocrine glands, but, in turn, the anterior pituitary's hormone production is controlled by hormones from the hypothalamus. The hypothalamus is a portion of the brain that can monitor hormone levels in the blood and secrete releasing or inhibitory hormones to control the production of pituitary hormones. This control mechanism is illustrated in Figure 25–2.

Posterior pituitary hormones, like hormones from the remainder of the endocrine organs, act directly on target tissues.

In general, hormones regulate the metabolism of the body and its most important constituents and control sexual maturation and pregnancy. Sex organs and their hormones will not be discussed in this chapter (see Chapters 16, 17, and 18). There are other important hormones, not mentioned in Table 25-1, such as the numerous hormones

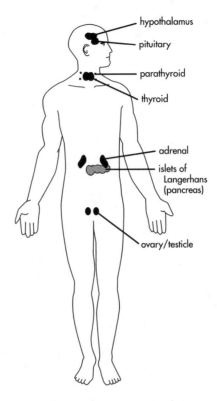

Figure 25–1. Endocrine organs and tissues.

of the gastrointestinal tract. In addition, there are still other hormones that appear to be of little importance or are poorly understood at the present time, such as melatonin of the pineal gland.

MOST FREQUENT AND SERIOUS PROBLEMS

Diabetes mellitus is the most common endocrine disease. It is estimated to affect 1 to 2 percent of adults and increases in frequency with age. Hypothyroidism is also quite common, particularly in women. Goiter (enlargement of the thyroid) may be associated with normal, hypo- or hyperfunction. Hyperparathyroidism is not uncommon and is found with parathyroid adenomas and hyperplasia or is secondary to chronic renal disease. Cushing's syndrome, caused by excess corticosteroids (glucocorticoids) is most commonly caused by the administration of corticosteroids for the treatment of various illnesses such as systemic lupus erthematosus, rheumatoid arthritis, and for the pre-

TABLE 25–1. SITE OF ORIGIN AND EFFECTS OF HORMONES

Site	Hormone (Synonyms, Abbreviations)	Effect
Anterior pituitary	Adrenocorticotropic hormone (corticotropin, ACTH)	Stimulates production of glucocorticoids by adrenal cortex
	Melanocyte-stimulating hormone (MSH)	Stimulates pigment production in skin
	Growth hormone (somatotropin, GH)	Promotes growth of body tissues
	Thyroid-stimulating hormone (thyrotropin, TSH)	Stimulates production and release of thyroid hormones
	Follicle-stimulating hormone (FSH)	Initiates maturation of ovarian follicles Stimulates spermatogenesis
	Luteinizing hormone (LH)	Causes ovulation and stimulates ovary to produce estrogen and progesterone Stimulates androgen production by interstitial cells of testis
	Prolactin	Stimulates secretion of breast milk
Hypothalamus	Releasing hormones	Act on anterior pituitary to cause release of specific hormones
	Inhibitory hormones	Act on anterior pituitary to cause inhibition of release of specific hormones
Posterior pituitary	Antidiuretic hormone (vasopressin, ADH)	Causes conservation of body water by promoting water resorption by renal tubules
	Oxytocin	Stimulates smooth muscle contraction in breast to aid in milk ejection
Thyroid	Thyroxine (tetraiodothyronine, T4)	Increases rate of cellular metabolism Nutritional effects on brain and other organs
	Triiodothyronine (T3)	Same as thyroxine
	Calcitonin	Promotes retention of calcium and phosphorus in bone
Parathyroid	Parathyroid hormone (parathormone, PTH)	Regulates metabolism of calcium and phosphorus Promotes resorption of calcium and phosphorus from bone
Adrenal cortex	Glucocorticoids, mostly cortisol-(hydrocortisone) with some corticosterone	Antagonizes effects of insulin Inhibits inflammatory response and fibroblastic activity Many other effects
	Mineralocorticoid, mainly aldosterone	Promotes retention of sodium by renal tubules
	Androgens	Masculinization
Adrenal medulla	Catecholamines (epinephrine and norepinephrine)	Regulation of blood pressure by effects on vascular smooth muscle and heart
Islets of Langerhans and gastrointestinal tract	Insulin	Promotes utilization of glucose and lipid synthesis
	Glucagon	Promotes utilization of glycogen and lipid

(continued)

TABLE 25–1. *Continued*

Site	Hormone (Synonyms, Abbreviations)	Effect
Ovaries	Estrogens	Cause development of female secondary sex characteristics
		Necessary to maintain menstrual cycle and pregnancy
	Progesterone	Preparation of endometrium for implantation and maintenance of pregnancy
Placenta	Human chorianic gonadotropin (HCG)	Maintains corpus luteum and progesterone production in pregnancy
	Human placental lactogen	Stimulates growth of breasts and has growth hormone-like effects
Testes	Testosterone	Causes development of male secondary sex characterisitics

vention of transplant rejections. The syndrome can also be caused by small tumors of the pituitary gland or the adrenal cortex. Hormone-producing neoplasms are relatively uncommon but cause specific syndromes and are often treatable.

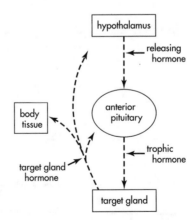

Figure 25–2. Negative feedback control mechanisms for hormones governed by the hypothalamus and anterior pituitary. A stimulating hormone of the hypothalamus causes increased production of the corresponding anterior pituitary hormone, which, in turn, causes the target organ to produce its hormone. The target organ's hormone inhibits the production of stimulating hormone of the hypothalamus, thus shutting off the stimulation until blood levels of the target organ's hormone drop.

SYMPTOMS, SIGNS, AND TESTS

Most endocrine disorders are manifest by hypersecretion or hyposecretion of a hormone. The diagnosis depends upon correctly matching the patient's symptoms and signs with hormone dysfunction and with laboratory confirmation of overproduction or underproduction of a particular hormone. For example, overproduction of insulin will decrease blood sugar levels and the patient will present acutely with measurable hypoglycemia manifested by hunger, pallor, shakiness, and decreased ability to perform mental tasks. All these manifestations result from the body's cells being unable to perform metabolic tasks due to the lack of glucose. On the other hand, too little insulin (diabetes mellitus) leads to elevated blood sugar levels, and the patient presents with excessive urination (polyuria) and excessive drinking (polydipsia). These symptoms occur because the excess glucose along with water is excreted by the kidney. The resultant loss of water leads to dehydration and thirst. Laboratory demonstration of excess glucose in the blood and/or glucose in the urine affords a diagnosis of diabetes mellitus.

The names of the conditions caused by deficiency or excess of the various hormones are given in Table 25–2. The causes and manifestations of the most important ones will be discussed under Specific Diseases.

The only endocrine gland accessible to physical examination is the thyroid gland. Generalized enlargement (goiter) can be nodular

TABLE 25–2. DISEASES ASSOCIATED WITH DEFICIENCY AND EXCESS OF VARIOUS HORMONES

Hormone	Hormone-Deficiency Diseases	Diseases Associated with Excess Hormone
Adrenocorticotropic hormone	Addison's disease	Cushing's syndrome
Growth hormone	Pituitary dwarfism	Gigantism; acromegaly
Antidiuretic hormone	Diabetes insipious	Inappropriate ADH-secretion syndrome
Thyroid hormones	Cretinism; hypothyroidism	Hyperthyroidism
Parathyroid hormone	Hypoparathyroidism	Hyperparathyroidism
Glucocorticoids	Addison's disease	Cushing's syndrome
Mineralocorticoids	May occur as part of Addison's disease	Conn's syndrome (hyperaldosteronism)
Insulin	Diabetes mellitus	Insulin shock

or diffuse; localized nodules, cysts, and masses can also be felt. Neoplasms of other endocrine organs are detected by the effects of the mass, by the effects of hormones produced by the neoplasm (functional neoplasm), or by hypofunction if the neoplasm replaces the normal glandular tissue.

The major hormones or their breakdown products can be measured directly in the blood or urine by laboratory analysis. These include the thyroid hormones; various steroid hormones of the adrenal cortices, ovaries, and testes; the catecholamines of the adrenal medulla; and growth hormone and prolactin of the pituitary. Indirect assessment of endocrine function may be accomplished by measuring blood or urine chemicals that are affected by a particular hormone. For instance, the presence of too little insulin may be inferred by finding too much glucose in the blood and urine. The status of the parathyroid glands may be evaluated by measurements of blood and urine calcium and phosphorus levels, because the metabolism of these substances is regulated by parathormone.

SPECIFIC DISEASES

Diseases of the Pituitary Gland

The anterior lobe of the pituitary is composed of epithelial cells that secrete various hormones. The posterior lobe is an extension of the brain composed of nerve fibers with neurosecretory granules. Disease of the anterior lobe consists of destructive conditions and adenomas. Disease of the posterior lobe is caused by destructive lesions.

Panhypopituitarism
Destruction of the anterior pituitary gland leads to panhypopituitarism. The most common causes of this rare condition are neoplasms of the pituitary that are large enough to destroy the gland, postpartum pituitary necrosis, and surgical removal of the pituitary for treatment of tumors. The pituitary is hyperplastic during pregnancy and thus more susceptible to infarction caused by an episode of hypotension as a result of excess bleeding from childbirth. Persons with panhypopituitarism have atrophy of the thyroid, adrenal cortex, and gonads, with variable secondary effects of hypothyroidism, adrenal insufficiency, and decreased libido or secondary sex characteristics, depending on the age of onset. There may be growth retardation from growth hormone deficiency. Although lethal if not treated, panhypopituitarism is readily treated by replacing trophic hormones.

PANHYPOPITUITARISM 25-1

causes	lesions	manifestations
Pituitary neoplasms Postpartum hypotension Surgical removal Other destructive processes	Infarct, replacement or pressure atrophy Inflammation	Decreased sexual function Hypothyroidism Adrenocortical insufficiency Decreased pigmentation Decreased lactation postpartum Decreased growth in children

Gigantism and Acromegaly

Excess growth hormone (GH) leads to enlargement of all tissues; however, bone enlargement is the most prominent clinical finding. In children, bones can grow longer as well as wider, leading to gigantism. In adults, excess GH causes thickening of soft tissue and bones—a condition called acromegaly. Patients suffer early debilitation because of bone and joint disease and die prematurely of cardiac dysfunction. Acromegalics have large hands and prominent coarse facial features (Figure 25–3). Gigantism and acromegaly are caused by pituitary adenomas that secrete GH and are treated by removal of the neoplasm,

GIGANTISM AND ACROMEGALY 25-2

cause	lesion	manifestations
Growth-hormone- secreting pituitary adenoma	Enlargement of body tissues, especially bones and soft tissues	Rapid increase in height of children (gigantism) Enlarged hands and coarse facial features in adults (acromegaly) Enlarged pituitary fossa by x-ray Increased serum growth hormone

causes	lesion	manifestations
Neoplasms	Destruction of posterior	Polyuria
Inflammation	pituitary and/or	Polydipsia
Histiocytic infiltration	hypothalamus	Special tests for
Trauma		hormone function
Surgical complications		

DIABETES INSIPIDUS **25-3**

by drugs that inhibit GH secretion (somatostatin analogues) or by radiation to decrease the size of the neoplasm.

Diabetes Insipidus

Destruction of the posterior pituitary and/or hypothalamus leads to decreased antidiuretic hormone and, thus, to diabetes insipidus. Diabetes insipidus is excessive urination due to failure of water reabsorption in the kidney, resulting from deficiency of antidiuretic hormone. The excess urination (polyuria) leads to excess thirst (polydipsia). This rare condition is caused by infiltrative processes such as neoplasms, and meningitis; by head injury; and, sometimes, by surgical operations in the area. Prognosis depends on the nature of the cause. Hormone replacement therapy is available.

Pituitary Tumors

Adenomas of the anterior pituitary and craniopharyngiomas are the most common types. Many pituitary adenomas do not secrete enough hormone to produce endocrine effects; they more often grow slowly and eventually compress the optic nerve to produce visual field defects. Functioning pituitary adenomas may produce gigantism, acromegaly, Cushing's syndrome, lactation, or amenorrhea, depending on the cell type of the neoplasm. Craniopharyngioma is a benign but locally aggressive tumor containing squamous cell elements that are derived from the embryonic remnant of Rathke's pouch. Craniopharyngiomas are most common in children, while pituitary adenomas are usually found in adults. Pituitary tumors can be cured if they can be removed, but this is often difficult because of their infiltration into surrounding vital structures. Some can be managed by drugs that suppress hormone hypersecretion and may cause tumor shrinkage.

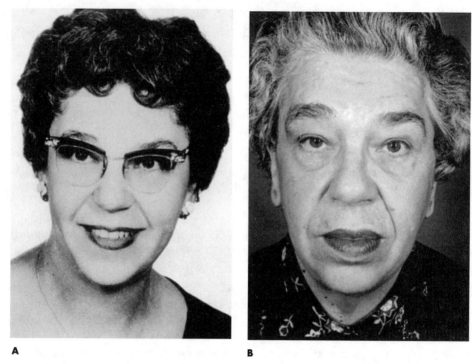

A   **B**

Figure 25–3. Face before (A) and after (B) development of acromegaly.

Diseases of the Thyroid Gland

The thyroid gland, which consists of two lobes connected by an isthmus, lies in the neck anterior and lateral to the trachea. It consists of acini that secrete a colloid substance containing thyroid hormones. Calcitonin-secreting C cells are present in the stroma but are not conspicuous. Idiopathic hypothyroidism, Hashimoto's disease, Graves' disease, nodular goiter, adenoma, and papillary carcinoma are the most common conditions of the thyroid gland.

Hypothyroidism

Hypothyroidism is much more commonly due to destruction or atrophy of the thyroid gland than it is to thyroid-stimulating hormone deficiency (hypopituitarism). Destruction of the thyroid gland most commonly results from treatment of hyperthyroidism with radioactive iodine. Destruction of the thyroid gland may be necessary to control hyperthyroidism; the resultant hypothyroidism can be treated by administering thyroid hormone to the patient.

The most common natural form of hypothyroidism is associated with atrophy and fibrosis. Atrophy and fibrosis may be idiopathic or may be part of the syndrome called *Hashimoto's disease.* Hashimoto's disease is generally considered to be an autoimmune disease, with destruction of thyroid due to lymphocytes reacting to the body's own tissue. In the early stages of Hashimoto's disease, the thyroid gland is enlarged but usually maintains normal function. It is thought that Hashimoto's disease progresses with time to atrophy and fibrosis, but more patients present with end-stage disease with hypothyroidism than present in the early stage with enlarged thyroid and euthyroidism (normal function). Thus, the most common cause of spontaneous hypothyroidism is variously referred to as idiopathic or Hashimoto's disease. The atrophy and fibrosis are thought to be caused by destruction of the thyroid epithelial cells by lymphocytes sensitized to thyroid epithelial cells. Hypothyroidism is occasionally caused by severe iodine deficiency and other rare conditions of the thyroid.

The results of hypothyroidism are similar regardless of cause. Since the normal action of thyroid hormone is to stimulate cellular metabolism, it is not surprising that patients with hypothyroidism present with slowness in muscular action and slowness in intellectual processes. In addition, they usually feel cold much of the time and have a sallow complexion, dry hair, and dry skin. Patients with prolonged hypothyroidism may develop deposits of mucopolysaccharides in skin, muscle, and viscera, producing a doughy edema called *myxedema*. Diagnosis of hypothyroidism is suspected from the clinical findings and confirmed by one or more laboratory tests that indicate a low level of circulating thyroid hormone, an elevated TSH level, or an abnormally low uptake of radioactive iodine-131.

As with other thyroid diseases, women are much more frequently affected than men. The severity of hypothyroidism varies greatly among patients, and diagnosis depends on careful consideration of laboratory data and clinical observations. In most cases, little can be done about the cause, but replacement therapy with thyroid hormone is effective.

HYPOTHYROIDISM   25-4

causes	lesions	manifestations
Treatment of hyperthyroidism	Destruction, atrophy, fibrosis	Decreased activity
Hashimoto's disease (autoimmune thyroiditis)	Lymphocytic infiltration (Hashimoto's disease)	Intolerance to cold Dry hair and skin Myxedema
Iodine deficiency (some cases)	Changes in connective tissue	Decreased T3 and T4 Decreased I^{131} uptake
Idiopathic		

Hyperthyroidism

Hyperthyroidism may occasionally occur with nodular goiter or a secreting thyroid neoplasm, but the majority of cases are due to Graves' disease.

Graves' disease is a condition of unknown cause but is thought to be due to stimulation of the thyroid by an antibody to the TSH receptor because the antibody mimics TSH and stimulates the thyroid to produce hormones. Graves' disease is characterized by one or more of the following features: hyperthyroidism with diffuse goiter, ophthalmopathy, or dermopathy (Figure 25–4). Hyperthyroidism is the most

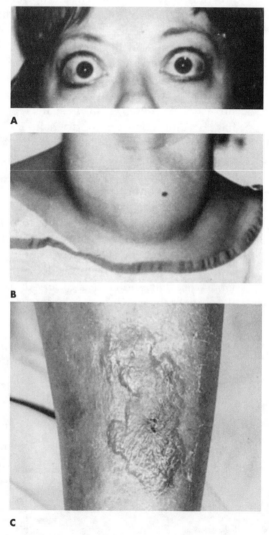

Figure 25–4. Graves' disease with exophthalmos (A), goiter (B), and pretibial myxedema (C).

common. In Graves' disease, the thyroid gland undergoes hyperplasia, and there is an associated lymphocytic infiltration. The hyperplastic gland secretes thyroid hormone despite the fact that production of thyroid-stimulating hormone in the pituitary is suppressed by the high serum levels of thyroid hormone.

Common manifestations of hyperthyroidism, regardless of cause, include tremor of extended fingers and tongue, increased nervousness, emotional instability, excessive sweating, heat intolerance, rapid heartbeat, increased motor activity, and weight loss. The increased metabolic activity associated with hyperthyroidism may lead with time to heart failure and muscle degeneration (thyrotoxic myopathy).

The ophthalmopathy and dermopathy of Graves' disease are not associated with other causes of hyperthyroidism. The eye changes are due to swelling of the soft tissues of the orbit, leading to protrusion of the eye (exophthalmos) and weakness of the eye muscles. The skin changes consist of localized raised thickening of the skin of the dorsum of the legs called *pretibial myxedema*. Graves' disease most commonly begins in young adult women and is progressive, although variable in severity.

Hyperthyroidism must be differentiated from anxiety states, which may mimic many of the nervous symptoms. The measurement of the thyroid hormone blood level is the best test for the demonstration of hyperthyroidism.

Treatment of hyperthyroidism may involve drugs to suppress thyroid function or reduction in thyroid tissue by surgical removal or administration of radioactive iodine. Iodine is selectively taken up by thyroid tissue, so radioactive damage can be safely limited to the thyroid.

 HYPERTHYROIDISM   **25-5**

causes	lesions	manifestations
Graves' disease	Diffuse hyperplasia and	Tremor
Toxic nodular goiter	lymphocytic infiltration	Nervousness
Thyroid neoplasms	(Graves' disease)	Emotional instability
(some)	Hyperplastic nodule or	Heat intolerance
	secretory neoplasm	Rapid heartbeat
		Weight loss
		Enlarged thyroid
		Muscle weakness
		Heart failure (late)
		Increased T3 and T4
		Increased I^{131} uptake
		Exophthalmos in
		Graves' disease

Nontoxic Goiter

Generalized enlargement of the thyroid with normal or low thyroid function is termed *nontoxic goiter.* Nontoxic goiter is very common in inland and mountainous areas of the world where there is a deficiency of iodine in the soil and water. Iodine deficiency produces a prolonged, low-grade hyperplasia of the gland that may lead to massive enlargement. The use of iodized salts greatly reduces the prevalence of goiter, but does not eliminate it. Nontoxic goiter in the United States is most often idiopathic or due to Hashimoto's disease.

Idiopathic goiter may be diffuse with increased colloid secretions in the acini (colloid goiter) or nodular due to irregular proliferation with fibrosis (nodular goiter). The nodules of nodular goiter may become large enough to require biopsy to differentiate them from neoplasms. Occasionally, nodules may become functional, resulting in toxic nodular goiter.

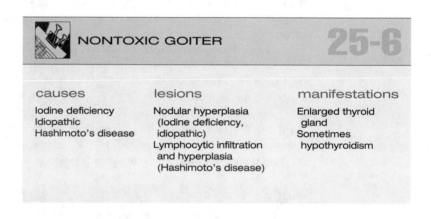

NONTOXIC GOITER   **25-6**

causes	lesions	manifestations
Iodine deficiency	Nodular hyperplasia	Enlarged thyroid
Idiopathic	(Iodine deficiency,	gland
Hashimoto's disease	idiopathic)	Sometimes
	Lymphocytic infiltration	hypothyroidism
	and hyperplasia	
	(Hashimoto's disease)	

Thyroid Neoplasms

Adenoma of the thyroid has a variable frequency in different geographic locations. It is a solitary nodule of thyroid acini surrounded by a fibrous tissue capsule. Similar-appearing nodules are found in some nodular goiters. Thyroid adenomas are removed to differentiate them from thyroid carcinoma and occasionally because they are functional. Thyroid carcinoma differs from most other carcinomas in that it occurs predominantly in young adult women and is most often well differentiated, with a papillary growth pattern. Surgical removal often results in a cure. A small percentage of thyroid carcinomas can be causally linked to radiation of the neck region in childhood. A rare type of thyroid carcinoma, called *medullary carcinoma* because the cells occur in solid masses rather than producing glands, arises from the calcitonin-secreting cells of the thyroid.

Diseases of the Parathyroid Glands

Two to six (usually four) tiny glands composed of epithelial cells that secrete parathormone are located adjacent to the inferior and superior aspects of each thyroid lobe. Hyperfunction from adenoma or hyperplasia is the main disease of the parathyroid.

Hypoparathyroidism

Most cases of hypoparathyroidism result from surgical removal of all four parathyroid glands, an uncommon complication of the treatment of hyperparathyroidism or of surgical removal of the thyroid gland. Hypoparathyroidism leads to decreased serum calcium, which, in turn, is manifested by increased irritability of muscle (tetany) and convulsions. Treatment consists of calcium supplements and a synthetic vitamin D derivative.

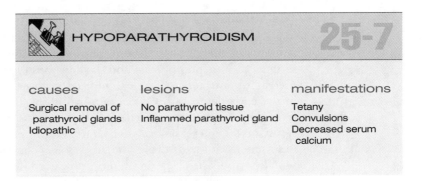

HYPOPARATHYROIDISM		25-7
causes	**lesions**	**manifestations**
Surgical removal of parathyroid glands Idiopathic	No parathyroid tissue Inflamed parathyroid gland	Tetany Convulsions Decreased serum calcium

Hyperparathyroidism

Hyperparathyroidism is a relatively common and important disease that may be mild and go undetected for a long time. Primary hyperparathyroidism occurs when the cause of increased parathyroid hormone production lies in the parathyroid glands and production is not controlled by normal feedback mechanisms. The causes are adenoma (80%), hyperplasia (18%), and carcinoma (2%). Secondary hyperparathyroidism occurs with conditions associated with low serum calcium, most often chronic renal failure or vitamin D deficiency. The metabolic changes in secondary hyperparathyroidism are quite complex and will not be further discussed.

In primary hyperparathyroidism, the excess parathyroid hormone causes increased breakdown of bone, increased absorption of calcium by the intestine, increased reabsorption of calcium by the kidney, and increased loss of phosphate in the urine. The net effect is to increase serum calcium and decrease serum phosphate. Urine calcium is also

HYPERPARATHYROIDISM   25-8

causes	lesions	manifestations
Primary	Resorption of bone	Flank pain from renal
Adenoma	Renal calculi	calculi
Hyperplasia	Causative lesion	Bone pain and
Carcinoma		pathologic fracture
Secondary		Increased serum
Chronic renal disease		calcium and alkaline
Vitamin D deficiency		phosphatase
		Decreased serum
		phosphate

increased, because the increase in glomerular filtration of calcium is greater than the increase in reabsorption by the renal tubules.

As osteoblasts attempt to repair the bone destruction, increased amounts of the enzyme alkaline phosphatase are released into the serum. Calcium, phosphorus, and alkaline phosphatase are commonly used as routine biochemical screening tests; thus, there has been a rise in the early detection of hyperparathyroidism. If not discovered by screening, the disease most commonly presents with renal calculi as a result of the increased calcium and phosphorus excretion. Bone destruction with pathologic fracture is a less common mode of presentation and is associated with more advanced disease.

The bone lesions are characterized by the presence of giant multinucleated osteoclasts and fibrosis, sometimes with cyst formation (osteitis fibrosa cystica). The bone resorption is commonly detected by x-rays of the hands and teeth, where subperiosteal resorption of bone and loss of the lamina dura are seen. Primary hyperparathyroidism is treated by removal of the adenoma, hyperplastic glands, or carcinoma.

Diseases of the Adrenal Glands

The two adrenal glands are located deep within the abdomen embedded in adipose tissue above each kidney. Cortical epithelial cells secrete glucocorticoids, mineralocorticoids, and androgens, while the neural-derived chromaffin cells of the medulla secrete hormones involved in control of the vascular system. Lesions of the adrenal are relatively uncommon and consist of destructive diseases of the cortex, hyperplasias and neoplasms that produce hypersecretion, and two neoplasms of the medulla, neuroblastoma in children and pheochromocytoma in adults.

Addison's Disease

Addison's disease is an uncommon condition characterized by insufficient production of adrenocortical hormones. The most common cause is idiopathic atrophy, thought by some to be autoimmune because of the lymphocytic infiltration of the adrenal cortex, presence of antibodies to adrenal tissue, and association with other presumed autoimmune diseases. Tuberculosis of the adrenal glands was formerly the most common cause. The deficient production of corticosteroids leads to increased release of the stimulatory hormone ACTH. ACTH also causes an MSH-like effect, which accounts for the increased skin pigmentation characteristic of Addison's disease. Other symptoms are often gradual in onset and not specific for Addison's disease, so the diagnosis is easily overlooked. These symptoms include tiredness, anorexia, nausea, weight loss, fainting due to hypotension or hypoglycemia, loss of body hair, and depression. Hormone levels can be measured to confirm the diagnosis. Symptoms may become acute and life threatening, with diarrhea, weakness, and hypotension. Acute insufficiency is likely to be precipitated by stress or infection. Immediate treatment with glucocorticoids and intravenous fluids containing salt and sugar are needed. The chronic condition can be controlled by corticosteroid therapy.

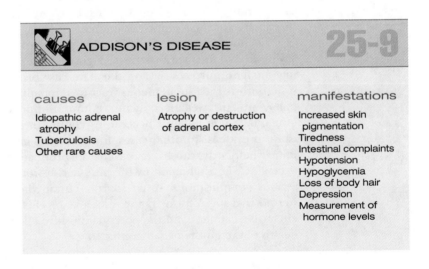

ADDISON'S DISEASE   25-9

causes	lesion	manifestations
Idiopathic adrenal atrophy	Atrophy or destruction of adrenal cortex	Increased skin pigmentation
Tuberculosis		Tiredness
Other rare causes		Intestinal complaints
		Hypotension
		Hypoglycemia
		Loss of body hair
		Depression
		Measurement of hormone levels

Cushing's Syndrome

Cushing's syndrome is the result of excess corticosteroids, predominantly glucocorticoids, regardless of whether due to excessive stimulation of the adrenals by ACTH, to primary overproduction by the adrenals, or to exogenous administration of corticosteroids. The most common cause is iatrogenic, the use of corticosteroids in the treat-

CUSHING'S SYNDROME 25-10

causes	lesions	manifestations
Increased pituitary production of ACTH	Obesity	Obesity of face and trunk
Cortisol-secreting adrenal adenoma or carcinoma	Osteoporosis	Purple striae
		Easily bruised
ACTH-secreting carcinoma		Hypertension
Iatrogenic corticosteroids or ACTH		Osteoporosis leading to fractures
		Hirsutism
		Psychosis
		Muscle weakness
		Hyperglycemia
		Special lab tests

ment of other diseases. Noniatrogenic Cushing's syndrome may be caused by adrenal hyperplasia resulting from production of ACTH by pituitary hyperplasia or tumor, by corticosteroid-secreting adenomas or carcinomas of the adrenal cortex, or by ACTH-secreting carcinomas such as bronchogenic carcinoma.

The most obvious effect of Cushing's syndrome is a peculiar obesity limited to the face and trunk (Figure 25–5). Other common findings include purple striae on the skin, easy bruising, hypertension, osteoporosis with spontaneous fractures, hirsuitism (increased body hair), muscle weakness, acne, immunosuppression, and hyperglycemia. Some patients become psychotic. In iatrogenic cases, the cause is evident. In other cases, function tests can be used to determine whether the cause is excess cortisol production by the adrenal or excess ACTH production by the pituitary. It would appear that such serious complications would sharply curtail the use of exogenous steroid therapy. Yet, for many diseases, steroids are by far the most effective treatment and the potential positive effects on the patient's health outweigh the negative effects.

Conn's Syndrome

Primary overproduction of mineralocorticoids (aldosterone) leads to Conn's syndrome. The cause is usually an aldosterone-secreting adenoma of the adrenal cortex. There is excess excretion of potassium and retention of sodium. The decreased serum potassium levels are associated with increased urine output and muscular weakness. Salt retention is associated with hypertension. The rare cases of Conn's syn-

CONN'S SYNDROME

25-11

cause	lesion	manifestations
Aldosterone-secreting adrenal adenoma	Adenoma of adrenal cortex	Muscle weakness Increased urination Hypertension Low serum potassium High serum sodium Other special tests

drome must be distinguished from the more common causes of secondary aldosterone overproduction, which include heart failure, cirrhosis of the liver, nephrotic syndrome, renal ischemia, and essential hypertension. Removal of the adenoma is curative in Conn's syndrome.

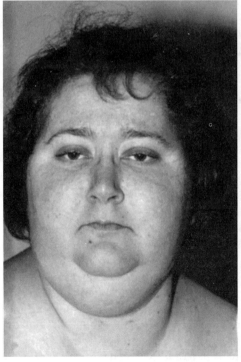 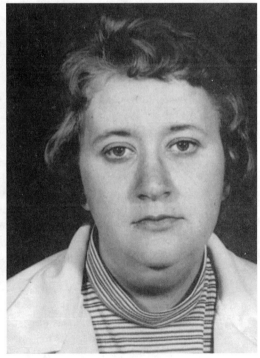

A **B**

Figure 25–5. A. Facial obesity and swelling of Cushing's syndrome. B. Same patient after removal of functional adrenal adenoma.

Pheochromocytoma

This is a neoplasm of the chromaffin cells of the adrenal medulla that produces catecholamines with resultant hypertension. It is usually a benign neoplasm but is occasionally malignant. Although it is a rare cause of hypertension, it is important to diagnose, because removal will cure the hypertension. Episodes of sweating and nervousness often accompany the hypertension. Measurement of a catecholamine breakdown product—vanilmandelic acid (VMA)—in the urine is helpful in diagnosis.

Neuroblastoma

Neoplasms of neural cells are particularly common in the adrenal in children under 5 years of age. Poorly differentiated neoplasms are called neuroblastoma, and they usually metastasize widely and kill the patient.

Diseases of the Pancreatic Islets of Langerhans

Myriads of small clusters of endocrine cells that develop from pancreatic ductules are scattered throughout the pancreas, particularly in the tail. The various cell types in the islets secrete different hormones— glucagon (A cell), insulin (B cell), somatostatin (D cell), and pancreatic polypeptide (PP cell). Diabetes mellitus is the major disease related to insulin secretion of the islets. Pancreatic endocrine tumors, although uncommon, are of interest because they become manifest due to excessive secretion of any one of several hormones.

Diabetes Mellitus

Diabetes mellitus is a disease condition in which there is more or less persistent hyperglycemia with loss of glucose homeostasis. Since insulin helps determine blood glucose levels, partly by controlling cellular uptake of glucose, diabetes mellitus is sometimes defined as a relative or absolute deficiency of insulin.

Insulin is normally produced by the B cells of the pancreatic islets of Langerhans. Lack of insulin may result from diminished production of insulin, faulty release of insulin, antibodies to insulin, and abnormalities of the body's cells precluding normal action of insulin. All cases of diabetes cannot be explained by any one of these mechanisms.

Occasional cases of diabetes are due to destructive diseases of the pancreas such as chronic pancreatitis or hemochromatosis, but the vast majority fall into one of two types called insulin-dependent diabetes mellitus (IDDM) or type I (formerly called juvenile-onset diabetes) and non–insulin-dependent diabetes mellitus (NIDDM) or type II (formerly called adult-onset diabetes).

The major differences between type I and type II diabetes mellitus are shown in Table 25–3. Both types have a multifactorial etiology

TABLE 25–3. INSULIN-DEPENDENT AND NON–INSULIN-DEPENDENT DIABETES MELLITUS

	IDDM (Type I)	NIDDM (Type II)
Age	Usually in children or young adults	Usually after age 25 Frequency increases with age
Onset	Generally abrupt Often triggered by infection	More often insidious Patients often obese
Treatment	Insulin	Often controlled by diet
Complications	Occur early Often severe, especially retinal, renal, and heart disease	Full range of complications Tend to develop more slowly and be less severe

involving both genetic and nongenetic factors. Neither type exhibits a Mendelian-type inheritance pattern. IDDM appears to be less dependent on genetic factors—if one identical twin has the disease, the other one only has a 50 percent chance of developing it, compared to 90 percent with NIDDM. However, IDDM is associated with certain histocompatibility antigens (HLA types) and antibodies to pancreatic islet cells; whereas, NIDDM is not. A person with NIDDM is more likely to have relatives with the disease than one with IDDM.

Nongenetic etiologic factors are also different for the two diseases. With IDDM, insulin production becomes deficient abruptly over a few days to weeks. At onset, most patients are under age 30, but may be older. An immunologic or viral injury is postulated as the cause in susceptible individuals. The initial lesions involve reduction in the number of insulin-producing B cells in the islets of Langerhans in the pancreas. Later, some patients have hyalinized islets, others appear relatively normal by light microscopy, but special studies can demonstrate the decrease in insulin-producing cells.

In contrast to the absolute lack of insulin in IDDM, with NIDDM there is only a relative lack of insulin and this is associated with inappropriate insulin release and peripheral cellular resistance to the effects of insulin. Major nongenetic factors producing NIDDM are those that stress glucose metabolism such as obesity, pregnancy, infections, and corticosteroid therapy. NIDDM has a gradual onset, usually in persons over 40 years of age, and responds to treatment that decreases stress on glucose metabolism.

The clinical manifestations of diabetes mellitus are initially due to abnormalities of glucose metabolism. Years later complicating lesions develop. Normally, insulin regulates the uptake and utilization of glucose by cells. The diabetic, therefore, has high levels of blood glucose and deficient cellular glucose. Because of this, the diabetic relies on lipids for energy, with excessive production of acetylcoenzyme A and ketone bodies resulting in acidosis. Coenzyme A enhances the production of cholesterol, which, in turn, may be partially responsible for the increased frequency of severe atherosclerosis in diabetics.

Classically, patients with diabetes present with polydipsia (excessive drinking) and polyuria (increased urination) as the initial manifestations of the disease. This is due to the hyperosmolality of the blood, which results from the increased glucose levels. Generalized weakness, increased tendency to infection, and poor wound healing are also commonly present in the initial stages. These symptoms of diabetes are related to excess blood glucose and also to increased breakdown of lipids, resulting in acidosis. Severe acidosis is characteristic of IDDM and if not treated with insulin the patient will die. After diagnosis, patients may maintain a relatively normal life if glucose metabolism is controlled by therapy (insulin for IDDM, dietary manipulation for NIDDM).

Complications of diabetes mellitus are the same for both types and are predominantly vascular. Complications tend to be more severe with IDDM, probably because the disease is more severe and begins at a much earlier age. The severity and time of development of these complications are not very predictable. They develop over many years.

Most diabetics die from the effects of atherosclerosis, but so do most nondiabetics. Persons with IDDM may die from myocardial infarcts or other atherosclerotic lesions at an early age, which is clearly beyond the norm. Persons with NIDDM die from atherosclerosis at ages that overlap with those of nondiabetics, but statistically they die younger and have more severe atherosclerosis. Myocardial infarct is the most common complication of atherosclerosis in diabetics, but it should be noted that diabetics have a disproportionate amount of vascular disease in the lower extremities leading to gangrene and amputation. The latter is often referred to as "diabetic gangrene," although it is no different than that occurring in nondiabetics.

In addition to accelerated atherosclerosis, diabetics have a more specific microangiopathy characterized by basement membrane thickening and other changes in small vessels. Angiopathy tends to develop in the retina and renal glomeruli at about the same time, leading to blindness and renal failure, respectively (see Chapters 16 and 20). Diabetic neuropathy, which is thought to be due in part to angiopathy involving nerves, has a variable distribution and may result in loss of sensation, neuromuscular weakness, or involvement of the autonomic nervous system with symptoms of delayed emptying of the stomach or bladder and impotence.

Many other conditions have been associated with diabetes. Increased susceptibility to infection is probably the most important.

The infections are not different than those that occur in nondiabetics except for frequency and severity.

The diagnosis and treatment of IDDM, which accounts for only 10 percent of patients with diabetes, is relatively straightforward. The abrupt onset calls attention to the disease, urinary and blood glucose levels are distinctly abnormal, and the response to insulin therapy is predictable. Management of the disease requires education of the patient and careful monitoring of therapy. The long-term goal is to prevent the development of complications. Clinical studies have shown that fight control of glucose metabolism prevents the late vascular complications. Implantable devices are being developed to automatically measure blood glucose levels and release the appropriate amount of insulin. The possibility of islet cell transplantation is also under investigation.

Diagnosis of NIDDM is more arbitrary and treatment less specific. When a patient develops symptoms of diabetes, spills glucose in the urine, and has a fasting blood glucose level over 140 mg/dl, the diagnosis of NIDDM is not difficult. The diagnostic problem relates to defining normal glucose levels, which vary with age, and deciding whether patients with chemical abnormalities should be labeled as diabetics.

The diagnostic test for borderline cases is the glucose tolerance test. Serum glucose is measured in the fasting state and 1, 2, and 3 hours after ingesting a defined amount of glucose. Table 25–4 shows a point system for making a diagnosis of diabetes developed by the U.S. Public Health Service. Only about half of asymptomatic diabetics diagnosed by these chemical criteria develop overt decompensation of carbohydrate metabolism within 10 years. NIDDM can often be controlled by a reduction in food intake, since most of these patients are overweight. Some diabetics of intermediate severity are treated with sul-

TABLE 25–4. DIAGNOSIS OF DIABETES BY GLUCOSE TOLERANCE TEST

Time	Plasma Glucose, mg/dl	Points[a]
Fasting	>130	1
1 hour	>195	½
2 hours	>140[b]	½
3 hours	>130	1

[a]Total of 2 or more – diabetes. Total of 1 or more but less than 2 – possible diabetes.
[b]Add 10 for each decade over 50.

fonylurea compounds, which enhance the release of insulin from pancreatic beta cells and also lessens the insulin resistance. In any diabetic, treatment consists of careful monitoring of the blood sugar, food intake, and insulin requirements as well as anticipation and treatment of complications of the disease.

Pancreatic Endocrine Tumors

Insulinomas are uncommon neoplasms of B cells that secrete insulin. They are manifest by attacks of confusion, stupor, and loss of consciousness associated with low blood sugar and relieved by eating. In most instances, surgical removal of a solitary adenoma effects a cure, but occasional multiple adenomas or malignant pancreatic endocrine tumors are encountered. Gastrinomas are pancreatic endocrine tumors that secrete gastrin, a hormone normally secreted by the stomach to increase its acid production. The ectopic hormone production causes Zollinger-Ellison's syndrome, which is characterized by severe, recurrent peptic ulcers. Gastrinomas are more often malignant than benign. Rarer types of pancreatic endocrine tumors are glucagonoma and somatostatinoma, which produce a diabetic-like illness, and vipoma, which produces diarrhea, hypokalemia (potassium loss), and achlorhydria.

Endocrine Syndromes

Multiple Endocrine Tumors

There are at least two familial syndromes in which tumors of several endocrine organs occur in family members. In type I, there are commonly adenomas of pituitary, parathyroid, adrenal cortex and pancreatic islets. The pancreatic endocrine neoplasms frequently secrete gastrin, a hormone that causes increased gastric acid production, leading to peptic ulcers. The inheritance pattern is incomplete dominant, and the clinical presentation may relate to one or more of the neoplasms present. In type II, there commonly are medullary carcinomas of the thyroid, less frequently pheochromocytomas, parathyroid hyperplasia, and rare neuromas. Type II syndromes are dominantly inherited and are due to mutations of a gene on chromosome 10 called *fet*. Screening for mutations in children of these families can prevent the development of potentially lethal medullary thyroid carcinoma because the thyroid gland can be removed prophylactically.

Ectopic Hormone-Producing Cancers

Endocrine cells are widely distributed throughout the body in tissues that are not classical endocrine organs. Cancers arising from these cells can produce hormones. A poorly differentiated form of bronchogenic carcinoma, called oat cell or small cell carcinoma because of its small, uniform cells, is sometimes associated with ectopic hormone production. Other types of cancer are more rarely involved. Hormone production may be responsible for the initial manifestations of the cancer or may be a problem to be dealt with in the treatment of a known cancer. ACTH, the most common ectopic hormone produced by cancers, leads to Cushing's syndrome.

Certain neoplasms, especially bronchogenic carcinomas of the lung, produce antidiuretic hormone (inappropriate antidiuretic hormone secretion), which leads to water intoxication by causing excess reabsorption of water by the kidneys. Water intoxication is associated with depression, lethargy, mental confusion, irritability, anorexia, nausea, and weakness. Electrolytes (sodium, potassium, and chloride) are lost in the urine while water is reabsorbed, resulting in dilute serum and relatively concentrated urine. Serum sodium levels are very low.

Many other hormones can be produced by endocrine cancers throughout the body, and more than one hormone can be produced by a particular cancer.

ORGAN FAILURE

Failure of each of the major endocrine organs has been mentioned under hypofunction in the preceding sections. Acute failure that is life threatening occurs with lack of parathyroid hormone, adrenocorticosteroids, and insulin. Failure of the pituitary and thyroid lead to more gradual changes that may cause premature death.

Review Questions

1. What are the most common endocrine disorders?
2. What are the names applied to syndromes of excess or deficiency of ACTH, growth hormone, antidiuretic hormone, thyroid hormones, parathyroid hormone, glucocorticoids, mineralocorticoids, and insulin?
3. Why are hormones sometimes measured directly and other times measured indirectly?
4. What are the causes, lesions, and manifestations of hyposecretion and hypersecretion of the pituitary, thyroid, parathyroid, and adrenal glands and the islets of Langerhans?
5. What are the neoplasms of the endocrine system that are commonly functional? What are the usual manifestations of nonfunctional types?
6. How do insulin-dependent and noninsulin-dependent diabetes differ in cause, presenting manifestations, and complications?
7. What do the following terms mean?
   Craniopharyngioma
   Hashimoto's disease
   Myxedema
   Graves' disease
   Exophthalmos
   Pretibial myxedema
   Goiter
   Ganglioneuroma
   Inappropriate antidiuretic hormone secretion

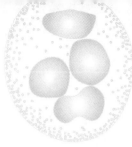

MULTIPLE ORGAN SYSTEM DISEASES

The purposes of this section are (1) to discuss groups of diseases that frequently involve more than one organ system and (2) to provide a broader overview of some of the diseases that have been encountered in Section III. Chapters 26 through 29 cover many diseases and are organized by cause or causative mechanism (infections, immune reactions, physical injury, chemical injury). Chapter 30 reviews diseases caused by under- and over-nutrition.

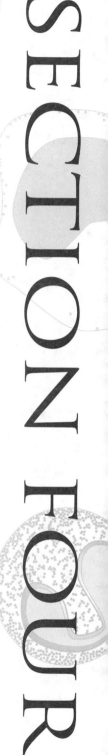

SECTION FOUR

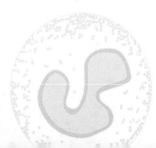

26.

Infectious Diseases

INFECTION AND THE BODY'S DEFENSE MECHANISMS

Saprophytes • Normal Flora • Pathogens • Infection • Vectors • Structural Barriers • Inflammatory Process • Immune System

MOST FREQUENT AND SERIOUS PROBLEMS

Overall Impact of Infectious Disease
Respiratory Illnesses • Pneumonia • Secondary (Opportunistic Infections)

Bacterial Infections
Abscesses, Pneumonia, and Wound Infections • Venereal Diseases

Viral Infections
Upper Respiratory Illnesses • Gastroenteritis • Influenza • Cold Sores • Infections of Childhood • Infectious Mononucleosis • Hepatitis • Squamous Papillomas • AIDS

Rickettsial Infections

Fungal Infections
Superficial • Primary Disseminated Infections • Opportunistic Infections

Protozoal Infections
Malaria • Trichomonas Vaginitis • Cryptosporidiosis

Helminth Infections
Schistosomiasis • Tapeworm Disease • Pinworm Infestation • Ascaris Infestation

SYMPTOMS, SIGNS, AND TESTS
Acute Presentation • Rashes • Cardinal Signs of Inflammation • Cultures • Smears • Immunologic Tests • Nonspecific Tests

SPECIFIC DISEASES

Bacterial Infections in General

Pyogenic Bacterial Infections
Staphylococcal Infections
Group A Streptococcal Infections

Streptococcus viridans Infection
Streptococcus Pneumoniae (Pneumococcus) Infection
Meningococcal Meningitis
Hemophilus influenzae Infection
Legionellosis
Enteric Bacterial Infections
Anaerobic Bacterial Infections
Sexually Transmitted Bacterial Infections
Sexually Transmitted Disease in General
Gonorrhea
Nongonococcal Urethritis
Syphilis
Bacterial Infections Mediated by Exotoxins
Tetanus
Botulism
Gas Gangrene
Diphtheria
Miscellaneous Bacterial Infections
Whooping Cough
Mycoplasma Disease
Lyme Disease
Plague
Tularemia
Typhoid Fever
Brucellosis
Leprosy (Hansen Disease)
Tuberculosis
Chlamydial Infections
Urethritis • Lymphogranuloma Venereum • Trachoma • Inclusion Body Conjunctivitis • Psittacosis
Viral Infections in General
Viral Diseases of Childhood
Measles (Rubeola)
Rubella (German Measles)
Varicella (Chicken Pox) and Zoster (Shingles)
Mumps
Smallpox (Variola)
Postviral Encephalitis
Other Common Viral Infections
Influenza
Infectious Mononucleosis
Herpes Simplex Infections
Human Papilloma Virus Infections
Cytomegalic Inclusion Disease
Viral Hepatitis
Human Immunodeficiency Virus Infection
Rickettsial Infections
Typhus • Rocky Mountain Spotted Fever

Fungal Infections
  Primary Systemic Fungal Infections
  Opportunistic Systemic Fungal Infections
  Cutaneous Fungal Infections
Protozoal Diseases
  Malaria
  Toxoplasmosis
  Cryptosporidiosis
  Giardiasis
Helminthic Infections
  Pinworm Infestation
  Trichinosis
  Tapeworm Disease
  Ascariasis
  Trichuriasis
  Filariasis

REVIEW QUESTIONS

INFECTION AND THE BODY'S DEFENSE MECHANISMS

The world is inhabited by myriad plant and animal species, most of which have no direct contact with man. Some microorganisms, especially certain bacteria, specialize in biodegrading dead animals or other organic material. Such microorganisms are called *saprophytes*. Other microorganisms, again mostly bacteria, live on the skin and in the alimentary tract of man without producing ill effects and sometimes are helpful. These are called *normal flora*. Finally, some microorganisms produce disease when they elaborate a toxin or gain entrance to a host tissue; hence, they are called *pathogens*. The degree to which an organism is a pathogen is termed its *virulence*. Any disease directly caused by pathogens is classified as an infection. Microorganisms that produce infection in man fall into several classes of small plant-like organisms (bacteria, fungi, rickettsiae), animals (protozoa and helminths), and viruses. It should be noted that the word *infection* is also used to describe the process of organisms gaining entrance to the body regardless of whether disease is produced. In this chapter, *infection* will be used synonymously with *infectious disease*.

Microorganisms may play various roles depending on circumstances. For example, *Clostridium perfringens* is an anaerobic (grows without oxygen) bacterium that is a normal member of the colonic flora. After death of the host animal, it becomes a saprophyte by participating in the postmortem degradation of the tissues. *Clostridium perfringens* may become a pathogen either by releasing potent toxins or by invading necrotic tissue.

Many of the common, mildly pathogenic bacteria, such as staphylococcus and *Escherichia coli*, are part of the normal flora of the skin, mouth, or intestines. Strongly pathogenic organisms, including many viruses, all rickettsiae, and many bacteria, require some method of spreading from person to person such as direct contact, environmental contamination, or a *vector* (another organism such as an insect that transports the pathogen to the host). When a pathogen is present in or on the body without causing disease, the host is said to be a *carrier*, meaning that the host can "carry" the disease to another host.

The body has evolved to provide continual defense against attack by foreign organisms. The most obvious defense mechanism is the structural barrier provided by the epithelium of the skin and internal passageways exposed to external contamination.

The second major line of defense is the inflammatory response. It protects against microorganisms that have penetrated the epithelial barrier. Microorganisms are walled off initially by fibrin deposition, later by fibrous tissue and are engulfed and destroyed by phagocytes (neutrophils and macrophages).

The third major line of defense, the immune system, requires previous or prolonged exposure to the offending agent and operates by enhancing the effectiveness of the inflammatory process. The immune defense mechanism consists of two distinctive systems—the humoral system, in which there are free antibodies in the blood, and the cellular immune system, in which the reaction is mediated by lymphocytes. Both of these systems aid in killing microorganisms and will be discussed in greater detail in the next chapter.

Antibodies are highly effective in neutralizing certain bacterial toxins such as tetanus toxin and diphtheria toxin, in enhancing phagocytosis of bacteria such as *Streptococcus pneumoniae* and *Bordetella pertussis* (the bacterium that produces whooping cough), and in preventing dissemination of certain viruses such as rabies virus and poliovirus. Routine immunization of infants protects against tetanus, diphtheria, whooping cough, poliomyelitis, measles, rubella, and mumps. Immunization for smallpox (vaccination) has been discontinued because of the remarkable elimination of this disease worldwide. Immune sera are available for selected other diseases when conditions warrant their use. For example, antirabies sera is used after a person has been bitten by a rabid animal.

In summary, the major defense mechanisms against infection are mechanical barriers, inflammation, and the immune reactions. There are obviously other defense mechanisms, but these are generally less well understood. For example, viral infection of cells causes release of a cytokine known as *interferon*, which limits viral replication. There is no known deficiency of, or way to enhance its action although it is now available therapeutically. For unknown reasons, pathogens often show a specific predilection for a part of the body where they can best live. For example, gonococci live on mucous membranes and grow less readily at other sites.

MOST FREQUENT AND SERIOUS PROBLEMS

Overall Impact of Infectious Disease

As presented in Chapter 2, respiratory illnesses, which are most frequently viral infections, account for about 50 percent of all acute illnesses, and other infections account for an additional 10 percent of acute illnesses. Very few chronic illnesses are primarily due to infection, notable exceptions being tuberculosis, leprosy, syphilis, and hepatitis B and C. Pneumonia, which is almost always due to infection, is a common cause of death. Pneumonia may occur as a primary illness, but more often it occurs in persons seriously ill with other diseases, in which case it is termed *secondary* or *opportunistic* because the other disease predisposed to the pneumonia. There are numerous other kinds of secondary infections. Significant predisposing factors to secondary infections are obstructions in body cavities, which enhance secondary bacterial infection, and deficient immunity, such as occurs in patients with chronic debilitating illness. Patients with advanced cancer or AIDS are susceptible to various bacterial, fungal, viral, and protozoal infections.

Respiratory infections, including upper respiratory infections, influenza-like infections, pneumonia, and bronchitis, account for over 80 percent of infections. Common childhood infections (mostly viral) and other viral diseases account for about half of the remaining infections. These statistics probably do not include many forms of secondary infection.

Of the primary infections that are on the required list of reportable infections, gonorrhea is by far the most common. Table 26–1 shows the relative frequency of reportable infections in the United States. Unreported sexually transmitted infections, however, may be more common (e.g., genitourinary infections due to chlamydia and human papilloma virus). Human immunodeficiency virus infection is more serious.

Bacterial Infections

Secondary infections and sexually transmitted diseases are the most common types of bacterial infection. Common secondary infections include abscesses, pneumonia, and wound infections. One of the most potent predisposing factors to secondary bacterial infection is the

TABLE 26–1. NUMBER OF NEW CASES OF REPORTABLE INFECTIOUS DISEASES IN THE UNITED STATES 1995

Disease	No. of Cases
Chlamydia	477,638
Gonorrhea	392,848
Varicella (chickenpox)	120,624
AIDS	71,547
Syphillis, total all stages	68,953
Hepatitis A, B, & C	46,963
Salmonellosis	45,970
Shigellosis	32,080
Tuberculosis	22,860
Lyme disease	11,700
Pertussis (whooping cough)	5,137
Meningococcal disease	3,243
Escherichia coli	2,139
Malaria	1,419
Legionellosis	1,241
Haemophilus influenzae, invasive	1,180
Mumps	906
Chancroid	606
Rocky Mountain spotted fever	590
Typhoid fever	369
Measles (rubeola)	309
Toxic-shock syndrome	191
Hansen disease (leprosy)	144
Rubella (German measles)	128
Brucellosis	98
Botulism, total	97
Psittacosis	64
Tetanus	41
Trichinosis	29
Cholera	23
Plague	9
Rubella, congenital syndrome	6
Rabies, human	5
Poliomyelitis, paralytic	2

Data from *Morbidity and Mortality Weekly*, Report by the Centers for Disease Control and Prevention. Public Health Service, Vol. 44, No. 53, October 25, 1996.

presence of dead tissue. Dead tissue is a growth medium for bacteria and lacks a blood supply to bring in phagocytes and antibodies. The most common predisposing factor for secondary bacterial infection is obstruction of a body passageway. For example, urinary tract obstruction predisposes to pyelonephritis, nasal obstruction leads to sinusitis, pharyngeal obstruction of eustachian tubes leads to otitis media. Obstruction allows normal flora to proliferate to concentrations at which they become pathogenic. Table 26–2 lists the common sites of obstruction and the resulting types of infection.

The classic sexually transmitted infections are gonorrhea and syphilis, with gonorrhea being far more frequent and syphilis much more serious; however, papilloma and herpes viruses and chlamydia infections appear to be more common, and human immunodeficiency virus infection leading to acquired immune deficiency syndrome (AIDS) is now the leading cause of death in adults between the ages of 25 and 49 in the United States. Most of the classic bacterial infections that will be presented in this chapter are uncommon or rare and are important because they must be kept in that status. Bacterial meningitis is an uncommon but serious problem that must be diagnosed early if treatment is to be effective.

Viral Infections

Upper respiratory illnesses, caused by several types of viruses, far outnumber all other infections. Viral gastroenteritis is less common but often occurs in epidemics. Cold sores due to *Herpes simplex* are a common type of recurrent viral infection that affects 50 percent of the population. Disseminated viral infections of childhood have greatly

---

TABLE 26–2. SITES OF OBSTRUCTIONS AND ASSOCIATED INFECTIONS

Site of Obstruction	Type of Infection
Sebaceous gland	Furuncle and acne
Eustachian tube	Otitis media
Nasal sinus openings	Sinusitis
Bronchus	Pneumonia
Urethra	Cystitis
Ureter	Pyelonephritis
Bile ducts	Cholangitis
Appendix (fecalith)	Acute appendicitis

decreased in frequency as vaccines have been developed for measles, rubella, polio, and mumps. There is no immunization available for chicken pox, and it is still quite common. Infectious mononucleosis and viral hepatitis are moderately common, with peak frequency in adolescents and young adults. Viral encephalitis is a rare but serious viral disease, usually spread by mosquitoes in summer epidemics. Human immunodeficiency virus (HIV) infection, the cause of acquired immune deficiency syndrome (AIDS), has become the most important viral infection worldwide because of its lethal outcome.

Rickettsial Infections

These are rare but serious disseminated infections caused by organisms intermediate between bacteria and viruses. Rocky Mountain spotted fever occurs sporadically in the United States. Typhus is even rarer. Ehrlichiosis is a newly discovered, tick-transmitted disease seen in the south-central and upper midwest parts of the United States.

Fungal Infections

Superficial fungal infections of the skin, such as athlete's foot and ringworm, are quite common but rarely serious. Superficial infection of skin and mucous membranes by candida, called mucocutaneous candidiasis, occurs particularly in diabetics and persons with neutropenia or on prolonged antibiotic therapy. Primary disseminated fungal infections, such as histoplasmosis and coccidioidomycosis, are geographically common as asymptomatic infections but uncommon as significant clinical illnesses. Species of *Candida, Aspergillus,* and *Mucor* may produce opportunistic infections in persons debilitated by chronic underlying disease.

Protozoal Infections

One of the most prevalent worldwide infections, malaria, is caused by a small protozoan that invades and destroys red blood cells. In the United States, malaria is uncommon except in those who have returned from tropical and subtropical areas of the world. Possibly the most prevalent protozoan is *Trichomonas vaginalis,* which may cause vaginal and lower urinary tract discomfort but only rarely is associated with significant morbidity.

Giardiasis is an intestinal protozoan infection usually acquired by drinking contaminated water. It causes profound watery diarrhea and weight loss if severe and prolonged. *Pneumocystis carinii* is an organism of uncertain type that has been variously classified as a protozoan or fungus and causes pneumonia in immunosuppressed persons.

Helminth Infections

Helminths comprise the primitive roundworms and flatworms. Worldwide, helminthic infestation is extremely common. Schistosomiasis is one of the most important infections in the world, because it produces chronic liver disease and urinary bladder cancer in areas of the world such as Asia, Africa, and South America. Many types of helminths infest (live in) the intestinal tract and occasionally produce disease. All types of tapeworm (beef, pork, dog, rat, and fish) can cause disease in man. Pork and dog tapeworm disease are most serious. Pinworm and ascaris are the most common helminths encountered in the United States. In general, helminth infections are uncommon in the United States.

SYMPTOMS, SIGNS, AND TESTS

The long list of infectious diseases produced by microorganisms includes many with distinctive clinical presentations and others that present as nonspecific syndromes. The common syndromes, such as upper respiratory infection, gastroenteritis, cystitis, and meningitis, have been discussed in previous chapters. The clinical presentations of selected specific diseases will be presented in the next section.

Symptoms common to many but not all infectious diseases include rapid onset, achiness, fatigue, fever, rapid pulse, and a feeling of tiredness and ill health (malaise). Physical examination of the lesions may, in many instances, be sufficient for diagnosis. For example, the rash of measles or chicken pox is distinctive, and the parotid swelling of mumps or pus draining from an abscess is usually all that is required for diagnosis. Since most lesions of infectious diseases are inflammatory in nature, they likely will exhibit the cardinal signs of inflammation—heat, redness, swelling, and pain.

The laboratory is essential for the diagnosis of most infectious diseases. Direct culture of organisms from the lesion is the most definitive test, although on occasion contaminants or normal flora may be cultivated while pathogens fail to grow. Culture is most commonly used for bacteria, and it is also the method of choice for diagnosis of many fungal diseases. Many viruses can be cultured, but the lack of effective therapy, time lapse, and high cost limit the use of culture for diagnosis of viral disease. Helminths and most protozoa are not cultured but are often identified by direct microscopic examination. Rickettsiae are dangerous to culture. The bulk of bacterial cultures are from throat, urine, sputum, and purulent lesions. When indicated, blood and spinal fluid cultures provide critical information for treatment of *septicemia* (generalized infection involving the blood) and meningitis. Significant pathogens isolated in culture are usually tested for their *sensitivity* to selected antibiotics so that the most appropriate therapy can be administered (Figure 26–1).

Microscopic examination of direct smears with or without staining are still of great value diagnostically. Gram-stained bacterial preparations are used to identify gram-positive (blue-staining) and gram-negative (red-staining) bacteria and to subdivide them into cocci (round) and bacilli (elongated) types. This information obtained from spinal fluid in a patient with meningitis is sufficient to start antibiotic treatment while results of culture and sensitivity testing are pending. Gonococci can be identified by gram-stained smear in pus dripping from the male urethra. Smears are generally useful in identifying the larger, more varied types of organisms, including fungi, protozoa, and eggs of the helminths.

In some instances, specific antibodies can be used to detect organisms in samples obtained by swabbing or scraping a lesion. For example, antibodies to group A streptococci attached to latex particles can be mixed with material from a throat swab; agglutination of the particles is interpreted as streptococcal pharyngitis. This is a very rapid and useful test to decide whether a patient with a sore throat should

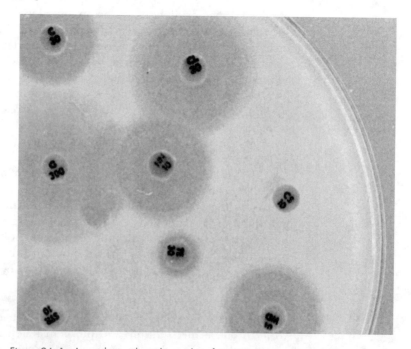

Figure 26–1. Agar plate with antibiotic discs for sensitivity test. Note inhibition of growth on the surface of the medium around some of the antibiotic discs.

be treated with penicillin. Another technique involves the use of fluorescent-tagged antibodies mixed with tissue sample and examined under a fluorescent microscope. This technique can be used for rapid diagnosis of herpes simplex type I and II infections, *Legionella* pneumonia, and urethritis due to chlamydia.

Immunologic reactivity of the host to an infection can be evaluated by measurement of serum antibodies or by skin testing to assess cellular immunity. In either case, the positive result only indicates previous exposure to the organism and may not mean active disease. Furthermore, antibodies or skin reactivity may not be present in early stages of a disease.

Tests for antibodies in the patient's serum are called serologic tests. Serology is commonly employed for the diagnosis of syphilis, systemic fungal disease, several bacterial diseases (brucellosis, leptospirosis, typhoid fever, Lyme disease, tularemia), many viral diseases, rickettsial disease, and some parasitic diseases. Skin tests are most commonly employed as a screening test for tuberculosis.

Recently, exciting progress has been made in developing rapid and highly accurate tests for microorganisms, especially viruses, that rely on detection of specific RNA or DNA.

The most commonly used tests for infectious disease are not really specific for infectious diseases. These tests include measurement of body temperature, white blood cell total and differential counts, and examination of a smear of urine sediment. An elevated body temperature (fever) occurs with many bacterial, viral, and rickettsial infections. An elevated white blood count, particularly when associated with increased numbers of neutrophils, suggests a bacterial infection. Viral infections may have elevated, normal, or low white blood counts, and often the proportion of lymphocytes is increased. Eosinophils are frequently increased with helminthic infections. White blood cells in the urine sediment suggest urinary tract infection, and if white blood cell casts are present, it suggests kidney involvement, since casts are formed in renal tubules.

SPECIFIC DISEASES

Bacterial Infections in General

Bacteria are small microbial agents distributed ubiquitously throughout nature. Humans normally harbor certain bacteria on the skin, in the oral and nasal cavities, the anterior urethra, the female genital tract, and throughout the intestinal tract. The body provides a home for these bacteria, which comprise the *normal flora*, and in some instances they even provide benefits for the host, an example being the production of vitamin K by intestinal bacteria. At certain times, because of imbalances in either host or bacteria, the bacteria invade body tissues and cause disease by proliferating in an unnatural location. Bacteria invade the body via the lungs, intestine, nasal sinuses, genitourinary tract, or through breaks or tears in the skin. They can localize in particular areas or organs, or they may gain access to the circulation and be disseminated throughout the body. Once inside the body, most bacteria proliferate in the interstitial tissue, although some prefer to proliferate in the host's cells. The response of the host to bacterial invasion is acute inflammation as outlined in Chapter 4. Different bacteria damage or destroy the host's tissues by different mechanisms; for example, some of the most virulent bacteria, such as *Clostridium botulinum*, secrete exotoxins that are proteinaceous poisons. Some exotoxins kill cells directly, others block nerve impulses or inhibit vital intracellular processes. Other bacteria, such as staphylococci, produce enzymes that enhance their invasiveness by dissolving connective tissue or fibrin. Still other bacteria are surrounded by thick capsules that retard phagocytosis by the host's phagocytes, an example being pneumococcus. Most pathogenic bacteria are *pyogenic*, meaning that they elicit a neutrophilic inflammatory response with purulent exudate. In most cases, the tissue damage in the patient is caused more by the patient's inflammatory and immune responses than by the direct action of the bacteria.

Pyogenic Bacterial Infections

Staphylococcal Infections

Of the several varieties of staphylococci, the most virulent is *Staphylococcus aureus*. *Staphylococcus aureus*, a member of the normal flora, can enter the body by any route and infect any organ; it has a particular propensity to cause abscesses. Most skin abscesses are staphylococcal, and abscesses in other sites are also commonly caused by staphylococci. Abscesses under the skin are referred to as *furuncles* (boils). A collection of furuncles is called a *carbuncle*. Another reason *S. aureus* is such an important pathogen is that many strains develop resistance to therapy with penicillin and other antibiotics. This can lead to particularly dangerous situations in hospitals, where resistant strains of *S. aureus* can infect debilitated patients, causing pneumonia and septicemia. Staphylococcal species can also cause impetigo of the skin, pneumonia, food poisoning, and endocarditis. Staphylococcus is readily cultured, and sensitivity tests are valuable because of the considerable resistance of many strains to various antibiotics.

STAPHYLOCOCCAL INFECTIONS 26-1

cause	lesions	manifestations
Staphylococcus aureus	Abscesses Furuncles Carbuncles Pneumonia Septicemia	Cardinal signs of inflammation Fever Leukocytosis Purulent drainage from abscess Toxic shock

In the late 1970s, there was a nationwide outbreak of severe illness mainly involving women using a hyperabsorbent tampon. The illness was named *toxic shock syndrome* (TSS) and was shown to be caused by a strain of *S. aureus* that produced a powerful exotoxin that was absorbed through the vaginal wall, resulting in shock. TSS still occurs, but is readily treatable by removal of the tampon, fluid replacement, and antibiotic therapy.

Group A Streptococcal Infections

Numerous varieties of streptococci exist and are classified into groups according to antigens they possess. Group A streptococci are the most virulent because many possess enzymes that allow them to spread rapidly through tissues via lymphatic vessels—a condition known as *cellulitis.* Acute pharyngitis (strep throat) is the most common disease produced by group A streptococci. Scarlet fever is an uncommon systemic streptococcal infection so named because the effect of one of the bacteria's toxins on blood vessels produces a scarlet rash. Impetigo

 GROUP A STREPTOCOCCAL INFECTIONS 26-2

cause	lesions	manifestations
Group A streptococci	Cellulitis Scarlet fever Acute pharyngitis Impetigo Remote: Rheumatic fever Glomerulonephritis	Cardinal signs of inflammation Fever Leukocytosis Purulent, often without abscess formation

is a superficial skin infection caused by group A streptococci (see Chapter 19). The immunologic sequelae of group A streptococcal infections in terms of production of rheumatic fever and poststreptococcal glomerulonephritis are discussed in Chapters 8 and 16.

There has been a recent pandemic of life-threatening invasive streptococcal infections caused by strains elaborating an exotoxin. Symptoms include bacteremia, severe soft tissue damage, and shock (streptococcal toxic shock syndrome). Antibiotic treatment and early surgical debridement are essential for survival.

Streptococcus Viridans Infection

Streptococcus viridans is part of the normal flora of the mouth and is the most common cause of bacterial endocarditis and dental caries. These organisms of low virulence occasionally get into the bloodstream, where they can infect damaged heart valves (such as following rheumatic fever) and slowly destroy the valves, resulting in congestive heart failure (Figure 26–2). Most strains of streptococcus can be readily cultured and identified in the laboratory, and fortunately, most streptococci are highly susceptible to penicillin and other antibiotics.

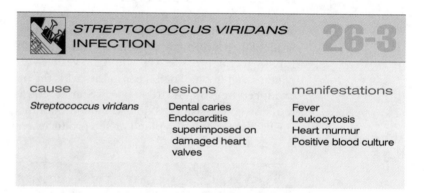

STREPTOCOCCUS VIRIDANS INFECTION 26-3

cause	lesions	manifestations
Streptococcus viridans	Dental caries Endocarditis superimposed on damaged heart valves	Fever Leukocytosis Heart murmur Positive blood culture

Streptococcus Pneumoniae (Pneumococcus) Infection

Pneumococcus pneumoniae, a normal member of the throat flora, is the most common cause of pneumonia, otitis media, meningitis, and rarely other local or generalized infections. Pneumococcus used to be highly susceptible to penicillin and related antibiotics; however, over the past decade, there has been a marked increase in infections of antibiotic-resistant strains, resulting in a major change in the management of pneumococcal diseases.

STREPTOCOCCUS PNEUMONIAE INFECTION

26-4

cause	lesions	manifestation
Streptococcus pneumoniae	Otitis media Pneumonia Sinusitis Endocarditis Meningitis	Local and systemic manifestations of inflammation

Meningococcal Meningitis

Neisseria meningitidis, a small gram-negative intracellular organism, causes endemic and epidemic meningitis, especially in children and young adults. It is transmitted via the oral route, most commonly in late winter to early spring. The disease usually starts with pharyngitis, fever, and a stiff neck. The myocarditis and disseminated intravascular coagulation caused by these organisms are more rare but also serious complications of meningococcal infection.

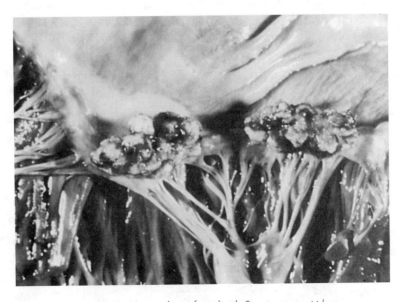

Figure 26–2. Heart valves infected with *Streptococcus viridans.*

Haemophilus Influenzae Infection

Haemophilus influenzae used to be the major cause of bacterial meningitis in children and also caused otitis media and pneumonia, but has become a rare cause of childhood disease with the availability of a highly effective vaccine—now given to all children.

Legionellosis

Legionella pneumophilia is a ubiquitous gram-negative bacterium that lives in water reservoirs and cooling units for air conditioners, but requires special media for culture. In retrospect, it was the cause of severe pneumonia in the past, but was only discovered after a severe epidemic at an American Legion convention in Philadelphia in 1976. The lesions are mainly confined to the lung and only occur when large numbers of organisms are inhaled. The disease is more common in summer and can be acquired in the community or in the hospital. It can be treated with erythromycin or tetracycline.

Enteric Bacterial Infections

Enteric bacteria are those bacteria that normally inhabit the intestinal tract of man and includes species of *Escherichia* (*E. coli*), *Klebsiella*, *Proteus*, *Pseudomonas*, *Salmonella*, and *Shigella*. Different strains of *E. coli* are found in virtually everyone's intestinal tract, while only a small percentage of people will harbor one or more types of the other organisms. Specific intestinal diseases produced by salmonella and shigella are discussed in Chapter 12. The rest of these bacteria can produce disease only if allowed to invade body tissues, and all are especially pathogenic in debilitated patients. Enteric bacteria generally cause abscesses. *E. coli* is a common cause of meningitis in newborns, and

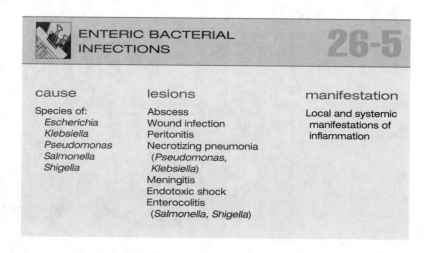

ENTERIC BACTERIAL INFECTIONS		26-5
cause	**lesions**	**manifestation**

Species of:
  Escherichia
  Klebsiella
  Pseudomonas
  Salmonella
  Shigella
	Abscess
	Wound infection
	Peritonitis
	Necrotizing pneumonia
	  (Pseudomonas,
	  Klebsiella)
	Meningitis
	Endotoxic shock
	Enterocolitis
	  (Salmonella, Shigella)
		Local and systemic
		  manifestations of
		  inflammation

certain strains can cause diarrhea (see Chapter 12). *Pseudomonas aeruginosa* commonly contaminates wounds and is characteristically associated with green pus. *Pseudomonas* and *Klebsiella* also cause a severe necrotizing pneumonia. Patients with a bacteremia from gram-negative enteric organisms often lapse into severe shock, which is caused by a cell wall material called *endotoxin* from gram-negative bacteria. This type of shock is referred to as *endotoxic shock* or *gram-negative shock* and has a 30 to 50 percent mortality rate. *Pseudomonas* is an increasingly common cause of hospital-acquired infections.

Anaerobic Bacterial Infections

It is now recognized that abscesses and wound infections may be caused by any of a wide variety of anaerobic bacteria derived from the intestinal tract, genital tract, or mouth. Anaerobes in the lower alimentary tract and in the mouth outnumber aerobes by more than 1000 to 1. These bacteria cannot grow in the usual culture conditions in which oxygen is present, so they are overlooked unless anaerobic culture techniques are used. The most distinctive feature of infections due to these anaerobes is the foul odor due to the gases produced. Otherwise, anaerobic infection will appear similar to that produced by *E. coli* or staphylococcus. Some anaerobic bacteria produce powerful exotoxins; these bacteria will be discussed as a group later in this chapter.

Sexually Transmitted Bacterial Infections

Sexually Transmitted Disease in General

Sexually transmitted (formerly called venereal) diseases are those diseases spread by genital contact, usually intercourse. However, they may also be spread by oral–genital or genital–rectal activity; oral–oral spread is rare. Table 26–3 lists the sexually associated diseases.

Neisseria gonorrhoeae, Chlamydia trachomatis, and *Ureaplasma urealyticum* all produce sexually transmitted disease similar to that classically described for gonorrhea. Chlamydia infections are more common than gonorrhea. Ureaplasma infection may also be more common than gonorrhea, but is difficult to diagnose and study. Human papilloma virus and HIV infections are discussed under viral infection.

In large metropolitan areas, sexually transmitted disease clinics have been established to efficiently handle diagnosis and to help identify sexual contacts who should also be treated to limit the spread of the disease. However, sexually transmitted diseases are the least well controlled epidemic diseases in the United States today.

TABLE 26–3. SEXUALLY ASSOCIATED DISEASES

Diseases exclusively transmitted via sexual activity	Non exclusively sexually transmitted disease
Gonorrhea (bacterial)	AIDS (viral)
Syphilis (bacterial)	Trichomoniasis (protozoal)
Chancroid (bacterial)	Candidiasis (fungal)
Lymphogranuloma venereum (chlamydial)	Herpes (viral)
Granuloma inguinale (bacterial)	Condyloma acuminatum (viral)
	Chlamydial infections (chlamydial)
	Ureaplasma infection (bacterial)
	Molluscum contagiosum (viral)
	Nonspecific urethritis (multiple microbes)
	Scabies (insect)
	Pediculosis (insect)
	Hepatitis A and B (viral)

Gonorrhea

Gonorrhea, commonly called "clap," or "the drip," is caused by *Neisseria gonorrhoeae* and is the number two reported communicable disease in the United States. Gonorrhea outnumbers syphilis by 6 to 1. Gonorrhea affects men and women differently.

Males usually note burning on urination (dysuria) and purulent urethral discharge (drip) within 3 to 5 days after exposure and seek treatment for these symptoms. Therefore, the most severe sequelae are usually avoided. In the asymptomatic male (5 to 7%) or those inadequately treated, later sequelae usually involve the urinary tract, leading to urinary strictures, or involvement of the prostate gland and the epididymus, leading to sterility.

The infected female seldom has symptomatic urethritis; 90 percent are asymptomatic in the acute stage of the disease. The predominant effect in the female is sterility due to fallopian tube involvement. Gonococci cross the cervical barrier during menstruation and work their way up to the fallopian tubes, where they produce infection (salpingitis) leading to scar formation. Narrowing of the fallopian tubes by scar mechanically interferes with migration of ova, although sometimes sperm can traverse the stricture, resulting in ectopic pregnancy. Another major problem in females is the continuation of purulent infection, with abscess formation at the tuboovarian juncture and peritonitis. Purulent gonococcal infection is commonly referred to as *pelvic inflammatory disease.*

GONORRHEA

26-6

causes	lesions	manifestations
Neisseria gonorrheae Usually transmitted sexually	Males: acute urethritis, chronic urinary strictures Females: urethritis, salpingitis Both: pharyngitis, conjunctivitis, bacteremia, arthritis, endocarditis	Dysuria (males) Purulent exudate (males) Sterility (mostly female) Ectopic pregnancy Positive Gram stain (male) Culture

Males and females are equally susceptible to pharyngeal gonorrhea and adult gonococcal conjunctivitis; however, females have disseminated gonococcal infection (septicemia, arthritis, and endocarditis) twice as often as males.

Diagnosis of gonorrhea is by clinical history combined with judicious application of laboratory procedures. The gram-stained smear is the test of choice in the symptomatic male. Smears are of little value in the female, the asymptomatic male, and pharyngeal gonorrhea. In all cases, culture must be attempted. Care must be taken in obtaining specimens for cultural diagnosis, as gonococcus is very susceptible to cold and drying and needs to be cultured in a carbon dioxide atmosphere. Over the past two decades, gonococci have shown an alarming increase in resistance to penicillin and other antibiotics; consequently, other, newer antibiotics are preferred.

Nongonococcal Urethritis

The minority of cases of acute urethritis in males is due to gonococcus. Most are due to chlamydial or possibly ureaplasma infections. The clinical illness is the same as gonorrhea but the treatment is different. Gonorrhea usually responds to potent antibiotic therapy; tetracyclines are typically used to treat chlamydial and ureaplasma infections. The diagnosis of chlamydial infection has been improved by the availability of tests for antigenic material or DNA in exudates and cell culture techniques. The laboratory diagnosis of ureaplasm infection is more difficult and not widely used.

Infections in the female are also similar to gonorrhea. During childbirth, chlamydia may infect the infant, causing conjunctivitis or pneumonitis.

Syphilis

Syphilis is caused by the spirochete *Treponema pallidum*, a long slender, spiral organism that is a motile bacterium. Syphilis, or the great pox, used to be a devastating disease. It produced chronic sequelae that in the past killed many people. Syphilis has a lower incidence and rate of infection than gonorrhea and chlamydia, because there is a simple and highly reliable diagnostic serologic test and because no antibiotic-resistant strains have emerged. The disease is only transmitted during the first two stages of the disease (about 1 year), while gonorrhea can be transmitted indefinitely. The 3-week incubation period of syphilis allows for therapy to be initiated before the patient can spread the disease. Also, syphilis can be cured by antibiotic therapy given for other diseases, such as streptococcal sore throat, without anyone being aware of its existence.

Unlike gonorrhea, syphilis affects the male and female with equally tragic results. In addition, a woman can transmit the disease to her unborn child even when she is in the chronic stages and no longer capable of transmitting the disease sexually. The frequency of congenital syphilis has decreased markedly due to routine serologic testing of pregnant women. The disease is not transmitted from mother to fetus until after midpregnancy, so that maternal penicillin therapy before this time prevents congenital syphilis.

Syphilis has three stages. In the first stage (primary syphilis), an ulcerated lesion called a *chancre* appears where the spirochete entered the body (Figure 26–3A). The chancre usually develops on or about the genitalia but is not limited to that area. It is a painless shallow ulcer resembling a fever blister and can be mistaken for herpes if on the lip. After the chancre appears, the serologic tests for syphilis become reactive, especially the highly specific fluorescent treponemal antibody test (FTA).

Without treatment, the chancre heals (resolves) in 2 to 3 weeks, and a period of quiescence ensues that can last from 6 weeks to as long as a year. During that time, the spirochete rests for a time, then goes into a rapid growth and multiplication phase, culminating in the production of the secondary stage of syphilis. Again, this stage is basically painless, but a syphilitic rash appears (Figure 26–3B). The rash may mimic everything from chicken pox to ringworm. The serologic tests for syphilis are at their highest titer during this stage, and serodiagnosis is no problem. The lesions are infective, but not as infective as the chancre. If the patient is not treated, the organisms withdraw into the body for the last time, selecting single or multiple sites within the host where they remain in a dormant state for varying lengths of time (latent stage). The latent stage of the disease is the most potentially dangerous, as the possibility of tertiary syphilitic sequelae exists.

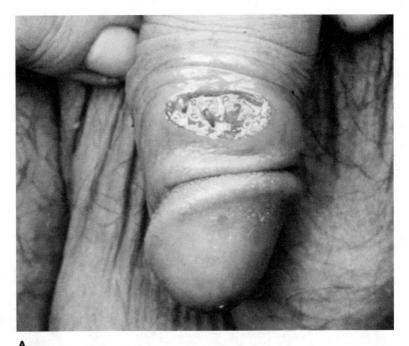

A

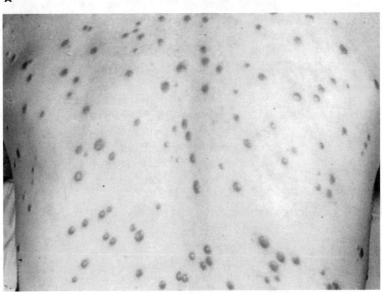

B

Figure 26–3. A. Syphilitic chancre of the penis. B. Rash of secondary syphilis.

SYPHILIS 26-7

causes	lesions	manifestations
Treponema pallidum Sexual transmission	Primary: chancre at site of entry Secondary: bacteremia, rash Tertiary: vasculitis of aorta, necrosis in brain and spinal cord; gummas of any organ	Primary: chancre, positive FTA (late) Secondary: rash, FTA almost always positive Tertiary: thoracic aorta aneurysms, paralysis, insanity, blindness, positive serology

Primary and secondary stages may be mild or unrecognized (subclinical) and go undetected, only to be inferred by finding a positive serology at a later time. Of those diagnosed in the primary or secondary stage, it is estimated that about one-third would resolve spontaneously, one-third would remain serologically positive without tertiary disease, and one-third would progress to a symptomatic tertiary stage. Tertiary syphilis may manifest itself in a variety of ways, involving almost any organ system of the body. Cardiovascular disease, with thoracic aortic aneurysm and secondary heart disease, is most common. Central nervous system disease, with paralysis, insanity, or blindness, is second most common. The basic lesions of syphilis are vasculitis that commonly involves the aorta, meninges, brain, and spinal cord and variable-sized, granuloma-like lesions in any organ. Tertiary syphilis, with its severe effects, may occur as early as 3 years or as late as 25 years after the primary stage. Syphilis is diagnosed by the clinical signs or symptoms complemented by laboratory diagnostic procedures, which include darkfield microscopy to visualize the organisms scraped from a lesion, simple screening serologic tests, with confirmatory fluorescent treponemal antibody tests.

Bacterial Infections Mediated by Exotoxins

Tetanus

Clostridia are very important and feared organisms because of the exotoxins they may produce. *Clostridium tetani* is found in the soil, and because it is anaerobic, it can grow silently in deep wounds where there is necrotic tissue. Toxin produced in the infected wound diffuses throughout the body, acting on the nerve-muscle junction, with resultant painful contractions of muscles throughout the body. The organisms are confined to the necrotic wound, so debridement of necrotic tissue helps in prevention of the disease. Generalized tetanus, commonly referred to as "lockjaw," has a high mortality rate. The best treatment of tetanus is prevention by an inoculation of tetanus toxoid to stimulate antibody production against the toxins. Every person should be immunized in childhood with booster immunizations every ten years.

Botulism

Although *Clostridium botulinum* does not produce classic invasive infection, it does secrete a powerful exotoxin that paralyzes the body's muscles by blocking the nerve-muscle junction, leading to rapid death from respiratory failure. *Clostridium botulinum* proliferates and produces toxin in improperly canned vegetables and meats. Adequate sterilization of canned foods prevents the disease.

Gas Gangrene

Several types of clostridial organisms cause gas gangrene, the most common being *C. perfringens*. Clostridia are harbored in the soil and intestinal tract. When introduced into wounds containing necrotic tissue, they proliferate well in the anaerobic conditions. The organisms ferment carbohydrates in the dead tissue to produce gas. The gas distends the tissue to produce compression of blood vessels, which in turn produces more tissue anoxia, tissue necrosis, and a foul smell. Clostridia also produce enzymes that destroy adjacent tissues to produce more tissue necrosis, thus allowing organisms to proliferate further. Primary treatment is aimed at breaking this perpetual cycle by removal of all dead tissue (debridement). In addition, antibiotics directed against the bacteria, antitoxins directed against the necrotizing enzymes produced by the bacteria, and oxygen therapy to inhibit growth of the bacteria may be helpful. Gas gangrene most commonly occurs after severe wounds but may also occur in the uterus following

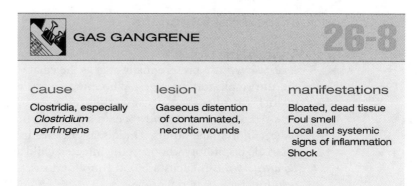

GAS GANGRENE   **26-8**

cause	lesion	manifestations
Clostridia, especially *Clostridium perfringens*	Gaseous distention of contaminated, necrotic wounds	Bloated, dead tissue Foul smell Local and systemic signs of inflammation Shock

traumatic nonsterile abortions. Gas gangrene is distinguished from simple gangrene by the production of the necrotizing enzymes (exotoxins). *Simple gangrene* refers to the invasion of dead tissue by a variety of saprophytic anaerobic bacteria that decompose dead tissue. Simple gangrene occurs most commonly in the legs and intestines following vascular occlusion.

Diphtheria

Corynebacterium diphtheriae produces pharyngitis with secondary toxemia. The bacterium is infected with a virus, which causes it to produce a powerful exotoxin. The toxin causes a local superficial necrotizing reaction in the pharynx called a *pseudomembrane* and is also absorbed into the blood to produce serious systemic disease. Myocarditis and peripheral nerve degeneration occurs in many cases, resulting in congestive failure and paralysis. Although the disease diphtheria is not as dreaded as it once was, there are still occasional outbreaks in this country resulting in loss of life. The disease can be prevented by immunization against the toxin.

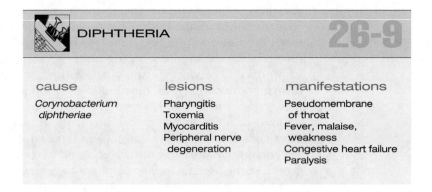

DIPHTHERIA 26-9

cause	lesions	manifestations
Corynobacterium diphtheriae	Pharyngitis Toxemia Myocarditis Peripheral nerve degeneration	Pseudomembrane of throat Fever, malaise, weakness Congestive heart failure Paralysis

Miscellaneous Bacterial Infections

Whooping Cough

Bordetella pertussis preferentially attacks the ciliated epithelial cells lining the respiratory passages. Whooping cough is no longer as prevalent as it once was, because children are routinely immunized, although there has recently been a significant increase especially in older children and adults. The disease derives its name from a characteristic inspiratory whoop as the infected child attempts to breathe. *Bordetella pertussis* elicits a blood lymphocytosis, which is an unusual response for a bacterial disease.

Mycoplasma Disease

Mycoplasma organisms are bacteria-like but do not possess rigid cell walls. They are the primary cause of an infection referred to as *primary atypical pneumonia*, which may smolder for many months with low-grade symptoms such as coughing, shortness of breath, and fatigue, commonly in children and adolescents. Primary atypical pneumonia is often referred to as "walking pneumonia." Ureaplasma is a similar organism that is implicated as a cause of nongonococcal urethritis.

Lyme Disease

This recently discovered, important disease is caused by infection with a spirochete, *Borrelia burgdorferi*, which is carried by a variety of small deer ticks. The site of the tick bite may be identified by a small "bulls eye" lesion and accompanied by fever and lymphadenopathy. In the second stage of the disease, the organisms spread throughout the body, resulting in skin lesions, muscle pain, arthritis, lymphadenopathy, cardiac arrhythmias, meningitis, and severe lethargy. Stage 3 occurs 2 to 3 years after initial infection and is characterized by severe arthritis and mild to severe encephalitis. Lyme disease is one of the causes of "chronic fatique syndrome." It appears to be increasing in incidence; as many as 50 percent of deer ticks in the northeast United States are infected with *B. burgdorferi*. Treatment with tetracycline can be very effective if initiated in the first stage of the disease.

Plague

This very serious disease caused by *Yersinia pestis* infection is endemic in wild animals in certain parts of the world but rarely causes disease in the United States. The organism is capable of rapidly spreading throughout the body and causes extensive necrosis and hemorrhage. At certain times in the middle ages, plague annihilated much of the population of Europe.

Tularemia

Tularemia is an uncommon disease caused by *Francisella tularensis* infection and is contracted from a wild animal reservoir, especially muskrats and rabbits. Tularemia can also cause pneumonia as well as a severe systemic infection, but is usually responsive to tetracycline treatment.

Typhoid Fever

Typhoid is a severe systemic disease caused by *Salmonella typhosa* infection but differs from other forms of salmonellosis in that the organism infects only humans and the disease is a more subacute disease than salmonella gastroenteritis. After entry into the gastrointestinal tract from contaminated water or food, the organism spreads throughout the mononuclear phagocytic system, where it grows, causes a histiocytic reaction, and produces bacteremia. The most serious complications are hemorrhage and perforation of lymphoid patches in the small intestine. Carriers harbor the organism in their gallbladder and are the source of outbreaks of the disease. Typhoid is relatively rare in the United States.

Brucellosis

Three different species of *Brucella* can cause brucellosis—*B. abortus, B. suis,* and *B. melitensis.* Brucellosis is a chronic systemic disease, often referred to as *undulant fever* because of the waxing and waning of febrile episodes in the patient. The bacteria are harbored in cows, sheep, hogs, and goats and human disease is acquired by ingestion of infected meat or milk or by contact with the animal. The organisms live intracellularly in macrophages, which spill the organisms into the bloodstream every few days to cause the febrile episodes. Brucellosis is rare but still endemic in the midwestern and western United States because of the large cattle and swine populations. Although *Brucella* organisms are difficult to culture, patients with the disease will develop antibodies to the organism, which can render a presumptive diagnosis.

Leprosy (Hansen Disease)

Mycobacterium leprae, a tuberculosis-like organism, preferentially invades skin and peripheral nerves, causing palpable lumps of granulomatous inflammation over the nerves. Over the course of many years, much disfigurement results from the bacterial infiltration in the skin and breakdown of tissue that has lost its nerve supply. Leprosy is uncommon but does occur in the United States, particularly in the South. The availability of effective drugs for treatment has obviated the need for quarantine.

Tuberculosis

Tuberculosis is discussed in Chapter 12.

Chlamydial Infections

Chlamydia are obligate intracellular parasites, now considered to be bacteria, that lack the ability to survive in the absence of a host-derived energy system. Overall, chlamydial infections are the number one reported communicable disease in the United States (see Table 26–1). They are susceptible to tetracycline and erythromycin. Various strains of *Chlamydia trachomatis,* a pathogen limited to humans, cause nongonococcal urethritis, lymphogranuloma venereum, trachoma, and inclusion body conjunctivitis and pneumonia in newborns. Nongonococcal urethritis has been discussed. Lymphogranuloma venereum is a less common form of sexually transmitted disease characterized by small genital ulcers and lymph node inflammation in males and, much less commonly, by anal strictures as a late lesion in females. Trachoma is spread by direct contact in areas of the world with poor living conditions. It produces a chronic progressive conjunctivitis and is the leading cause of blindness in areas where it occurs. Inclusion body conjunctivitis is a milder ocular disease that is more widespread and commonly seen in the United States, but rarely leads to blindness.

Chlamydia psittisi is transmitted from birds, especially imported pet birds, to man and rarely causes pneumonitis and generalized disease.

Viral Infections in General

Viruses are particles of genetic material (DNA or RNA) coated by protein and can only replicate inside host cells (*obligate intracellular parasites*). Most are invisible with the light microscope, although some viruses aggregate into inclusion bodies that then become visible in the nucleus or cytoplasm of cells. Viruses cannot reproduce (replicate) by themselves but are capable of inducing the host's cells to produce the ribo- or deoxyribonucleic acid and protein necessary for replication. Some viruses will infect many cells in the body and, after proliferating, exit from those cells into the blood, producing viremia with subsequent infection of other cells. Other viruses lay dormant in cells for years and only reappear following diminished host immunity or stimuli such as stress. Still others slowly destroy cells over a period of years (Figure 26–4).

Viruses are known to cause certain neoplasms in animals, and have been linked to some human cancers. Examples include hepatoma (hepatitis B and C virus), cervical carcinoma (human papilloma virus), anal carcinoma (herpes simplex virus) and Burkitt's lymphoma (Epstein–Barr virus). Some viruses probably live a long

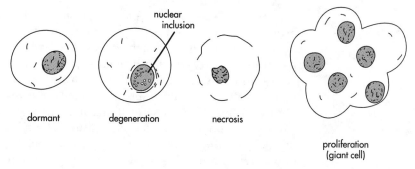

Figure 26–4. Possible reactions of cells to viral infection.

time in host cells without doing harm. These viruses are called *commensals* and are analogous to normal bacterial flora. Routes of viral invasion are oral, nasal, respiratory, gastrointestinal, and through bites. Often, the exact route of viral entry cannot be determined but is assumed.

The body's response to viral infection may be inflammatory in terms of vascular congestion and leakage of exudate, but pus formation seldom attends a viral infection. Immune response to viruses occurs readily, and evidence of this response is the collection of lymphocytes in infected tissues. In addition, the body's cells produce a protein called *interferon*, which acts to prevent viral replication. Viral diseases do not respond to antibiotic therapy; consequently the treatment must be supportive, as in a head cold, or preventive by immunization. Adequate immunizations in the past have helped to almost eradicate such feared viral diseases as poliomyelitis, yellow fever, and smallpox. Immunization programs in the past few years have helped to control epidemics of influenza and curtail mumps, measles, and rubella.

Viral Diseases of Childhood

Viral diseases of childhood, including measles, rubella, varicella, and mumps, have certain attributes in common. They affect children who have no immunity to them, although they may also readily affect adults who have not had the disease. Once a person has been infected with one of these viruses, antibodies usually confer lifetime immunity. Diagnosis generally is made on the basis of a characteristic clinical picture. In cases where the exact diagnosis is in doubt, serologic tests for antibodies may be performed. Some of these viruses can also be grown in tissue cultures. However, the results of either serologic tests or culture often come too late to aid the individual patient.

Measles (Rubeola)

Measles virus is a small RNA virus transmitted by droplet infection through the mouth and nose. It is highly infectious. After an incubation period of about 10 days, the disease begins with conjunctivitis and photophobia (excessive sensitivity to light). Within a few days, a rash ensues, which is characterized by small red spots over the face or behind the ears, gradually spreading over the trunk and extremities (Figure 26–5A). Measles is usually accompanied by a cough and fever, and a severe pneumonia may also result. The symptoms of measles indicate that the measles virus infects many cells in the body, with destruction of some. As the patient begins to produce antibodies, the disease slowly abates. Measles is far less common since the employment of measles immunization.

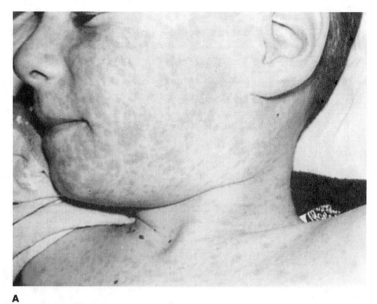

A

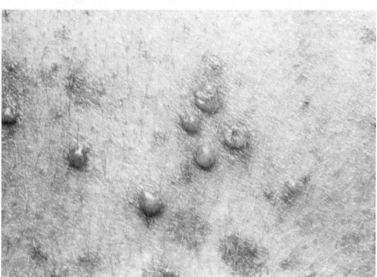

B

Figure 26–5. A. Macular rash of measles. B. Papular rash of chicken pox.

Rubella (German Measles)

Rubella virus is also a small RNA virus transmitted via the respiratory route and causes a very mild disease characterized by a light rash, low-grade fever, and lymphadenopathy. The importance of rubella lies in the fact that it is teratogenic and can cause congenital heart defects and other defects in the infant when acquired by the mother within the first trimester of pregnancy. In recent years, massive immunization has lessened tremendously the impact of rubella.

Varicella (Chicken Pox) and Zoster (Shingles)

Varicella–zoster is a DNA virus and is transmitted through the respiratory tract. After an incubation period of 2 weeks, chicken pox starts with malaise and fever followed by a rash that is much different than that of measles, being composed of large red bumps that develop blisters (vesicles) and later form a crust. A patient will show the rash in different stages of development on different areas of the body at the same time (Figure 26–5B). Chicken pox runs its course in a week or two, and treatment consists only of rest and prevention of secondary bacterial infections in the rash. After an attack of chicken pox, or even without a history of chicken pox, the virus remains dormant in nerve ganglia for many years. If the virus becomes activated in adults, it produces zoster (shingles). In zoster, the virus spreads along the course of a spinal nerve causing a painful eruption in the area of skin supplied by the nerve. In immunocompromised patients, it commonly proceeds to a severe, generalized infection. The difference between chicken pox and shingles, both caused by the same virus, depends on the level of immunity in the patient. Early treatment with acyclovir or related antiviral drugs significantly reduces the painful neuralgia of zoster.

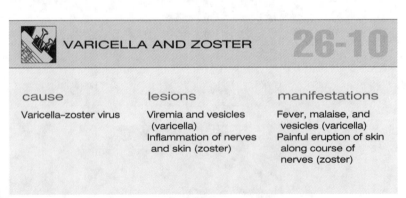

VARICELLA AND ZOSTER 26-10

cause	lesions	manifestations
Varicella–zoster virus	Viremia and vesicles (varicella) Inflammation of nerves and skin (zoster)	Fever, malaise, and vesicles (varicella) Painful eruption of skin along course of nerves (zoster)

Mumps

Mumps is an RNA virus acquired by the respiratory route that preferentially infects the salivary glands and sometimes the ovaries, testes, and pancreas. After an incubation period of 2 to 3 weeks, the disease starts with malaise and fever and is usually followed by painful swelling of the parotid glands. Male patients occasionally experience painful inflammation of the testes (orchitis). Widespread use of mumps vaccine has greatly reduced the incidence of mumps in recent years.

Smallpox (Variola)

This disease is no longer encountered in the United States and is the first human infectious disease now considered to be eliminated from the world because vaccination has been so successful. Smallpox occupies an important place in history, as epidemics in centuries past have devastated populations. The virus is highly contagious and causes a rash much like that of chicken pox, although when it heals it leaves deep, pitted scars. Focal necrotizing lesions occur in many organs, especially lungs and intestinal tract, leading to death in 10–20 percent of cases.

Postviral Encephalitis

All of the viral diseases thus far mentioned may cause an encephalitis that is usually mild and follows the acute phase of the disease. It is attributed to production of T-lymphocytes or antibodies against the virus that cross-react with brain antigens (autoimmunity). Children who manifest this illness have symptoms of altered sensorium.

Other Common Viral Infections

Influenza

Influenza A is a human viral pathogen that causes respiratory disease occurring in small or large epidemics during the winter months. Strains having mutated antigens arise in Asia and sweep the world every 2 or 3 years, causing disease that has a rather high mortality rate among the elderly and the debilitated. The symptoms of influenza range from those of a head cold with malaise to high fever with severe muscular aches and pains and pneumonia. Relative resistance to Influenza A depends upon yearly vaccination with the mutated strains. It must be remembered that all the disease states that we call *flu* are

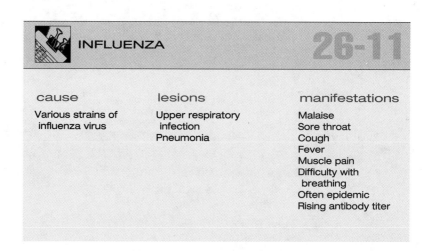

INFLUENZA		26-11
cause	lesions	manifestations
Various strains of influenza virus	Upper respiratory infection Pneumonia	Malaise Sore throat Cough Fever Muscle pain Difficulty with breathing Often epidemic Rising antibody titer

not necessarily caused by the influenza A virus. There are many viruses that cause various upper respiratory infections, malaise, muscle aches, and colds; some of them are well known, such as adenoviruses and rhinoviruses, but many others are nameless. These viruses do not cause large-scale epidemics of disease as do the influenza viruses. Most of these viruses will probably remain nameless for some time, because they are difficult to culture and the diseases they cause are usually of minor consequence to the individual patient. True influenza, although encompassing a spectrum of severity, can cause severe pneumonia with death of the patient. The mechanism of death is usually that of superimposed (secondary) bacterial pneumonia. Other viruses in this general category of agents that cause flu-like syndromes also cause more or less specific illnesses that can be significant; for example, one type of Coxsackie virus causes a myocarditis, and certain strains of echo-viruses cause gastroenteritis.

Infectious Mononucleosis

The agent of infectious mononucleosis is the Epstein–Barr virus, another of the human herpes viruses. This interesting disease characteristically affects teenagers and young adults and generally starts with a sore throat and extreme tiredness. Most victims have splenomegaly and lymphadenopathy, and some may get significant hepatitis. Some patients may get over the disease within a few weeks, but others are ill for many months with fatigue, and physical exertion often exacerbates the symptoms. It appears that the older the patient, the more devastating the disease. The peripheral blood in patients with infectious mononucleosis will show increased numbers of lymphocytes, many of which have atypical morphology. Serum from these patients will react on a glass slide with horse red blood cells, causing them to agglutinate.

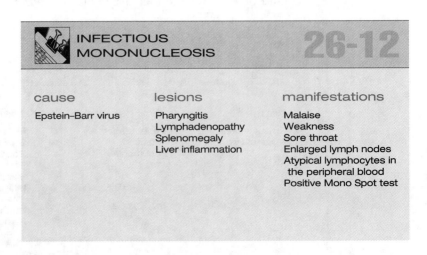

INFECTIOUS MONONUCLEOSIS   26-12

cause	lesions	manifestations
Epstein–Barr virus	Pharyngitis Lymphadenopathy Splenomegaly Liver inflammation	Malaise Weakness Sore throat Enlarged lymph nodes Atypical lymphocytes in the peripheral blood Positive Mono Spot test

This is the basis of the Mono Spot test, which is used to diagnose the disease in patients with the appropriate symptoms.

Herpes Simplex Infections

Herpes simplex is a DNA virus. Two serotypes (I and II) produce a variety of infections. Type I causes most of the oral and skin lesions and is transmitted by direct contact. Type II causes most of the genital lesions and is transmitted by sexual contact. The vesicular lesions that occur on or near the lips, the most common site of type I lesions, are called cold sores or fever blisters, because they are precipitated by febrile illness or other stress such as overexposure to sunlight. After the initial infection, the virus lies dormant in nerves, particularly the trigeminal ganglion in the head, until an episode of stress causes the virus to spread down the nerve with recurrence of the skin lesions. Herpes virus type I occasionally causes a severe and often fatal encephalitis. Herpes simplex virus II may be transmitted during childbirth and produce a fatal disseminated neonatal infection. Administration of acyclovir is highly effective in ameliorating the course of primary herpes simplex infection and may be lifesaving in encephalitis or disseminated infection of the neonate.

Human Papilloma Virus Infections

The 50 or more genetically distinct human papilloma viruses cause or are causally related to proliferative lesions of squamous epithelium including common skin warts (verruca vulgaris), plantar warts (verruca planus), condyloma acuminata (venereal warts), laryngeal polyps, premalignant dysplasias and carcinomas of the cervix and vulva, and squamous carcinoma of skin in immunosuppressed individuals. Different strains are associated with different lesions, e.g., types 2, 4, and 7 with skin warts; 6 and 11 with venereal warts; and 16, 18, and 33 with carcinoma of the cervix. See Chapters 17 and 19 for further details on these lesions.

Cytomegalic Inclusion Disease

This disease is caused by cytomegalic inclusion virus (CMV) another of the human herpes viruses, which is so named because infection with the virus results in giant cells having large intranuclear inclusions. The disease affects infants in utero or neonatally, causing severe brain destruction with mental retardation similar to toxoplasmosis. Cytomegalic inclusion disease is a rare systemic infection in normal adults, but a common infection in immunosuppressed individuals, especially transplant and AIDS patients. The diagnosis is presumptively made upon finding the typical large cells with inclusions in brain, kidney, liver, lung, intestinal tract, or other organ and presence of serum antibodies. DNA testing allows rapid and sensitive detection and the antiviral drug gancyclovir is an effective treatment in most cases.

Viral Hepatitis

This disease is discussed in Chapter 14.

Human Immunodeficiency Virus Infection

Human immunodeficiency virus (HIV) infection is the cause of acquired immune deficiency syndrome (AIDS), which is a disease defined as recurrent opportunistic infections, or Kaposi's sarcoma, or a high-grade lymphoma of the brain in a patient with a positive antibody test for HIV. HIV infection can be diagnosed with very high reliability by serology, culture of the virus, or detection of HIV RNA in blood. The virus must be present for 3 to 17 weeks before the disease can be detected by a screening antibody test. The disease is characterized by a very long latent period of 2 to 8 years or more before symptomatic AIDS becomes manifest. Generalized lymphadenopathy, fever, weight loss, diarrhea, and decreased CD4+ T lymphocytes precede the development of AIDS.

AIDS was first recognized in the early 1980s and is caused by the retrovirus HIV. It was soon recognized that HIV is transmitted both sexually and by direct inoculation through the use of contaminated needles (mainly by drug addicts) and by transfusion of blood products.

Within 2 to 12 weeks after exposure, an acute clinical illness ensues in most persons and is characterized by fever, night sweats, lymphadenopathy, rash, myalgias, arthralgias, headache, and persistent lethargy. Mood changes, irritability, diarrhea, and anorexia may also be seen. Some HIV-infected persons never develop this initial acute clinical illness. The initial illness is not considered AIDS because the patient usually recovers and has a more or less symptom-free period for years (average 8 years) before developing full-blown AIDS. AIDS is heralded by persistent generalized lymphadenopathy followed by fevers, weight loss, diarrhea, fatigue, night sweats, and encephalopathy with dementia, the latter occurring in 60 to 90 percent of all patients with clinical AIDS. Once full-blown AIDS has developed, the prognosis for longterm survival is very poor. More than half of patients with AIDS develop pneumonia due to *Pneumocystis carinii*, an organism that does not cause disease in normal adults. Other opportunistic infections include toxoplasmosis, salmonellosis, tuberculosis, candidiasis, cytomegalovirus infection, herpes simplex, and histoplasmosis and coccidioidomycosis in endemic areas.

The symptoms of AIDS and its complications are related to acquired deficiency in the immune system, particularly the cellular immune system. HIV infects cells by attaching to a receptor called

CD4. Although found on many types of cells, the CD4 receptor is most prevalent on T helper lymphocytes. Thus, the infection of T helper lymphocytes over a period of years results in the gradual destruction of these cells, which are of paramount importance in orchestrating the immune response of other immunocompetent cells, particularly B lymphocytes. It is this insidious and persistent destruction of the cellular immune system that allows opportunistic organisms such as CMV, herpes simplex, toxoplasma, and candida to proliferate and produce devastating disease.

Within a few weeks to months after initial infection, HIV antibodies appear in the patient's serum. Because the standard serologic test can be falsely positive, a more definitive test (called *Western blot*) for the presence of HIV is used to confirm a positive test. Another test that can be used to predict whether the virus is causing significant damage to the immune system is the CD4 helper T cell count—values below 400 cells per microliter are considered abnormal. The concentration of HIV RNA circulating in the peripheral blood (the "viral load") can also be determined.

The lesions in AIDS are mostly nonspecific or related to opportunistic infections. The lymph nodes may demonstrate a simple increase in lymphocytes. The wasting resulting from AIDS is manifest as a loss of adipose tissue and organ atrophy. The opportunistic infections are generally similar to opportunistic infections in patients with other serious illnesses such as cancer or organ transplant. In the brain, however, there is a specific lesion that is virtually diagnostic for AIDS, namely multinucleated giant cells scattered around blood vessels in gray and white matter associated with nonspecific proliferation of glial cells. Some patients with AIDS develop unusual neoplasms, especially lymphomas of unusual type with brain involvement and Kaposi's sarcoma. Kaposi's sarcoma is a neoplastic proliferation of blood vessels that is seen in a relatively high proportion of people with AIDS but rare in other people, and appears to be caused by another human herpes virus.

Millions of people in the United States and around the world are infected with HIV. Homosexual men and intravenous drug users make up the largest proportion in the United States. Blood testing has greatly reduced the risk for patients with hemophilia who are routinely treated with concentrated blood products or transfusion. Heterosexual transmission is the rule in Africa and rapidly increasing in other areas of the world, especially where there are concentrations of prostitutes.

As yet there is no vaccine to protect an individual against the virus once it has been transmitted. Currently available antiviral drugs such as HIV protease inhibitors and reverse transcriptase inhibitors used in combination may slow the replication of the virus and prolong the

HUMAN IMMUNODEFICIENCY VIRUS INFECTION 26-13

cause	lesions	manifestations
Retrovirus (HIV)	Decreased CD4+ lymphocytes	+ Antibody test
	Opportunistic infections	+ Western blot test
	Kaposi's sarcoma	Nonspecific wasting
	Rare lymphoma	Pneumocystis
	Giant cell brain lesion	pneumonia
		Other Infections
		Dementia
		Skin tumors (Kaposi's)

latent period and reduce the severity of the illness. Prevention of transmission is difficult from an educational and biologic standpoint. The primary means to prevent transmission include testing of blood products before use, elimination of the use of potentially contaminated needles by drug users, and prevention of contact between semen and superficial injuries. The virus is present in macrophages in the semen of male carriers and can gain access to male or female sexual partners through minor tears during intercourse. The transmission rate is higher with anal intercourse. Male-to-female transmission is much more likely than the reverse. Condoms provide protection most of the time, but are not always fail-safe. Intrauterine transmission to the fetus also occurs. Ordinary contact with carriers is not considered to be dangerous, and the risk of health care workers being infected by their patients is very small. Transmission of the virus from health care worker to patient is exceedingly rare.

The AIDS epidemic rages on with no signs of abatement. Health costs for treatment, prevention, and research continue to escalate.

Rickettsial Infections

Rickettsia are very small organisms intermediate between bacteria and viruses like chlamydiae. Rickettsia must live within cells (obligate intracellular organisms), and they preferentially attack the endothelial cells of blood vessels.

Rickettsia cause several types of serious and often fatal infectious diseases in man. Among them are typhus, in which the rickettsia are transmitted to man by the body louse, and Rocky Mountain spotted fever, in which the organism is transmitted to man by the tick. Most rickettsial infections cause a skin rash, which is due to small blood vessel involvement in the skin with hemorrhages from these vessels.

RICKETTSIAL DISEASE		26-14
cause	**lesions**	**manifestation**
Various species of rickettsia	Invasion of blood vessel endothelial cells, resulting in small hemorrhages	Skin rashes plus systemic symptoms

Ehrlichiosis is a newly recognized infection caused by a rickettsial-like organism acquired by tick bites that is being encountered with increasing frequency in the United States. It is characterized by fever and lymphadenopathy, but without a rash.

Fungal Infections

Throughout the world, there are numerous fungi that cause disease in man. In the United States, there are several important pathogenic fungi that repeatedly cause disease and others that only rarely cause disease in healthy people but may infect debilitated patients (opportunistic fungi). An infection by a fungus is called a *mycosis* or a *mycotic infection*. Some fungi prefer to invade tissues in the yeast (bud) phase, while others proliferate as hyphae (stems) in the body. A very general way to classify fungal disease is into systemic and cutaneous forms.

Primary Systemic Fungal Infections

Certain fungi invade the interior of the body, usually via a respiratory route although other routes are possible. These fungi can be either primary pathogens or they can be opportunistic, which means that the body has some form of diminished resistance. Some of the important primary systemic mycoses are histoplasmosis, coccidioidomycosis, blastomycosis, and cryptococcosis, caused by *Histoplasma capsulatum, Coccidioides immitis, Blastomyces dermatitidis,* and *Cryptococcus neoformans,* respectively. These diseases share the common features of proliferation of fungi in the yeast phase (Figure 26–6) which usually elicit a granulomatous response from the body. All these diseases can affect the whole body or can be concentrated in one organ. Histoplasmosis is prevalent in parts of the Mississippi and Ohio River valleys and usually causes a subclinical (inapparent) infection. Often, persons get this disease after cleaning chicken coops since the fungal agent is carried in bird droppings. Coccidioidomycosis is prevalent in the San Joaquin Valley in California and parts of Texas, New Mexico, and Arizona.

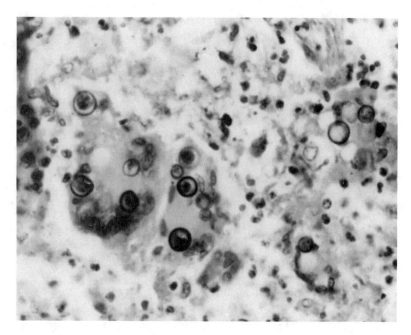

Figure 26–6. Blastomyces in yeast phase (contrast with Aspergillus in hyphal phase, Figure 26–7).

It may cause a subclinical, a severe systemic infection or pneumonia or a characteristic meningitis. The fungal agent is harbored in the soil, and individuals have encountered the disease simply by driving through these endemic areas. Blastomycosis and cryptococcosis can be acquired in most locations. Blastomycosis causes a very destructive lung disease or may present with chronic skin ulcers. Cryptococcosis

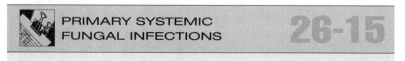

PRIMARY SYSTEMIC FUNGAL INFECTIONS 26-15

causes	lesion	manifestations
Histoplasma capsulatum *Coccidioides immitis* *Blastomyces dermatitidis* *Cryptococcus neoformans*	Granulomatous inflammation of numerous organs (fungus in yeast phase)	Subacute or chronic systemic illness (all) Chronic skin ulcers or lung infection (*Blastomyces, Histoplasma*) Chronic meningitis (*Cryptococcus*)

usually causes a chronic meningitis, often in immunocompromised patients. These diseases follow a slow, protracted course, and diagnosis depends on demonstrating antibodies to the particular organism in the patient's serum by serologic tests, or by detecting an antigen of the organism. Treatment is with intravenous amphotericin B, an antibiotic that can have severe side effects, or by one of the newer oral azole antifungal agents.

Opportunistic Systemic Fungal Infections

These fungal infections usually occur with the fungus in the hyphal phase (Figure 26–7) and elicit an acute inflammatory response rather than a granulomatous one. Some of the more important opportunistic mycoses are candidiasis, aspergillosis, and mucormycosis, caused by species of *Candida, Aspergillus,* and *Mucor* respectively. They occur in persons with impaired cellular immunity due to cancer, other chronic infections, or drugs such as steroids. These infections may be responsible for death or may only be found incidentally at autopsy. Mucormycosis and candidiasis tend to occur in diabetic patients who are out of control and in patients with leukemia. The infection with any of these fungi may be in one or many organs. Pneumonia is most common. Opportunistic infections of all types (fungal, viral, parasitic) have increased in recent years, because the powerful drugs used to prevent organ rejection or to treat cancer commonly suppress bone marrow and lymphatic tissues, thereby decreasing the patient's ability to produce white blood cells and antibodies.

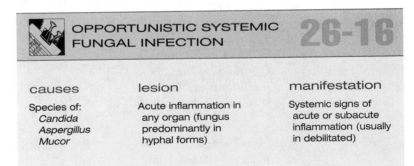

OPPORTUNISTIC SYSTEMIC FUNGAL INFECTION		26-16
causes	**lesion**	**manifestation**
Species of: Candida Aspergillus Mucor	Acute inflammation in any organ (fungus predominantly in hyphal forms)	Systemic signs of acute or subacute inflammation (usually in debilitated)

Cutaneous Fungal Infections

These mycoses produce bothersome skin lesions that are not a serious threat to the patient. Examples of cutaneous fungi are the tineas, which cause athlete's foot, and numerous varieties of organisms that cause ringworm. New antifungal drugs have greatly improved the treatment of these infections.

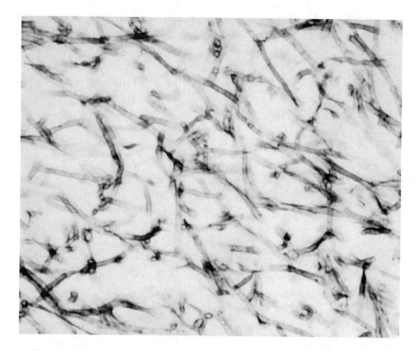

Figure 26–7. Hyphae of Aspergillus in the lung of a patient who died of leukemia.

Protozoal Diseases

Protozoa are unicellular organisms. Pathogenic species are of various types, some invade and live in the blood or tissue cells, while others live on body surfaces. The major blood diseases, malaria and trypanosomiasis, are not endemic in the United States, but are major world health problems. Chagas' disease, found in South America, is a chronic destructive disease that causes severe damage to the heart and esophagus. Leishmaniasis includes forms with involvement of the mononuclear phagocytic systems and skin, but occurs in the United States only rarely, near the Mexican border. Toxoplasmosis is widespread and will be discussed below. Of the surface diseases, trichomoniasis is a vaginal infection (see Chapter 17); amebiasis is due to an intestinal organism that invades and produces colonic ulcers and occasionally liver abscesses (see Chapter 14); and giardiasis is a diarrheal illness due to intestinal infection.

Malaria

There are four types of malaria, caused by *Plasmodium falciparum, P. vivax, P. ovale,* and *P. malariae.* All are transmitted by varieties of Anopheles mosquitoes, mainly throughout Africa, Asia, and Central and South America. *P. falciparum* is the most important type of malaria because it results in the death of up to 1.5 million persons per year. Approximately 1,500 cases of all species are reported in the United States each year and some are transmitted by transfusions and drug use.

The bite of a *P. falciparum* infected mosquito results in the release of sporozoites into the blood of the victim which rapidly invade hepatic cells and multiply. Rupture of the hepatic cell results in the release of 20,000 or more asexual merozoites that invade erythrocytes, multiply and break out of the erythrocytes in cyclic waves that are concomitant with clinical symptoms of chills, fever, severe headaches, sweating, and profound malaise. Anemia, renal failure (blackwater fever), pulmonary edema, and diarrhea can all occur acutely. Children, who have not made antibodies to *P. falciparum*, are particularly susceptible to cerebral malaria because the parasite binds to the endothelium of cerebral microvessels resulting in clogging of the vessels by parasite-infested erythrocytes with hemorrhages, cerebral edema, and neuronal death. Adults are relatively resistant to cerebral malaria, but after repeated bouts of infection develop fibrotic, pigmented livers, and spleens.

Malaria is diagnosed in suspected patients by microscopic examination of blood smears for the parasite. Serum antibodies can be detected by serology but do not distinguish between current or past infection. Chloroquine has been the time-honored treatment but development of resistant strains has resulted in the use of mefloquine or doxycycline. The prognosis for *P. ovale, P. malariae,* and *P. vivax* is generally good but *P. falciparum* is a dangerous disease, even with prompt treatment.

Toxoplasmosis

Toxoplasma gondii organisms are found in the soil and are harbored in small animals, particularly the house cat. Most infections are caused by eating undercooked meat. Toxoplasmosis rarely occurs in healthy adults but causes chronic inflammation as an opportunistic agent in debilitated patients (especially in AIDS) or causes congenital brain

TOXOPLASMOSIS		26-17
cause	**lesions**	**manifestations**
Toxoplasma gondii	Chronic systemic inflammation in debilitated patients	Systemic signs of inflammation in debilitated adults
	Brain infection in newborns	Mental and motor retardation in infants infected transplacentally

infection in newborns. In the case of infants, the organism is transmitted from the mother to the fetus across the placenta, causing a severe infection with destruction of the brain. It is estimated that many retarded individuals in institutions were victims of toxoplasmosis, but the actual incidence is not known. Subclinical toxoplasmosis is prevalent; 50 percent of people in some geographic areas of the United States have antibodies to the organism. Pyrimethamine is usually the drug of choice.

Cryptosporidiosis

Cryptosporidium parvum is a pathogen that is harbored in water systems and causes epidemics of diarrheal illness and a debilitating diarrhea in patients with AIDS. Contamination of water reservoirs has resulted from huge manure piles containing the organism leaking into surface water sources used by municipalities. In 1993, 400,000 residents of Milwaukee, Wisconsin became ill with cryptosporidiosis following contamination of the city's water system.

Giardiasis

Giardia lamblia is a flagellate that lives in the intestinal lumen of man and animals such as cats and beavers. Humans acquire the organism from contaminated water. Most infections are probably asymptomatic, but diarrhea and malabsorption may occur. Metronidazole is highly effective for treating symptomatic diarrhea.

Helminthic Infections

Helminths are primitive round- and flatworms. Most proliferate in the gastrointestinal tract. Those helminths that cause the more severe diseases are generally those that also invade tissues outside the intestinal tract.

Pinworm Infestation

Enterobius vermicularis (pinworm) can cause annoying anal itching but otherwise does not cause serious disease. These small white worms are rapidly spread among members of a family by contact and poor hygiene. They most often cause symptoms in children and can sometimes be seen crawling about the anal orifice where they lay their eggs at night. Cellophane tape is used to dislodge the eggs from the anus for easy diagnosis by viewing the tape under a microscope.

Trichinosis

Trichinella spiralis causes trichinosis. The organism is acquired by ingestion of inadequately cooked meat, especially pork or occasion-

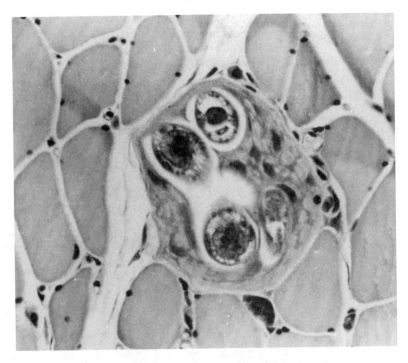

Figure 26–8. Trichinella larvae encysted in skeletal muscle.

ally, bear, because the larval stage of this worm encysts in the animal's muscles (Figure 26–8). After humans eat the meat, the larvae mature and produce more larvae, which disseminate and encyst in the muscles of the human. Other larvae are passed by the human and end up in the garbage, where they may be eaten by swine, thereby repeating the cycle. Just about any muscle can be affected in humans, including the heart. The brain is sometimes involved. Patients have severe muscle pain, fever, and marked eosinophilia in the blood. Occasional deaths result from involvement of heart or respiratory muscles.

TRICHINOSIS   26-18

cause	lesion	manifestations
Trichinella spiralis	Larval cysts in human muscle, including heart (myositis)	Muscle pain Fever Eosinophilia

Tapeworm Disease

Cestodes (tapeworms) include beef, pork, rat, fish, and dog tapeworms. They may cause intestinal disease in man. All are acquired by ingestion of poorly cooked meat or fish. They can cause abdominal pain and diarrhea. The most important of these cestodes is the pork tapeworm (*Taenia solium*), which causes cysticercosis secondary to encystment of the taenia larvae (cysticerca). Unlike most of the other tapeworms, the cysticerca larvae can invade the intestinal wall and disseminate to other organs, especially the brain. The dog tapeworm (*Echinococcus granulosus*) is also capable of causing a similar larval disease (echinococcosis) in which large cysts, called *hydatid cysts*, develop in the involved organs, especially in the liver. The diagnosis of cestode infection is made by finding segments of the worms or ova in the stool. Diagnosis of disseminated cysts in the case of dog or pork tapeworm disease follows a high index of suspicion. Patients may also have blood eosinophilia.

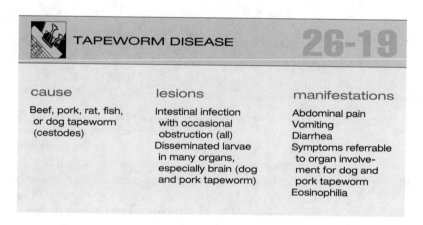

TAPEWORM DISEASE 26-19

cause	lesions	manifestations
Beef, pork, rat, fish, or dog tapeworm (cestodes)	Intestinal infection with occasional obstruction (all) Disseminated larvae in many organs, especially brain (dog and pork tapeworm)	Abdominal pain Vomiting Diarrhea Symptoms referrable to organ involvement for dog and pork tapeworm Eosinophilia

Ascariasis

Ascaris lumbricoides is a large roundworm measuring up to 30 centimeters long. The worm is acquired by ingestion of ova present in soil contaminated by feces. Larvae enter the blood vessels and migrate through the lungs, where they can cause pneumonitis. They are then coughed up and swallowed. After maturing in the intestines, adult worms can cause intestinal obstruction.

Trichuriasis

Trichuris trichuria (whipworm) is fairly common in some parts of the United States. The eggs are ingested from fecally contaminated sources and mature into adults in the lower intestinal tract. Heavy infestations of these worms may cause abdominal pain due to distention and anemia due to bleeding.

Filariasis
This is a tropical disease caused by several species of filarial worms that are acquired by mosquito bites and invade and obstruct lymphatics, causing swelling of the affected part of the body. This swelling may be massive and is called *elephantiasis.*

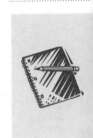

Review Questions

1. What are the body's major defenses against infection by microorganisms?
2. What are the classes of microorganisms that produce infection?
3. What are the major types of bacterial and viral infections?
4. What are the local and systemic signs of inflammation secondary to infection?
5. How are each of the following tests or procedures helpful in the diagnosis of infectious disease?
    Culture
    Gram-stained smear
    Skin tests
    Serologic tests
    Body temperature
    White blood cell count
    Blood eosinophil count
6. How does the laboratory diagnosis of a bacterial infection differ from that of a viral infection?
7. What are the causes, lesions, and major manifestations of each of the specific infectious diseases discussed in this chapter?
8. What are the common diseases caused by staphylococcus? By streptococcus?
9. How do gonorrhea and syphilis differ in terms of chronicity, complications, and means of diagnosis?

10. Which harmful bacterium does not produce an inflammatory response?

11. How are viral diseases controlled?

12. What are the possible complications of each of the viral diseases of childhood?

13. How does influenza differ from various other illnesses labeled as *flu*? What are some of the causes of these other flu-like illnesses?

14. How do primary and secondary systemic fungal infections differ in terms of common organisms causing each, condition of the respective hosts, and type of inflammatory response elicited by each?

15. Why are pork and dog tapeworm infections more serious than other tapeworm infections?

16. What do the following terms mean?
    Saprophyte
    Normal flora
    Pathogen
    Virulence
    Infection
    Anaerobic
    Vector
    Carrier
    Primary infection
    Secondary (opportunistic) infection
    Septicemia
    Exotoxin
    Pyogenic
    Endotoxin
    Endotoxic shock
    Chancre
    Fluorescent treponemal antibody test (FTA)
    Lockjaw
    Primary atypical pneumonia
    Undulant fever
    Obligate intracellular parasite
    Commensal
    Shingles
    Flu
    Yeast
    Hyphae
    Cysticercosis
    Elephantiasis

27.

Immunologic Diseases

REVIEW OF STRUCTURE AND FUNCTION

Antigens and Antibodies
B Lymphocytes • T Lymphocytes • Immunoglobulins • Major Histocompatability System

CLASSIFICATION OF IMMUNOLOGIC DISEASES

Immune Deficiency Diseases
Allergy (Hypersensitivity)
Anaphylactic-Atopic Allergy • Cytotoxic Hypersensitivity • Immune Complex Reactions • Delayed Hypersensitivity
Autoimmunity
Allergic Versus Nonallergic Reactions

MOST FREQUENT AND SERIOUS PROBLEMS

Atopic Allergies
Hayfever • Asthma
Anaphylactic Reactions
Urticaria
Cytotoxic Reactions
Transfusion Reactions • Erythroblastosis Fetalis
Delayed Hypersensitivity Reaction
Contact Dermatitis
Immune Deficiencies

SYMPTOMS, SIGNS, AND TESTS

Electrophoresis • Immunodiffusion • Skin Tests • Coombs' Test • Tissue Immunofluorescence • Antinuclear Antibody Test

SPECIFIC DISEASES

Immune Deficiency Diseases
Acquired Immune Deficiency Syndrome (AIDS)
Anaphylactic-Atopic Allergies (Type I)
Allergic Rhinitis (Hay Fever) and Asthma
Urticaria (Hives) and Angioedema

Systemic Anaphylaxis
Gastrointestinal Food Allergies
Cytotoxic Hypersensitivities (Type II)
Erythroblastosis Fetalis
Blood Transfusion Reactions
Autoimmune Hemolytic Anemia and Thrombocytopenia
Immune Complex, or Arthus-Type, Hypersensitivities
(Type III)
Arthus Reaction
Serum Sickness
Glomerulonephritis
Polyarteritis Nodosa
Delayed, or Cell-Mediated, Hypersensitivities (Type IV)
Contact Dermatitis
Infections Manifest Primarily as Delayed Hypersensitivity
Reactions
Graft Rejection
Autoimmune Diseases
Systemic Lupus Erythematosus (SLE)

REVIEW QUESTIONS

REVIEW OF STRUCTURE AND FUNCTION

Immunity is a term that means the resistance to or protection from an individual's environment. Certain forms of protection, such as the skin and the inflammatory response, have been discussed in other chapters. The immune system is an internal chemical system whose purpose is to enhance reactivity to material that is foreign to the body. Material recognized as foreign by the immunologic system is called an antigen. Most antigens are introduced from outside of the body, but some are altered endogenous materials that are treated as if they were foreign. The immunologic system recognizes antigens by producing *antibodies* or specialized lymphocytes specific for each antigen (Figure 27–1). Large foreign particles, such as bacteria, contain several antigens and may elicit the production of several different antibodies. Also, several different foreign substances may contain the same antigen; for example, some persons have the same antigen in heart muscle that exists in group A streptococci.

Antigens are classified as either complete or incomplete. Complete antigens both induce immune responses and react with the antibodies produced by the immune response. Incomplete antigens can react with antibodies but cannot induce an immune response unless chemically coupled to another antigen. Incomplete antigens are also called *haptens*.

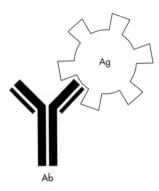

Figure 27–1. Schematic representation of antigen (Ag) and antibody (Ab).

Antibodies are produced within the cytoplasm of plasma cells, which in turn are derived from lymphocytes. Antibodies produced by plasma cells are released into the blood, where they circulate freely as part of the gamma-globulin fraction of serum proteins and are called *immunoglobulins.* The lymphocytes that are capable of developing into plasma cells to produce immunoglobulins are called *B lymphocytes* or *B cells* after the bursa of Fabricius of chickens. In chickens, the bursa is the primary site of development of B cells. In humans, B cells originate from lymphoid tissue of the alimentary tract and bone marrow.

A second type of lymphocyte is the *T lymphocyte* or *T cell,* so named because its production is programmed by the thymus in both humans and lower animals. T lymphocytes and B lymphocytes are similar morphologically in ordinary tissue sections; specialized tests are required to distinguish them. They are both capable of recognizing specific antigens.

There are several known functions of T cells and subtypes of T cells are named to reflect their function. Some *T-helper cells* physically deliver information about antigens to B cells in order to aid B cells in the production of antibodies, whereas other T cells primarily aid macrophages in carrying out delayed hypersensitivity functions. *T-suppressor cells* suppress B cells in order to prevent the production of excess antibody; they also prevent the production of antibodies to the body's own tissues. *Cytotoxic T cells* can directly kill other cells that process foreign or altered antigens, such as neoplastic cells or cells infected with viruses. Another class of lymphocytes, *natural killer cells* (NK cells) destroy other cells in the absence of any known antigenic stimulation, possibly by reacting with glycoproteins on the target cells' surface. It is hypothesized that the body continually develops neoplastic cell lines but NK cells destroy these neoplastic cells before they can accumulate to form neoplasms. This type of police action by NK cells is termed *immune surveillance.* There is probably some overlap in function of each of the T-cell types.

Antigens are usually broken-down (processed) and then presented to T cells by macrophages or other specialized cells collectively called *antigen-presenting cells.* Once a T cell with a specific receptor for a particular antigen receives the antigen, it will either help program a group of B cells to produce antibody, suppress the production of antibody, or directly kill a foreign cell, depending upon whether it is a helper, suppressor, or cytotoxic T cell. The concept of specific antigenic receptors on T cells implies that there must be countless different T cells in the normal body in order to accommodate the almost infinite number of potential antigens. This indeed appears to be the case and is a very functional aspect of immunity, because, if the possibility of T cell cross-reactivity with different antigens were great, then the possibility of self-reactivity would also be great, resulting in autoimmune phenomena.

In addition to the regulatory mechanisms already outlined, T cells work in cooperation with B cells in other ways to increase the specificity of the immunoglobulin to the antigen. T cells also elaborate numerous cytokines with various functions in acute and chronic inflammation, including recruitment of other cells.

About 10 days after the first encounter with an antigen, antibodies become detectable. Subsequent encounters with the same antigen are associated with a more rapid production of antibodies called the *secondary response.* Certain lymphocytes serve as *memory cells,* which means that they are long-lived, and are programmed to proliferate rapidly after a second encounter with that antigen.

Immunoglobulins carry out their function in several ways, depending on the structure of the antigen and the class of antibody involved. Immunoglobulins are divided into five classes (IgA, IgG, IgM, IgD, and IgE) based on their biologic properties and major differences in their protein structure. IgG and IgM, the most common, are schematized in Figure 27–2.

IgG, the most abundant immunoglobulin, can combine with antigens such as bacterial exotoxins to neutralize their activity, or it can adhere to antigen on the surface of larger foreign materials such as bacteria to promote their phagocytosis by leukocytes. IgG is particularly important to infants, who because of their age have an immature immune system. IgG antibodies are transmitted across the placenta to the fetus from the mother; thus, the infant is protected during its first 6 months of life from diseases previously encountered by the mother. The combination of IgG with antigen sometimes employs another reaction, called *complement activation.* Complement is a group of spe-

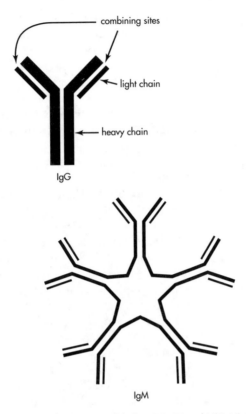

Figure 27–2. Basic structures of immunoglobulins G (IgG) and M (IgM). IgM is the equivalent of five IgG molecules.

cial serum proteins that often take part in antigen-antibody reactions. Activation of complement is a complex series of enzymatic reactions that has at least three important effects: proteins are produced that may lyse (rupture) cells, mediators are released that may in turn cause release of histamine from mast cells, and chemotactic agents are produced that may attract leukocytes. The first effect can destroy cells that are recognized as foreign; the other two effects initiate the vascular and cellular components of acute inflammation, respectively.

IgM antibodies are noteworthy for their large size, which is five times that of IgG antibodies (Figure 27–2). IgM antibodies do not readily pass into the tissues or across the placenta. They develop more quickly than IgG antibodies following antigenic stimulation, and they are important in controlling bacteria that enter the bloodstream and in agglutination (clumping) of large foreign substances such as incompatible red blood cells. IgM antibody reactions may also activate complement.

IgA is noteworthy because it is secreted into body fluids such as tears, milk, saliva, bronchi, and the intestinal tract, where it may interact with antigens before they can enter the body's tissues.

IgE acts in a very specific manner. IgE becomes attached to basophils in the bloodstream and mast cells in tissues. When antigen reacts with IgE on the surface of basophils or mast cells, the cells release vasoactive substances such as histamine. For unknown reasons, IgE reactions are often associated with increased numbers of eosinophils in tissue and blood.

IgD serves as an antigen receptor on the surface of mature B cells (along with IgM).

Thus, immunoglobulins can protect the body from antigenic foreign materials in a variety of ways, including precipitating or neutralizing the chemical action of small foreign materials, agglutinating larger foreign materials so they can be phagocytosed, and lysing foreign cells (Figure 27–3). Immunoglobulins can also initiate an acute inflammatory reaction to control the spread of and destroy certain foreign agents, and they can combine with foreign substances on body surfaces to prevent their entry into the body.

The major histocompatibility system genetically controls the expression of both self- and foreign antigens on cell surfaces of most cells in the body. This system in man is located on genes in the sixth chromosome and is very similar to the ABO system in which different individuals express different erythrocyte surface antigens. Just as it is important to insure that transfused blood is given to recipients who are of the same ABO type as the donor, likewise, organ transplants such as kidney, skin, or bone marrow must share similar major histocompatibility antigens between donor and recipient. If the antigens are not similar, the recipient's immune system will recognize a trans-

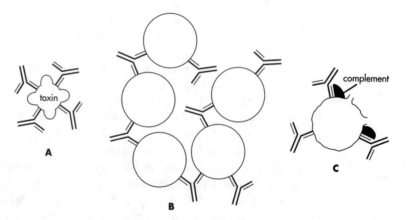

Figure 27–3. Neutralizing (A), agglutination (B), and lysing (C) actions of immunoglobulins.

planted kidney, for example, as foreign and produce antibodies and cytotoxic T cells to destroy the kidney. Conversely, donor lymphocytes, transplanted with an organ into an incompatible host, can, under certain circumstances, mount an attack against the recipient's tissues. This phenomenon is referred to as *graft vs. host disease.*

T cells cannot process antigen unless it is presented to the T cells in conjunction with products of the histocompatibility system. For example, a macrophage presenting antigen to a T cell must carry on its surface with the foreign antigen, certain major histocompatibility antigens which the T cells can recognize as similar to their own. Otherwise, the T cell cannot recognize the antigen as foreign. This is referred to as major histocompatibility complex restriction. The reasons for this restriction are not entirely known, but it must serve as a link in programming B cells to produce antibodies.

CLASSIFICATION OF IMMUNOLOGIC DISEASES

Immune reactions are generally protective and helpful. However, in certain circumstances, they can be more harmful than helpful, in which case they produce disease. Immune diseases fall into two major categories: *immune deficiency diseases,* in which there is too little response to foreign agents, and allergy or hypersensitivity reactions, in which there is too much response to antigens. The term *hypersensitivity* is slightly broader than the term *allergy* and may include some exaggerated responses that are not antigen-antibody mediated or are of unknown cause. Hypersensitivity reactions to the body's own components mediated by the immune system are called *autoimmune diseases.*

Immune deficiency diseases are subdivided into inherited and acquired forms and into deficiencies of the T-cell and B-cell immune systems or both.

The four major types of allergy (hypersensitivity) are divided on the basis of mechanisms. The first three types involve immunoglobulins, and the fourth type involves T lymphocytes.

Type I, called anaphylactic-atopic allergy, includes those reactions mediated by IgE antibody and involving release of vasoactive chemicals from tissue mast cells or blood basophilic leukocytes (Figure 27–4). The reaction occurs within minutes; hence, it is sometimes designated as immediate. It is virtually the same reaction as the initial stage of the acute inflammatory reaction.

Type II, called *cytotoxic-type hypersensitivity,* involves destruction of host cells either by agglutination and phagocytosis or by lysis of the cell membrane as a consequence of complement fixation (Figure 27–5). Red blood cells are commonly targets of this type of hypersensitivity,

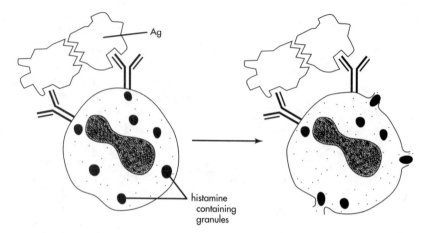

Figure 27–4. Pathogenesis of type I allergic reaction. Antigen reacts with antibody attached to mast cells by cross-linking two IgE molecules (or receptors) to cause release of histamine-containing granules.

and the antigens are either the red blood cell membrane itself or a foreign chemical, such as a drug, that adheres to the red cell membrane as a hapten. The reaction may be either immediate or prolonged.

Type III, called *immune complex* or *Arthus-type hypersensitivity* is defined as a complement-mediated reaction to precipitates of antigen and antibody (antigen–antibody complexes). The antigen–antibody complexes lodge in vessel walls, and the activation of certain inflammation-inducing components of complement (C3a, C5a) results in release of vasoactive substances from mast cells and attraction of polymorphonuclear leukocytes to the site (Figure 27–6). The

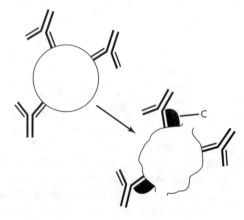

Figure 27–5. Type II allergic reaction with lysis of red blood cells. Antibody reacts with cell surface antigens, resulting in complement fixation (c) and cell lysis.

blood vessel wall

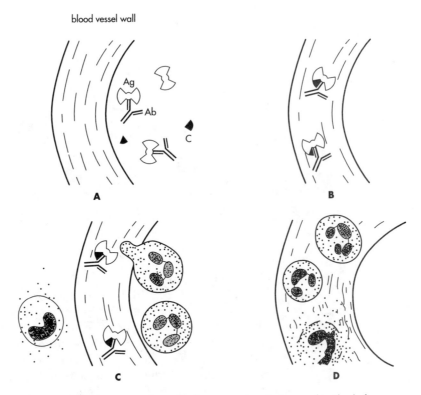

Figure 27–6. Pathogenesis of type III allergic reaction. Antigen and antibody form complexes (A) in the presence of excess antigen. The complexes are deposited in the vessel wall and fix complement (B). Activated components of complement cause release of vasoactive materials from mast cells and chemotaxis of polys (C). The end result is acute inflammation and destruction of the vessel wall (D).

acute inflammatory reaction takes several hours to develop and may be prolonged if the amount of antibody is small. Antigen excess over antibody is required to produce the reaction, because complete binding of all antigens by antibodies inhibits complement activation.

Type IV, called *delayed hypersensitivity* or *cell-mediated hypersensitivity*, is the harmful destruction of tissue by T lymphocytes and macrophages (Figure 27–7). Lymphocyte-mediated reactions are slow to develop, usually requiring 1 to 2 days to reach a peak, hence the name *delayed hypersensitivity*.

There are numerous other allergic diseases that cannot be subclassified on the basis of mechanism because the mechanism is not known. Many autoimmune diseases and drug reactions fall into the unclassifiable category.

The principal criteria that separate allergic from nonallergic reactions to foreign substances are as follows:

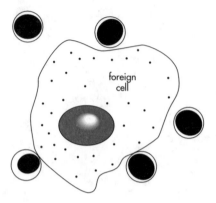

Figure 27–7. Pathogenesis of type IV allergic reaction. Sensitized T lymphocytes attack foreign cells.

1. The initial reaction in an allergic disease requires approximately 10 days, the time required for antibody production; subsequent responses will recur immediately for immunoglobulin-mediated allergies and in 1 to 2 days for cell-mediated allergies. The reaction time for nonallergic responses to foreign materials will be constant and dependent on the nature of the offending agent rather than on an allergic mechanism. For example, chemical injuries may be immediate, inflammatory reactions may take several hours, and hyperplastic responses may take days to weeks.

2. Allergic diseases tend to occur only in selected susceptible individuals, while other foreign substances tend to affect people without bias. Multiple genetic and environmental factors appear to be involved in the selected susceptibility to allergens (antigens). Most people have the protective responses, but few have the harmful responses to antigens.

3. In allergic diseases there is usually a poor relationship between dose of allergen and severity of the reactions, whereas with other agents, the dose-injury relationship is usually quite predictable.

MOST FREQUENT AND SERIOUS PROBLEMS

Of type I hypersensitivity reactions, atopic allergies are most frequent, affecting about 10 percent of the population. The most common example is hay fever (allergic rhinitis). Atopic diseases are chronic reactions, because they are caused by exposure to antigens in the environment, e.g., ragweed pollen, house dust, or animal danders. Allergic asthma, another atopic reaction caused by the same antigens, affects approximately 3 percent of the population. Anaphylactic reactions are acute reactions following a distinct reexposure to an antigen. Urticaria (hives) is a common form and may be the result of food allergy or drug reaction. A more severe and immediately life-threatening form of type I hypersensitivity is anaphylactic shock, a condition in which vasoactive substances are released systemically. Drugs and insect stings are the most common causes of anaphylactic shock.

The most common types of cytotoxic (type II) hypersensitivity reactions are transfusion reactions, in which antibodies to transfused blood cells are present in the recipient, and erythroblastosis fetalis, in which maternal antibodies cross the placenta to cause destruction of the infant's red blood cells.

Immune complex hypersensitivities (type III) are common and very complicated and vary considerably in terms of exact mechanisms, tissue involved, and severity. Frequent types are serum sickness, which is usually a drug reaction, and some types of glomerulonephritis. Polyarteritis nodosa is a rare but potentially fatal immune complex hypersensitivity. Rheumatoid arthritis and lupus erythematosus are probably immune complex hypersensitivities.

Allergic contact dermatitis is the most common type of delayed hypersensitivity (type IV) reaction, and poison ivy is the most common specific cause. Graft rejection, following a skin graft or renal transplant, are examples of delayed hypersensitivity in which the donor and recipient tissue antigens are incompatible.

Immune deficiencies are much less common than allergies. Inherited immune deficiencies, whether of the B cell or T cell immune systems, are rare but particularly significant because they lead to repeated, severe infections in the first few years of life and are often fatal. Acquired immune deficiencies are more common than inherited forms and vary in severity from mild to severe. Causes include disseminated hematopoietic diseases such as leukemia or lymphoma, cancer chemotherapy, and immunosuppressive drug therapy, which is used to protect transplanted organs from being rejected as foreign tissue. Acquired immune deficiency syndrome (AIDS) is frequent, and due to a virus.

SYMPTOMS, SIGNS, AND TESTS

The clinical manifestations of immune disease are quite varied and often unique to the specific types of diseases as well as to the organ system involved. Consequently, clinical manifestations will be discussed in relation to specific diseases.

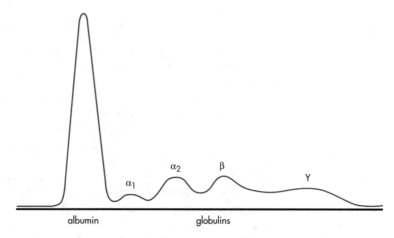

Figure 27–8. Normal serum proteins as measured by serum electrophoresis test.

Many laboratory tests have been devised to aid in the diagnosis of immune diseases. The amount of gamma globulin in the blood can be measured by *electrophoresis of serum* (Figure 27–8). The five specific types of immunoglobulin can be measured by *immunodiffusion* tests in which prepared antibodies are reacted against IgG, IgA, IgM, IgE, and IgD. The reaction product precipitates in a gel medium and can then be stained and measured. These tests are most important in the evaluation of relative and absolute immune deficiencies.

The components of complement can also be measured by immunodiffusion. A decreased level of complement is inferential evidence that a type II or III reaction has taken place.

The most important tests for diagnosing type I anaphylactic–atopic allergies are *skin tests,* in which a suspected antigen, such as a drug, house dust, cat hair, seafood, dander, or ragweed pollen, is injected into the skin. Allergy to a specific antigen is manifested immediately as a small inflammatory reaction at the site of injection. Hundreds of different antigens have been isolated and can be used for such skin tests.

Cytotoxic (type II reactions) antibodies on erythrocytes are demonstrated by the *direct Coombs' test* in which antihuman gamma globulin is added to a test tube of washed erythrocytes. If the erythrocytes have been coated with cytotoxic or other antibodies, they will agglutinate upon addition of the antihuman gamma globulin (Figure 27–9). The *indirect Coombs' test* will detect serum antibodies having the potential to react with erythrocytes. In this test, the patient's serum is first incubated with another person's erythrocytes in a test tube to allow the antierythrocyte antibodies to coat the erythrocytes. The test then proceeds in the same fashion as the direct Coombs' test. Similar tests are less commonly performed to demonstrate antibodies to white cells or platelets.

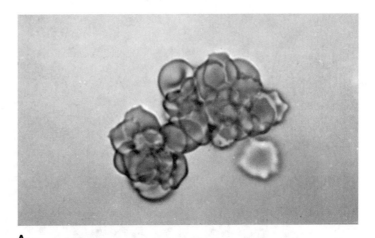

A

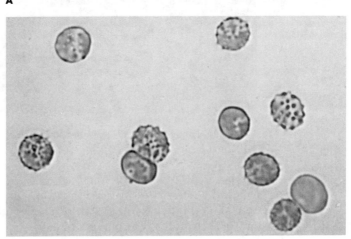

B

Figure 27–9. Positive (A) and negative (B) direct Coombs' test.

Immune complex (type III) diseases are often diagnosed on the basis of history plus the clinical picture of the disease. However, the deposition of antigen–antibodies and complement in tissues may be tested for by *immunofluorescence.* In this test, a section of tissue (biopsy) from a diseased organ is overlain with fluorescent-tagged antibodies to specific immunoglobulin or complement. The fluorescent-tagged antibody will form a complex with the deposited immunoglobulin or complement (usually in vessels) and fluoresce a bright yellow-green color under special blue light (Figure 27–10). This test is used routinely on kidney biopsies in order to separate the various types of glomerulonephritis.

Delayed (cell-mediated) hypersensitivity to microorganisms such as occurs in tuberculosis and fungal diseases can be evaluated by skin

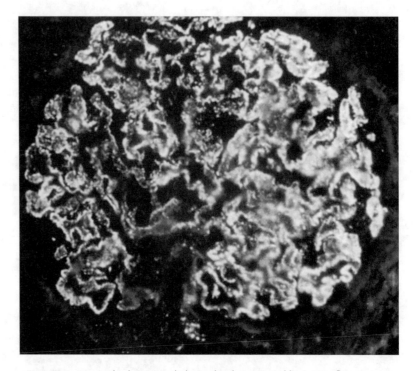

Figure 27–10. Antibodies in renal glomerulus demonstrated by immunofluorescence.

tests in which the antigen (killed microorganisms) is injected into the skin and a delayed (48 to 72 hours) inflammatory reaction ensues. Contact dermatitis is most often diagnosed by good detective work, but suspected allergens may be tested by placing them on the skin (patch test).

Autoimmune diseases are so varied that most are difficult to diagnose as such. An exception is systemic lupus erythematosus (SLE), for which the *antinuclear antibody test* (ANA) has been devised. Persons with SLE have antibodies directed against the nuclei of their own cells, and this is demonstrated by the ANA test. In rheumatoid arthritis, the laboratory demonstration of the *rheumatoid factor* (RF) may aid in diagnosis.

SPECIFIC DISEASES

Immune diseases are the result of excessive or deficient antibody or cellular immune response. They can take many forms including developmental, inflammatory, and neoplastic conditions involving various organ systems. Specific diseases in this chapter will be classified into the immune deficiencies and the four basic types of allergy.

Immune Deficiency Diseases

Immune deficiencies are manifest by an increased susceptibility to infections, i.e., more frequent and severe infections. If the deficiency is in the immunoglobulins (B cell system), infections produced by pyogenic bacteria, such as pneumonia, will occur. If the deficiency is in the cell-mediated immune system, infections produced by a variety of weak pathogens, including bacteria, fungi, viruses, and protozoa, will occur. Inherited deficiency of the immunoglobulin system can be substantiated by finding very low levels of serum gamma globulin (*agammaglobulinemia*). In acquired forms, the levels are not usually as low (*hypogammaglobulinemia*). Deficiencies of the T cell immune system are demonstrated by absence of skin reactivity to substances that commonly cause a delayed hypersensitivity reaction. A delayed hypersensitivity skin test is performed by placing the antigen in or on the skin and checking in 1 to 2 days for the typical raised, firm delayed hypersensitivity reaction. A person with a positive skin test for tuberculosis may later revert to a negative skin test following an acquired deficiency of T cell-mediated immunity. T cell deficiencies can also adversely affect antibody production if the deficiency involves T-helper cells.

Acquired Immune Deficiency Syndrome (AIDS)

Acquired immune deficiency syndrome (AIDS) is now the most important and severe form of acquired immune deficiency. It is discussed in Chapter 26.

Anaphylactic–Atopic Allergies (Type I)

Anaphylactic–atopic allergies are caused by the release of chemicals called vasoactive amines. These substances include histamine from mast cells or blood basophils, which produces the most immediate reaction, and other substances which cause slightly more delayed reactions. As a group, these substances produce the following effects: (1) contraction of most nonvascular smooth muscle, producing effects such as bronchial constriction leading to asthmatic breathing; (2) vasodilation, which locally leads to increased blood flow and systemically may lead to shock; (3) increased vascular permeability, which leads to edema such as is seen in the raised wheals of urticaria of the skin or the swollen nasal mucosa of hay fever; and (4) stimulation of secretory activity of some glands, such as the increased mucus secretion in the bronchus in asthma and increased nasal secretions in hay fever. A typical laboratory finding in this group of diseases is an increase in eosinophils in the blood or tissue. Thus, eosinophilia suggests atopic allergy, but it also may be found in some immune complex diseases. Potential atopic allergens may be evaluated by skin testing. A raised edematous lesion with red border (wheal and flare) reaches a maximum about 15 minutes after intradermal injection of the allergen being tested.

Allergic Rhinitis (Hay Fever) and Asthma

Because many allergens are airborne, the respiratory tract is a common site for hypersensitivity reactions to them. The portion of the tract affected presumably reflects individual differences of unknown nature. Both rhinitis and asthma can be triggered by nonallergic mechanisms in susceptible individuals. Asthma involves the lungs and produces three effects: (1) bronchoconstriction, resulting from the contraction of the smooth muscle layers of bronchial and bronchiolar segments of the tract; (2) edema, resulting from vasodilation and increased permeability of bronchial vessels; and (3) increased secretion of thick, tenacious mucoid material. If secretions are not removed by expectoration, their accumulation can impede air flow. The chief mechanical difficulty experienced in bronchial asthma is increased resistance to air flow manifested by wheezing. Generally, attacks are episodic, but the occasional asthma patient may experience a persistence of symptoms for 24 hours or more and fail to respond to medication. This condition of prolonged and unresponsive asthmatic distress is termed *status asthmaticus*. The patient exhibits very labored breathing with great respiratory effort, dyspnea, harassing cough, and sometimes cyanosis. Anxiety is great, and sleeplessness, extreme fatigue, exhaustion, dehydration, and disorientation develop.

When allergic rhinitis is of short duration (days to a few weeks) and seasonal, the term *hay fever* is used. The allergens of hay fever are seasonal plant pollens including ragweed pollen (late summer and early autumn) and tree and grass pollens (spring and early summer). Ubiquitous allergens, such as those found in house dust, may produce a chronic condition lasting the year round that may be aggravated by

ASTHMA		27-1
cause	**lesions**	**manifestations**
Type I allergy	Spasm of bronchi	Wheezing
	Thickened bronchi with	Dyspnea
	increased mucus and	Cough
	eosinophils	Positive skin test to
		allergen (some cases)

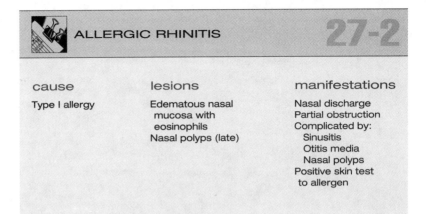

ALLERGIC RHINITIS

27-2

cause	lesions	manifestations

Type I allergy	Edematous nasal mucosa with eosinophils
	Nasal polyps (late)
		Nasal discharge
		Partial obstruction
		Complicated by:
		  Sinusitis
		  Otitis media
		  Nasal polyps
		Positive skin test to allergen

factors such as high humidity, irritating vapors, and upper respiratory tract infections. Allergic rhinitis is marked by edema and hypersecretion by the mucosal lining of the nasopharyngeal cavities that produces partial blockage of the airways and intense nasal and postnasal discharge. The involved nasopharyngeal mucosa appears pale and swollen. Edema may affect the mucosa of the paranasal sinuses, reducing their drainage, and it may close the eustachian tube. Secondary infection and inflammation of the sinuses (sinusitis) and the middle ear (otitis media) may result. After many years, allergic nasal polyps may develop. These are masses of redundant edematous mucosa, which may obstruct breathing, and occur more frequently with nonallergic (intrinsic) rhinitis and asthma.

Urticaria (Hives) and Angioedema

Urticaria is a type I allergy that is recognized on the skin by slightly raised, flat, well-demarcated, edematous patches with a congested border (wheal and flare) (Figure 27–11). Urticaria develops rapidly after exposure to an allergen and is associated with pruritus. Urticaria may be caused by an anaphylactic reaction in the skin to allergens that may have been introduced into the skin (injected drugs or insect stings) or, more often, by allergens that have been ingested and distributed throughout the body after alimentary absorption. A great variety of foods are known to cause urticaria, shellfish, strawberries, and tomatoes being common examples. Some contain histamine or histamine-releasing substances, thus causing urticaria by a nonspecific rather than an IgE-mediated mechanism. Mosquito bites cause a wheal due to nonspecific irritants in the saliva of the mosquito, whereas, stinging insects (mainly *trymenoptera*) inject allergens into the skin with rear stingers rather than mouth parts. Most chronic urticaria is idiopathic. *Angioedema* is a more extreme skin manifestation of immediate hyper-

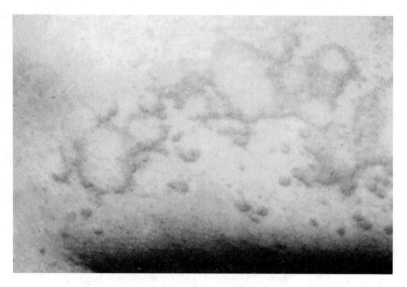

Figure 27–11. Urticaria.

sensitivity than urticaria. It also is an edematous eruption, but it is more widespread and involves the deep dermis. Often it affects the lips, tongue, face, or even the pharynx, perhaps blocking the airway. Its causes are similar to those of urticaria.

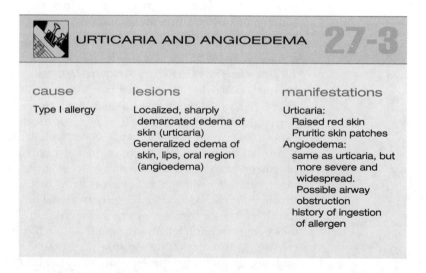

URTICARIA AND ANGIOEDEMA 27-3

cause	lesions	manifestations

Type I allergy	Localized, sharply demarcated edema of skin (urticaria)
	Generalized edema of skin, lips, oral region (angioedema)
		Urticaria:
		  Raised red skin
		  Pruritic skin patches
		Angioedema:
		  same as urticaria, but more severe and widespread.
		  Possible airway obstruction
		  history of ingestion of allergen

Systemic Anaphylaxis
This is one of the true medical emergencies. Within seconds to minutes after exposure to the allergen, the patient feels an itching of the scalp, tongue, and throat followed by generalized flushing and

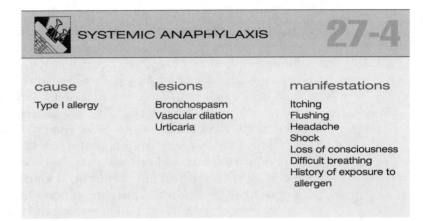

SYSTEMIC ANAPHYLAXIS **27-4**

cause	lesions	manifestations
Type I allergy	Bronchospasm Vascular dilation Urticaria	Itching Flushing Headache Shock Loss of consciousness Difficult breathing History of exposure to allergen

headache. Difficulty in breathing begins and is joined shortly thereafter by precipitous drop in blood pressure and body temperature. Shock and loss of consciousness occur within a short time. If early reversal is not instituted, the train of events may lead to death from shock within 15 minutes of allergic exposure. Treatment is immediate subcutaneous administration of epinephrine, which causes vasoconstriction, thereby reversing systemic shock. The more common allergens that cause anaphylaxis are pollens, foods, chemicals, venoms from stinging insects, foreign sera such as diphtheria or tetanus antitoxins, and drugs such as penicillin.

Gastrointestinal Food Allergies

Primary allergic reactions in the gastrointestinal tract are less common than skin reactions. A gastrointestinal reaction begins shortly after eating specific foods to which the person is allergic. Symptoms include diarrhea, vomiting, and cramps. Shellfish contain common allergens that can produce this reaction.

Cytotoxic Hypersensitivities (Type II)

Cytotoxic hypersensitivity reactions are usually manifested by low levels of blood cells, because this type of reaction is often directed against blood cells. Antibodies may form against red blood cells, platelets, or white blood cells and produce anemia, thrombocytopenia, or leukopenia, respectively. The direct Coombs' test is used to detect antibodies on the surface of red blood cells.

Erythroblastosis Fetalis

This hemolytic disorder of the newborn is caused by immunologic incompatibility between mother and child and usually involves the Rh antigen of red blood cells. This antigen is expressed as an autosomal dominant trait present on the erythrocytes of 85 percent of the population. When the fetus is Rh positive and the mother Rh negative, the mother will develop anti-Rh antibodies, because some of the fetal erythrocytes will enter the mother's circulation at the time of birth. Consequently, the first pregnancy of a woman with an Rh incompatible fetus is uncomplicated. If the sensitized mother has a subsequent pregnancy with an Rh-positive child, the transplacental passage of IgG immunoglobulins brings anti-Rh to the child's blood. By the time of birth, the child has suffered from continuous hemolysis and may be jaundiced from excess bilirubin, anemic, and edematous. The hemolysis is often accentuated just after birth, at which time the infant no longer has the help of the placenta in removing bilirubin. Consequently, blood of the infant is often exchanged for Rh-negative blood (exchange transfusion). Erythroblastosis fetalis can be prevented by injecting mothers with human gamma globulin containing anti-Rh antibodies within 72 hours after delivery of the first and subsequent Rh-positive children. This binds the antigens on the fetal red blood cells so that the mother's immune system does not recognize them as antigenic and, therefore, does not produce antibodies. Because of this now routine preventive measure, erythroblastosis fetalis is not nearly so common as it once was.

ERYTHROBLASTOSIS FETALIS 27-5

causes	lesion	manifestations
Type II allergy (cytotoxic) Development of anti-Rh antibodies in an Rh-negative mother directed against Rh-positive fetal red cells	Hemolyzed red cells in the fetus	Anemia Edema Jaundice Positive Coombs' test Elevated serum bilirubin

Blood Transfusion Reactions

There are many different antigen systems in red blood cells of which the ABO and Rh systems are most important. An Rh-negative individual does not have anti-Rh antibodies unless previously sensitized. A person with the A antigen on red blood cells has anti-B antibody as a natural phenomenon. Thus, persons with blood group B have anti-A antibodies, those with O blood have both anti-A and anti-B, and those

	BLOOD TRANSFUSION REACTIONS	27-6

cause	lesion	manifestations
Incompatible ABO or Rh blood systems	Hemolysis of recipient's red cells	Chills Fever Renal failure Positive Coombs' test

with AB have neither antibody. Because the antibodies are normally present, transfused blood with an ABO incompatibility will produce immediate hemolysis of the transfused red blood cells, resulting in fever, chills, and possible renal failure. These reactions are prevented by typing and cross-matching of blood before transfusion. *Typing* refers to checking for major (ABO and Rh) blood groups to make sure that they are not incompatible, and *cross-matching* refers to mixing samples of donor and recipient blood to see if an in vitro (test tube) reaction occurs due to an unsuspected antibody.

Autoimmune Hemolytic Anemia and Thrombocytopenia

Many spontaneously occurring hemolytic anemias and thrombocytopenias are cytotoxic-type hypersensitivity reactions. The reactions may be mild, with agglutinated cells being prematurely removed by the spleen. In mild types, splenectomy may control the disease. Autoimmune hemolytic anemias can be detected by the direct Coombs' test, in which red cells coated with an antibody will be observed to agglutinate in vitro with the addition of antihuman globulin serum. Sometimes drugs attach to the cell surface and become part of the antigen, in which case the drug is a hapten.

Immune Complex, or Arthus-Type, Hypersensitivities (Type III)

Immune complex hypersensitivity reactions produce vasculitis and, as a secondary phenomenon, edema because of the release of vasoactive substances. The frequent involvement of renal glomeruli in immune complex diseases is often associated with loss of protein and red blood cells in the urine and variable degrees of renal failure. Involvement of joint surfaces leads to joint swelling. More severe forms result in a generalized vasculitis with involvement of many organs.

Arthus Reaction

This is the prototype of immune complex hypersensitivity reactions and is an experimental reaction and not a naturally occurring disease. Local injection of soluble antigen in an animal previously sensitized by the same antigen produces an acute inflammation at the site of inoculation. Histologically, the reaction shows evidence of cell necrosis, infiltration with neutrophils, and vasculitis, all sequelae of the acute inflammatory reaction.

Serum Sickness

This is the prototype of a systemic Arthus-type or immune complex reaction. Classically, it occurred after injection of horse serum. The horse serum was used as a source of antibodies to toxins such as tetanus toxin; however, the protective effect was often offset by the harmful effect produced when the patient developed antibodies to the horse serum. The horse serum (antigen) circulates in the patient's blood for a long time. As antibodies begin to develop after about 10 days, antigen-antibody complexes form, lodge in small vessels, and elicit the immune complex reaction at many sites. Although horse serum is rarely used anymore, the same reaction is seen with drugs such as penicillin. The name serum sickness has been retained, although it is no longer appropriate. Symptoms are fever, painful joints, enlarged lymph nodes and spleen, and frequently an allergic urticaria. Usually, after suspending administration of the offending material, the patient recovers with no permanent damage.

SERUM SICKNESS 27-7

causes	lesion	manifestations
Type III allergy (immune complex) Medicated by horse serum or drugs	Immune complex deposition in small vessels, with acute vasculitis	Fever Painful joints Enlarged lymph nodes and spleen Urticaria

---

Glomerulonephritis

Some forms of acute and chronic glomerulonephritis are mediated by immune complex reactions due to lodging of antigen–antibody complexes in the basement membrane of glomeruli. One form of glomerulonephritis, poststreptococcal glomerulonephritis, develops in association with the immune response to infection by group A streptococci. The renal disturbance is first seen 1 to 4 weeks after apparent recovery from the acute streptococcal infection. Immune complexes are caught on the glomerular basement membrane, where they fix complement and promote an inflammatory process that compromises the filtering function of the glomerulus. The disease predominantly affects children, but some adults are also affected. Recovery is the rule, probably because the antigenic stimulation of the streptococcal infection subsides. Chronic glomerulonephritis results from a variety of antigens and is often low grade but persistent, eventually leading to renal failure. Glomerulonephritis is also discussed in Chapter 16.

Polyarteritis Nodosa

This is a severe but rare form of immune complex reaction producing widespread, multifocal, necrotizing vasculitis (Figure 27–12). It usually leads to fatal complications as a result of occlusion or rupture of vessels. The antigen is usually not identified, although hepatitis virus B is implicated in about 35 percent of cases and penicillin is occasionally implicated.

Delayed, or Cell-Mediated, Hypersensitivities (Type IV)

Delayed hypersensitivity reactions are manifest as subacute or chronic inflammation, with infiltration of the tissue by lymphocytes and

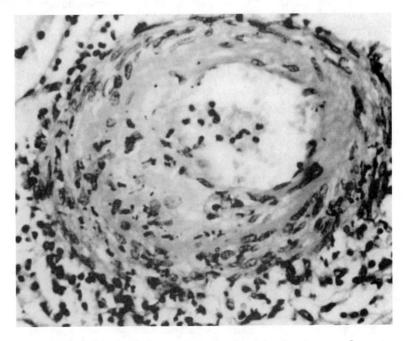

Figure 27–12. Polyarteritis nodosa, with necrosis of vessel wall and intense inflammation.

macrophages and variable degrees of necrosis. The tuberculin skin test is an example of a typical subacute reaction, with development of a red, firm lump at the site of injection of tuberculin in a sensitized individual. The reaction reaches a peak at 2 days and gradually disappears. Contact dermatitis to a piece of jewelry is an example of a chronic reaction, the appearance being that of a thickened, slightly red irregular lesion of the skin at the site of contact. The lesion persists until the antigen is removed. Internal delayed hypersensitivity reactions are quite variable in appearance but are all characterized by a chronic inflammatory cell reaction, with predominance of lymphocytes and with variable degrees of tissue destruction. These are often seen by the pathologist in tissues invaded by malignant neoplasms. The neoplastic cells carry antigens recognized as foreign that elicit delayed hypersensitivity.

Contact Dermatitis

This is an acute or chronic delayed-type hypersensitive response to allergens placed on the skin surface. A notable example is *poison ivy*. However, the range of agents that cause contact dermatitis is very large and includes many topically applied drugs, cosmetics, paints, dyes, plastics, plants, and jewelry. The lesion varies from simple erythema discretely localized to the area of allergen contact to the more edematous, pruritic, vesicular dermatitis seen with poison ivy. It is sometimes difficult to distinguish the reaction caused by direct irritants from that produced by allergens. Furthermore, it may be difficult to discover the allergen or to remove it from the environment once discovered.

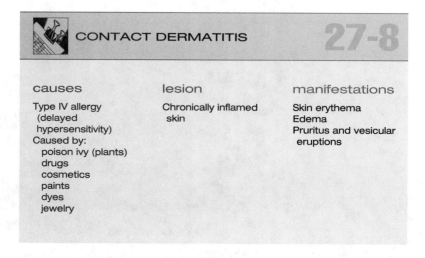

CONTACT DERMATITIS 27-8

causes	lesion	manifestations
Type IV allergy (delayed hypersensitivity) Caused by: poison ivy (plants) drugs cosmetics paints dyes jewelry	Chronically inflamed skin	Skin erythema Edema Pruritus and vesicular eruptions

Infections Manifest Primarily as Delayed Hypersensitivity Reactions

Some microorganisms tend to stimulate cell-mediated immunity. Examples are the bacteria causing tuberculosis and leprosy, many fungi, and some viruses. A marshalling of sensitized T lymphocytes and macrophages into an infected tissue produces a picture of either chronic or granulomatous inflammation. In tuberculosis and fungal infection, the caseous necrosis is thought to be mediated by sensitized T lymphocytes. Manifestations of viral infections may be due in part to delayed hypersensitivity reactions. Encephalitis occurring after a viral infection may also be a delayed hypersensitivity reaction.

Graft Rejection

The rejection of skin or a kidney grafted from one person to another is in large part due to a delayed hypersensitivity reaction. Different naturally occurring tissue antigens cause the development of sensitized lymphocytes in the person receiving the graft. The lymphocytes then cause necrosis of the graft. Such a reaction does not occur in identical twins because they have the same tissue antigens. Tissue typing, which is analogous to blood typing, is now used to match donor and recipient as closely as possible.

Autoimmune Diseases

Intolerance to self as a disease phenomenon requires an autoimmunization process in which sensitized lymphocytes or antibodies are developed against self-antigens. A number of relatively uncommon diseases appear to evolve as a result of such autoimmunization and its hypersensitive expression. Autoimmunity probably encompasses all four categories of hypersensitivity, but the most common types appear to be immune complex (type III) and hypersensitivity (type IV). Autoimmune hemolytic anemias are good examples of cytotoxic (type II) autoimmunity. A partial list of diseases thought to be autoimmune is given in Table 27–1. One example is discussed.

Systemic Lupus Erythematosus (SLE)

This moderately common systemic disease may affect a number of different organ systems. A characteristic skin lesion, the butterfly rash, is an erythematous dermatitis that covers the bridge of the nose and extends bilaterally onto the cheeks (Figure 27–13). The skin is generally photosensitive; thus, rashes may appear after excessive exposure to sunlight. The joints may also be involved, producing complaints of arthritis. Muscles may become weak and atrophic. The kidneys develop a glomerulonephritis. Degenerative changes in heart valves also may occur. The blood may show hypergammaglobulinemia, ane-

TABLE 27–1. AUTOIMMUNE DISEASES

Disease	Organ or Tissue	Antigen
Hashimoto's thyroiditis	Thyroid	Thyroglobulin
Pernicious anemia (vitamin B_{12} deficiency)	Gastric mucosa	Intrinsic factor
Goodpasture's syndrome	Kidney glomeruli and lung	Basement membrane
Autoimmune hemolytic anemia	Red cells	Red cell surface
Idiopathic thrombocytopenic purpura	Platelets	Platelet surface
Myasthenia gravis	Skeletal muscle	Acetylcholine receptors on muscle cells
Rheumatoid arthritis	Synovial membranes	Altered IgG
Systemic lupus erythematosus	Synovial membranes, kidney, skin, blood vessels	Many: DNA, DNA protein, RNA cardiolipin, microsomes

mia, leukopenia, and thrombocytopenia. Lupus erythematosus predominantly affects young to middle-aged women and usually has a protracted course, which ends with renal insufficiency, bacterial endocarditis, cardiac failure, sepsis, or pneumonia. A number of different autoantibodies occur in lupus. The primary tissue damage is probably due to cytotoxic antibodies and immune complexes, as well as to

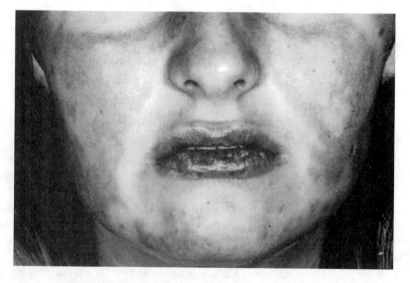

Figure 27–13. Butterfly rash of systemic lupus erythematosus.

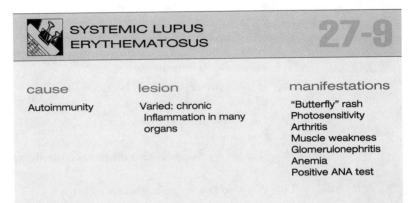

cause	lesion	manifestations
Autoimmunity	Varied: chronic Inflammation in many organs	"Butterfly" rash Photosensitivity Arthritis Muscle weakness Glomerulonephritis Anemia Positive ANA test

SYSTEMIC LUPUS ERYTHEMATOSUS

27-9

delayed hypersensitivity. Infiltrates of chronic inflammatory cells (lymphocytes and plasma cells) are found in many organs. Antinuclear antibody, an antibody directed against the body's own cell nuclei, provides the basis for the diagnostic antinuclear antibody (ANA) test.

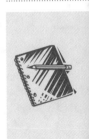

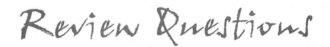

Review Questions

1. What are antigens and antibodies?
2. How do B lymphocytes and T lymphocytes differ in terms of origin and function?
3. What are the major functions of each of the five classes of immunoglobulins?
4. What are the four major types of allergy?
5. How are each of the following tests or procedures helpful in evaluation of a patient with allergy or immune deficiency?
   Serum electrophoresis
   Serum immunodiffusion
   Immunofluorescent tests
   ANA test
   Skin tests
   Complement fixation test
   Coombs' test

6. What are the causes, lesions, and major manifestations of each of the specific immune diseases discussed in this chapter?

7. How do deficiencies of the immunoglobulins differ from those of the T cell immune system?

8. What is the relationship between hay fever and asthma in terms of cause, lesions, manifestations, and complications?

9. How are transfusion reactions diagnosed? How are they prevented?

10. What is the basic lesion common to the delayed hypersensitivity diseases?

11. What do the following terms mean?
    Hapten
    Secondary response
    Complement
    Agammaglobulinemia
    Hypogammaglobulinemia
    Rh antigen
    ABO red blood cell antigens
    Typing and cross-matching
    Tissue typing
    Butterfly rash

28.

Physical Injury

MOST FREQUENT AND SERIOUS PROBLEMS
Trauma • Automobile Accidents • Thermal Burns • Sunburn • Chronic
Skin Changes from Sunlight • X-ray and Gamma Ray Injury

MECHANICAL INJURIES
Types of Simple Wounds
Contusion (Bruise) • Abrasion • Laceration • Incision • Puncture Wound
Missile Wounds
Types of Major Body Trauma
Abdominal Injury
Chest Injury
Spinal Injury
Head Injury

THERMAL INJURY
Burns
Electrical Burns
Excessive Heat Exposure
Frostbite
Excessive Cold Exposure

RADIATION INJURY
Sun Radiations
X-radiation and Gamma Radiation

REVIEW QUESTIONS

MOST FREQUENT AND SERIOUS PROBLEMS

Major external agents causing physical injury fall into three general categories—mechanical, thermal, and radiation. The term *trauma* refers to injury caused by extrinsic forces, particularly when associated with an accident or violence. Overall, trauma is the fourth leading cause of death in the United States and is the most common cause of death in persons under 38 years of age. Trauma accounts for about 7 percent of patient visits to a physician, with half of these visits involving fractures and lacerations. Automobile accidents are the most frequent cause of serious traumatic injury. The mortality rates of various types of accidents is shown in Figure 28–1.

Thermal injuries most commonly occur as burns. Extensive thermal burns produce a serious threat to life and result in a long course of treatment.

Sunlight is the most common source of radiation injury. Radiation from sunlight affects all people, but fair-skinned, outdoor people are more susceptible to sunburn and chronic skin changes. X-ray and gamma-ray injuries are most often encountered as a complication of cancer therapy.

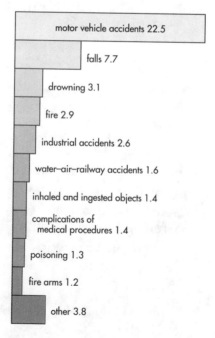

motor vehicle accidents 22.5

falls 7.7

drowning 3.1

fire 2.9

industrial accidents 2.6

water–air–railway accidents 1.6

inhaled and ingested objects 1.4

complications of
  medical procedures 1.4

poisoning 1.3

fire arms 1.2

other 3.8

Figure 28–1. Mortality rate (deaths per 100,000 persons per year) from accidents.

MECHANICAL INJURIES

Types of Simple Wounds

The cause of simple wounds can often be determined by their appearance. Common types include contusion, abrasion, laceration, incision, and puncture wounds.

A *contusion*, or *bruise*, is a crushing, dislocation, or disruption of subsurface tissue caused by a blunt instrument that does not penetrate or break the surface. Blood released from broken vessels has no outlet and pools in the damaged tissue causing gross discoloration. A "black eye" is a typical example.

An *abrasion* is a scraping or scuffing of the skin surface without full-thickness loss of skin.

A *laceration* is a tear in the surface caused by shearing of tissue, leaving irregular, ragged wound margins. Vessels and nerves tend to bridge the gap, because they stretch rather than tear in response to the shearing force.

An *incision* is a clean cut caused by a sharp instrument such as a knife and differs from a laceration in that it has clean, regular edges. The underlying tissue, including blood vessels, is divided by the edge of the instrument. Thus, an incision has more bleeding and less tissue injury than a laceration.

A *puncture wound* is a deep, narrow injury caused by a sharp-pointed instrument that penetrates through tissue.

Missile Wounds

A missile wound is a wound caused by a flying object such as a stone, arrow, or bullet. Gunshot wounds are the most common type. Injury by metallic objects thrown from rotary mowers are also common. The nature of the injury produced by missiles depends on the mass of the object and the square of its velocity. Large, slow-moving missiles produce much surface destruction and do not penetrate very deeply. High-velocity, small missiles may have a small entrance wound while producing much internal injury.

Types of Major Body Trauma

Major accidents, such as automobile accidents, often cause characteristic patterns of injury in various parts of the body. Injuries to the abdomen, chest, spine, and head will be discussed. Injuries to the bones and joints are discussed in Chapter 21.

Abdominal Injury

Severe blows, sometimes even without any penetration, can produce significant injury to abdominal viscera. The most important effects of abdominal trauma are hemorrhage, which is often unrecognized and delayed; perforation of the intestines leading to peritonitis; and rupture of the urinary bladder. Hemorrhage is most commonly due to laceration of the spleen but may also be from a lacerated liver or kidney. Because of its muscularity, mobility, and serosal covering, the intestine may slide away from relatively slowly penetrating instruments like needles, swords, and knives. If the intestines are ruptured, spillage of gastrointestinal contents into the peritoneal cavity causes an intense inflammatory reaction (peritonitis) and the motility of the tract is depressed (ileus). Air may leak out of the ruptured viscus and accumulate under the diaphragm, where it may be detected by an abdominal x-ray. Fluid-filled and distended organs, such as the bladder and the pregnant uterus, are prone to rupture with rapid pressure changes such as occur in automobile accidents. Since these serious abdominal injuries are likely to be fatal if not treated promptly, abdominal operations are often performed as a part of the diagnostic work-up when serious abdominal injury is suspected.

Chest Injury

Major effects of chest trauma include fatal hemorrhage and interference with breathing. Fatal hemorrhage occurs from tears in the heart or great vessels produced by stab wounds or gunshot wounds and sometimes by rapid deceleration, as in an automobile accident when the chest hits the steering wheel. Difficulty in breathing is produced by three mechanisms—obstruction of the tracheobronchial tree, fluid in the pleural space compressing the lungs, and multiple rib fractures resulting in an inability to move the chest cage (*flail chest*). Obstruction of the tracheobronchial tree may be due to accumulation of blood, to an inhaled foreign body, or to compression of the trachea. Tracheostomy (making an opening through the neck to the trachea) and suction are used to open the airway. Fluid in the pleural space may be air (pneumothorax), blood (hemothorax), or watery fluid (pleural effusion). Hemothorax is due to rupture of a vessel. Pleural effusion is due to heart failure or pleural inflammation rather than trauma. Pneumothorax is most important because it can be treated but may be fatal if untreated. Open chest wounds must be closed to prevent sucking of air into the pleural space. A tube is placed in the pleural cavity under a water seal so that air is forced out of the pleural space with inhalation and cannot reenter the pleural space during expiration. Multiple rib fractures (flail chest) require fixation of the sternum by wiring it to something overhead in order to prevent collapse of the chest with each inspiration. Artificial breathing may also be necessary.

Most deaths following automobile accidents are the result of chest trauma.

Spinal Injury

Fractures or extreme dislocations of vertebrae can shear the spinal cord, interrupting all neural connections below the damaged site. Injury to the lower cord causes *paraplegia*—loss of control over the lower limbs and, usually, loss of bladder function. Injury of the spinal cord in the neck causes *quadriplegia*—loss of control over all limbs. Major long-term complications of spinal cord injury include neurogenic bladder with superimposed cystitis and pyelonephritis. With repeated bouts of pyelonephritis, kidney stones often form, and renal failure may lead to death. Decubitus ulcers (bed sores) form in the severely disabled from pressure of skin against bone. Frequent changes of position through good nursing care prevent these ulcers from occurring over pressure points. Difficulty in breathing and pneumonia are major complications of quadriplegia.

Head Injury

The brain is encased in a nonexpansive bony vault, the skull. If tissue contents of the cranial cavity enlarge, the skull cannot accommodate for the increased mass. The two major mass-producing lesions of trauma are edema and hemorrhage. Edema may be localized or widespread, but, in either case, the increasing mass of the brain causes increased pressure throughout the cranial cavity. The increased pressure may affect neuronal function and compromise blood flow. Herniation of the brain through the foramen magnum into the spinal column causes secondary hemorrhages into the respiratory center of the brain stem, leading to death. See Chapter 23 for further discussion of brain hemorrhage and trauma.

THERMAL INJURY

Burns

Minor small burns are very common and heal by regeneration of the surface epithelium without residual effects. The damage produced by larger burns (Figure 28–2) depends on two major factors—the depth of the burn and the percentage of body surface involved. The depth of the burn can be estimated by inspection and determined accurately by biopsy. First-degree burns are limited to the epidermis and are red, painful, and dry. Regeneration occurs rapidly from remaining epidermal cells.

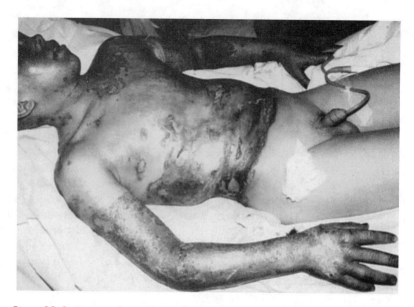

Figure 28–2. Extensive thermal burns of varying severity. Note catheter in urethra to monitor urine output as an index of adequate fluid replacement.

Second-degree burns destroy the epidermis and upper dermis and are red, moist, and often blister. Regeneration of the epidermis can occur because epithelial cells from sweat glands, sebaceous glands, and hair follicles in the dermis can proliferate and, with time, form new epidermis and remodel these skin appendages.

Third-degree burns destroy epidermis and dermis down to the subcutaneous tissue and are charred and dry. Pain sensation is reduced because of destruction of sensory nerve endings in the skin. Since all epithelial cells are destroyed, regeneration of epidermis can only occur from the margins of the burn, and this type of regeneration can only proceed for a few centimeters into the injured area. Thus, third-degree burns cannot regenerate new epithelium, and skin grafting is required if the area is larger than a few centimeters. After the body has formed granulation tissue under the charred surface and the necrotic tissue is removed, postage stamp-sized pieces of skin are removed from a normal area of the body and placed on the granulation tissue. The graft will grow, and the adjacent grafts will fuse to form a new surface. The donor site will also regenerate, because only a split thickness of skin is removed, leaving skin appendages behind to accomplish the regeneration of the donor site. The grafted sites will not be normal, because the burn will have provoked considerable scarring in the dermis and because the new epidermis will not be capable of regenerating skin appendages. Sometimes excessive scarring occurs (Figure 28–3).

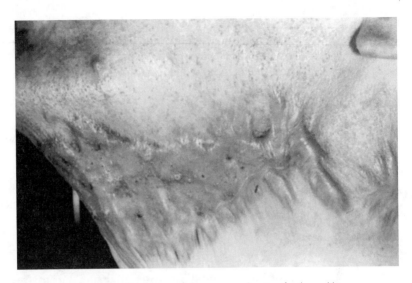

Figure 28–3. Excessive scar formation at the site of a thermal burn.

The amount of body surface involved by second- and third-degree burns correlates roughly with the chances of survival. The general health of the patient and quality of medical care are also very important determinants of survival with extensive burns. As a crude estimate, 30 percent body burns are serious and 60 percent body burns are fatal most of the time. The major complications of extensive burns are fluid loss from the exposed surface leading to shock and infection developing in the burned skin and spreading to the bloodstream. Pseudomonas is a bacterium notorious for its occurrence in burns and its ability to produce fatal septicemia in patients with burns. Severely burned patients should be transferred to major treatment centers, where the skilled personnel and proper facilities are available to carry out the meticulous care needed to prevent dehydration and infection and to provide skin grafting and follow-up care.

Electrical Burns

Electricity produces two major effects—burns at entry and exit sites and electrical conduction changes, such as cardiac arrest. The amount of local injury depends on the amount of electrical energy and amount of electrical resistance in the tissue. Dry tissue, such as skin, is a poor conductor and, therefore, accumulates the energy and is burned. The effect of the electrical energy as it flows through the body in the shortest pathway from entry to exit site depends on the amount of energy absorbed at the entrance site and the location of entry and exit sites. As the electricity encounters resistance at the exit site, a burn also occurs there. The outcome is likely to be either sudden death or survival with burns at entry and exit sites. Artificial respiration and cardiac resuscitation may be life saving. The burned tissue may be extensive and needs to be debrided to prevent secondary infection.

Excessive Heat Exposure

Prolonged exposure to hot weather can have two possible effects. Excessive sweating can cause dehydration and salt depletion leading to shock. Salt and water replacement are indicated. The other effect is called *malignant hyperpyrexia* and is due to a failure of sweating. The skin is hot and dry and failure to lose heat by vaporization of sweat leads to a progressive rise in body temperature and death.

Frostbite

Frostbite is simply necrosis of tissue due to freezing. It occurs on exposed parts, such as feet, hands, and ears. The dead tissue demarcates from adjacent viable tissue in a few days and is either sloughed or removed surgically so that the remaining viable tissue can heal.

Excessive Cold Exposure (Hypothermia)

The body can tolerate moderate degrees of hypothermia for a considerable time; however, when hypothermia is excessive (less than 33°C for a prolonged time), death occurs. Death is much more rapid in water and occurs with temperatures above the freezing level, because water rapidly conducts heat from the body. In air, conduction of heat away from the body occurs more slowly.

RADIATION INJURY

Sun Radiations

The acute effects of sun radiations are sunburn, a mild superficial injury of epidermis with vascular congestion. Much of the sunburn effect is due to ultraviolet radiation, which can be reduced by certain types of lotions. The chronic effects of sun exposure include a general deterioration in collagenous tissue of the skin termed *senile elastosis*. This accounts for the wrinkling and drooping of facial and hand skin. Sun exposure also relates to the frequency of premalignant skin lesions (senile or actinic keratoses) and skin cancers (basal cell carcinoma, squamous cell carcinoma, and malignant melanoma).

X-Radiation and Gamma Radiation

The basic effect of X-rays and gamma rays on cells is on the nucleus, with resultant death of the cells or interference with its ability to divide. Thus, continuously dividing cell lines are most susceptible to radiation injury. These include bone marrow, small intestinal epithelium, testes, and epidermis. Lymphocytes and ova are also very radiosensitive (easily killed by radiation). Conversely, cells least capable of cell division are least susceptible to radiation injury. Thus, very high doses are required to injure the brain or muscle. Other tissues are intermediate in their radiosensitivity. The relationship of radiosensitivity to proliferative activity also holds for most neoplasms. In general, rapidly dividing, poorly differentiated malignant neoplasms are radiosensitive; well-differentiated malignant neoplasms are moderately radiosensitive or radioresistant. Benign neoplasms approach their tissue of origin in their degree of radiosensitivity.

In addition to the effects on specific tissues, radiation causes gradual changes in connective tissue and microvasculature that require months to years to develop. These effects include increased density of collagenous tissue, vascular changes leading to decreased blood supply, and ulceration of epithelial surfaces overlying the areas of connective tissue change.

The treatment of cancer by radiation therapy is based on the cancer being more radiosensitive than surrounding normal tissue. The radiologist who performs radiation therapy is an expert at delivering the maximum dose of radiation to the cancer with as little damage to surrounding tissue as possible. Radiation therapy is provided in four forms. High-energy radioactive cobalt sources are available in major treatment centers and are used to deliver penetrating doses to deep-lying cancers. X-ray therapy machines are more widely available and are also used for treatment of solid cancer masses, although the lesser penetration of x-rays results in more tissue damage to the normal tissue lying in the treatment pathway. Radioactive substances that emit less-penetrating gamma rays are selectively implanted near the cancer. For example, applicators containing radioactive cesium are implanted into the uterus for treatment of cervical and endometrial cancer, and radioactive gold is inserted into the prostate for treatment of prostatic cancer. Finally, radioactive compounds with particular chemical properties may be injected so that they will be localized in the target tissue. For example, radioactive iodine localizes in the thyroid gland and thus can be used to selectively treat hyperplasia of the thyroid or the occasional functional thyroid cancer.

Although most radiation injury is encountered as a complication of radiation therapy for serious disease, the effects of radiation used for diagnosis and of radiation encountered in the environment are of constant concern to society. The damaging effects of diagnostic x-rays appears to be very limited because of careful controls and knowledge gained from previous experiences. Radiologists no longer develop skin cancers on their hands, because protective gloves are worn. Radiation of the chest and neck of children for benign conditions has been stopped because of the high frequency of thyroid cancers that develop some years after such treatment.

Injury from environmental radiation is of much greater long-range concern because of the massive number of people that might be involved and because radiation contamination of the environment might last for years. A background level of atmospheric radiation is present from cosmic rays. The role of cosmic radiations in relation to the spontaneous occurrence of cancer and genetic defects is unknown. In principle, we know that radiation can alter genes and that genetic change is involved in carcinogenesis. There is current concern that alteration of the stratosphere may lead to an increase in the background cosmic radiation. An increase in radioactive fallout from nuclear bombs or accidents would have an effect similar to an increase in cosmic radiation, except that some of the fallout would be in the form of radioactive chemicals that might be selectively concentrated in the biologic chain. From experimental research, it can be predicted that the long-term effects of a generalized increase in environmental radioactivity will be an increase in the frequency of congenital anomalies and of cancer. Many years would be required to gather statistics to prove that an effect had occurred.

Massive high dose exposure to radiation occurs with nuclear bombs and nuclear reactor accidents. Bombs produce injury from mechanical trauma, burns, and superficial injury from beta-particle radiation, as well as from gamma rays. A nuclear accident exposure is more likely to be pure gamma radiation. When the whole body is exposed to gamma rays, the bone marrow is the most sensitive organ involved in fatal injury. About 500 roentgens will destroy the bone marrow beyond its ability to regenerate before fatal infection and anemia occurs in a few weeks from loss of white and red blood cells. Doses of 1000 R or more will produce death in 4 to 7 days from injury to the intestine. Doses of over 50,000 R will produce death in a few hours from brain injury.

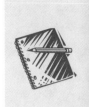

Review Questions

1. What are three major categories of physical injury?
2. What is the most common cause of fatal accidents? What are other important causes?
3. What is the pathogenesis and appearance of contusions, abrasions, lacerations, incisions, and puncture wounds?
4. What factors determine the appearance and amount of damage caused by missile wounds?
5. What are the typical injuries and their complications for abdomen, chest, spine, and head injuries?
6. How do the depth and extent of burns affect the course and treatment of burns?
7. What are the two major effects of electrical injury?
8. What are the effects of frostbite and excessive general exposure to hot and cold environments?
9. What are the acute and chronic effects of sunlight?
10. What are the similarities and differences in the effects of exposure to x-rays and gamma rays?
11. Which tissues and neoplasms are most and least sensitive to injury by radiation?
12. What are four forms of radiation therapy? What are the advantages of each?
13. What are the likely effects of a gradual rise in environmental radioactivity and of a massive nuclear accident?
14. What do the following terms mean?
    Trauma
    Flail chest
    Paraplegia
    Quadriplegia
    First-degree burn
    Second-degree burn
    Third-degree burn
    Radiosensitive
    Radioresistant

29.
Chemical Injury

MODES OF CHEMICAL INJURY
*Drug Overdose • Accident, Homicide, and Suicide •
Environmental Exposure*

MOST FREQUENT AND SERIOUS PROBLEMS
*Drug Overdose • Drug Abuse • Accidents in Children under 6 Years
of Age • Carbon Monoxide Poisoning • Environmental Agents •
Cigarettes • Alcohol*

SYMPTOMS, SIGNS, AND TESTS
*History of Exposure • Vomiting • Burns • Effects on Nervous System •
Renal or Liver Damage • Nonspecific Tests for Injury •
Chemical Assay for Specific Agents*

SPECIFIC DISEASES
Adverse Drug Reactions
Drug Abuse
Accidental Poisonings
Carbon Monoxide Poisoning
Agricultural Chemical Injury
Injury by Other Agents

REVIEW QUESTIONS

MODES OF CHEMICAL INJURY

The wide variety of chemical agents that are potentially harmful to man produce diverse types of injury that are difficult to classify. Knowledge of the effects of each chemical agent is needed to provide the best treatment. However, it is impossible for any one person to be familiar with all potential injurious compounds. Application of general principles along with knowledge of common agents is needed to make appropriate initial decisions in cases of chemical injury. Poison control centers provide ready access to information regarding more rarely encountered agents.

The mode of exposure to chemical injury provides the first clue to the likely agents involved. Three modes of chemical injury will be considered: (1) overdose of a drug that a person is purposely taking for its effects; (2) exposure of an individual by accident or because of suicidal or homicidal intent; and (3) potential exposure of many people because of environmental pollution or accident.

Most drugs are potentially harmful if taken in sufficient dose. Often, the harmful dose is close to the therapeutic dose, so that deleterious effects occur as a side effect of therapy. A second mode of drug overdose is miscalculation of the dose or misunderstanding by the patient of how much to take. Drug abuse, which involves self-administration of drugs for their psychological effects, is another mode of drug overdose.

Accidental exposure of an individual to harmful chemicals may occur by ingestion, by inhalation, or by contact with corrosive chemical agents. Agents selected for suicidal or homicidal purposes are likely to be strong agents that can be easily ingested, such as barbiturate drugs.

Environmental accidents and pollution may be either acute or chronic. Carbon monoxide poisoning from car exhaust or fires is an example of acute environmental poisoning. Lead poisoning from eating paint or burning storage batteries is an example of chronic poisoning from environmental exposure.

The likely means of discovery of chemical injury relates to the mode of exposure. Drug overdose as related to therapy will be reported by the patient or observed by the physician. Drug abuse is a social problem that comes to the surface in many ways, sometimes medical, sometimes criminal, and sometimes social in nature. Accidental poisoning brings patients to emergency rooms or poison control centers. Suicide and homicide are investigated by police, medical examiners, and forensic pathologists. Unsuccessful suicide and homicide attempts present as emergency medical problems. Acute environmental exposures are likely to be handled in emergency rooms and may involve enough people to be considered a disaster. Chronic environmental injury is likely to go undetected until pilot cases are identified and the mechanism of exposure is brought to public attention.

MOST FREQUENT AND SERIOUS PROBLEMS

Drug overdose in the form of side effects is very common. Another major and common problem resulting in drug overdose occurs when patients receive prescriptions from multiple physicians and multiple pharmacies for similar or additive drugs, and thus take a drug overdose. This is particularly likely to occur with patients who take tranquilizers, sedatives, and analgesics. Drug abuse with barbiturates, opiates, cocaine, and other drugs is a major medical and social problem involving millions of individuals and in recent years has caused an increase in fatal poisonings in young adults. Drug abuse is the most common type of drug-related death followed by accidental drug poisoning and suicide.

The frequency of poisoning is based on data reported to poison control centers. It gives an approximation of emergency medical care problems relating to chemicals regardless of the mode of injury or potential injury. Most persons seeking medical care for poisoning are asymptomatic and few die (Table 29–1). Of the many agents that cause poisoning, drugs are collectively most common (Table 29–2). Over 70 percent of reported poisonings occur in children under age 6 (Table 29–3).

The importance of environmental injury by chemicals is difficult to assess, because data are difficult to gather and effects may go undetected. Among acute cases of environmental chemicals causing death, carbon monoxide poisoning is common whereas fatal poisoning from plants, such as mushrooms, is rare in the United States (Table 29–4). Pesticides and herbicides are widely used and may produce acute injury when spilled on the skin or ingested. The long-term effects of many of these compounds in humans are unknown. Air pollutants, particularly hydrocarbons, producing smog in large metropolitan areas, increase the frequency and severity of emphysema and other chronic lung diseases.

Examples of uncommon, but serious exposure to gases include silo filler's disease and ammonia burns. In silo filler's disease, nitrogen dioxide produced in silos by fermentation is inhaled and results in

TABLE 29–1. MEDICAL OUTCOME BY REASON FOR EXPOSURE IN HUMAN POISONING CASES

	Unintentional (%)	Intentional (%)
No Effect	26	20
Minor Effect	19	29
Moderate Effect	3	14
Major Effect	0.1	3
Death	0.1	0.3
No follow-up or unrelated effect	52	34

TABLE 29–2. SUBSTANCES MOST FREQUENTLY INVOLVED IN HUMAN POISON EXPOSURES

Substance	No.	%
Cleaning substances	208,843	10.3
Analgesics	196,805	9.7
Cosmetics and personal care products	171,426	8.5
Cough and cold preparations	105,947	5.2
Plants	104,187	5.1
Bites/envenomations	87,628	4.3
Pesticides (includes rodenticides)	84,346	4.2
Foreign bodies	75,021	3.7
Topicals	72,124	3.6
Food products, food poisoning	67,084	3.3
Antimicrobials	66,274	3.3
Hydrocarbons	65,143	3.2
Sedatives/hypnotics/antipsychotics	63,271	3.1
Antidepressants	56,285	2.8
Alcohols	52,119	2.6
Chemicals	51,508	2.5
Vitamins	45,952	2.3

1995 Annual Report of the American Association of Poison Control Centers. *American Journal of Emergency Medicine* 4:5, 1996.

acute and sometimes chronic damage to the lung. Ammonia burns skin, eyes, and respiratory tract when leakage occurs from tanks of liquid ammonia.

Pneumoconioses are chronic pulmonary diseases due to inhalation of particulate matter such as silica, asbestos, and plant fibers (see Chapter 12 for further discussion).

Another large category of chronic environmental chemical injury relates to chemicals that induce cancer. Cigarette smoke is the most well established and has the greatest impact, because it is related to the development of lung cancer, squamous cell cancers of the oral region and esophagus, and transitional cell carcinoma of the bladder. Our knowledge of cancer-causing chemicals is limited, although epidemiologic evidence suggests that they play a role in the development of some cancers.

Probably the most important injurious chemical is alcohol. It does not fit well into the categories discussed above, and, because of its importance, alcohol injury will be discussed separately in Chapter 30.

TABLE 29–3. SUBSTANCES MOST FREQUENTLY INVOLVED IN PEDIATRIC POISON EXPOSURES (CHILDREN UNDER 6 YEARS)		
Substance	No.	%
Cosmetics and personal care products	127,419	11.9
Cleaning substances	118,332	11.1
Analgesics	81,643	7.6
Plants	74,829	7.0
Cough and cold preparations	70,862	6.6
Foreign bodies	53,972	5.0
Topicals	53,875	5.0
Pesticides (includes rodenticides)	44,150	4.1
Antimicrobials	39,718	3.7
Vitamins	36,553	3.4
Gastrointestinal preparations	34,922	3.3
Hydrocarbons	26,723	2.5
Arts/crafts/offices supplies	26,421	2.5
Antihistamines	18,330	1.7
Hormones and hormone antagonists	18,291	1.7

1995 Annual Report of the American Association of Poison Control Centers. *American Journal of Emergency Medicine* 4:5, 1996.

SYMPTOMS, SIGNS, AND TESTS

The manifestations of chemical injury are obviously dependent upon the route of exposure, the dose, the amount of absorption, the site of metabolism, the degree of excretion, and the specific chemical action of the agent involved. A discussion of these aspects of chemical injury is beyond the scope of this text; specific characteristics of individual agents will be mentioned as needed.

Some broad generalizations can be made about presentation of chemical injuries. From the data presented in the previous section, it is clear that the most common mode of presentation is the child under 5 years of age who has swallowed something and is brought to the emergency room. Examples of signs and symptoms of chemical injury include vomiting, burns, behavioral changes, and unconsciousness. The most important historical information is identification of the chemical agent to which the person was exposed. With knowledge of

TABLE 29–4. DRUG OR POISON CATEGORIES WITH LARGEST NUMBERS OF DEATHS

Category	Death	% of All Exposures in Category
Analgesics	235	0.119
Antidepressants	168	0.298
Cardiovascular drugs	115	0.347
Stimulants and street drugs	108	0.319
Sedative/hypnotics/antipsychotics	97	0.153
Alcohols	82	0.157
Gases and fumes	48	0.113
Chemicals	23	0.045
Asthma therapies	20	0.103
Insecticides/pesticides (includes rodenticides)	18	0.021
Automotive products	17	0.125
Cleaning substances	17	0.008
Hydrocarbons	14	0.021

1995 Annual Report of the American Association of Poison Control Centers. *American Journal of Emergency Medicine* 4:5, 1996.

the agent, the physician can look for the specific signs and laboratory abnormalities caused by the agent and select the proper treatment.

Signs of chemical injury are usually not specific but may provide helpful clues. Nausea, vomiting, and diarrhea are observed with intestinal injury. Dyspnea occurs after inhalation of noxious fumes. Careful neurologic examination may detect changes caused by injury to the nervous system. Decreased urine output suggests severe renal injury.

Laboratory tests may be used to suggest whether or not injury has occurred, the likely site of injury, and sometimes the type and amount of the agent involved. General laboratory tests that may suggest whether injury has occurred include elevation of the white blood count, alteration in serum electrolytes, and elevation of serum enzymes, such as aspartate aminotransferase. Elevated blood urea nitrogen and creatinine levels suggest renal injury, high aspartate aminotransferase levels are found with liver damage, and altered levels of blood gases are associated with altered oxygen-carbon dioxide exchange in the lungs.

Many chemicals can be measured in samples of blood, urine, feces, or tissues. However, the laboratory needs a clue as to which chemical to look for among the myriads of possibilities. Extensive search for a poison is only indicated when the information will be of value in treatment or in criminal investigation.

SPECIFIC DISEASES

The emphasis in this section will be on representative specific agents and the type of injury they produce. Agents will be grouped for discussion by mode of injury and/or similarities in patterns of injury. Effects of chemical agents on specific organs that have been previously discussed, such as pneumoconioses, will not be repeated here. Other texts should be consulted for more comprehensive coverage of specific types of chemical injury.

Adverse Drug Reactions

Adverse drug reactions are reactions caused by drugs during the usual course of therapy of a patient. In many instances, the adverse drug reaction is due to hypersensitivity, usually due to an allergic reaction. Other mechanisms include use of drugs with a toxic dose range close to the therapeutic dose range, an enzyme deficiency that accentuates the effective dose of the drug, and renal or liver failure with decreased excretion of the drug.

The most common types of fatal adverse drug reactions are shown in Table 29–4. Penicillin is a common cause of anaphylaxis although anaphylaxis may be caused by many other drugs. Patients admitted to hospitals and patients given drugs as outpatients should be routinely asked about their sensitivity to drugs, although most cases of anaphylaxis occur in patients not known to be sensitive to a drug. Fatal drug-induced liver injury is most often due to halothane, a commonly used anesthetic. A wide variety of other drugs may cause liver cell injury or bile stasis, but most reactions are of mild degree and reversible upon discontinuance of the drug. Bone marrow suppression leading to leukopenia, thrombocytopenia, and/or anemia may occur as a hypersensitivity reaction to the antibiotic chloramphenicol or as a predictable action of anticancer drugs. Renal tubular injury is a complication of treatment with several antibiotic agents as well as other drugs. Other specific reactions worthy of special mention include hemorrhage resulting from anticoagulant drug therapy and malignant hyperthermia due to a rare enzyme defect that is manifested when patients are given succinylcholine, a muscle relaxant, in combination with halothane or certain other general anesthetic agents.

Drug Abuse

Agents involved in drug abuse include opiates, barbiturates, tranquilizers, hallucinogens, muscle relaxants, and stimulants such as amphetamines and cocaine. As mentioned earlier, these agents probably account for about 50 percent of drug-related deaths and for the high incidence of drug overdoses in adolescents and young adults. Death may occur because of overdose as a direct result of the pharmacologic effects of the drug, or it may be due to other complications. The drugs themselves do not produce lesions, and most cause death by their effects on respiration and cardiac function.

Opiates are frequently taken intravenously, leaving telltale lesions on the skin and occasionally leading to severe complications. Local lesions in drug addicts consist of inflammation at the injection sites due to a granulomatous reaction to the talc or starch in the injection mixture or due to infection from failure to use sterile technique. Injected talc or starch is carried to the small vessels of the lung, where a granulomatous reaction occurs in small arterioles and may eventually lead to pulmonary hypertension and heart failure (cor pulmonale) because of the arteriolar obstruction.

Allergic reactions may occur to other ingredients in the injection mixture, such as central nervous system damage resulting from a reaction to quinine. Systemic infections, such as bacterial endocarditis and viral hepatitis, are more frequent in addicts, presumably because of direct injection of organisms into the bloodstream.

Symptoms of amphetamines and cocaine abuse include hypertension, acidosis, anxiety, agitation, psychosis, and, if severe, seizures, hyperthermia and myocardial infarction from coronary artery spasm. Diagnosis is established by finding metabolites of these drugs in the urine.

Accidental Poisonings

Since most accidental poisonings occur in children under 5 years of age, it is not surprising that the agents involved are those that are commonly found around the house (Table 29–3). Aspirin has been a common drug involved, although aspirin poisonings have decreased since childproof caps have been used on bottles and other drugs have been substituted. The major harmful effects of aspirin are metabolic, with an initial alkalosis due to hyperventilation and later severe acidosis. Accidental or suicidal ingestion of sleeping tablets containing barbiturates produces central nervous system and respiratory depression. Mothers of young children frequently take oral iron medications; accidental ingestion of these iron compounds by a child leads to corrosive damage to the stomach and small intestine, but more importantly, the absorbed iron may lead to fatal shock.

Next to drugs, cleaning agents are the next most common cause of accidental poisoning (see Tables 29–2 and 29–3). Most of these agents cause direct caustic damage to tissue by coagulation of protein. The result is a chemical burn. Benzene and toluene are common ingredients of paint removers, dry cleaning solutions, and glues. Acutely, they cause central nervous system poisoning. Chronic benzene poisoning is noted for its destructive effect on the bone marrow. Carbon tetrachloride is a common solvent that may be inhaled or ingested and leads to severe liver and kidney damage.

Carbon Monoxide Poisoning

Carbon monoxide is produced by incomplete combustion, and when inhaled, it preferentially combines with oxygen-carrying sites on hemoglobin molecules of red blood cells, so that there is a resultant systemic anoxia. The anoxia may be fatal or may lead to permanent brain damage. Automobiles are a common source of carbon monoxide. Most deaths in cases of fire are due to carbon monoxide poisoning rather than burns. Carbon monoxide is particularly dangerous because it is odorless and because initial symptoms of impaired mental function are not apparent to those affected. The effects of chronic low-level carbon monoxide poisoning resulting from smoking, smog, or automobile fumes have not been quantitated. It is possible that mental impairment from mild carbon monoxide poisoning may cause some accidents.

Agricultural Chemical Injury

A number of chemicals encountered in farming cause rather specific types of damage. Nitrogen dioxide, produced by fermentation of silage, may be inhaled to produce severe, acute injury to the lining cells of the pulmonary alveoli. In mild cases of this condition, called *silo filler's disease*, the damage is gradually resolved, but in severe cases, damage to the alveolar walls leads to permanent fibrosis of the lungs and residual decreased breathing capacity.

Fertilizers, herbicides, and insecticides are man-made agricultural poisons. Liquid ammonia, when spilled, may lead to severe burns of the skin, eyes, and respiratory tract. Paraquat is a commonly used weed killer that causes damage to the pulmonary alveoli regardless of whether it is ingested or inhaled. Acute damage may be fatal or may lead to pulmonary fibrosis. Many insecticides contain cholinesterase inhibitors, which may lead to depression of the central and autonomic nervous systems and motor nerve endings.

Injury by Other Agents

Cyanide poisoning may result from inhalation of hydrocyanic acid or ingestion of soluble inorganic cyanide salts or cyanide-releasing substances. Modes of cyanide poisoning include industrial accidents, ingestion of certain plants, suicide, homicide, and execution. Cyanide combines with cytochrome oxidase of cells throughout the body to prevent cellular oxygen utilization. Cyanide is extremely toxic and rapid in its effects.

Methyl alcohol (methanol, wood alcohol) is widely used as a solvent and denaturing agent for ethyl alcohol. The major effect of nonfatal doses is the production of blindness. Methyl alcohol is metabolized to formaldehyde, which in turn causes damage to the retina and optic nerve. Severe acidosis occurs in fatal methyl alcohol poisoning as a consequence of its metabolism to formic acid.

Lead poisoning is usually chronic and often occurs in children who eat paint. It may also follow exposure to burning lead batteries. Lead poisoning affects the brain, peripheral nerves, and bone marrow. Abdominal cramps or colic is a characteristic symptom of peripheral nerve involvement. Encephalopathy of varying degrees, with convulsions and behavioral changes, results from the brain damage. There may be permanent mental incapacity. The mild anemia is recognized as being due to lead poisoning by a peculiar basophilic stippling of the red blood cells. A black line due to deposition of lead sulfide along gingival margins is a characteristic physical finding.

Poisoning with mercuric chloride by ingestion leads to corrosive damage to the oral region and esophagus. The absorbed mercury is excreted by the renal tubules and colonic mucosa, where it produces renal tubular necrosis, leading to acute renal failure, and ulceration of the colon, leading to bloody diarrhea.

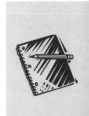

Review Questions

1. What are three general modes of chemical injury?
2. Under what circumstances may drugs lead to injury?
3. What chemical agents account for the most serious and common medical and social problems?
4. What percent of apparent poisonings lead to symptoms? To death?
5. What are the most frequent classes of agents involved in poisoning?
6. What is the age distribution of poisonings?
7. What chemical agent is most important as a cause of cancer?
8. What steps are involved in the evaluation of a person suspected of having injury due to a chemical agent?
9. What roles do laboratory tests play in diagnosis of poisoning?
10. What type of injury is associated with each of the following agents, and under what circumstances do they occur?
   Penicillin
   Halothane
   Chloramphenicol
   Anticancer drugs
   Anticoagulants
   Succinylcholine
   Opiates
   Amphetamines
   Cocaine
   Barbiturates
   Aspirin
   Iron compounds
   Cleaning agents
   Benzene
   Carbon tetrachloride
   Carbon monoxide
   Nitrogen dioxide
   Ammonia
   Paraquat

Cholinesterase inhibitors
Cyanide
Lead
Mercury

11. What do the following terms mean?
Drug abuse
Therapeutic drug monitoring
Silo filler's disease
Adverse drug reaction

30.
Nutritional Disorders and Alcoholism

REVIEW OF FUNCTION
Guidelines for Nutrition • Major Foods • Energy Derived from Foods • Vitamins

MOST FREQUENT AND SERIOUS PROBLEMS
Obesity • Alcoholism • Generalized Undernutrition • Vitamin Deficiencies

SYMPTOMS, SIGNS, AND TESTS
Serum Levels of Certain Vitamins and Minerals • Obesity • Alcoholism

SPECIFIC DISEASES
Deficiency Diseases
Generalized Undernutrition
Vitamin Deficiencies
Mineral Deficiencies
Dietary Excess
Obesity
Specific Dietary Excesses
Vitamin Toxicity
Mineral Excesses
Alcoholism

REVIEW QUESTIONS

REVIEW OF FUNCTION

Nutrition plays a significant role in health. Other parameters of good health in the individual that are important include heredity, personality, attitude, and environment. Even when these health constituents are normal, a person cannot be healthy if he or she habitually eats too much or too little.

Humans are omnivores and can adapt to a wide variety of diets. Guidelines for good nutrition are difficult to outline because they are subject to various conditions. Infants and young children need relatively more calories for growth and minerals and vitamins to insure normal bone growth. The growth spurt and sexual characterizations at puberty also result in some special dietary needs. Pregnancy and lactation are very demanding situations in the life cycle in which the diet of the mother must be supplemented with nutrients to provide for growth of the fetus, as well as the production of milk. In the elderly, some specific nutritional requirements wane and problems sometimes arise in persuading elderly persons to maintain an adequate diet because of such factors as loss of taste for food and loss of appetite due to loneliness and inactivity. Some general dietary guidelines, good for most every person, would be to (1) maintain ideal weight; (2) eat a variety of foods in order to meet vitamin and mineral needs; (3) avoid excessive fat, saturated fat, and cholesterol; (4) eat food with adequate starch and fiber content; (5) avoid excessive sugar; (6) avoid excessive sodium; and (7) avoid alcohol, or drink only in moderation.

Normal nutritional requirements are a balance of the three major foods: carbohydrates, proteins, and fats (lipids), plus certain vitamins and minerals. Roughly 45 dietary entities are considered essential and these include 9 amino acids (the building blocks of protein), 2 lipids, the vitamins, and several minerals. Note that no carbohydrates are essential.

Energy is derived from carbohydrates, lipids (fats), and protein. There is very little caloric value in vitamins and none in minerals although both of these latter nutritive constituents are necessary for life.

Energy in foods is expressed in calories. A calorie (cal) is the amount of heat required to raise the temperature of 1000 g of water from 15° to 16°C. The caloric value of any food can be directly determined by oxidizing (burning) the food in a calorimeter chamber and measuring the amount of energy released. The energy released by this method is equivalent to the breakdown of the food in the human body although the body utilizes food in a much more prolonged and complicated process than simple oxidation.

The caloric content of each of the three major food categories differ. Overall, carbohydrates yield 4.1 cal per g, protein 4.3 cal per g, and lipids 9.3 cal per g. All three foods are utilized for building structural components of the body's cells, but carbohydrates are the main source of readily available energy in the form of sugars and complex chains of sugars referred to as starches. All carbohydrates can be synthesized in the body from proteins, lipids, or other carbohydrates. Proteins contribute heavily to the structural components of the cells, as well as to enzymes. Proteins are made up of variable-sized aggregates of individual amino acids that are essential, meaning that they are necessary for life. The amino acids can be synthesized in the body to some extent from carbohydrates and lipids, but there are a few essential amino acids that need to be ingested in at least small amounts. Whereas selective deficiencies of carbohydrates or lipids can be compensated by the body by synthesis of the necessary molecules from proteins, a diet selectively deficient in protein will result in a disease called kwashiorkor. Lipids are important components of all cell membranes as well as serving other roles. One or two naturally occurring lipids need to be ingested, but all the others can be synthesized from proteins. Lipids are an important source of energy because their metabolism in the body yields more than twice as many calories as either protein or carbohydrates.

Unlike proteins, carbohydrates and lipids, vitamins do not provide the body with a source of energy. Vitamins are special molecules utilized by the body in small amounts for many and varied specific functions (Table 30–1). Some vitamins are utilized as coenzymes, whereas others contribute to cell and tissue structure. Most vitamins are needed in small amounts and need to be ingested. A few are synthesized by intestinal bacteria, and a few are synthesized in the body by breakdown of other foods.

Of the minerals that are essential for life, large amounts of calcium and phosphorus are incorporated into bone. Iron is needed in relatively large amounts because it is a component of hemoglobin and myoglobin. Blood loss and pregnancy increase dietary iron needs.

TABLE 30–1. FUNCTION OF VITAMINS

Vitamin	Function
A	Maturation of various epithelia, necessary for retinal photosensitivity
D	Regulates serum calcium levels
E	Antioxidant (prevents oxidation of certain lipids)
K	Necessary for synthesis of coagulation factors
B_1 (thiamine)	Coenzyme involved in energy metabolism and neural function
B_2 (riboflavin)	Cofactor in cellular respiration
B_3 (niacin)	Coenzyme component for oxidative-reduction reactions
B_6 (pyridoxine)	Coenzyme involved in several metabolic reactions
B_{12} (cobalamine)	DNA synthesis, myelin synthesis
Folic acid	DNA synthesis
C	Collagen synthesis

Magnesium is important for nerve and muscle physiology but normal diets provide adequate amounts. Iodine is a necessary constituent of thyroid hormone, but the body can get along without renewed iodine supplies for relatively long times. Copper, chromium, boron, zinc, and manganese are important but are used in only trace amounts. Potassium and sodium are necessary electrolytes in cells and blood, but their functions are beyond the scope of this chapter.

MOST FREQUENT AND SERIOUS PROBLEMS

In the United States, overnutrition is recognized as a serious problem. Although there are varying criteria for what constitutes obesity, there is no question that there are millions of Americans in whom obesity contributes to an unhealthy lifestyle in terms of various physical and emotional problems. Extreme (morbid) obesity may also shorten a lifespan by its contribution to various disease states, the most important of which may be infections, cardiac problems, and atherosclerosis.

Alcoholism is also a serious physical and mental health problem. Alcoholism is found in at least 2 percent of the United States population and is a heavy contributor to accidental death (particularly automobile accidents), loss of work, break-up of families, suicide, and hospitalization for the various secondary effects of alcohol abuse.

Undernutrition is divided into primary malnutrition, in which there is a lack of a balanced diet and decreased total caloric intake, and secondary malnutrition, in which undernutrition results from a disease condition such as cancer, anorexia nervosa, depression, alcoholism, or any chronic disease. As a world-wide phenomenon, undernutrition is extremely significant in terms of scope and individual suffering.

Vitamin deficiencies may result in specific disease states, but they are usually secondary to general undernutrition and are uncommonly seen as isolated deficiencies of specific vitamins.

SYMPTOMS, SIGNS, AND TESTS

Potassium, phosphorus, sodium, and calcium are referred to as electrolytes and their blood levels can be easily and quickly measured. Copper, iodine, and iron can also be measured in blood. Most vitamins can also be measured in the blood if a specific vitamin deficiency is suspected.

Obesity is usually obvious by physical examination, but the degree may be determined by referring to standard charts of body weight and height. The symptoms and signs of alcohol abuse are many and varied. Symptoms of acute alcoholic excess include flushed face, tachycardia, and vomiting. Alcoholism often leads to absence from work, loss of interest in activities, interpersonal difficulties, and divorce. More severe chronic alcohol abuse results in increased incidence of infections, cardiac arrhythmias, peripheral neuropathy, heavy drinking to relieve anger, insomnia, or depression. In its most severe manifestations, alcoholism may result in tremors, withdrawal seizures, delirium tremens, cirrhosis, pancreatitis, gait disturbances, and cardiomyopathy.

Undernutrition manifests with specific signs and symptoms discussed under the specific diseases.

SPECIFIC DISEASES

Many of the disease states resulting from deprivation of essential foods have already been covered in this book because the major manifestations are focused on particular organ systems such as iron-deficiency anemia or rickets due to vitamin D deficiency. This chapter will focus on deficiencies and excesses that have not been adequately covered.

Deficiency Diseases

Generalized Undernutrition

Undernutrition means that the body weight is under that of an accepted standard for height, age, and body build. Undernutrition may result from insufficient diet or from excessive catabolic activity. Undernutrition implies a caloric deficiency of carbohydrates, lipids, and proteins. It is generally stated that up to 75 percent of humanity is undernourished. The true incidence of undernutrition in the United States is not really known. Throughout the world, endemic undernutrition results from several contributing factors, which include poor natural resources, poverty, large families, and lack of knowledge regarding production and preparation of food. Contributing factors to undernutrition include alcoholism, illiteracy, and unstable family situations.

Severe malnutrition in children, such as occurs in many areas of Africa, is divided into two types. *Marasmus* refers to a total caloric malnutrition with severe wasting but without specific effects of serum protein deficiency. *Kwashiorkor* is a severe protein deficiency, with or without caloric deficiency, characterized by generalized edema (due to low serum proteins) and fatty liver (due to insufficient production of lipoproteins).

In general, undernutrition is manifested in children by stunted growth, delayed bone maturation, slowed mental processes, and retarded puberty. Severely undernourished children often have diarrhea, which further complicates the problem. Mental retardation will result from early-onset undernutrition with consequent failure of proper brain development. Children who are undernourished are very susceptible to infections, and most severely undernourished children die by this means.

In adults, undernutrition may not be easily recognizable unless carried over from childhood, in which case short stature will be obvious. Otherwise, a decrease in adipose tissue and muscle mass may be the only obvious physical manifestations. In milder undernourished conditions, there is little desire to improve living conditions, and more primitive forms of gratification surface, such as alcoholic intake and sexual drive. Since the gonads are not involved in milder undernutritional states, the number of pregnancies may increase, much to the detriment of women and their offspring. More severe adult undernourishment is manifested by skin rashes, diarrhea, disappearance of body hair, hepatomegaly, polyneuropathy, and numerous endocrine manifestations. Sexual activity is usually decreased markedly at this stage and is accompanied by gonadal atrophy. Anemia is very common. Superimposed vitamin and mineral deficiencies and infections are common.

Vitamin Deficiencies

Vitamin deficiencies are outlined in Table 30–2. Deficiency of fat-soluble vitamins can be caused by severe fat malabsorption (such as might occur with celiac disease or chronic pancreatitis), but most patients with malabsorption syndrome do not exhibit these deficiencies. A severely restricted diet, such as occurs in some areas of the world, may cause deficiency of vitamins A, thiamine, riboflavin, niacin, and folic acid. Dietary deficiency of vitamins E, K, pyridoxine, and cobalamine are extremely unlikely, although a diet consisting entirely of processed foods potentially may cause a deficiency of pyridoxine. Dietary supplementation with vitamin D has largely eliminated rickets, a disease that occurred in children with reduced exposure to sunlight during the cold season. Vitamin C deficiency is unlikely except with diets deficient in citrus fruits and vegetables for a prolonged period such as formerly occurred in sailors.

In the United States, dietary vitamin deficiency is uncommon and is most likely to occur in alcoholics, the elderly, poor persons, or persons with severe disease that are living on a very restricted diet. Vitamin B_{12} deficiency is most often due to an autoimmune gastritis (pernicious anemia), a disease that destroys the cells that produce the intrinsic factor needed for vitamin B_{12} absorption. Lifelong injections of vitamin B_{12} prevent further difficulties. Folic acid deficiency, most often found in alcoholics with poor dietary intake, mimics pernicious anemia in its hematologic effects but does not cause the neuropathy

TABLE 30–2. VITAMIN DEFICIENCIES

Vitamin	Deficiency	Causes of Deficiency
A	Night blindness, skin changes	Dietary deficiency, malabsorption
D	Rickets, osteomalacia	Lack of sun exposure, dietary deficiency, malabsorption
E	None (lipofuscin and ceroid pigment accumulation)	Malabsorption syndrome
K	Hemorrhagic diathesis	Newborn, prolonged antibiotic therapy, malabsorption syndrome
B_1 (thiamine)	Beriberi (neuropathy, cardiomyopathy)	Dietary deficiency
B_2 (riboflavin)	Skin and mucosal lesions	Dietary deficiency
B_3 (niacin)	Pellagra (dermatitis, diarrhea, dementia)	Dietary deficiency
B_6 (pyridoxine)	Dermatitis, neuropathy, anemia	Diet of processed foods
GB_{12} (cobalamine)	Megaloblastic anemia, subacute combined degeneration	Intrinsic factor deficiency, malabsorption
Folic acid	Megaloblastic anemia	Dietary deficiency, malabsorption, cancer chemotherapy, increased need (pregnancy)
C	Scurvy (hemorrhagic diathesis, poor wound healing, retarded bone and tooth growth)	Dietary deficiency

of pernicious anemia. Folic acid is well absorbed in the face of malabsorption syndrome, so oral therapy followed by adequate diet is sufficient for treatment. In summary, one can say that healthy persons on a balanced diet have adequate vitamin intake, except, perhaps, for the need for vitamin D supplements for children in winter.

Mineral Deficiencies

Dietary iodine deficiency in inland and mountainous areas is easily corrected by use of iodized salt. Iron deficiency usually occurs in situations of increased need (infancy, pregnancy, blood loss) in association with low dietary intake; malabsorption can also lead to iron deficiency. A relative deficiency of calcium may occur, especially during the period of rapid bone growth (childhood). It has been suggested that increased calcium intake may retard the development of osteoporosis. Deficiencies of trace elements, such as magnesium, copper, selenium, and zinc, have been described.

Dietary Excess

Obesity

Obesity means having excess body adipose tissue. Although usually associated with being overweight, a person such as an athlete may be overweight and still not be obese because of increased muscle rather than adipose tissue. Obesity results from an imbalance in calories ingested versus calories expended. Although different persons utilize calories at different rates for a given amount of physical activity, it is a simple fact that obese persons eat too much food relative to their personal metabolic demands and their level of physical activity. Mild obesity is usually tolerated fairly well, but extreme obesity (greater than 20 percent above the standard average body weight at a given age and height) is associated with numerous serious health hazards that collectively reduce life expectancy. Obesity is associated with diabetes mellitus, gout, gallbladder disease, pulmonary emphysema, hypertension, atherosclerosis, and chronic bronchitis.

Treatment of obesity is accomplished by correcting the causative factors. In the cases of habitual overeating and psychogenic problems, the individual must be strongly motivated to decrease caloric intake and exercise properly. Operations that reduce the size of the stomach have been used to treat extreme obesity, but are not without hazard.

Specific Dietary Excesses

Diets high in saturated fatty acids and cholesterol are associated with increased risk for atherosclerotic disease such as myocardial infarct. Excessive protein intake may be deleterious to renal function, especially in patients with chronic renal failure. Excess sugar intake stresses mechanisms that control blood sugar and may lead to overt diabetes mellitus. Complex carbohydrates, such as those found in bread, pasta, rice, and potatoes, help stabilize blood glucose levels.

Vitamin Toxicity

Most vitamins are not toxic, but excessive dietary supplementation with vitamins A and D can lead to problems. Vitamin A toxicity produces a variety of problems with skin, bone, brain, and liver; mental disturbances mimicking psychoses may occur. Excessive doses of vitamin D may lead to hypercalcemia and to renal calculi.

Mineral Excesses

Excessive exogenous iron from iron tablets, blood transfusions, or production of alcoholic beverages in iron containers can lead to hemochromatosis. Excessive intake of sodium contributes to the development of hypertension. In general, the body regulates the intake of minerals to meet its needs.

Alcoholism

Ethanol is a natural food but may also be considered as a toxic compound when taken in excess over prolonged periods. It must be recognized that psychological and social factors powerfully predispose the potential victim. The term *alcoholism* refers to the pattern of continued alcohol abuse and the biologic and behavioral antecedents and consequences of this pattern. An important ingredient in alcoholism is the poorly understood physiologic dependence (addiction) on ethanol that drives the victim to continued intake. There are probably several different types of alcoholism, each with its own psychophysiologic focus. However, all types of alcoholism have the common denominator of interfering with the person's health, interpersonal relations, and economic and social position. By conservative estimates, over 2½ percent of the population of the United States is alcoholic.

Ethanol absorption starts in the stomach and continues in the duodenum and jejunum. It distributes with body water and rapidly appears in urine, spinal fluid, and pulmonary alveolar air. Alcohol is metabolized by oxidation to acetaldehyde and acetic acid and then to carbon dioxide and water. The main immediate target of ethanol is the brain, where relatively small amounts will depress mental functions, including judgment. Nearly every major organ system in the body is affected, major lesions occurring in the gastrointestinal system (including liver and pancreas), the central nervous system, and the cardiovascular system.

The liver is the most important organ affected by chronic alcoholic intake. Alcoholic changes in the liver caused by ethanol vary from fatty change in hepatocytes, a reversible process, to alcoholic cirrhosis, which is irreversible. Cirrhosis is the most common organic cause of death in alcoholics. The consequences of cirrhosis are discussed in Chapter 14. The acute clinical effects of alcohol intoxication also cause many deaths among alcoholics as well as among innocent bystanders involved in automobile accidents caused by alcoholics. Chronic pancreatitis develops in some chronic alcoholics and may lead to severe disability from pain, malabsorption with weight loss, and diabetes mellitus secondary to destruction of islets of Langerhans. The major, although infrequent, effect on the cardiovascular system by alcohol is cardiomyopathy. Direct toxic injury to heart muscle fibers results in slow accumulation of fibrous scarring and loss of function, first on the right side and then the left. Thiamine deficiency also occurs in alcoholics and causes a similar cardiomyopathy called *beriberi heart disease.*

Excessive alcohol intake may affect the nervous system in several ways. *Wernicke's encephalopathy* involves degeneration of several regions in the center of the brain, producing incoordination and mental confusion. Thiamine deficiency is likely a factor in Wernicke's encephalopathy, as high thiamine doses can reverse the process.

Chronic degenerative changes in the thalamus of alcoholics cause *Korsakoff's dementia*, a condition accompanied by severe memory loss and organic psychosis. Degenerative changes may also occur in the cerebellum, producing ataxia and tremor of the extremities. *Delirium tremens* (DTs) occur in the withdrawal period from acute, excessive alcoholic intake. DTs are manifested by a state of delirium in which the patient experiences frightening visual hallucinations. There is no demonstrable organic lesion in the brain of patients who die after experiencing delirium tremens.

Numerous treatment modalities for alcoholism have been attempted; these include tranquilizers, drugs that make one sick if alcohol is taken following the drug, and criminal incarceration. The only long-term treatment of alcoholism that has proven effective is Alcoholics Anonymous-type organizations, where persons with drinking problems may receive psychological support from other persons with similar problems. In modern society, the issue of alcoholism has shifted from that of a moral problem to one of a disease process and an affliction of society.

Review Questions

1. How do the manifestations of undernutrition in children differ from those in adults?

2. How do the functions and deficiencies of fat-soluble vitamins differ from those of water-soluble vitamins?

3. What is the usual cause and effect of deficiency for each of the vitamins?

4. What are the major causes and complications of obesity?

5. What is the treatment of obesity?

6. What are the major effects of alcoholism on the liver, pancreas, heart, and brain?

7. How is alcoholism best treated?

INDEX

Page numbers followed by *f* and *t* indicate figures and tables, respectively.

Abdominal injury, 608
ABO red blood cell antigens, 596–597
Abortion
  septic, 333, 343
  spontaneous, 333, 342
Abrasion, 607
Abscess, 59, 60*f*, 60–61, 535, 539
  cerebral, 460
  dental, 241
  enteric bacterial, 546
  pulmonary, 219
  skin, 363, 363*f*, 368–370, 369*f*, 542
  staphylococci in, 542
Academic pathologists, 2
Accidents
  chemical injury in, 618
  deaths from, 606, 606*f*
Accommodation, visual, 404
Accumulations, 43–46
Acetabulum, malformation of,
    416–417, 417*f*
Achlorhydria, 260
Achondroplasia, 415, 418, 419*f*
Acinus, pulmonary, 210, 210*f*
Acne, 361, 367–368, 368*f*
Acquired immune deficiency
    syndrome, 564, 566, 587. *See
    also* Human immuno-
    deficiency virus
Acquired injuries, 5
Acral-lentiginous melanoma, 383–385
Acromegaly, 512–513, 514*f*
Actin, 442
Actinic keratosis, 362, 379–380, 380*f*,
    385, 612
Activated partial thromboplastin time,
    202–203
Activity level, and atherosclerosis, 154
Acute, definition of, 14
Acute inflammatory demyelinating
    polyradiculoneuropathy, 455
Acute necrotizing ulcerative gingivitis,
    242
Acute poststreptococcal
    glomerulonephritis, 315–317,
    316*f*

Acute renal failure, 327
Acute respiratory distress syndrome,
    228
Acute toxic psychoses, 491
Acute tubular necrosis, 310, 327
Addison's disease, 521
Adenoids, 245
Adenomas
  adrenal, 522–523
  pituitary, 484–485, 513
  thyroid, 518
  tubular, 278–279, 280*f*
  villous, 278–279, 280*f*
Adhesion, 48, 196
Adolescence
  definition of, 102
  diseases of, 109
Adrenal cortex, 506, 508*t*
  diseases of, 520
Adrenal glands, diseases of, 520–524
Adrenal medulla, 506, 508*t*
  neoplasms of, 520
Adrenocorticotropic hormone, 506,
    508*t*
  deficiency or excess, disorders
    associated with, 510*t*, 521–522
Adult polycystic kidney disease, 313*f*,
    313–314
Adventitia, 142, 142*f*
Adverse drug reactions, 622*t*, 623
Adynamic ileus, 259
Affective disorders, 490–491, 494,
    497–498
Aflatoxin, 89
Agammaglobulinemia, 591
Age
  and atherosclerosis, 154
  and cancer types, 88*f*
Age-dependent disease, 17
Age-related disease, 17
Agglutination tests, 540–541
Aggregation, 196
Aging, 16–18
Agnosia, 493*t*
AIDS. *See* Acquired immune deficiency
    syndrome

Airway obstruction, 245, 250
Albinism, 364
Alcohol, 620
  and oral/upper respiratory cancer,
    248
Alcohol abuse. *See also* Alcoholism
  and congenital anomalies, 107, 115
Alcoholic hepatitis, 295
Alcoholism, 491, 632, 637–638
  cirrhosis in, 289
  definition of, 627
  liver disease in, 294–295
  pancreatitis in, 299–300
  pathophysiology of, 637–638
  signs and symptoms of, 633
  treatment of, 638
Aldosterone, excess, 522–523
Alimentary tract, 253–283
  cancer, 277–278
  diseases of, 257–258
    genetic/developmental, 260–263
    hyperplastic/neoplastic, 277–281
    inflammatory/degenerative,
        263–277
    signs and symptoms, 258–260
    tests for, 258–260
  layers of, 255, 256*f*
  malformations of, 261*f*, 261–262
  obstruction of, 259
  organ failure, 282
  segments, removal of, 257
  structure and function of, 254, 255*f*
Alkaline phosphatase, 290
Allergic rhinitis, 246, 586, 592–593
Allergy, 41, 583–586
  anaphylactic-atopic (type I), 583,
    586, 591–595
Alopecia, 364
Alpha-1-antitrypsin deficiency, 227
ALS. *See* Amyotrophic lateral sclerosis
Alveoli, 210
  diffuse damage, 228
Alzheimer disease, 460, 478–479, 495
Amblyopia, 398
Amebiasis, 266, 267, 570
Amines, vasoactive, 591

Amino acids, 630–631
Ammonia
  burns caused by, 620
  injury caused by, 625
Amnesia, 493t
Amniocentesis, 109, 110f
Amphetamines, abuse, 624
Amyloid, 44
Amyotrophic lateral sclerosis, 453
Anaerobic bacterial infections, 547
Anaphylactic reactions, 587
Anaphylactic shock, 587
Anaphylatoxins, 50
Anaphylaxis, 623
  systemic, 594–595
Anasarca, 166
ANA test, 590, 603
Anatomic pathology, tests and
        procedures in, 27–29
Androgens, 508t
Anemia, 172–173, 177–178
  aplastic, 185
  cancer and, 93
  of chronic disease, 185
  classification of, 177t
  with decreased red blood cell
        production, 183–185
  detection of, 173–176
  iron-deficiency, 184, 334
    in infants, 108–109
  sickle-cell, 111, 180, 180f
Anencephaly, 464
Aneurysm, 131
  atherosclerotic, 151, 151f
  saccular (berry), 470–471, 471f, 472f
Angina pectoris, 122
Angioedema, 593–594
Angiography, 124
  cerebral, 462–463
Angiomas, 147–148
Angiotensin, 309
Ankylosing spondylitis, 421, 434
Ankylosis, 432
Annulus fibrosus, 422
Anoxia, 40
Anthracosis, 229
Antibiotics, adverse reaction to, 623
Antibiotic susceptibility testing, of
        microorganisms, 540, 540f
Antibodies, 534, 578–579, 579f
  in diagnosis of infection, 540–541
Anticancer drugs, adverse reaction to,
        623
Anticoagulants, adverse reaction to,
        623
Antidiuretic hormone, 508t
  deficiency or excess, disorders
        associated with, 510t
  inappropriate secretion of, 529

Antigen, 578, 579f
  complete, 578
  incomplete, 578
  processing, 580
Antigen-presenting cells, 580
Antinuclear antibody test, 590, 603
Antithrombin III, 199, 205–206
Anuria, 310
Anus
  diseases of, 258
  imperforate, 261f, 262
Anxiety, 493t, 494
Anxiety disorders, 491, 498–499
  in childhood, 501
Aorta, atherosclerosis of, 152, 152f
Aortic stenosis, 133, 133f
Aphasia, 470, 493t
Aphthous stomatitis, 243, 244f
Aplastic anemia, 185
Apnea, 212
Apocrine glands, 360f, 361
Apoptosis, 38
Appendicitis, acute, 258, 260, 264,
        272–274, 273f
Appendix, 255, 272, 273f
Aqueous humor, 393, 399
Arteries, 142
Arteriography, 145, 146f
Arterioles, 142, 142f
Arteriolosclerosis, 148
Arteriosclerosis, 148, 148f
Arteriosclerotic heart disease, 128–132
Arthritis, 413. See also Rheumatoid
        arthritis
  acute, 427
  degenerative, 413, 421, 431, 432f,
        433f
  gouty, 413, 432f, 433f, 434–435
  infectious, 427
    signs and symptoms of, 414
  juvenile, 434
  signs and symptoms of, 414
Arthus reaction, 598
Asbestosis, 229
Ascariasis, 574
Ascaris lumbricoides, 539, 574
Ascending colon, 254, 255f
Ascites, 297
Aspartate aminotransferase, 290
Aspergillosis, 569, 570f
Aspergillus, 569, 570f
Aspiration pneumonia, 218
Aspirin, poisoning, 624
Asthma, 212, 223–224, 502
  allergic, 586–587, 592–593
Astigmatism, 393, 405
Astrocytes, 460, 472
Astrocytomas, 483
Asymptomatic disease, care of, 22
Atelectasis, 222f, 222–223
  definition of, 214

Atherosclerosis, 11–12, 144, 148f,
        148–156, 149f–150f
  in diabetes, 526
  prevention of, 155–156
  risk factors for, 153–155
  treatment of, 155
Atherosclerotic heart disease, 121
Atherosclerotic plaques, 12
Athlete's foot, 371
Atrial septal defect, 125, 125f
Atrophy, 43–46
Attention deficit disorder, 500–501
Audiometry, 239
Auscultation, 123
Autism, 500, 502
Autistic thinking, 493t
Autoimmune disease, 583, 601–603,
        602t
  diagnosis of, 590
Autoimmune hemolytic anemia, 597,
        602t
Autoimmune inflammatory
        myopathies, 451–452
Autoimmune reaction, 41
Autonomic nervous system, 444
Autopsy, 29
Autosomal inheritance, 104
Axons, 444, 445f, 458, 460
Azotemia, 328

Bacteria
  enteric, infections, 546–547
  exotoxins, 542, 552–554
  pyogenic, 542
Bacterial endocarditis, 134–135
Bacterial infections, 541–542
  anaerobic, 547
  enteric, 546–547
  mediated by exotoxins, 552–554
  most frequent and serious, 535–537
  pyogenic, 542–543
  secondary, 535–537
  sexually transmitted, 547–552
Baldness, 364
Band neutrophil, 171
Barbiturates, abuse, 624
Barium enema, 260, 281, 281f
Barr bodies, 102, 102f
Barrel chest, 227
Barrett's esophagus, 267
Bartholin's glands, 332
Basal cell carcinoma, 383, 385–388,
        386f, 387f
Becker's dystrophy, 448
Benign, definition of, 5
Benign neoplasms, 72
  morphologic features of, 77f, 77–78
  nomenclature for, 74t

Benign prostatic hyperplasia, 322–324, 324f
Benzene, accidental poisoning with, 625
Beriberi heart disease, 637
Berylliosis, 229
Bile ducts, 286, 288
Bile salts, production of, 287
Biliary atresia, 291
Bilirubin, 170–171
  excretion of, 287–288
Biopsy specimens, 27–28
Bipolar disorder, 497
Bladder, 306f, 309
  catheterization of, 312
  infection, 310
Bladder cancer, 310
  transitional cell, 325–326, 326f
Blastomyces dermatitidis, 567–568, 568f
Blastomycosis, 567, 568
Bleeding. *See also* Hemorrhage
  abnormal uterine, 333
  from mouth, 239
Bleeding disorders, 195–208
  detection of, 200–203
Bleeding time, 202
Blindness
  causes of, 406
  congenital, 406
  in infancy, 406
  legal, 406
Blister, 363, 363f
Blood
  coagulation. *See* Coagulation
  type and cross-match, 597
  vascular system, 141–143
Blood-brain barrier, 460
Blood-loss anemias, 178–179
Blood pressure, 123, 142
  high. *See* Hypertension
  low, signs and symptoms of, 145
Blood smear, 174, 174f
Blood transfusion reactions, 596–597
Blood urea nitrogen, 312
B lymphocytes, 579, 580
Body temperature, in infectious disease, 541
Boils, 368, 542
Bone formation, 410–412
  endochondral, 411–412
  intramembranous, 411
Bone marrow
  biopsy of, 175
  failure of, 191
  functions of, 171–172
Bones and joints, 409–439
  cancer metastatic to, 413–414
  diseases, 414–437
    genetic/developmental, 414–420
    hyperplastic/neoplastic, 435–437

inflammatory/degenerative, 420–435
  signs and symptoms of, 414
  tests for, 414
injuries, 420–421
major, 410, 411f
most frequent and serious problems of, 413–414
organ failure, 437
structure and function of, 410–413
Bordetella pertussis, 554
Boron requirements, 632
Borrelia burgdorferi, 555
Botulism, 265, 553
Brain, 458f, 458–460, 459f
  atrophy, in Alzheimer disease, 478, 479f
  blood flow to, 459–460
  contusion, 473–474
  destructive lesions of, 464–465
  hemorrhage in, 470, 471f
  malformations, 463–464
  most frequent and serious problems, 460
  neoplasms of, 482–485
  organ failure, 485
  penetrating injuries, 475–476
  trauma, 473–476
  tumors metastatic to, 485
Brain death, 485
Brain stem, 458, 458f
Breast, 347–358
  development of, 348
  diseases of
    genetic/developmental, 351
    hyperplastic/neoplastic, 352–357
    inflammatory/degenerative, 351–352
    signs and symptoms of, 350–351
    tests for, 350–351
  epithelial hyperplasia, 349
  fat necrosis, 349, 351
  fibroadenoma, 349, 352, 352f
  fibrocystic disease, 349, 352–354, 353f
  infection, 349
  intraductal papilloma, 354
  in lactation, 348
  male, lesions of, 357
  most frequent and serious problems of, 349, 349f
  painless masses, 349f, 350
  in pregnancy, 348
  structure and function of, 347–348, 348f
Breast cancer, 349, 354–357
  clinical course of, 357
  hormone receptor status, 356
  infiltrating, 355, 356f
  in situ, 355
  of male breast, 357
  metastases of, 355–356

signs and symptoms of, 349f, 350, 350f, 354, 354f
  treatment of, 355
Breast tissue, accessory, 351
Bronchi, 211, 211f
Bronchial carcinoid, 233
Bronchiectasis, 223, 224–225, 225f
Bronchitis, 211–212
  chronic, 223, 225–227
Bronchoalveolar carcinoma, 233
Bronchogenic carcinoma, 230–233, 231f, 232f, 528–529
Bronchopneumonia, 216–219, 217f
Brown atrophy, 46, 362
Brucella abortus, 556
Brucella melitensis, 556
Brucella suis, 556
Brucellosis, 556
Bruise, 607
Buccal smear, 102, 102f
Buffy coat, 170
Burns, 362, 388, 606, 609–611, 610f
  electrical, 611–612
  first-degree, 609
  scarring with, 610, 611f
  second-degree, 610, 611
  survival, 611
  third-degree, 610, 611
Butterfly rash, of systemic lupus erythematosus, 601, 602f

Cachexia, in cancer, 93
Calcification, 45
Calcitonin, 508t
Calcium
  deficiency, 635–636
  requirements for, 631
Calculi
  renal, 310, 321–322, 322f, 323f
  staghorn, 321
Calories, 630
Calves, pseudohypertrophy of, in Duchenne muscular dystrophy, 448–449, 449f
Campylobacter enteritis, 267
Cancer, 5, 73, 74, 85–96. *See also* Malignant neoplasms
  alimentary tract, 277–278
  and anemia, 93
  bladder, 310
    transitional cell, 325–326, 326f
  breast, 349, 354–357
  cachexia in, 93
  carcinoma, 74, 86
  cervical, 333, 337, 340–341, 341f
    risk factors for, 563
    signs and symptoms of, 334
    tests for, 334, 335f
  chemicals causing, 620

Cancer (*cont.*)
  chemotherapy for, 95
  cigarette smoking and, 620
  colon, 258, 277, 280–281, 281*f*
  common, age peaks of, 88*f*
  diagnosis of, 93–94
  ectopic hormone production by, 528–529
  endometrial, 337, 339*f*, 339–340
  etiology of, 88–91
  frequency of, 86–88
  gastric, 278, 279*f*
  gastric, *Helicobacter pylori* and, 278
  grading, 82–83
  hemorrhage in, 92
  hormonal therapy for, 95–96
  hormone production in, 93, 528–529
  and infection, 92–93
  of kidneys, 326–327
  laryngeal, 248
  life history of, 80–81
  lung, 211, 212, 230–233
  manifestations of, 91–94
  metastases
    to bones and joints, 413–414
    to liver, 301, 302*f*
    to lung, 233
  most common types, 87*f*
  natural history of, 94
  oral/upper respiratory
    alcohol and, 248
    cigarette smoking and, 248
  ovarian, 333, 337, 341–342
  pancreatic, 289, 301
  pathologic fractures in, 92
  pharyngeal, 248
  prostate, 310, 324–325, 325*f*
  radiation-induced, 90
  radiation therapy for, 95
    sarcoma, 74, 86
  skin, 362, 385–388, 386*f*, 387*f*, 612.
    See also Melanoma
  types, relative frequencies of, 379, 379*f*
  spread of, 80–82, 83*f*
  staging, 82–83
  of testis, 327
  thyroid, 518
    medullary, 518
  treatment of, 94–96
  types, age and, 88*f*
  viruses linked to, 90–91, 557–558
  vulvar, 334, 337
Candida, 569
  vaginitis, 334, 337, 337*f*
Candidiasis, 569
  mucocutaneous, 538
  superficial, 371, 372
Canker sore, 243, 244*f*
Capillaries, 142, 142*f*
Capillary aneurysms, 402

Capsule, of benign neoplasm, 70*f*, 77*f*, 78
Carbohydrates
  accumulation of, 44
  dietary, 630–631
Carbon dioxide content, of arterial blood, 213
Carbon monoxide poisoning, 618, 619, 625
Carbon tetrachloride, poisoning with, 293, 625
Carbuncle, 370, 542
Carcinogens, 80
  identification of, 89
Carcinoid, bronchial, 233
  carcinoma, 86
    infiltrating ductal, 355
    infiltrating lobular, 355
Carcinoma in situ, 81, 82*f*
Cardiac arrhythmia, 120, 123
  and heart attack, 130
Cardiac catheterization, 124
Cardiogenic shock, 137, 165, 165*t*
Cardiomyopathy, 122
Cardiovascular diseases, percent as cause of death, 121*f*
Carotid angiography, 145, 146*f*
Carotid arteries, 459
Carrier, 534
Caseous necrosis, 42–43
Casts, urinary, 311, 311*f*, 319–320
Cataracts, 393–395, 398, 399*f*
  congenital, 398
  senile, 398, 406
Catecholamines, 508*t*
Causes of disease, 6–8
  endogenous, 6, 7*t*
  exogenous, 6, 7*t*
Cecum, 254, 255*f*
Celiac disease, 271–272, 272*f*
Cell-mediated hypersensitivity, 585. *See also* Delayed hypersensitivity
Cells, 34*f*, 34–35
  injury, continuum of, 41–42, 42*f*
  types in tissue, 35, 36*f*
Cellulitis, 543, 6061
Central core disease, 451
Central nervous system, 457–487
  diseases of
    degenerative, 476–482
    genetic/developmental, 463–465
    hyperplastic/neoplastic, 482–485
    inflammatory, 465–468
    signs and symptoms of, 460–463
    tests for, 460–463
    vascular, 468–476
  most frequent and serious problems, 460
  organ failure, 485
  structure and function of, 458*f*, 458–460, 459*f*
  trauma, 468–476

Central nuclear myopathy, 451
Cerebellum, 458, 458*f*
Cerebral infarct, 12
Cerebral palsy, 108, 464–465
Cerebrospinal fluid, 459
  analysis, 462
Cerebrovascular accident, 460, 468–472
  anoxia in, brain cell vulnerability to, 472
  causes of, 468, 469*f*
  outcome with, 471, 473*f*
  pathophysiology of, 468, 469*f*, 470*f*
Cerebrum, 458, 458*f*
Cervical cancer, 333, 337, 340–341, 341*f*
  risk factors for, 563
  signs and symptoms of, 334
  tests for, 334, 335*f*
Cervical intraepithelial neoplasia, 340
Cervix, uterine, structure and function of, 332, 332*f*
Cestodes. *See* Tapeworm
Chagas's disease, 570
Chancre, syphilitic, 336, 371, 550, 551*f*
Charcot-Marie-Tooth disease, 451
Chemical carcinogenesis, 89
Chemical injury, 617–628
  agricultural, 625
  deaths from, 619, 622*t*
  to liver, 293–294
  modes of, 617–618
  most frequent and serious problems, 618–620
  signs and symptoms of, 621–623
  tests for, 621–623
Chemotaxis, 48
Chemotherapy, for cancer, 95
Chest injury, 608–609
Chest radiography, 213
  in tuberculosis, 221–222
Chickenpox, 538, 539, 559*f*, 560
Childhood
  definition of, 102
  diseases of, 109
  generalized emotional disorders of, 500–501
Children
  poisoning in, 619, 621*t*
  undernutrition in, 633–634
  viral infections in, 558–561
Chlamydia, 537, 549
  infections, 333, 336, 556–557
Chlamydia psittaci, 557
Chlamydia trachomatis, 547, 556–557
Chloramphenicol, adverse reaction to, 623
Chocolate cyst, 338, 342
Cholecystitis, 298–299
  acute, 289
  chronic, 298–299

Cholecystography, 290
Cholesteatoma, 247, 250
Cholinesterase inhibitors, injury
    caused by, 625
Choriocarcinoma, 345
Choroid, 392
Christmas disease, 204
Chromium requirements, 632
Chromosomal diseases, 102, 106
    detection of, 110
    examples of, 112–113
Chronic, definition of, 14, 52
Chronic brain syndrome, 491
Chronic fatigue syndrome, 555
Chronic obstructive pulmonary
    disease, 223
Chronic renal failure, 327–328
Cigarette smoking
    and atherosclerosis, 154
    and cancer, 248, 620
    and lung disease, 211, 225, 227
Ciliary body, 392*f*, 392–393
Circle of Willis, 459, 470
Cirrhosis, 289, 295–297, 296*f*
    in alcoholic liver disease, 294–297
    postnecrotic, 295, 296*f*
CJD. *See* Creutzfeldt-Jakob disease
Cleaning agents, accidental poisoning
    with, 620*t*, 621*t*, 625
Cleft lip, 239–240, 240*f*
Cleft palate, 239–240, 241*f*
Clinical pathology, 29–30
Clinical procedures, 24
Clostridium spp., in gas gangrene, 43
Clostridium botulinum, 553
Clostridium difficile, 274
Clostridium perfringens, 533–534, 553–554
Clostridium tetani, 552–553
Clotting. *See* Coagulation
Clubfoot, 414, 415, 415*f*
Coagulation, 50, 197
    chemical reactions in, 198*f*, 198–199
Coagulation cascade, 198
Coagulation disorders, 195–208
    detection of, 200–203
    and hemorrhage, 204–206
    and thrombosis, 206–207
Coagulation factor deficiency, 205
Coagulation necrosis, 42
Coarctation of aorta, 127–128, 128*f*
Cobalamine. *See* Vitamin B$_{12}$
Cocaine abuse, 624
Coccidioides immitis, 567–568
Coccidioidomycosis, 222, 538, 567–568
Cognitive function, tests of, 461
Cold exposure, excessive, 612
Cold sores, 243, 243*f*, 537
Colon
    cancer of, 258, 277, 280–281, 281*f*
    structure and function of, 254

Colonoscopy, 260, 281
Coma, 461, 485
Comedomastitis, 351
Comedones, 367
Commensals, 558
Common bile duct, 288
Common cold, 238, 244
Complement, 50
    activation, 580, 584–585
    components, measurement of, 588
    immunofluorescent test for, 589
Complement fixation, 583–584, 584*f*
Complications, 8
Compound nevus, 382
Compulsion, 493*t*
Computed tomography, 25–26, 26*f*
    abdominal, 312
    of central nervous system, 463
Concussion, 473
Conduct disorders, 501
Conduction deafness, 250
Conduction system of heart, 119–120,
    120*f*
Condyloma acuminatum, 334,
    336–337, 365, 366*f*, 563
Cone biopsy, 335, 340
Confusion, 493*t*
Congenital, definition of, 103
Congenital anomalies, 5, 103
Congenital heart disease, 121, 124–128
Congenital myopathies, 451
Congestion, 143
Congestive heart failure, 137, 138*f*
Conjunctiva, 392, 392*f*
Conjunctivitis, 393, 396*f*, 396–397
    inclusion body, 556–557
Connective tissue, 37
Connective tissue cells, 70
Conn's syndrome, 522–523
Constipation, 257, 259
Consumption, 221
Consumption coagulopathy, 205
Contact dermatitis, 590, 600. *See also*
    Poison ivy
    and chronic inflammation, 55–56
Contrecoup lesions, 473
Contusion, 607
    cerebral, 473–474
Conversion disorder, 501
Coombs' test
    direct, 588, 589*f*, 595, 597
    indirect, 588
COPD. *See* Chronic obstructive
    pulmonary disease
Copper requirements, 632
Cornea, 392, 392*f*
Coronary arteries, 119, 119*f*
Coronary artery atherosclerosis,
    128–132
    and myocardial infarct, 129, 129*f*

Cor pulmonale, 121, 136, 136*f*, 230
Corpus luteum cyst, 342
Cortex, cerebral, 458, 459*f*
Corynebacterium diphtheriae, 554
Coryza, 244
Cotton wool patches, 400, 401*f*
Cough, 212
Coup lesions, 473
Cradle cap, 377
Craniopharyngiomas, 513
Creatine kinase, 446
Creatinine, 312
Creutzfeldt-Jakob disease, 477–478
Crohn's disease, 258, 264, 274*f*, 274–275
Cross-matching, 597
Croup, 245
Crust, 363, 363*f*
Cryptococcosis, 567–569
Cryptococcus neoformans, 567–568
    meningitis, 466
Cryptorchism, 314
Cryptosporidiosis, 572
CT. *See* Computed tomography
Culture, of microorganisms, 539–540,
    540*f*
Cushing's syndrome, 507–509,
    521–522, 523*f*, 529
Cyanide poisoning, 626
Cyanosis, 126, 212
Cyclopia, 395
Cysticercosis, 574
Cystic fibrosis, 111, 215
    of pancreas, 291
Cystic hygroma, 147
Cystitis, 310, 320
Cystograms, 312
Cystoscopy, 312
Cysts
    ovarian, 341–342
    periapical, 241–242
Cytokines, 51
Cytomegalic inclusion disease, 563–564
Cytomegalovirus, 563–564
Cytotoxic T cells, 579

Dandruff, 361
Deafness, 238, 239, 250
    causes of, 250
Debridement, 65
Decubitus ulcers, 609
Degeneration, 5, 38
Degenerative diseases
    of central nervous system, 476–482
    erythropoietic, 176–187
    of heart, 128–136
    vascular, 148–164
Degenerative joint disease. *See*
    Arthritis, degenerative

Delayed hypersensitivity, 585, 586*f*, 587, 599–601
  tests for, 589–590
Deletion, 100, 100*f*
Delirium, 491, 493*t*, 495
Delirium tremens, 295, 638
Delta agent, 293
Delusions, 493*t*, 494, 495
Dementia, 493*t*, 495
  definition of, 478, 492
Dendrites, 460
Dental caries, 238, 240–242
Dental plaque, 240
Depression, 491, 493*t*, 494
  clinical features of, 497
  definition of, 497
Dermatitis, 372–374, 373*f*
  atopic, 374, 374*t*, 375–376
  classification of, 374, 374*t*
  contact, 374*t*, 374–375
  definition of, 365, 372
  eczematous, 361
  exfoliative, 374, 374*t*
  light-induced, 374, 374*t*
  seborrheic, 361, 374, 374*t*, 377
Dermis, 360*f*, 360–361
Dermoid cyst, 341–342
Descending colon, 254, 255*f*
Developmental diseases, 4–5, 97–116
  of alimentary tract, 260–263
  of bones and joints, 414–420
  of breast, 351
  of central nervous system, 463–465
  erythropoietic, 176
  of eye, 395
  of female genital organs, 336
  of genitourinary system, 312–314
  of heart, 124–128
  of lung, 213–215
  of skin, 364–365
  vascular, 146–148
Developmental disorders, 501
Diabetes insipidus, 513
Diabetes mellitus, 111, 289, 507, 524–528, 525*t*
  and atherosclerosis, 154
  clinical features of, 525–526
  complications of, 526
  insulin-dependent (type I) (IDDM), 524–528, 525*t*
  non-insulin-dependent (type II) (NIDDM), 524–528, 525*t*
  renal damage in, 319
Diabetic neuropathy, 445, 455
Diabetic retinopathy, 402*f*, 402–403, 406
Diagnosis, 3
Diagnostic resources, 21–31
Diagnostic tests and procedures, 23–30
Dialysis, 319, 327, 328
Diaphragmatic hernia, 261, 261*f*

Diarrhea, 257, 259, 282
  infectious, 263, 264–265
DIC. *See* Disseminated intravascular coagulation
Dietary excess, 636–637
Differentiation, 82–83
Diffuse idiopathic pulmonary fibrosis, 230
Diffusion, definition of, 210
Digestive process, 257
Digestive system, structure and function of, 254–257
Dilation and curettage, 335, 342
Diphtheria, 554
Diplopia, 454
Disease(s)
  categories of, 4*t*
  definition of, 2–3
  frequency of, 14*t*, 14–15, 15*t*
    and family physician visits, 15–16, 16*t*
Disseminated intravascular coagulation (DIC), 206
Disuse atrophy, 43
Diuresis, 327
Diverticulosis, 258
  colonic, 264, 275–276, 276*f*
Dominant inheritance, 104, 105*f*
Doppler ultrasound, of renal blood flow, 312
Down syndrome, 106, 112–113, 464
Drugs
  abuse, 618, 619, 624
  detoxification, by liver, 288
  exposure, and congenital anomalies, 107
  hepatotoxicity, 293–294
  overdose, 618–619
Dry eyes, 396
Duchenne muscular dystrophy, 444, 448–449, 449*f*
Duodenum, 254, 255*f*
Duplication, 100, 100*f*
Dura, 459
Dysentery, 267
Dysesthesia, 461
Dysfunctional uterine bleeding, 334
Dysmenorrhea, 334, 338
Dysphagia, 259, 268
Dysplasia, 81
Dysplastic nevi, 383
Dyspnea, 212
Dystrophic calcification, 45
Dystrophies, 447–448, 448*f*
Dystrophin, 111, 448
Dysuria, 310, 320

Ear
  diseases of, 238
  structure and function of, 238

Eccrine glands, 360*f*, 361
ECG. *See* Electrocardiography
Echinococcosis, 574
Echinococcus granulosus, 574
Eclampsia, 343–344
Echocardiogram, 123
Ectopic pregnancy, 333, 342–343, 343*f*, 344*f*
Eczema, definition of, 372
Edema, 47, 143
EEG. *See* Electroencephalogram
Ehrlichiosis, 538, 567
Electrical burns, 611–612
Electrocardiography, 123
Electroencephalogram, 463
Electromyography, 446
Elephantiasis, 166, 575
Embolus, 41, 161, 163*f*
Embryonal, definition of, 72
Embryonic anomalies, 103, 107–108, 113–114
  detection of, 110
Embryonic development, 101
Emigration, 48
Emphysema, 211–212, 223, 225, 226*f*, 227–228
  centriacinar, 227
  irregular, 228
  panacinar, 227
  paraseptal, 227–228
Empyema, 59, 219
Encephalitis, 460, 466–467, 538
  in HIV-infected (AIDS) patients, 467
  postviral, 561, 601
Endarterectomy, 155
Endocardial thrombus formation, 131–132
Endocarditis, infective, 134–135
Endocrine atrophy, 43
Endocrine disease
  most frequent and serious, 507–509
  signs and symptoms of, 510–511
  tests for, 510–511
Endocrine syndromes, 528–529
Endocrine system, 505–530
  organ failure in, 529
  organs and tissues of, 506, 507*f*, 508*t*–509*t*
  structure and function of, 506–507
Endogenous, definition of, 6
Endometrial cancer, 337, 339*f*, 339–340
Endometriosis, 337–338
Endometritis, 345
Endometrium, 332
Endoscopic procedures, 260
Endotoxic shock, 547
Endotoxin, 547
Energy, in foods, 630
Enterobius vermicularis, 572
Enucleation, 406
Environmental exposure, chemical injury due to, 618

Enzymatic fat necrosis, 43
Enzymatic necrosis, 299
Eosinophil count, in infectious disease, 541
Eosinophilia, 591–592
Epidermis, 360f, 360–361
Epidermolysis, 388
Epidural hematoma, 474, 475f
Epilepsy, 460, 482
Epiphysis, 410, 412f
Epithelial cells, 70
Epithelioid cells, 57
Epithelium, of alimentary tract, 255, 256f
Epstein-Barr virus, 562–563
Erythroblastosis fetalis, 108, 114–115, 587, 595–596
Erythrocytes, 170
    decreased production of, anemias with, 183–185
    maturation of, 171, 172f
    measurements of, 174–175, 175t
    sickled, 180, 180f
Erythropoietin, 172
Escherichia coli, 534
    diarrhea caused by, 265
    infection, 546–547
    meningitis, 465
Esophageal atresia, 261, 261f
Esophageal varices, 163
Esophagitis, 263–264
Esophagus, structure and function of, 254, 255
Essential hypertension, 136, 144–145, 156
Estrogens, 509t
Etiology, 3
Euphoria, 493t
Excisional biopsy, 28
Exfoliative dermatitis, 362
Exogenous, definition of, 6
Exophthalmos, 516f, 517
Exotoxins, 542
    bacterial infections mediated by, 552–554
Extramedullary hematopoiesis, 185
Extravascular hemolysis, 177, 179
Exudate, 59
Eye, 391–407
    anatomy of, 392f, 392–393
    chemical injury, 395–396
    diseases of
        genetic/developmental, 395
        hyperplastic/neoplastic, 405–406
        inflammatory/degenerative, 395–405
        signs and symptoms of, 394–395
        tests for, 394–395
    most frequent and serious problems, 393
    organ failure, 406

structure and function of, 392–393
    trauma, 393–396

Factitious disorder, 501
Fallopian tubes, structure and function of, 332, 332f
Familial adenomatous polyposis, 280
Familial diseases, 103–104
Familial periodic paralysis, 454
Farsightedness. *See* Hyperopia
Fascicles, skeletal muscle, 442, 442f
Fascioscapulohumeral dystrophy, 451
Fats, dietary, 630–631
Fatty liver, 294, 295
Fatty metamorphosis (change), 44
Fecalith, 272, 273f
Feces, tests of, 260
Females, common cancers in, 87f
Femoral anteversion, 416
Fertility, 345
Fertilization, 98
Fetal alcohol syndrome, 115
Fetal development, 101
Fetal diseases, 108
    detection of, 110
    examples of, 114–115
Fever, in infectious disease, 541
Fibrin degradation products, 203
Fibrin fibers, 197, 197f
Fibrinogen, 49, 197
Fibrinolysis, 199, 203
Fibrinolytic system, 199
Fibrinous exudate, 59
Fibroid, uterine, 338
Fibroma, 74
Fibrosis, 61, 63, 64f
Fibrous connective tissue repair, 61, 63, 64f
Filariasis, 166, 575
Fine-needle aspiration (FNA), 28
Flail chest, 608
Flame hemorrhage, 400, 401f
Flank pain, 310, 321
Flare, 377
Flat bones, 410
Flight of ideas, 493t
Flu, 244, 561–562
Fluorescent treponemal antibody test, 550, 552
FNA. *See* Fine-needle aspiration
Folic acid
    deficiency, 184–185, 634–635, 635t
    function of, 631t
Follicle-stimulating hormone, 506, 508t
Follicular cyst, 342
Food allergy, gastrointestinal, 595
Food poisoning, 263, 264–265
    Salmonella, 265–267
    staphylococcal, 265–267

Foods, 630
Foramen magnum, 461, 462f
Foramen ovale, 125
Foreign bodies, and chronic inflammation, 54
Forensic pathology, 30
Fovea, 401f
Fractures, 413, 424–427, 426f, 427f
    closed, 424, 426f
    comminuted, 424, 426f, 426–427
    complete, 424, 426f, 427f
    compression, 424, 426f
    healing, 424–427
    incomplete, 424, 426f
    infection, 426
    nonunion, 425
    open, 424, 426, 426f
    osteoporotic, 430
    pathologic, 413, 424, 427
        in cancer, 92
    signs and symptoms of, 414
    sites, 424
    of skull, 462
    stable, 424, 425
    unstable, 424, 425
Fragile X-syndrome, 113
Francisella tularensis, 555
Freckles, 362, 385
Frostbite, 612
Functional bowel syndrome, 258
Functional diseases, 6, 6t
Funduscopic examination, 394
Fungal infections, 567–569, 601
    cutaneous, 569
    disseminated, 538
    most frequent and serious, 538
    opportunistic systemic, 569, 570f
    primary systemic, 567–569, 568f
    pulmonary, 222
    superficial, 371–372, 538
Furuncles, 60, 368, 369, 542

Galactorrhea, 350
Gallbladder
    most frequent and serious problems of, 289
    nonfunctioning, 302
    structure and function of, 286, 288
Gallstones, 289, 298f, 298–299
    pancreatitis with, 300
    signs and symptoms of, 289
    tests for, 290
Gamma radiation
    effects of, 613
    injury from, 613–614
Ganglion, 435
Gangrene (gangrenous necrosis), 43
    atherosclerosis and, 152, 153f
    in diabetes, 526
    simple, 554

Gas exchange, definition of, 210
Gas gangrene, 43, 553–554
Gastric analysis, 260
Gastric cancer, 278, 279f
Gastrin, 528
Gastrinomas, 528
Gastritis, 264, 268–269
    acute, 268
    chronic, 269
    fundic, 269
    Helicobacter, 269
Gastroenteritis, viral, 537
Gastrointestinal tract
    allergic reactions in, 595
    endocrine functions of, 506, 508t
    structure and function of, 254–257
Genes, 100–101
Genetic diseases, 4–5, 97–116. *See also*
        Developmental diseases
    definition of, 102
    examples of, 110–112
    incidence of, as percentage of live
        births, 107t
    signs and symptoms of, 109
    tests for, 109, 110f
Genital organs
    female, 331–346
        biopsy of, 335
        failure, 345
        genetic/developmental diseases
            of, 336
        hyperplastic/neoplastic diseases,
            337–342
        most frequent and serious
            problems of, 333
        structure and function of, 332f,
            332–333
    male, 305–329
        examination of, 311
        structure and function of, 306f,
            306–310
Genitourinary system
    diseases of
        genetic/developmental, 312–314
        hyperplastic/neoplastic, 322–327
        inflammatory/degenerative,
            314–321
        most frequent and serious problems
            of, 310
German measles. *See* Rubella
Gestational trophoblastic neoplasms,
        345
Ghon complex, 220, 220f
Giant hairy nevi, 383
Giardiasis, 538, 570, 572
Gigantism, 512–513
Gingivitis, acute necrotizing ulcerative,
        242
Glaucoma, 393, 395, 399–400, 406
    closed-angle, 399–400, 400f
    open-angle, 399, 400f
Glial scar, 472

Glioblastoma multiforme, 483, 483f
Glioma, 75
Globe
    of eye, 392
        retinal layer of, 392, 392f
        scleral layer of, 392, 392f
        uveal layer of, 392, 392f
Glomerular diseases, 315
Glomerulonephritis, 315, 587, 598–599
    acute poststreptococcal, 315–317, 316f
    chronic, 317–319
    immune complex, 315–317, 316f
    membranous, 318–319
        idiopathic, 318–319
Glomerulus, 307, 308f
    immune complex deposits in, 315,
        316f
    normal, components of, 315, 316f
Glucagon, 508t, 524
Glucagonoma, 528
Glucocorticoids, 507, 508t
    deficiency or excess, disorders
        associated with, 510t
Glucose-6-phosphate dehydrogenase
        deficiency, 182
Glucose tolerance test, 527, 527t
Gluten, 271
Goiter, 507, 510–511, 516, 516f
    colloid, 518
    nodular, 518
    nontoxic, 518
    toxic nodular, 518
Gonorrhea, 333, 336, 535, 537,
        547–549
Goodpasture's syndrome, 602t
Gout, 111–112, 362, 432f, 433f, 434–435
Grading, 82
Graft rejection, 601
Graft-versus-host disease, 583
Gram-negative shock, 547
Gram-stained smear, 540
Granulation tissue, 63, 65
Granulocytes, 171
Granuloma, periapical, 241
Granulomatous colitis, 275
Granulomatous inflammation, 57–59,
        58f
Graves' disease, 516f, 516–517
Gray matter, 458, 459f
Grief, 493t
Growth hormone, 506, 508t
    deficiency or excess, disorders
        associated with, 510t, 512–513
Guillain-Barré syndrome, 455
Gunshot wounds, 607
Gynecomastia, 357

Haemophilus influenzae
    infection, 546
    meningitis, 465

Hair disorders, 364
Hallucinations, 493t, 494, 495
Halothane, adverse reaction to, 293, 623
Hansen disease. *See* Leprosy
Haptens, 578, 597
Hashimoto's disease, 514–515
Hashimoto's thyroiditis, 602t
Hay fever, 246, 586, 592–593
    and chronic inflammation, 55
Headache, 460
Head injury, 609
Hearing loss. *See also* Deafness
    age-related, 247, 250
    drug-related, 250
    with otosclerosis, 247, 250
Heart, 117–139
    blood flow in, 118, 119f
    function of, 118–120
    structure of, 118f, 118–119, 119f
Heart attack, 120–121, 130
    first, survival time after, 121f
Heartburn, 260, 268
Heart disease, 11–12, 120–122
    congenital, 124–128
    detection of, 122–124
Heart failure, 137–138
Heart murmur, 123
Heat, in inflammation, 47
Heat exposure, excessive, 612
Helicobacter pylori, 269
    and gastric cancer, 278
Helminthic infestations, 572–575
    most frequent and serious, 539
Hemangiomas, 147f, 147–148, 364
Hematemesis, 258
Hematochezia, 259
Hematocrit, 174
Hematoma, 75, 201, 202f
Hematopoiesis, extramedullary, 185
Hematopoietic system, 169–193
Hematuria, 201, 310
Hemiparesis, 461
Hemochromatosis, 45–46
Hemoglobin electrophoresis, 176
Hemoglobinopathies, 180
Hemolytic anemias, 179–183
Hemophilia, 111, 204–205
Hemopoietic diseases, 172–173
    detection of, 173–176
Hemoptysis, 212, 232
Hemorrhage. *See also* Bleeding
    in cancer, 92
    cerebral, 470, 471f
    disorders with, 203–206
    gastrointestinal, 258–259
Hemorrhagic diathesis, 200
Hemorrhagic disease of the newborn,
        205
Hemorrhagic shock, 165, 165t
Hemorrhoids, 144, 258
Hemosiderosis, 45
Hemostasis, 196–199

Hemothorax, 608
Heparin, 205
Hepatitis
    alcoholic, 295
    viral, 289, 291–293
Hepatitis A, 292
Hepatitis B, 292–293
Hepatitis C, 293
Hepatocytes, 286–287, 287*f*
Hepatoma, 75
Hepatomegaly, 290
Hereditary motor and sensory,
    neuropathies, 451
Hereditary spherocytosis, 181–182
Hernia
    diaphragmatic, 261, 261*f*
    hiatal, 258, 267, 268*f*
    inguinal, 258, 264, 276–277, 277*f*
Herpes simplex virus, 537, 563
    cold sores, 243, 243*f*
    encephalitis, 467
    female genital infection, 333, 336
Herpes stomatitis, 243, 243*f*
Heterotropia. *See* Strabismus
Hip
    congenital dislocation of, 414,
        416–417, 417*f*
    fracture, 430
Hirschsprung's disease, 263, 264*f*
Hirsutism, 364
Histamine, 591
    in inflammation, 50
Histiocytes, 36
Histoplasma capsulatum, 567–568
Histoplasmosis, 222, 538, 567
History, 4
HIV. *See* Human immunodeficiency
    virus
Hives, 363, 363*f,* 377, 587, 593–594, 594*f*
Hodgkin's disease, 190
Homicide, 618
Hormonal therapy, for cancer, 95–96
Hormones, 506, 508*t*–509*t*
    assessment of, 511
    ectopic production, by tumors,
        528–529
    negative feedback regulation of, 506,
        509*f*
    production, in cancer, 93
Human chorionic gonadotropin, 509*t*
    measurement of, in pregnancy tests,
        334
Human immunodeficiency virus
    encephalitis, 467
    infection, 535, 537, 538, 564–566
        clinical features of, 564
        diagnosis, 564–565
        management of, 565–566
        prevention of, 566
        transmission, 564, 566
Human papilloma virus, 333, 336–337,
    340, 365, 537, 563

Hutchinson's freckle, 383
Hyalin, 44
Hyaline membrane disease, 213–215,
    214*f*
Hydatid cysts, 574
Hydatidiform mole, 345
Hydrocephalus, 464, 480–481, 481*f*
    acquired, 480–481
    congenital, 480–481
Hydronephrosis, 321, 322*f*
Hydrostatic pressure, 166
Hyperactivity, 493*t*
Hypercapnia, 213
Hyperemia, 46
Hyperkeratosis, 380
Hyperlipidemia, and atherosclerosis,
    153–154
Hypernephroma, 75
Hyperopia, 393, 394, 403–404, 404*f*
Hyperparathyroidism, 413, 429, 507,
    519–520
Hyperplasias, 5, 69–84, 72*f*
    definition of, 71
    morphologic features of, 76–77
Hypersensitivity, 583–586
    Arthus-type (type III), 584–585, 585*f,*
        587, 597–599
    tests for, 589, 590*f*
    cytotoxic-type (type II), 583–584,
        584*f,* 587, 595–597
    type I, 583, 584*f,* 586–587, 591–595
    type IV. *See* Delayed hypersensitivity
Hypersplenism, 179, 183, 204
Hypertension, 144–145, 156–159, 502.
        See also Pulmonary
        hypertension
    and atherosclerosis, 154
    causes of, 156–157
    detection of, 158
    effect on heart, 135*f,* 135–136
    signs and symptoms of, 145
    treatment of, 159
Hypertensive heart disease, 120–121,
    135–136
Hypertensive retinopathy, 400, 401*f*
Hyperthyroidism, 516*f,* 516–517
Hypertrophy, 71–72, 72*f*
    morphologic features of, 76–77
Hyphae, 567, 569, 570*f*
Hypoactivity, 493*t*
Hypochondria, 493*t*
Hypogammaglobulinemia, 591
Hypoparathyroidism, 519
Hypoplastic kidney, 113
Hypotension, 145
Hypothalamus, 506, 507*f,* 508*t,* 509*f*
Hypothermia, 612
Hypothyroidism, 514–515
Hypoxemia, 213
Hypoxia, 40

Iatrogenic, definition of, 8
Idiopathic, definition of, 8
Idiopathic hypertension. *See* Essential
    hypertension
Idiopathic thrombocytopenic purpura,
    186–187, 602*t*
Ileum, 254, 255*f*
Ileus, 259, 608
Illusions, 493*t*
Immune complex glomerulonephritis,
    315–317, 316*f*
Immune complex hypersensitivity,
    584–585, 585*f,* 587, 597–599
Immune deficiency disease, 583, 587,
    591
Immune hemolytic anemia, 182–183
Immune surveillance, 580
Immune system, 534
    and inflammation, 56–57
Immunity, 578
Immunizations, 534, 538, 558
Immunodiffusion, 588
Immunofluorescent tests, 589, 590*f*
Immunoglobulins, 579
    classes of, 580, 581*f*
    deficiencies of, 591
    functions of, 580–582, 582*f*
    IgA, 582
    IgD, 582
    IgE, 582, 583
    IgG, 580–581, 581*f*
    IgM, 581, 581*f*
    structure of, 580, 581*f*
Immunologic disease, 577–603
    classification of, 583–586
    most frequent and serious, 586–587
    signs and symptoms of, 587
    tests for, 588–590
Immunosuppressed patient,
    pneumonia in, 218–219
Imperforate anus, 261*f,* 262
Impetigo, 370*f,* 370–371, 544
Inborn error of metabolism, 109
Incidence, 13
Incision, 607
Incisional biopsy, 27–28
Incoherence, 493*t*
Infancy
    definition of, 101
    diseases of, 108–109
Infantile polycystic kidney disease, 314
Infarct, 40
Infections, 7. *See also* Infectious diseases
    associated with obstructions, 537, 537*t*
    bacterial, 541–542
        anaerobic, 547
        enteric, 546–547
        most frequent and serious,
            535–537
        pyogenic, 542–543
        secondary, 535–537
        sexually transmitted, 547–552

Infections (*cont.*)
of brain, 465–468
cancer and, 92–93
chlamydial, 333, 336, 537, 547, 549, 556–557
definition of, 533
in diabetics, 526–527
fungal, 567–569, 601
cutaneous, 569
disseminated, 538
most frequent and serious, 538
opportunistic systemic, 569, 570*f*
primary systemic, 567–569, 568*f*
pulmonary, 222
superficial, 371–372, 538
group A streptococcal, 543–544
and hematopoietic system, 187
and host defense mechanisms, 533–535
manifest as delayed hypersensitivity, 601
primary, 535
protozoal, 570–572
most frequent and serious, 538
pulmonary, 215–216
reportable, 535
relative frequencies of, 535, 536*t*
rickettsial, 538, 566–567
secondary, 535. *See also* Opportunistic infections
sexually transmitted, 333, 535, 537, 547, 548*t*
bacterial, 547–552
signs and symptoms of, 539–541
staphylococcal, 542–543
tests for, 539–541
upper respiratory, 244–245
venereal, 333
viral, 557*f*, 557–558, 601
and cancer, 90–91, 557–558
of childhood, 558–561
most frequent and serious, 537–538
Infectious diseases, 531–576. *See also* Infections
most frequent and serious, 535–539
overall impact of, 535
Infectious mononucleosis, 538, 562–563
Infertility, 345
Inflammation, 5, 38, 46–61, 539
acute, 46–52, 47*f*
cardinal signs of, 46–47
chronic, 52–57, 53*f*
granulomatous, 57–59, 58*f*
suppurative, 59
time frame of, 39*f*
Inflammatory bowel disease, 258, 264, 274–275
Inflammatory diseases, 5
of alimentary tract, 263–277
of bones and joints, 420–435

of breasts, 351–352
of central nervous system, 465–468
erythropoietic, 176–187
of eye, 395–405
of female genital organs, 336–337
of genitourinary system, 314–321
of heart, 128–136
of lung, 215–230
of mouth, 240–243
of skeletal muscle, 451–455
of skin, 365–388
vascular, 148–164
Inflammatory lesions, gross, 60–61
Inflammatory response, 534
Influenza, 561–562
Initiation, 80
Injury, 39–46
acute, 40–43
chemical, 617–628
agricultural, 625
deaths from, 619, 622*t*
to liver, 293–294
modes of, 617–618
most frequent and serious problems, 618–620
signs and symptoms of, 621–623
tests for, 621–623
chronic, 43–46
events following, 38–39
mechanical, 607–609
physical, 605–615
most frequent and serious problems, 606
radiation-related, 606, 612–614
thermal, 606, 609–612. *See also* Burns
Insecticides, injury caused by, 625
Insulin, 508*t*, 524
deficiency or excess, disorders associated with, 510, 510*t*
Insulinomas, 528
Intelligence, 492
Interferon, 534–535, 558
Intermittent claudication, 152
Interstitial nephritis, 320
Intervertebral disk, 413*f*
herniated, 421, 422, 423*f*, 424*f*
Intestinal flu, 258, 265, 266
Intestinal perforation, 258, 259
Intima, 142, 142*f*
Intoeing, 414, 416
Intoxication, 495
Intracranial pressure, increased, 461–462, 462*f*, 482–483, 609
Intradermal nevus, 382
Intraocular pressure, 400
Intravascular hemolysis, 177, 179
Intravenous urogram, 312
Invasion, 72, 78
Iodine
deficiency, 635
requirements for, 632

Iris, 392*f*, 392–393
Iron
deficiency, 635
excess, 636
requirements for, 631
Iron compounds, toxicity, 624–625
Iron-deficiency anemia, 184, 334
in infants, 108–109
Irritable bowel syndrome, 258
Ischemia, 40
Islets of Langerhans, 289, 506, 507*f*, 508*t*
diseases of, 524–528
Isoniazid, adverse reaction to, 293
ITP. *See* Idiopathic thrombocytopenic purpura

Jaundice, 288, 289, 291
neonatal, 290–291
in viral hepatitis, 291
Jejunum, 254, 255*f*
Jock itch, 371
Joints. *See* Bones and joints
Junctional nevus, 382
Juvenile arthritis, 434
Juxtaglomerular apparatus, 309

Kaposi's sarcoma, 565
Karyolysis, 39
Karyorrhexis, 39
Karyotyping, 102, 103*f*
Keratitis, 395
Kidneys, 305–329
agenesis, 113, 313
biopsy of, 312
cancers of, 326–327
dysplastic, 314
failure, 327–328
function, tests of, 312
hypoplasia, 313
most frequent and serious problems of, 310
multicystic, 314
polycystic, 313*f*, 313–314
structure and function of, 306*f*, 306–310, 307*f*
Kidney stones, 310, 321–322, 322*f*, 323*f*
Kinin system, 50
Klebsiella, infection, 546–547
Klinefelter syndrome, 113
Knee joint
injury, 421
structure and function of, 410, 412*f*
Korsakoff's dementia, 638
Kupffer cells, 287
Kwashiorkor, 631, 633
Kyphosis, 422–423, 425*f*

Laboratory abnormalities, 4
Laboratory medicine, 29–30
Laceration, 607
Laennec's cirrhosis, 295
Lamina propria, of alimentary tract, 255, 256*f*
Laparoscopy, 335, 342
Large intestine, structure and function of, 254
Laryngeal cancer, 248
Laryngitis, 244, 245
Larynx. *See also* Upper respiratory tract structure and function of, 238
Lead poisoning, 626
Left-sided congestive heart failure, 137, 138*f*
Legionella pneumophila, 546
Legionellosis, 546
Legionnaire's disease, 218
Leiomyoma of uterus, 333, 334, 337, 338*f,* 338–339
Leishmaniasis, 570
Lens, of eye, 392*f,* 392–393
Lentigo, 379
Lentigo maligna melanoma, 383
Lentigo senilis, 385
Leprosy, 445, 556
Lesions, 4
  inflammatory, gross, 60–61
Leukemias, 187–189
  relative frequency of, 173*f*
Leukocytes
  disorders of, 186
  measurements of, 175, 175*t*
Leukoplakia, 76
Leukotrienes, 51
Lewy body, 480
Limb-girdle dystrophy, 451
Lipid, accumulation of, 44
Lipofuscin, 46
Lipoid nephrosis, 317–318, 318*f*
Liquefaction necrosis, 42
Lithotripsy, 321
Liver
  biopsy of, 290
  chemical injury to, 293–294
  diseases of
    alcoholic, 294–295
    most frequent and serious, 289
    neonatal, 290–291
    signs and symptoms of, 289–290
  failure, 302
  histologic structure of, 286–287, 287*f*
  metastatic cancer of, 301, 302*f*
  structure and function of, 286*f,* 286–288
Liver function tests, 290
Lockjaw, 553
Long bones, components of, 410, 412*f*
Loss of function, in inflammation, 47

Lou Gehrig disease. *See* Amyotrophic lateral sclerosis
Low back pain, 413, 421
Lung, 209–235
  abscess, 219
  benign neoplasms of, 233
  cancer of, 211, 212, 230–233
  cancer metastatic to, 233
  function of, 210–211
  infections, 215–216
  organ failure, 234
  structure of, 210–211, 211*f*
Lung disease, 211–233
  death from, 234
  fungal, 222
  genetic/developmental, 213–215
  hyperplastic/neoplastic, 230–233
  inflammatory/degenerative, 215–230
  interstitial
    acute noninfectious, 228
    chronic noninfectious, 228
  signs and symptoms, 212–213
  tests for, 212–213
  vascular, 230
Luteinizing hormone, 506, 508*t*
Lyme disease, 555
Lymphangiomas, 147
Lymphatic system, 141, 144
  failure of, 166
Lymph node biopsy, 175–176
Lymphocytes, 171
Lymphocytic leukemia, 189
Lymphogranuloma venereum, 556–557
Lymphomas, 75, 188, 190
  relative frequency of, 173*f*

Macrophages, 36
  alveolar, 211
  in inflammation, 49
Macula, 401*f*
Macular degeneration
  age-related, 393, 394
  senile, 406
Macule, 362, 363, 363*f*
Magnesium requirements, 632
Magnetic resonance imaging, 26
  of central nervous system, 463
Major histocompatibility complex, 582–583
Major histocompatibility complex restriction, 583
Malabsorption syndrome, 264, 271–272, 272*f*
Malaise, 539
Malaria, 538, 570–571
Males, common cancers in, 87*f*

Malignant, definition of, 5
Malignant hyperpyrexia, 612
Malignant hypertension, 158
  vascular effects of, 158, 159*f*
Malignant hyperthermia, 623
Malignant melanoma. *See* Melanoma
Malignant neoplasms, 72. *See also* Cancer
  morphologic features of, 78–79, 79*f,* 80*f*
  nomenclature for, 75*t*
Malingering, 501
Malnutrition, 632
Malocclusion, 239
Malpighian zone, 360*f,* 361
Mammography, 350, 350*f*
Mammoplasty, 349
Manganese requirements, 632
Mania, definition of, 497
Manic-depressive psychosis, 497
Manifestations, 3–4, 4*t*
Marasmus, 633
Marfan's syndrome, 415, 420
Margination, 48
Mass, 91
Mast cells, in inflammation, 50
Mastication, loss of, 250
Mastitis, 349
  acute, 351–352
Mastoiditis, 247
MCHC. *See* Mean corpuscular hemoglobin concentration
MCV. *See* Mean corpuscular volume
Mean corpuscular hemoglobin concentration, 174–175
Mean corpuscular volume, 174
Measles, 538, 539, 558, 559*f*
Meckel's diverticulum, 114, 261, 261*f*
Media, 142, 142*f*
Medial sclerosis, 148
Medulloblastoma, 485
Meiosis, 98, 99*f*
  nondisjunction in, 98–100, 99*f*
Melanocytes, 361, 379
Melanocyte-stimulating hormone, 506, 508*t*
Melanocytic nevus, 381–383, 382*f*
Melanoma, 75, 362, 383–385, 384*f*
  acral-lentiginous, 383–385
  lentigo maligna, 383
  nodular, 384*f,* 385
  ocular, 405, 406
  superficial spreading, 383, 384*f*
Melatonin, 507
Melena, 258
Membranous glomerulonephritis, 318–319
Memory cells, 580
Meniere's syndrome, 247, 250
Meninges, 459

Meningioma, 483–484, 484*f*
Meningitis, 460, 464, 465–466, 539, 540
  enteric bacterial, 546
  meningococcal, 545
Meningococcal meningitis, 545
Meningomyelocele, 114, 464
Menisci, 410, 412*f*
Menorrhagia, 334
Menstrual cycle, 332–333
Menstruation, 333–334
Mental illness, 489–504
  characteristics of, 489–490
  classification of, 492–495, 494*t*
  disorders arising in childhood and
    adolescence, 499–501
  most frequent and serious problems,
    490–491
  and organic disease, associations
    between, 493–494
  signs and symptoms of, 491–492,
    493*t*
  with symptoms suggestive of organic
    disease, 501
  tests for, 491–492
Mental retardation, 492, 493*t*, 500
Mental status examination, 492
Mercuric chloride poisoning, 626
Mesentery, 256
Metaphysis, 410, 412*f*
Metaplasia, 76
Metastasis, 72
Metastatic calcification, 45
Metatarsus adductus, 416
Methyl alcohol poisoning, 626
Metrorrhagia, 334
Micelles, 257, 287
Microangiopathic hemolytic anemia,
    179, 183
Microhemorrhages, 402
Middle cerebral artery, 469*f*, 469–470
Migraine, 502
Mineralocorticoids, 508*t*
  deficiency or excess, disorders
    associated with, 510*t*, 522–523
Minerals
  deficiencies of, 635–636
  excess, 636–637
  requirements for, 631–632
Miosis, 393
Miscarriage, 333, 342
Missile wounds, 607
Mitosis, 98, 99*f*
Mitral stenosis, 133, 133*f*
Mixed tumor, of salivary glands, 248
Moles, 381–383
Monocytes, 171
Monocytic leukemia, 189
Monogenetic diseases, 104–105
Mononuclear phagocytic system, 171
Monosomy, 98

Mood disorders. *See* Affective disorders
Morbidity
  causes of, 13
  measures of, 13–14
Mortality
  causes of, 11–13, 12*t*
  measures of, 13–14
Mortality rate, 13
Mosaicism, 100
Motor system, examination of, 461
Mouth
  diseases of, 238
    genetic/developmental, 239–240
    hyperplastic/neoplastic, 248, 249*f*
    inflammatory/degenerative,
      240–243
  structure and function of, 238
MRI. *See* Magnetic resonance imaging
MS. *See* Multiple sclerosis
Mucor, 569
Mucormycosis, 569
Mucosa, of alimentary tract, 255, 256*f*
Multiple endocrine neoplasia, 528
Multiple myeloma, 188, 191, 414
  relative frequency of, 173*f*
Multiple sclerosis, 460, 476–477, 477*f*
Mumps, 538, 539, 560
Mural thrombosis, 131–132
Muscle cells, 70
Muscle fibers, 442, 442*f*
  type I, 442–444, 443*f*
  type II, 442–444, 443*f*
Muscle relaxants, abuse, 624
Muscular dystrophy, 111, 444
  signs and symptoms of, 446
Muscularis, of alimentary tract, 255,
    256*f*
Muscularis mucosae, of alimentary
    tract, 255, 256*f*
Mutation, 100
Myasthenia gravis, 453–454, 602*t*
Mycobacterium leprae, 556
Mycobacterium tuberculosis, in caseous
    necrosis, 42
Mycoplasma, infections, 555
Mycoplasma pneumoniae, 219, 555
Mycosis, 567
Mycotic infection, 567
Myelin sheath, 444, 445*f*, 458, 460
Myelitis, 468
Myeloblast, 171
Myelocyte, 171
Myelofibrosis, 185
Myelogram, 422, 423*f*
Myeloid metaplasia, 185
Myelophthisic anemia, 185
Myocardial infarct/infarction, 12, 130
  coronary artery atherosclerosis and,
    129, 129*f*
Myocardial rupture, 131

Myointimal cells, 152
Myopathy, 451
  congenital, 451
  metabolic, 454–455
Myopia, 393–395, 403, 403*f*
Myosin, 442
Myotonia, 449
Myotonic dystrophy, 449–450, 450*f*
Myxedema, 515
  pretibial, 516*f*, 517

Natural killer (NK) cells, 579–580
Nearsightedness. *See* Myopia
Necrosis, 5, 38
  acute, 40–43
  time frame of, 39*f*
Needle biopsy, 28
Negri bodies, 468
Neisseria gonorrhoeae, 547–549
Neisseria meningitidis, meningitis, 465,
    545
Nemaline myopathy, 451
Neoplasms, 5, 69–84
  categories and suffixes for, 74*f*
  classification of, 74–75
  definition of, 71
  of heart, 137
  hematopoietic, 173, 173*f*, 187–191
  malignant. *See* Cancer; Malignant
    neoplasms
  vascular, 164
Nephritis, 315
  interstitial, 320
Nephron, 307, 308*f*
Nephrotic syndrome, 310–311,
    317–319
Nerve conduction tests, 447
Nerve deafness, 250
Nervous tissue cells, 70
Neuroblastoma, 520, 524
Neurofibromas, 445, 455
Neurofibromatosis, 445, 455
Neurogenic shock, 165, 165*t*
Neurons, 460
  ischemic damage to, 472
Neuropathies, 444–445
  hereditary motor and sensory, 451
Neurosis, 498
Neutrophils, 35
  in inflammation, 48
Nevi, 361, 362. *See also* Nevus
  dysplastic, 383
  giant hairy, 383
  melanocytic, 381–383, 382*f*
Nevocellular nevus, 381–383
Nevus, 75. *See also* Nevi
  compound, 382
  intradermal, 382

junctional, 382
melanocytic, 381–383, 382*f*
nevocellular, 381–383
Niacin. *See* Vitamin B₃
Nipples, supernumerary, 351
Nitrogen dioxide, injury caused by, 619–620, 625
Nocturia, 310
Nodes of Ranvier, 444
Nodule, 363, 363*f*
Nondisjunction, 98–100, 99*f*
Non-Hodgkin's lymphoma, 190
Nonpenetrance, 101
Normal flora, 533, 534, 541–542
Normoblasts, 171
Nose. *See also* Upper respiratory tract
structure and function of, 238
Nosocomial, definition of, 8
Nuclear isotope scan, 27, 29*f*
Nucleus pulposus, 410, 413*f*, 422
Nutrition, 629–630
guidelines for, 630
most frequent and serious problems with, 632
Nystagmus, 394

Obesity, 632–633, 636
and atherosclerosis, 154
Obligate intracellular parasites, 556–557
Obsession, 493*t*
Obsessive-compulsive disorder, 491
Obsessive compulsive neuroses, 499
Obstruction, in cancer, 92
Obstructive pulmonary disease, 234
definition of, 210
Oculopharyngeal dystrophy, 451
Oligodendroglia, 460
ischemic damage to, 472
Oliguria, 310
Oncogenes, 81
Ophthalmoscope, 394
Opiates, abuse, 624
Opportunistic infections, 535, 538, 569
fungal, 569, 570*f*
in HIV-infected (AIDS) patients, 564, 565
Opsonins, 48
Optic disk, 401*f*
Optic nerve atrophy, 406
Oral region, structure and function of, 238, 254
Organ, 34
Organelles, 35
Organic brain disorder, 492
Organic brain syndromes, 490, 491
acute, 494
chronic, 494
versus functional disease, 495

Organic diseases, 4–5
Organic mental disorders, 490, 495–496
Organization. *See* Fibrous connective tissue repair
Organized thrombus, 199
Orthopnea, 212
Osmotic pressure, 166
Ossification, 410
Osteitis deformans. *See* Paget's disease of bone
Osteitis fibrosa cystica, 520
Osteoarthritis. *See* Arthritis, degenerative
Osteoblasts, 411, 412
Osteoclasts, 413
Osteogenesis imperfecta, 415, 419
Osteoid, 411
Osteomalacia, 413, 429, 430–431
Osteomyelitis, 428
Osteopenia, 413, 428
Osteoporosis, 413, 421, 428–430, 429*f*
Osteosarcoma, 414, 436*f*, 436–437
Otitis media, 238, 239, 245, 246–247, 248*f*, 593
Otosclerosis, 247, 250
Ovarian cancer, 333, 337
Ovarian cysts, 341–342
Ovarian tumors, 341–342
Ovaries, 506, 507*f*, 509*t*
structure and function of, 332, 332*f*
Overnutrition, 632
signs and symptoms of, 632
Oxygen, content, of arterial blood, 213
Oxytocin, 508*t*

Paget's disease of bone, 429, 435, 436
Pain. *See also* Low back pain
abdominal, 259–260
in cancer, 91
flank, 310, 321
with fracture, 414
in inflammation, 47
Palliative, definition of, 27
Pancreas
cancer of, 289, 301
cystic fibrosis of, 291
diseases of
signs and symptoms of, 289–290
tests for, 290
failure, 302
inflammation of, 289
structure and function of, 288–289
Pancreatic endocrine tumors, 528
Pancreaticobiliary tract, structure and function of, 254
Pancreatic polypeptide, 524
Pancreatitis, 289, 299–300
chronic, 272

Panhypopituitarism, 511, 512
Panic disorder, 491
Panic reactions, 499
Pannus, 432
Papilla of Vater, 286, 286*f*
Papilledema, 394
Papillomas, juvenile laryngeal, 365, 367
Pap smear, 334, 335*f*
Papule, 363, 363*f*
Paralysis, 455–456
Paramnesia, 493*t*
Paraplegia, 609
Paraquat, injury caused by, 625
Parathyroid glands, 506, 507*f*, 508*t*
diseases of, 519–520
Parathyroid hormone, 508*t*
deficiency or excess, disorders associated with, 510*t*
Paresis, 470
Paresthesia, 461
Parkinson's disease, 460, 480
Paronychia, 60, 368, 369*f*
Patch test, 374, 590
Patella, 410, 412*f*
Pathogenesis, 3
Pathogens, 533, 534
Pathologic fractures, 413, 424, 427
in cancer, 92
Pathologist, roles of, 2*t*
Pathology
definition of, 1–2
introduction to, 1–10
Pathophysiologic change, 6
Patient care, 8–9
approach to, 21–23
Pelvic examination, 334
Pelvic inflammatory disease, 333
gonococcal, 548
Pemphigus vulgaris, 388
Penicillin, adverse reaction to, 623
Peptic ulcer disease, 264, 269–271, 270*f*, 502
Percussion, 212
Perfusion, definition of, 211
Perinatal diseases, 108
Perinatal period, definition of, 101
Periodontal disease, 238, 242
Peripheral nerves
assessment of, 447
biopsy of, 447
structure and function of, 444, 445*f*
Peristalsis, 256
Peritonitis, 258, 259, 608
Perleche, 372
Pernicious anemia, 184, 602*t*, 634–635
Personality disorders, 491, 499, 500*t*
Petechiae, 201, 201*f*
Phagocytosis, 48, 49
Pharyngeal cancer, 248
Pharyngitis, 239, 244
streptococcal, 543

Pharynx. *See also* Upper respiratory tract
structure and function of, 238
Phenotype, 101
Phenylketonuria, 111
Pheochromocytoma, 157, 520, 524
Phlebothrombosis, 161
Phobias, 493*t*, 498
Phosphorus requirements, 631
Photophobia, 394, 396, 397
Physical examination, 4
Physical injury, 605–615
mechanical, 607–609
most frequent and serious problems, 606
thermal, 606, 609–612. *See also* Burns
Pia-arachnoid, 459
Pigeon toes deformity, 416
Pigmentation, disorders of, 364
Pilonidal abscess, 368, 370
Pink-eye, 393
Pinworm, 539, 572
Pituitary gland
anterior, 506, 508*t*, 509*f*
diseases of, 511–513
posterior, 506, 508*t*
tumors, 484–485, 513
Placenta, 506, 509*t*
Placental lactogen, 509*t*
Plague, 555
Plaque, 150, 363
Plasmodium falciparum, 570–571
Plasmodium malariae, 570–571
Plasmodium ovale, 570–571
Plasmodium vivax, 570–571
Platelet count, 202
Platelets, 171, 196
disorders of, 186–187
and hemorrhage, 203–204
and thrombosis, 206
measurement of, 175
Pleural effusion, 230, 608
Pneumococcus, 544
Pneumoconioses, 228–229, 620
definition of, 212
Pneumocystis carinii, 538
pneumonia, in HIV-infected (AIDS) patients, 564
Pneumocytes
type I, 210
type II, 210
Pneumonia, 215–216, 245, 535
aspiration, 218
definition of, 212
fungal, 222
in immunosuppressed patient, 218–219
interstitial, 217*f*, 219
Legionella pneumophila, 546

lobar, 216, 217*f*
neonatal, 556–557
opportunistic, 535
primary atypical, 219, 555
secondary, 535
viral, 219
Pneumonitis, 219
definition of, 212
Pneumothorax, 228, 608
Poisoning, 619, 619*t*
accidental, 621*t*, 624–625
substances most frequently involved in, 619, 620*t*, 621*t*
Poison ivy, 375, 376*f*, 587, 600
Poisons, detoxification, by liver, 288
Poliomyelitis, 468
Polyarteritis nodosa, 161, 587, 599, 599*f*
Polycythemia, 188
Polycythemia vera, 188
Polydipsia, 510, 513, 526
Polygenetic disorders, 105–106
Polymorphonuclear leukocytes (polys), 35
maturation of, 171–172, 172*f*
Polymyositis, 451
Polyps, 77–78
colonic, 258, 278–279, 280*f*
juvenile laryngeal, 365, 367
Polyuria, 510, 513, 526
Portal hypertension, 295–297
Port wine stains, 147, 147*f*, 364
Postnecrotic cirrhosis, 295, 296*f*
Post-traumatic stress disorder, 491, 499
Potential disease, care of, 22–23
Pregnancy, 332–333
diseases of, 342–345
ectopic, 333, 342–343, 343*f*, 344*f*
hyperpigmentation in, 362
most frequent and serious problems of, 333
Pregnancy tests, 334
Premature birth/prematurity, 108
and hyaline membrane disease, 213–215
and neonatal mortality, 215
Presbycusis, 247, 250
Presbyopia, 393, 404–405
Pressure atrophy, 43
Pretibial myxedema, 516*f*, 517
Prevalence, 13
Preventive medicine, 22–23
Primary atypical pneumonia, 219, 555
Primary union, wound repair by, 63–64, 65*f*
Prion, 477
Procedure, 23
Progeria, 17

Progesterone, 509*t*
Prognosis, 8, 83
Prolactin, 506, 508*t*
Promoter, 80
Propionibacterium acnes, 367–368
Prostacyclin, 196
Prostaglandins, 51
Prostate gland, 306*f*, 309–310
benign hyperplasia, 322–324, 324*f*
cancer of, 310, 324–325, 325*f*
transurethral resection of, 324
Prostate-specific antigen, 324
Prostatitis, 310, 321
Protamine, for heparin overdose, 206
Protein
accumulation of, 44
dietary, 630–631
Proteinuria, 310
Proteus infection, 546–547
Prothrombin time, 203, 290
Protozoal disease, 570–572
most frequent and serious, 538
Pruritus, 362
vulvar, 334
Pruritus ani, 258
Pseudohypertrophy of calves, in Duchenne muscular dystrophy, 448–449, 449*f*
Pseudomembrane, 554
Pseudomembranous enterocolitis, 264, 274
Pseudomonas infection, 546–547
Psoriasis, 362, 378, 378*f*
Psychiatric emergencies, 491
Psychiatrists, 490
Psychologists, 490
Psychophysiologic disorders, 494, 502
Psychosis, 494
organic, 495–496
Psychosomatic complaints, 501
Public health laboratories, 30
Pulmonary, definition of, 210
Pulmonary edema, 230
Pulmonary embolism, 161, 163*f*, 230
Pulmonary hypertension, effect on heart, 136, 136*f*
Puncture wound, 607
Pupil, of eye, 393
Purulent exudate, 42, 59
Pus, 42, 59
Pustule, 363, 363*f*
Pyelonephritis, 310, 319–320
chronic, 320
Pyknosis, 39
Pyloric stenosis, congenital, 262*f*, 262–263
Pylorus, 254, 256
Pyogenic, definition of, 48

Pyridoxine. *See* Vitamin B₆
Pyuria, 319

Quadriplegia, 609

Rabies, 467–468
Radiation-induced cancer, 90
Radiation injury, 606, 612–614
Radiation therapy, 613
  for cancer, 95
Radiologic procedures, 24*t*, 24–27
Radiology, 24–25
Radioresistance, 613
Radiosensitivity, 613
Rales, 213
Rashes, 361, 363
  of secondary syphilis, 550, 551*f*
Raynaud's phenomenon, 161
Recessive inheritance, 104, 105*f*
Rectum, 255, 255*f*
Red blood cells. *See also* Erythrocytes
  lysis, in allergic reaction, 583–584, 584*f*
Red cell fragility test, 176
Redness, 46
Reed-Sternberg cell, 190
Reflexes, testing of, 461
Reflux esophagitis, 267–268
Refractive error, 395
Regeneration, 61–63, 62*f*
Regional enteritis, 275
Regression, 81
Renal calculi, 310, 321–322, 322*f*, 323*f*
Repair, 5, 38, 61–66
  time frame of, 39*f*
Resection, 28
Resolution, 63
Resorption, 308
Respiratory distress syndrome of
    newborn, 213–215
Restrictive pulmonary disease, 234
  definition of, 210
Reticulocyte count, 175
Reticulocytes, 171
Reticulocytosis, 175
Reticuloendothelial system, 171
Retina, 392, 392*f*, 393, 401*f*
Retinitis, 395
Retinitis pigmentosa, 406
Retinoblastoma, 395, 405–406
Rhabdomyosarcoma, 455
Rh antigen, 595–597
Rheumatic fever, 132
Rheumatic heart disease, 132–134
  effects on valves, 132–133, 133*f*
  pathogenesis of, 134*t*

Rheumatic valvulitis, 132, 133, 134*t*
Rheumatoid arthritis, 413, 421, 432*f*,
    432–434, 433*f*, 451, 587, 590,
    602*t*
  juvenile, 434
  signs and symptoms of, 414
Rheumatoid factor, 433–434, 590
Rhinitis, 244
  allergic, 246, 586, 592–593
Riboflavin. *See* Vitamin B₂
Ribosomes, 35
Rickets, 413, 430–431
Rickettsial infections, 538, 566–567
Right-sided congestive heart failure,
    137, 138*f*
Ringworm, 371–372, 569
Rocky Mountain spotted fever, 538, 566
Roentgenogram, 25, 25*f*
Rubella, 559–560
  and congenital anomalies, 107
Rubeola. *See* Measles
Rubricytes, 171

Salivary glands
  mixed tumor of, 248
  structure and function of, 238
  tumors of, 248
Salmonella infection, 546–547
Salmonella typhosa, 555–556
Salpingitis, 334, 336
  gonococcal, 548
Saprophytes, 533, 534
Sarcoidosis, 228, 229–230
  and granulomatous inflammation,
    58
Sarcoma, 74, 86
Scale, 363, 363*f*
Scarlet fever, 543–544
Scarring, 61, 63, 64*f*
Schistosomiasis, 539
Schizophrenia, 491, 494, 496–497
  subtypes of, 496, 496*t*
Schwann cells, 444, 445*f*
Schwannomas, 445, 455
Sciatica, 422
Sclera, 392, 392*f*
Scoliosis, 422–423, 425*f*
Screening, 22, 23, 23*t*
Sebaceous gland, 360*f*, 361
Seborrheic keratosis, 361–362, 381,
    381*f*, 385
Secondary hypertension, 156
Secondary response, 580
Secondary union, wound repair by,
    64–65, 65*f*
Secretin test, 300
Secretion, 308

Seizures, 482
Seminoma, 327
Senile atrophy, 43
Senile cataracts, 398
Senile dementia, 460, 478–480, 479*f*
  definition of, 478
Senile elastosis, 612
Senile keratosis, 379–380, 612
Sensory system, examination of, 461
Separation anxiety, 501
Septic abortion, 333, 343
Septicemia, 539
Serologic tests, 541
Serosa, of alimentary tract, 255–256,
    256*f*
Serous exudate, 59
Serum, 170
Serum electrophoresis, 588, 588*f*
Serum enzyme levels, myocardial
    infarct and, 123–124, 124*f*
Serum immunodiffusion, 588
Serum proteins, production of, 288
Serum sickness, 587, 598
Sex
  and atherosclerosis, 154
  and cancer types, 87*f*
Sex-linked recessive inheritance, 104,
    106*f*
Sexually transmitted disease, 333, 535,
    537, 547, 548*t*
  bacterial, 547–552
Shigella infection, 546–547
Shigellosis, 266, 267, 546–547
Shingles, 560
Shock, 164–165, 165*t*
Sickle-cell anemia, 111, 180, 180*f*
Sickle-cell preparation, 176
Sigmoid colon, 254–255, 255*f*
Sigmoidoscopy, 260, 281
Signs, 4
Silicosis, 229
Silo filler's disease, 619–620, 625
Sinusitis, 238, 239, 245, 246*f*, 593
Sinusoids, 143
Skeletal muscle
  atrophy, 446
    neurogenic, 452, 452*f*
  biopsy of, 446, 446*t*
  diseases of
    autoimmune, 451–452
    hyperplastic/neoplastic, 455
    inflammatory/degenerative,
      451–455
    myopathic, 445, 446*t*
    neurogenic, 445, 446*t*
    signs and symptoms of, 445–447
    tests for, 445–447
  failure, 455–456
  fascicles, 442, 442*f*

Skeletal muscle (*cont.*)
most frequent and serious problems, 444–445
neurogenic disorders of, 452*f*, 452–453
structure and function of, 442*f*, 442–444, 443*f*
weakness, 444, 445
Skeletal system. *See* Bones and joints
Skin, 359–389
diseases of, 364–388
genetic/developmental, 364–365
hyperplastic/neoplastic, 379
inflammatory/degenerative, 365–388
most frequent and serious, 361–362
signs and symptoms, 362–363
tests for, 362–363
histologic components of, 360*f*, 360–361
organ failure, 388
solar degeneration, 379, 380*f*
structure and function of, 360–361
superficial fungal infections of, 371–372, 538
Skin cancer, 362, 385–388, 386*f*, 387*f*, 612. *See also* Melanoma
types, relative frequencies of, 379, 379*f*
Skin tests, 541, 588, 590–592
Skull fractures, 462
SLE. *See* Systemic lupus erythematosus
Slit-lamp, 394
Small intestine, structure and function of, 254, 255, 255*f*
Smallpox, 534, 561
Social phobia, 491
Social workers, 490
Sodium, excess, 636–637
Solar keratosis, 362, 379–380
Somatoform disorders, 501
Somatostatin, 524
Somatostatinoma, 528
Sore throat, 244
Spastic colon, 258
Speculum, 334
Spherocytosis, hereditary, 181–182
Spina bifida, 464
Spinal column, structure and function of, 410, 413*f*
Spinal cord, 458*f*, 458–460
crushing injuries, 476
inflammation, 468
neoplasms of, 482–485
penetrating injuries, 476
Spinal injury, 609
Splinter, and chronic inflammation, 54
Spontaneous abortion, 333, 342
Spontaneous thrombosis, 207

Sprains, 413, 420–421
Sputum, 212
Squamous cell carcinoma, 383
oral, 248, 249*f*
of skin, 379, 379*f*, 380, 385–388, 386*f*, 387*f*
Squamous metaplasia, 76
Staghorn calculi, 321
Staging, 82
Staphylococcal infections, 542–543
Staphylococcus aureus, 542–543
alpha hemolytic, 134–135
Status asthmaticus, 224, 592
Stenosis, esophageal, 268
Stethoscope, 212
Stomach
carcinoma of, 278, 279*f*
structure and function of, 254, 255
Stomatitis
aphthous, 243, 244*f*
herpes, 243, 243*f*
Strabismus, 393, 395, 397–398, 398*f*
Strains, 413, 421
Strep throat, 244, 543
Streptococci
group A, infections, 543–544
hemolytic
in endocarditis, 134
and rheumatic heart disease, 133–134
Streptococcus pneumoniae, 216
defense mechanisms of, 48
infection, 544–545
meningitis, 465
Streptococcus viridans infection, 544, 545*f*
Stress, and atherosclerosis, 154
Stress disorders, 499
post traumatic, 499
Stroke, 12. *See also* Cerebrovascular accident
Structural diseases, 4–5, 6*t*
Subcutaneous tissue, 360*f*, 361
Subcutis, 360*f*, 361
Subdural hematoma, 474–475, 475*f*
Sublethal cell injury, 5
Subluxation, 421
Submucosa, of alimentary tract, 255, 256*f*
Succinylcholine, adverse reaction to, 623
Sudden death, from heart disease, 121–122
Suicide, 491, 618, 619
Sunburn, 612
Sun radiations, effects of, 612
Superficial spreading melanoma, 383, 384*f*
Suppurative inflammation, 59
Surfactant, 210, 213–215
Surgical pathology, 27–28
Swallowing disorder, 250, 259

Swelling, 47
Symptomatic disease, care of, 21–22, 22*t*
Symptoms, 3–4
Syncope, 165
Syndrome of inappropriate antidiuretic hormone secretion, 529
Syndromes, 3
Syphilis, 336, 371, 537, 550–552
and chronic inflammation, 55
congenital, 108, 115
Systemic lupus erythematosus, 160, 362, 451, 587, 601–603, 602*f*, 602*t*
diagnosis of, 590

Tachypnea, 212
Taenia solium, 574
Talipes equinovarus. *See* Clubfoot
Tapeworm, 539, 574
dog, 574
pork, 574
Telangiectasia, 379
Teratomas, 72, 341–342
Test, 23
Testis, 306*f*, 309, 506, 507*f*, 509*t*
accessory glands of, 306*f*, 309
cancers of, 327
Testosterone, 509*t*
Tetanus, 552–553
Tetralogy of Fallot, 113, 126–127, 127*f*
Thalassemia, 181
T-helper cells, 579
Thermal injury, 606, 609–612. *See also* Burns
Thiamine. *See* Vitamin B₁
Throat culture, 239, 244
Thrombin, 198
Thrombocytopenia, 175, 186, 597
Thrombocytosis, 175
Thrombophlebitis, 161–163, 163*f*
Thrombosis, 197–198
disorders with, 206
spontaneous, 207
Thrombus/thrombi, 41, 197
endocardial, 131–132
formation of, 144
Thyroid gland, 506, 507*f*, 508*t*
carcinoma, 518
medullary, 518
diseases of, 514–518
examination of, 510–511
neoplasms of, 518
Thyroid hormones, deficiency or excess, disorders associated with, 510*t*
Thyroid-stimulating hormone, 506, 508*t*

Thyrotoxic myopathy, 517
Thyroxine, 508*t*
Tibial torsion, 416
Tinea, 371, 569
Tinea barbae, 371
Tinea capitis, 371
Tinea cruris, 371
Tinea pedis, 371
Tinnitus, 247
Tissue, 34
  components of, 35, 36*t*
Tissue typing, 601
T lymphocytes, 579, 580, 583
  deficiencies of, 591
Tobacco, and oral cancer, 248
Toluene, accidental poisoning with,
  625
Tonometer, 394
Tonsillitis, 244
Tophi, 434
Torticollis, 414, 417–418, 418*f*
Toxemia of pregnancy, 343–344
Toxic shock syndrome, 543
  streptococcal, 544
Toxoplasmosis, 570, 571–572
Trachea, 211, 211*f*
Tracheoesophageal fistula, 261, 261*f*
Trachoma, 395, 556–557
Tranquilizers, abuse, 624
Transformation, 81
Transfusion reactions, 587, 596–597
Transitional cell carcinoma of bladder,
  325–326, 326*f*
Translocation, 100, 100*f*
Transudate, 59, 166
Transurethral resection of prostate,
  324
Transverse colon, 254, 255*f*
Trauma, 6, 12
  abdominal, 608
  and acute injury, 41
  chest, 608–609
  deaths from, 606
  definition of, 606
  head, 609
  muscle injury in, 444
  nerve injury in, 444
  pancreatitis with, 300
  spinal, 609
  types of, 607–609
Traveler's diarrhea, 265, 266
Trench mouth, 242
Treponema pallidum, 550
Trichinella spiralis, 572–573, 573*f*
Trichinosis, 572–573, 573*f*
Trichomonas vaginalis, 334, 337, 337*f*, 538
Trichomoniasis, 570
Trichuriasis, 574–575
Triiodothyronine, 508*t*
Trisomy, 98

Trisomy 21. *See* Down syndrome
Trypanosomiasis, 570
T-suppressor cells, 579
Tuberculin skin test, 600
Tuberculosis, 215–216, 220–222, 601
  and granulomatous inflammation, 58
  meningitis due to, 466
  screening, 221
Tubular adenoma, 278–279, 280*f*
Tularemia, 555
Tumor, 73
Turner syndrome, 113
Typhoid fever, 555–556
Typhus, 538, 566

Ulcer, 61
Ulcerative colitis, 258, 264, 274*f*, 274–275
Ultrasound, 26–27, 28*f*
  abdominal, 312, 335
  of gallstones, 290, 298*f*
Undernutrition, 632, 633–634
  signs and symptoms of, 633
Undulant fever, 556
Unipolar disorder, 497–498
Upper gastrointestinal endoscopy, 260
Upper GI series, 260
Upper respiratory infection, 244–245,
  535
  viral, 537
Upper respiratory tract, diseases of,
  238
Urea nitrogen, 288, 312
Ureaplasma urealyticum, 547, 549, 555
Uremia, 328
Ureters, 306*f*, 309
Urethra, 306*f*, 309
Urethritis, 310
  nongonococcal, 548, 556–557
Urinalysis, 311
Urinary tract
  examination of, 311
  infection, 310
  lower, 305–329
    structure and function of, 306*f*,
    306–310
Urination
  frequency of, 310, 320
  urgency of, 320
Urine
  composition of, 307–309
  culture, 311
  formation of, 307–309
Urticaria, 365, 377, 587, 593–594, 594*f*
Uterus
  duplication, 336
  leiomyoma of, 333, 334, 337, 338*f*,
    338–339
  structure and function of, 332, 332*f*

Uvea, 392, 392*f*
Uveitis, 395

Vaccination, 534
Vagina, structure and function of, 332,
  332*f*
Vaginal spotting, 334
Vaginitis, 337, 337*f*
Vanillylmandelic acid, 524
Variable expressivity, 101
Varicella, 560. *See also* Chickenpox
Varicose veins, 163–164
Varicosities, 144
Variola. *See* Smallpox
Vascular disorders
  detection of, 145–146
  functional, 161
  and hemorrhage, 203
  and thrombosis, 206
Vascular system, 141–168
  failure of, 164–166
Vasculitis, 160–161, 162*f*
Vas deferens, 306*f*, 309
Vector, 534
Veins, 142
Ventilation, definition of, 210
Ventricular aneurysm, 131
Ventricular fibrillation, 121, 131
Ventricular septal defect, 125–126, 126*f*
Venules, 142, 142*f*
Verruca, 365–367, 366*f*
Verruca planus, 563
Verruca vulgaris, 361, 365–367, 366*f*, 563
Vertebrae, 410
Vertebral bodies, 410, 413*f*
Vertigo, 247
Vesicle, 363, 363*f*
Villous adenoma, 278–279, 280*f*
Vincent's infection, 242
Vipoma, 528
Viral enteritis, 258, 265, 266
Viral exanthems, 365
Viral infections, 557*f*, 557–558, 601
  of childhood, 558–561
  most frequent and serious, 537–538
Virulence, 533
Viruses
  and cancer, 90–91, 557–558
  and chronic inflammation, 55, 56
Vision, 20/20, 394
Visual acuity, 393
  decreased, 394
  normal (20/20), 394
  testing, 394
Visual field tests, 394, 395*f*
Vitamin A
  deficiency, 634, 635*t*
  function of, 631*t*
  toxicity, 636

Vitamin B₁
  deficiency, 634, 635*t*
  function of, 631*t*
Vitamin B₂
  deficiency, 634, 635*t*
  function of, 631*t*
Vitamin B₃
  deficiency, 634, 635*t*
  function of, 631*t*
Vitamin B₆
  deficiency, 634, 635*t*
  function of, 631*t*
Vitamin B₁₂
  deficiency, 184, 634, 635*t*
  function of, 631*t*
Vitamin C
  deficiency, 634, 635*t*
  function of, 631*t*
Vitamin D
  deficiency, 634, 635*t*
  function of, 631*t*
  toxicity, 636
Vitamin E
  deficiency, 634, 635*t*
  function of, 631*t*
Vitamin K
  and bleeding disorders, 205
  deficiency, 634, 635*t*
  function of, 631*t*

Vitamins, 631, 631*t*
  deficiencies, 632, 634–635, 635*t*
  toxicity, 636
Vitiligo, 379
Vitreous humor, 393
Vomiting, 259, 282
Von Willebrand's disease, 204
Vulva, 332
Vulvar carcinoma, 334, 337

Walking pneumonia, 555
Warfarin, 205
Warts, 361, 365–367, 366*f,* 563
  plantar, 563
  venereal, 336–337, 563. *See also*
    Condyloma acuminatum
Water intoxication, 529
Werdnig-Hoffman's disease, 453
Wernicke's encephalopathy, 637–638
Western blot, in diagnosis of HIV
  infection, 565
Wheal, 363, 363*f,* 377
Whiplash injury, 420
Whipworm, 574–575
White blood cell count, in infectious
  disease, 541
White blood cells. *See also* Leukocytes
  types of, 35–37, 37*f*

White matter, 458, 459*f*
Whooping cough, 554
Wilms tumor, 326
Wound infection, 535
Wound repair, 63–66, 65*f*
Wounds
  gunshot, 607
  missile, 607
  simple, types of, 607
Wry neck. *See* Torticollis

Xanthomas, 362
Xeroderma pigmentosum, 364
X-radiation
  effects of, 613
  injury from, 613–614

Yeast, 567, 568*f*
Yersinia pestis, 555
Youth, cancers common in, 88*f*

Zinc requirements, 632
Zollinger-Ellison syndrome, 528
Zoster, 560